P9-BYE-963

3 1299 00757 6714

DICT
MEDICAL TERMS
Fifth Edition

Mikel A. Rothenberg, M.D.
Emergency Care Educator
North Olmsted, Ohio

Charles F. Chapman
Former Coordinator, Editorial Office
Louisiana State University
School of Medicine
New Orleans, Louisiana

BARRON'S

All inquiries should be addressed to:
Barron's Educational Series, Inc.
250 Wireless Boulevard
Hauppauge, New York 11788
www.barronseduc.com

Library of Congress Catalog Card No. 2005058873

ISBN-13: 978-0-7641-3463-0
ISBN-10: 0-7641-3463-9

Library of Congress Cataloging-in-Publication Data
Rothenberg, Mikel A.
    Dictionary of medical terms / Mikel A. Rothenberg, Charles F.
Chapman—5th ed.
        p.   cm.
    Includes bibliographical references.
    ISBN-13: 978-0-7641-3463-0 (alk. paper)
    ISBN-10: 0-7641-3463-9 (alk. paper)
        1. Medicine—Dictionaries. I. Chapman, Charles F., 1929–
        II. Title

R121.R854 2006
610.3—dc22

                                                    2005058873

PRINTED IN UNITED STATES OF AMERICA

9 8 7 6 5 4 3 2

CONTENTS

PREFACE TO THE FIFTH EDITION

Effective communication is vital for successful interpersonal relationships. This is true whether these associations be social, business, or professional. Nowhere is the need for clear and mutual understanding more important than in dealing with one's health.

The language of medicine is viewed by many nonmedical persons as complex and unintelligible. Unfortunately, the profession itself is at times responsible for perpetuating this situation. All too often, laypersons are not able to grasp fully the implications of something they have read or have been told by a health care professional because it was expressed in complicated technical terms.

It is my firm belief that there is no medical term or procedure that cannot be described in plain English. I have tried to keep this in mind as I prepared the Fifth Edition. Countless changes have been made, not only to update the content, but to make the format as easy to use as possible. Illustrations, tables, and appendices help to clarify definitions and to further the reader's understanding of a topic. Many definitions have been updated, expanded, and simplified. Several terms have been revised, many new ones added, and a few deleted from the previous edition. Detailed new additions cover current "hot topics," such as avian influenza ("bird flu"), erectile dysfunction, fibromyalgia, and mad cow disease. References to medications have been updated and include the very latest preparations for heart disease, high blood pressure, diabetes, human immunodeficiency virus infection (AIDS), and other common conditions. Much of the new drug information is summarized in table form in the Appendix (see pp. 652–696). The *Dictionary* now includes appendices of "Over-the-Counter (OTC) Medications" and "How to Find More Medical Information." I have added many new clearly marked cross references to other words in the *Dictionary* (see "How To Effectively Use This Dictionary," pp. vi).

In undertaking this revision, I was pleased to have the highly successful framework of the first four editions as the base for my work. Without it, the Fifth Edition would not have been possible. The proliferation of available information, particularly on the Internet, made my task both formidable and intellectually fascinating at the same time. Terms regarding "alternative and complementary therapies," managed care, and herbal medications are commonplace in our daily experiences. With this in mind, I have included several summary tables in the appendices specifically aimed at these topics (see pp. 697).

I truly enjoyed the revision process. It is my sincere hope that readers will refer to this *Dictionary* frequently and will find in it all the information they seek.

I wish to thank my wife, Diane, and my children, Kara and Marc, for their patience and support. I love you more than words can say.

Mikel A. Rothenberg, M.D.

HOW TO EFFECTIVELY
USE THIS DICTIONARY

Overall View: To obtain an overall view of this book that will enable you to use it effectively, follow these steps:

1. Refer to the Table of Contents and turn to each section, familiarizing yourself with the general content and purpose of each.
2. Read the Preface to the Fifth Edition.
3. Study the Table of Abbreviations to avoid misinterpretations.
4. Read several main entries in the alphabetical listings. Note that all main entries are singular, except as indicated. Each entry lists the part of speech; provides a clear and concise definition of the term, often with an example; and where appropriate provides related parts of speech and plural forms. Pronunciation is included for many of the main entries.

Alphabetization: Note that all entries have been alphabetized word by word as much as possible, rather than letter by letter.

Cross References: Cross references appear both in the definition, such as: "**adrenaline** see EPINEPHRINE," or, if they occur at the end of a definition: "*See also* EPINEPHRINE."

The appearance of a word in regular type does not preclude the possibility of its having been included as a separate entry. Many terms that represent basic and commonly understood concepts or substances—for example, bone and muscle—are often printed in regular type, though they are listed as separate entries.

TABLE OF ABBREVIATIONS

Abrev.	abbreviation
approx.	approximately
ADJ.	adjective
ADV.	adverb
comb. form	combining form
colloq.	colloquialism
e.g.	(*exempli gratia*) for example
esp.	especially
i.e.	(*id est*) that is
N.	noun
pert.	pertaining
pl.	plural
sing.	singular
V.	verb

The material presented in this dictionary is for informational purposes only. Nothing in this book should be construed as endorsing any product, or representing or intending to represent medical advice to the reader. The only source for this type of information should be your personal health care provider.

PRONUNCIATION KEY

The pronunciation symbols are listed in the column headed **Symbols**. In the column headed **Examples** a word or words illustrates how the symbol is pronounced.

Symbols	Examples	Symbols	Examples
ă	sat	s	source, confess
ā	may	sh	shell, fish, mission
âr	scare	t	taught, attack, plate
ä	father	th	think
b	bib	*th*	then, this
ch	change, march	ŭ	but
d	deed, filled	ûr	urgent, term, firm
ě	net	v	vile, hive
ē	see	w	wet, away
f	fire, life, phone, tough	y	yet
g	gag	z	zone, xylem
h	hit	zh	vision, measure, garage
ĭ	sit	ə	about, item, edible, gallop, circus
ī	lie, try	ər	batter
j	job, judge		
k	kick, cook, ache, pique		
l	last, little, fool		
m	moon, lumber, hum		
n	now, hidden, town		
ng	sing, linger		
ŏ	top		
ō	foe		
ô	taught, saw, all		
oi	coin, employ, poise		
ŏŏ	book		
ōō	boot		
ou	out		
p	pepper, sip		
r	rear, heard		

A

a-, an- prefixes meaning without, not (e.g., aspecific, not specific, not associated with a specific cause or organism).

A blood type N. one of four blood groups (the others being AB, B, and O) in the ABO blood group system for classifying human blood based on the presence or absence of antigen A and/or B on the surface of red blood cells (erythrocytes). A person with type A blood produces antibodies against B antigens that cause the blood cells to agglutinate, or clump together. A person with type A blood must receive blood transfusions only from others with type A or type O blood. *See also* BLOOD TYPING.

A vitamins N. fat-soluble chemicals (retinol, dehydroretinol, and carotene) essential for the development and proper function of the eyes and epithelium; found in liver, cream, butter, egg yolk, and some green and yellow vegetables; deficiency can result in night blindness and xerophthalmia. *See also* VITAMIN; TABLE OF VITAMINS.

AA *see* ALCOHOLICS ANONYMOUS.

ab- prefix meaning from, away from (e.g., abduct); departing from (e.g., abnormal).

AB blood type N. one of four blood groups (the others being A, B, and O) in the ABO blood group system based on the presence or absence of two antigens A and B on the surface of red blood cells (erythrocytes); it is the least common of the four groups in the U.S. population. A person with type AB blood has both antigens and does not produce antibodies against either. A person with type AB blood can receive blood transfusions from any other type (A, B, or O) and is sometimes called the universal recipient. If the donor and recipient are inappropriately matched, a transfusion reaction may occur. *See also* BLOOD TYPING.

abarticulation N. dislocation of a joint (e.g., a pulled-out shoulder). V. articulate.

abasia N. inability to walk. ADJ. abasic, abatic

abate V. to make or become less severe, strong, or intense; often used in regard to a patient's symptoms (e.g., her abdominal pain has abated).

abdomen N. that part of the body between the chest and the pelvis; the belly, including the abdominal wall, stomach, liver, intestines, and other organs called the viscera. ADJ. abdominal.

MAJOR MUSCLES OF THE
HUMAN ABDOMINAL WALL

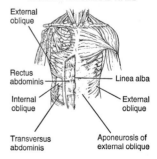

External oblique

Rectus abdominis

Linea alba

Internal oblique

External oblique

Transversus abdominis

Aponeurosis of external oblique

abdominal breathing N. breathing in which the abdominal muscles perform the major part of the respiratory effort. Such breathing may be seen in various abnormal conditions (cerebrovascular accident, spinal cord injury, coma). Singers practice this method to enhance their vocal performance.

abdominal delivery N. delivery of a child through an incision in the abdomen. *See also* CESAREAN SECTION.

abdominal pregnancy N. pregnancy in which the conceptus develops in the abdominal cavity, not in the uterus; occurs in about 2% of ectopic (extrauterine) pregnancies and usually results in fetal death. *See also* ECTOPIC PREGNANCY.

abdomino- comb. form indicating an association with the abdomen (e.g., abdominothoracic, pert. to the abdomen and chest).

abdominocentesis (ăb-dŏm′ə-nō-sĕn-tē′sis) N. surgical puncture into the belly, generally to remove fluid or other material for diagnosis. *See also* PARACENTESIS.

abdominovesical ADJ. pert. to the abdomen and urinary bladder.

abducens muscle N. lateral rectus muscle of the eyeball, responsible for turning the eye outward.

abducens nerve N. one of a pair of motor nerves, the sixth cranial nerves, that originates in the brainstem and supplies the lateral rectus muscles of the eye.

abduct V. to move a body part (e.g., an arm) away from the center line of the body, as in testing range of motion or general function (*compare* ADDUCT).

abduction N. moving of a part away from the body, as a limb being drawn away from the center of the body.

abductor N. muscle that causes a body part to abduct.

aberrant ADJ. deviating from the typical or normal state (e.g., having an abnormal chromosome number); wandering (e.g., in relation to a person's speech).

aberration N. imperfection, deviation from normal; mental disorder.

abetalipoproteinemia (ā-bā′tə-lĭ pō-prō′tē′mē-ə) N. rare, inherited disorder of fat metabolism characterized by severe deficiency or total absence of beta-lipoproteins, abnormally low cholesterol levels, and the presence of abnormal red blood cells. Symptoms include malnutrition, growth retardation, degeneration of the retina, and progressive neurological dysfunction (*compare* HYPOBETALIPOPROTEINEMIA).

abient ADJ. avoiding a stimulus (e.g., in relation to a research animal avoiding a flash of light).

abiotrophy (ā′bī-ŏt′rə-fē) N. loss of vitality, degeneration of cells and tissues, esp. those involved in hereditary degenerative disorders.

ablactation N.
1. weaning; accustoming a child to take nourishment in some way other than breast feeding.
2. cessation of milk secretion.

ablate (ă-blāt′) V. to remove, esp. by suction or cutting, or a combination of the two (as is sometimes done in removing part of an organ, e.g., damaged tissue in the brain). N. ablation

ablepharia (ā'blĕ-fár'ē-ə) N. condition in which the eyelids are small or absent; also called ablephary. ADJ. ablepharous

abnormal ADJ. unusual in placement, development, structure, or condition.

ABO blood group system N. the most important of several systems for classifying human blood, used in blood transfusion therapy. Based on the presence or absence of two antigens, A and B, on the surface of red blood cells (erythrocytes), the system classifies blood into four groups: type A, which contains antigen A and antibodies against antigen B; type B, which contains antigen B and antibodies against antigen A; type AB, which contains both antigens; and type O, which contains neither antigen but has antibodies against both. *See also* BLOOD TYPING.

abocclusion N. condition in which, in biting, the upper jaw teeth do not touch the lower jaw teeth.

aboral ADJ. away from, furthest from, or opposite the mouth.

abortifacient N. agent that produces abortion.

abortion N. termination of pregnancy; expulsion or removal of the embryo or fetus before it has reached full development and can normally be expected to be capable of independent life. It may be spontaneous or induced. ADJ. abortive

    habitual abortion N. repeated spontaneous expulsion of the products of conception in three or more pregnancies, often for no known cause.

    imminent abortion N. appearance of symptoms, including bleeding from the vagina and colicky pains, that signal impending loss of the products of conception.

    incomplete abortion N. termination of pregnancy in which some of the products of conception are not expelled but rather are retained in the uterus. It usually leads to heavy bleeding, is occasionally complicated by infection, and almost always requires surgical interven-

ABO BLOOD GROUP SYSTEM

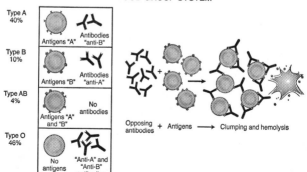

Type A 40%	Antigens "A"	Antibodies "anti-B"
Type B 10%	Antigens "B"	Antibodies "anti-A"
Type AB 4%	Antigens "A" and "B"	No antibodies
Type O 46%	No antigens	"Anti-A" and "Anti-B" antibodies

Opposing antibodies + Antigens → Clumping and hemolysis

tion. Also called partial abortion.

induced abortion N. deliberate termination of pregnancy. The conception product may be removed by suction, curettage (scraping of the uterus), the induction of uterine contractions, or hysterotomy (cutting into the uterus).

spontaneous abortion N. noninduced, natural loss of the products of conception. Common causes include faulty development of the embryo; abnormality of the placenta; or disease, injury, or trauma in the expectant mother. Symptoms include bleeding from the vagina and abdominal pain. Also called miscarriage.

therapeutic abortion N. legal, induced abortion done for medical reasons, as when the pregnancy threatens the pregnant woman's life.

threatened abortion N. appearance of symptoms, including bleeding from the vagina and sometimes abdominal cramps, that signal that the products of conception may be lost. Rest and careful medical observation are usually advised.

abortion pill *See* RU 486.

abortus (ə-bôr′təs) N. fetus whose weight is below ½ kilogram (a little more than 1 pound) at the time it is removed or expelled from the mother's body.

abrachia (ə-brā′kē-ə) N. condition of having no arms. *See also* PHOCOMELIA.

abrade (ə-brād′) V. to rub off, as a skin or covering layer, deliberately or accidentally.

abrasion N.
1. rubbing or wearing away by some frictional, mechanical process.
2. area of body surface that has lost its outer layer of skin or mucous membrane because it has been rubbed off or worn away, as in scraping the knee in a fall. ADJ. abrasive

abreaction N. esp. in psychoanalysis, working out a repressed disagreeable experience or emotion by reliving it in speech and action; this release may be accomplished through psychotherapy, hypnosis, or the use of certain drugs (*see also* CATHARSIS). If feelings are worked out through muscular (motor) use, the process is called motor abreaction.

abruptio placentae (ə-brŭp′shē-ō′ plə-sĕn′-tē′) N. disorder of pregnancy in which the placenta prematurely separates from attachment to the wall of the uterus; marked by hemorrhage (concealed or evident), pain, and fetal distress.

abscess (ăb′sĕs′) N. accumulation of pus that results from a breakdown of tissues (a common problem being tissue breakdown around a tooth, producing an abscessed tooth).

absolute threshold N. lowest level of stimulus that can be sensed (e.g., the lowest intensity of a sound that a person can hear).

absorbance N. ability of a substance to absorb light or X rays. Materials with high absorbance for X rays are termed radiodense or radiopaque.

absorption (əb-sôrp′shən) N. incorporation of matter by other matter, as in the dissolving of a gas in a liquid or the taking up of a liquid by a

porous solid; the passage of substances into tissues, as in the passage of digested food into the intestinal cells (*compare* ADSORPTION).

abstinence (ăb′stə-nəns) N. voluntary act of going without something such as food, alcohol, tobacco, or sex.

acanthocyte (ə-kăn′thə-sīt′) N. abnormal red blood cell (erythrocyte) with irregular projections of protoplasm, giving it a spiny or thorny appearance.

acanthocytosis (ə-kăn′thə-sī-tō′sĭs) N. presence of acanthocytes in the blood, as in abetalipoproteinemia.

acantholysis N. breakdown of the thorny-cell layer of the epidermis (e.g., in the skin disorder pemphigus).

acanthoma (ăk′ən-thō′mə) N. tumor of outer-skin cells.

acanthosis (ăk′ăn-thō′sĭs) N. overdevelopment and thickening of the prickle-cell layer of the outer skin, as in psoriasis. ADJ. acanthotic
acanthosis nigricans N. skin disease characterized by hyperpigmentation and warty lesions of the body folds; can be benign or malignant.

acapnia (ā-kăp′nē-ə) N. condition in which the carbon dioxide level in the blood is less than normal, sometimes caused by very deep or very rapid breathing; also called hypocapnia. ADJ. acapnic, acapnial

acardia (ā-kär′dē-ə) N. congenital absence of the heart, as in some monsters.

acariasis (ăk′ə-ri′ə-sĭs) N. infestation with mites (e.g., the itch mite, which causes scabies); also called acaridiasis, acariosis.

acaryote (ā-kăr′ē-ōt′) *see* PROKARYOTE.

acataleptic ADJ.
1. mentally deficient.
2. uncertain or doubtful.

acataphasia (ā-kăt′ə-fā′zē-ə) N. condition in which a central nervous system lesion leaves one unable to express thoughts in an organized manner.

acathexia (ăk′ə-thĕk′sē-ə) N. inability to retain bodily secretions. ADJ. acathectic

acathexis (ăk′ə-thĕk′sĭs) N. abnormal psychological condition in which objects, thoughts, and memories that ordinarily have great significance to an individual arouse no emotion.

accessory (ăk-sĕs′ə-rē) ADJ. aiding or serving to supplement; for example, the eyebrow is an accessory of the eye, helping to protect it.

accessory nerve N. one of a pair of motor nerves, the eleventh cranial nerves, that supply muscles involved in speech, swallowing, and certain movements of the head and shoulders.

accident N. unexpected happening, esp. one that results in injury. *See also* CEREBROVASCULAR ACCIDENT.

accident-prone ADJ. having a greater-than-average incidence of accidents.

acclimation (ăk′lə-mā′shən) N. state of adaptation to new conditions or environment; also called acclimatization.

Accolate N. *See* TABLE OF COMMONLY PRESCRIBED DRUGS—TRADE NAMES.

accommodation (ə-kŏm′ə-dā′shən) N. adjustment of the eye for various distances.

accommodation reflex N. reflex consisting of the changes that enable an object to be focused on the retina. In adjusting for near vision, the pupils constrict, the lenses become more convex, and the eyes converge; in adjusting for far vision, the reverse changes occur. The ability of the eye to accommodate decreases with age.

accretio N. abnormal joining of parts that are normally separate (e.g., two fused organs).

accretion (ə-krē′shən) N. addition of new material, resulting in growth; accumulation.

Accupril N. See TABLE OF COMMONLY PRESCRIBED DRUGS—TRADE NAMES.

ACE inhibitors N. abbrev. for angiotensin converting enzyme inhibitors.

acebutolol N. oral beta blocker (trade name Sectral) used in the treatment of hypertension and also capable of stimulating the cardiovascular system. Adverse effects include fatigue and exacerbation of asthma or angina.

acellular (ā-sĕl′yə-lər) ADJ. not containing cells; not having a cell structure.

acephalia N. absence of the head, as in the development of some monsters; also, acephalism, acephaly.

acetabulum (ăs′ĭ-tăb′yə-ləm) N. cup-shaped hollow in the hipbone into which the head of the thighbone (femur) fits and rotates in a ball-and-socket joint. ADJ. acetabular

acetaminophen (ə-sē′tə-mĭn′ə-fən) N. widely used nonprescription drug, sold under many trade names (e.g., Tylenol, Liquiprim, Panadol, Tem-pra, Anacin III) that relieves mild to moderate pain (analgesic) and reduces fever (antipyretic); it is frequently used in place of aspirin because it is less likely to cause gastrointestinal upset. Overdosage, either acute or chronic, may cause severe liver or kidney disease, which can be fatal.

acetaminophen/codeine N. See TABLE OF COMMONLY PRESCRIBED DRUGS—GENERIC NAMES.

acetazolamide N. drug (trade name Diamox) that inhibits an enzyme, carbonic anhydrase. Formerly used as a diuretic, and now used in the treatment of high altitude pulmonary edema and glaucoma.

acetone (ăs′ĭ-tōn′) N. colorless liquid with a characteristic sweet, fruity odor present in small amounts in normal urine but in increased amounts in the blood and urine of persons with faulty glucose and fat metabolism (e.g., in diabetes mellitus and certain other metabolic disorders). Commercially available specially treated paper and sticks that turn a certain color when wet with urine containing acetone are used by some persons with diabetes mellitus to test for acetone production as an indication of the course of their disorder.

acetone bodies See KETONE BODIES.

acetonemia (ăs′ĭ-tō-nē′mē-ə) N. presence of large amounts of acetone in the blood.

acetonuria (ăs′ĭ-tōn-yŏōr′ē-ə) See KETONURIA.

acetylcholine (ə-sēt′l-kō′lēn′) N. chemical that is an important neurotransmitter in the body, functioning in the transmission of impulses between nerve

cells and between nerve cells and muscle.

acetylcholinesterase N. enzyme that stops the action of acetylcholine by chemically altering it; present in several body tissues including muscle, nerves, and red blood cells.

acetyl Co-A N. high-energy organic molecule formed during metabolism of carbohydrates (sugars), amino acids (proteins), and fats; a major source of metabolic energy and the main precursor for body synthesis of cholesterol and other steroids. Also called acetyl Coenzyme-A.

acetylsalicylic acid *See* ASPIRIN.

achalasia N. failure of a muscle, particularly a sphincter (muscular ring or valve), to relax, esp. in the gastrointestinal tract (e.g., the cardiac sphincter of the stomach). *See also* CARDIOSPASM.

ache (āk) N. a dull, usually moderately intense, persistent pain as in headache.

Achilles tendon N. large tendon that connects the calf muscles to the heel bone.

achlorhydria (ā′klôr-hī′drē-ə) N. abnormal condition characterized by the absence of hydrochloric acid in the gastric juice, often associated with pernicious anemia, other severe anemias, and cancer of the stomach. ADJ. achlorhydric

acholia (ā-kō′lē-ə) N.
1. condition in which little or no bile is secreted.
2. condition in which the normal flow of bile into the digestive tract is obstructed.

achondroplasia (ā-kŏn′drō-plā′zhə) N. inherited disorder in which a defect in cartilage and bone formation results in a form of dwarfism characterized by short limbs on a normal trunk; also called chondrodystrophy. ADJ. achondroplastic

achromasia (ăk′rō-mā′zē-ə) N. condition in which there is less pigment in the skin than is normal; pallor. *See also* ALBINISM; VITILIGO.

achromatism N. state of seeing gray tones instead of colors; colorlessness.

achromia (ā-krō′mē-ə) N. absence of normal color, as in albinism. ADJ. achromic

Achromycin N. trade name for the antibiotic tetracycline.

achylia (ā-kī′lē-ə) N. absence or severe deficiency of hydrochloric acid, pepsinogen, or other digestive secretions. ADJ. achylous

acid N.
1. chemical that has at least one hydrogen atom, tastes sour, turns litmus paper pink or red, and forms a salt when combined with a base (hydrochloric acid is normally a part of the digestive juice produced in the stomach).
2. colloquialism for lysergic acid diethylamide (LSD), a drug that causes hallucinations (a person using LSD is called an acid head). ADJ. acidic

acid poisoning N. poisoning resulting from the ingestion of a toxic acidic compound, such as hydrochloric acid, sulfuric acid, or nitric acid, many of which are found in cleaning products; for emergency treatment, contact a local poison control center for advice.

acid-base balance N. normal equilibrium between acids and alkalis (bases) in the body maintained by buffer systems in the blood and the regulatory activities of the lungs and kidneys in excreting wastes to prevent the buildup of excessive acids (acidosis) or alkalis (alkalosis) in the blood and other tissues. With a normal acid-base balance in the body, the blood is slightly alkaline, registering 7.35–7.45 on the pH scale (where 7 is neutral and above 7 alkaline).

acidemia (ăs′ĭ-dē′mē-ə) N. condition in which there is an increased concentration of hydrogen ions in the blood and hence the blood is more acid than normal (below 7 on the pH scale.)

acid-fast ADJ. pert. to microorganisms whose stained color resists decolorization after treatment with an acid solution, esp. the tubercle bacillus *Mycobacterium tuberculosis*.

acidity (ə-sĭd′ĭ-tē) N. condition of having an acid content, or of being an acid, or of tasting sour.

acidophil N.
  1. cell that readily stains with acids.
  2. microorganism that grows in acidic materials; also called acidophile. ADJ. acidophilic

acidophilus milk (ăs′ĭ-dŏf′ə-ləs) N. preparation of milk that has been acted on (fermented) by a bacterium (*Lactobacillus acidophilus*), used in treating some intestinal disorders.

acidosis (ăs′ĭ-dō′sĭs) N. disturbance in the normal acid-base balance of the body in which the blood and body tissues are more acidic than normal. It may result from respiratory causes leading to retention of carbon dioxide, as in breathing disorders; from metabolic causes such as prolonged or severe diarrhea, from impaired kidney function, as a complication of diabetes, or as a result of several common poisonings (salicylate, cyanide, isoniazide, methanol).

aciniform ADJ. grape-shaped, as some tumors.

acinus (ăs′ĭ-nəs) N., *pl.* acini, general term for a small saclike structure, esp. that found in a gland, ADJ. acinar, acinic, acinose, acinous

acne (ăk′nē) N. inflammatory disease of the sebaceous glands of the skin, usually on the face and upper body, characterized by papules, pustules, comedones (blackheads) and in severe cases by cysts, nodules, and scarring. The most common form, acne vulgaris, usually affects persons from puberty to young adulthood. Treatment includes topical and oral antibiotics (e.g., tetracycline but not before age 12), topical vitamin A derivatives, dermabrasion, and cryosurgery. *See also* ROSACEA.

acne rosacea *See* ROSACEA.

acneiform ADJ. resembling or like acne.

acorea (ăk′ə-rē′ə) N. absence of the pupil in an eye.

acou- comb. form indicating an association with hearing (e.g., acousma, hallucination that strange sounds are heard).

acoustic nerve (ə-kōō′stĭk) N. *See* AUDITORY NERVE.

acquired (ə-kwīrd′) ADJ. resulting from outside factors; not inherited or congenital; for example, dislikes for some odors and foods are acquired.

acquired immune deficiency syndrome (AIDS) N. serious,

often fatal condition in which the immune system breaks down and does not respond normally to infection. The victims commonly develop Kaposi's sarcoma and recurrent severe infections. The disease became epidemic in the early 1980s, affecting almost exclusively male homosexuals, intravenous drug users, and hemophiliacs. It has now spread to heterosexual populations and is known to be transmitted through sexual contact or the use of contaminated drug apparatus. The cause has been identified as a virus (human immunodeficiency virus—HIV). No treatment has yet proven effective. The best defense against AIDS is prevention. *See also* SAFE SEX.

acquired immunity N. any form of immunity (insusceptibility to a particular disease) not innate but obtained during life. It may be natural, actively acquired by the development of antibodies after an attack of an infectious disease (e.g., chicken pox) or passively acquired, as when a mother passes antibodies against a specific disease to a fetus through the placenta or to an infant through colostrum, or it be may be artificial, acquired through vaccination. *See* HIV.

acquired reflex N. *See* conditioned reflex.

acritical (ā-krĭt'ĭ-kəl) ADJ. without a crisis, as of some diseases; not critical.

acro- comb. form indicating an association with a limb (an extremity) or an extreme state (e.g., acroanesthesia, loss of sensation in the extremities).

acrocyanosis (ăk-rō-sī'ə-nō'sĭs) N. abnormal condition characterized by bluish discoloration and coldness of the extremities, esp. the hands, caused by spasm of the blood vessels brought about by exposure to cold, emotional stress, or other factors; also called Raynaud's sign.

acrodermatitis (ăk'rō-dûr'mə-tī'tĭs) N. inflammation or dermatitis of the skin of either the arms or the legs.

acromegaly (ăk'rō-měg'ə-lē) N. hormonal disorder occurring in middle-aged people and characterized by progressive enlargement and elongation of the hands, feet, and face, often accompanied by headache, muscle pain, and visual and emotional disturbances. It is caused by an overproduction of growth hormone by the anterior pituitary gland (due to a tumor) and is treated by radiation or surgery of the pituitary. Also called acromegalia. ADJ. acromegalic

acromicria N. condition of having underdeveloped fingers and toes and other parts; also called acromikria.

acromion (ə-krō'mē-ŏn') N. high point of the shoulder; an extension of the spinous part of the scapula. ADJ. acromial

acromphalus (ə-krŏm'fə-ləs) N. abnormal protrusion of the navel, sometimes marking the start of umbilical hernia.

acromyotonia (ăk'rō-mī'ō-tō'nē-ə) N. abnormal pulling of the muscles that move the hand or foot, causing a contraction deformity; also called acromyotonus.

acrophobia (ăk'rə-fō'bē-ə) N. abnormal fear of high places.

ACTH *See* ADRENOCORTICOTROPIC HORMONE.

Actifed N. trade name for a fixed-combination drug containing an antihistamine and a decongestant. It is used in the treatment of minor allergic and upper respiratory conditions.

actin (ăk′tĭn) N. protein in muscle that, along with myosin, makes up the contractile elements of muscles. *See also* TROPONIN, SARCOMERE.

acting out N.
1. in psychiatry, indulging or manifesting some forbidden or detrimental behavior by a patient in treatment who experiences trouble in talking about a conflict in a therapeutic session.
2. more broadly, unconsciously showing feelings, not in words but in actions (as in impulsively breaking something without admitting anger).

actino- prefix indicating an association with a ray or radiation (e.g., actinotherapy, treatment of disease by means of special rays, such as ultraviolet radiation).

actinomycosis (ăk′tə-nō-mī-kō′sĭs) N. disease of cattle and humans (in humans, caused by the bacteria *Actinomyces israeli*) characterized by the appearance of lumpy abscesses that exude pus through long sinuses. The most common and least severe form of the disease (cervicofacial actinomycosis) affects the face and neck region and is often called lumpy jaw. Less common, more serious forms affect the chest (thoracic actinomycosis) and abdomen (abdominal actinomycosis). Fever, chills and sweats, and weakness may occur in all forms of the disease. Treatment includes incision and drainage of the abscesses and administration of penicillin. ADJ. actinomycotic

action potential (ăk′shən) N. change in electrical charge (activity) developed in a muscle or nerve cell after stimulation that leads to its discharge or contraction. Occurs as a result of the movement of various chemicals such as sodium, potassium, and calcium between cells. *See* DEPOLARIZATION, RESTING POTENTIAL.

THE ACTION POTENTIAL
IN A NERVE CELL

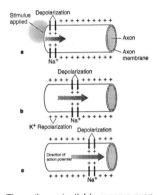

The action potential in a nerve axon consists of a transient change in electrical charge between the inside and the outside of the axon. At baseline, the outside of the axon is more positively charged than the inside. During depolarization (passage of the action potential), the inside becomes more positive, due to the inward movement of sodium (Na^+) and the outward movement of potassium (K^+) ions. The region then repolarizes (returns to the baseline state) when movements of Na^+ and K^+ reverse. This process takes place sequentially, moving like a "wave" from one end of the nerve to the other.

Activase N. trade name for the commercially available form of the thrombolytic agent recombinant tissue plasminogen activator.

activated charcoal N. purified powder form of charcoal used as a potent antidote in the treatment of some forms of poisoning. Given orally, usually as a slurry, it aids in the adsorption of many different agents.

activation N.
1. stimulation of the brain by way of the brainstem (reticular activating system).
2. stimulation of activity in an organism, body part, or chemical.

active immunity N. form of acquired immunity in which the body produces its own antibodies against disease-causing antigens. It can occur naturally after infection or artificially after vaccination (*compare* PASSIVE IMMUNITY).

active transport N. carrying of a substance (e.g. drug, amino acid) across a cell membrane against the concentration or pressure gradient, requiring the expenditure of energy (*compare* OSMOSIS; PASSIVE TRANSPORT).

acuity (ə-kyoo′ĭ-tē) N. clarity or sharpness; the degree of being distinct, such as in visual acuity.

acupressure (ak′yə-prĕsh′ər) N. compression of various points on the body leading to stimulation of nerves and physiologic effects; for example, pressure on the inside of the wrist will result in a decrease in motion sickness. *See also* MOTION SICKNESS BANDS.

acupuncture (ăk′yoo-pŭngk′ chər) N. method of producing analgesia or treating disease by inserting very thin needles into specific sites on the body along channels, called meridians, and twirling, energizing, or warming the needles.

acute (ə-kyoot′) ADJ.
1. coming on suddenly and severely.
2. sharp, as an acute pain (*compare* CHRONIC).

acute childhood leukemia N. progressive, malignant disease of the blood-forming tissues that is the most common type of cancer in children, *See also* ACUTE LYMPHOCYTIC LEUKEMIA.

acute lymphocytic leukemia (ALL) N. rapidly progressive malignancy of the blood-forming tissues, characterized by proliferation of immature lymphoblastlike cells in the bone marrow, spleen, lymph nodes, and circulating blood. Most common in children, particularly from ages two to ten, it has a sudden onset with fever, pallor, loss of appetite, fatigue, hemorrhage, and recurrent infections. Treatment involves chemotherapy, blood transfusions, and treatment of secondary infections. Since the mid-1970s there have been improved survival rates. Also called acute lymphoblastic leukemia.

acute myelocytic leukemia (AML) N. malignant disease of blood-forming tissues characterized by uncontrolled proliferation of granular leukocytes (a type of white blood cell). It may occur at any age but is most frequent in adolescents and young adults. Onset, which often is gradual, is marked by spongy, bleeding gums; anemia; fatigue; bone pain; and recurrent infection. Treatment includes chemotherapy, repeated blood transfusions, immunotherapy, and bone marrow transplants. Also called myeloid leukemia.

acute organic brain syndrome N. sudden confusion and disorientation in an otherwise mentally normal person, resulting from drugs, infections, head injury, or other factors.

acute stress response *See* FIGHT OR FLIGHT RESPONSE.

acyclovir (ā-sī′klō-vîr) N. oral antiviral (trade name Zovirax) used in the treatment of herpes genitalis, and indicated for the management of both initial and recurrent episodes. Although it does not cure the disease, clinical symptoms are reduced, as is the frequency of recurrence. Adverse effects include nausea, vomiting, and headache.

ad- prefix meaning toward (e.g., adduction), sticking to (e.g., adhesion), increase of (e.g., adjunct).

-ad suffix meaning toward a given part (e.g., cephalad, toward the head).

ad nauseam N. literally, of such a degree as to produce nausea; rarely used other than colloquially for needless repetition.

adactyly (ā-dăk′tə-lē) N. absence of fingers and/or toes. Also called adactylia, adactylism. ADJ. adactylous

Adalat N. *See* TABLE OF COMMONLY PRESCRIBED DRUGS—TRADE NAMES

adamantine ADJ.
  1. pert. to tooth enamel.
  2. hard-surfaced.

Adams-Stokes syndrome N. condition characterized by recurrent sudden attacks of unconsciousness, with or without convulsions, caused by transient heart block; also called Stokes-Adams syndrome.

Adam's apple N. bulge at the front of the neck formed by the thyroid cartilage of the larynx.

adaptation (ăd′ăp-tā′shən) N.
  1. ability of an organism or body part to adjust to changes in its environment.
  2. adjustment of the eye to changing light in the surroundings. *See* LIGHT ADAPTATION.
  3. decrease in the frequency of nerve response under conditions of constant stimulation (*compare* HABITUATION).

Adderall N. *See* TABLE OF COMMONLY PRESCRIBED DRUGS—TRADE NAMES.

addict (ə-dĭkt′) N. person whose use of a particular substance (e.g., heroin, alcohol) is such that abrupt deprivation of the substance produces characteristic withdrawal symptoms.

addiction (ə-dĭk′shən) N. condition of strong or irresistible dependence on the use of a particular substance (e.g., heroin, alcohol) such that abrupt deprivation of the substance produces characteristic withdrawal symptoms.

Addison's disease N. disease caused by failure of function of the cortex of the adrenal gland, resulting in deficiency of adrenocortical hormones and disturbance of the normal levels of glucose and minerals in the body. Symptoms, often gradual in onset, include weakness, anorexia, fatigue, increased pigmentation, weight loss, and reduced tolerance to cold. Treatment includes administration of adrenocortical hormones and maintenance of normal levels of glucose and electrolytes in the blood. Many people with Addison's disease wear a Medi-

Alert ID. Also called Addison's syndrome; hypoadrenalism.

additive N. something added as a flavoring or dye to food, either natural or artificial.

adduct (ə-dŭkt′) V. to pull a part toward the body (*compare* ABDUCT).

adduction N. moving of a part toward the body (esp. toward a line that would pass through the body's center from head to foot); for example, returning an outstretched arm to the side of the trunk.

adductor (ə-dŭk′tər) N. muscle that, when flexed, pulls a part toward the body or the body's vertical midline.

aden-, adeni-, adeno- comb. forms indicating an association with a gland or glands (e.g., adenectomy, surgical removal of a gland; adenalgia, pain in a gland).

adenine (ăd′n-ēn′) N. chemical (a purine) contained in DNA (deoxyribonucleic acid) and RNA (ribonucleic acid) and also found in tea; important in carrying genetic information in cells.

adenitis (ăd′n-ī′tĭs) N. inflammation of a lymph node or gland, often associated with infection, as in neck adenitis in cases of throat infection.

adenocarcinoma (ăd′n-ō-kär′sə-nō′mə) N. malignant tumor of a gland, or tumor in which the cells form a glandular structure.

adenohypophysis (ăd′n-ō-hī-pŏf′ĭ-sĭs) N. *See* ANTERIOR PITUITARY GLAND.

adenoid (ăd′n-oid′) N. lymphatic tissue in the back of the nasal passage, on the wall of the nasopharynx. Adenoids may become enlarged and cause difficulty in breathing through the nose after repeated infection. Also known as pharyngeal tonsils. ADJ. adenoid, glandlike. *See* TONSIL.

ANATOMICAL LOCATION
OF THE ADENOIDS

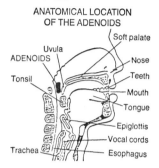

adenoidectomy (ăd′n-oi-dĕk′tə-mē) N. surgical removal of the adenoids. This operation was once commonly performed along with tonsillectomy (removal of the tonsils) but is now much less common, usually performed only when pharyngeal complications are present.

adenoma (ăd′n-ō′mə) N. benign epithelial tumor in which the cells are derived from glandular tissue or have a glandular structure. An adenoma may cause the affected gland to become overactive.

adenomalacia N. condition in which a gland or glands become soft.

adenomatosis (ăd′n-ō′mə-tō′sĭs) N. condition in which many glandlike growths develop.

adenomegaly N. gland enlargement.

adenomyomatosis N. condition in which many nodules develop in the tissues of or around the uterus.

adenomyosis N. condition in which the endometrium (lining of the uterus) grows into the uterine muscle tissue; also called adenomyometritis.

adenopathy (ăd′n-ŏp′ə-thē) N. general term for gland disease and enlargement, esp. of the lymph glands.

adenosclerosis N. glandular hardening.

adenosine (ə-děn′ə-sēn′) N. compound that is a major constituent of many biologically important molecules, including the hereditary materials DNA (deoxyribonucleic acid) and RNA (ribonucleic acid), the energy-storage compounds ATP (adenosine triphosphate) and AMP (adenosine monophosphate), and many enzymes; also used as an anti-arrythmic drug.

adenosine diphosphate (ADP) (dī-fŏs′fāt′) N. compound consisting of adenosine, ribose, and two phosphate (phosphorous-containing) groups and involved in the storage and transfer of energy in cells, esp. in muscle.

adenosine monophosphate (AMP) (mŏn′ŏ-fŏs′fāt′) N. body chemical found in muscle and important in metabolism; cyclic AMP (cAMP) is involved in nervous system, hormone, and cell functions.

adenosine triphosphate (ATP) (trī-fŏs′fāt′) N. compound consisting of adenosine, ribose, and three phosphate (phosphorous-containing) groups and involved in the storage and transfer of energy in cells, esp. in muscle.

adenosis (ăd′n-ō′sĭs) N. general term for a disease of the glands, esp. the lymph glands.

adenovirus (ăd′n-ō-vī′rəs) N. any of a large group of viruses, many of which are responsible for upper respiratory tract infections (e.g., the common cold) and other common infections.

ADH *See* ANTIDIURETIC HORMONE.

adhesion (ăd-hē′zhən) N. band of fibrous tissue that causes normally separate structures to stick together. Adhesions are most common in the abdomen where they frequently follow surgery, injury, or inflammation. If they cause pain or other symptoms or interfere with normal functioning, surgical intervention is necessary.

adient ADJ. having a tendency to move toward a stimulation source, such as light or warmth.

adipo- (ăd′ə-pō) comb. form indicating an association with fat or fatness (e.g., adipogenesis, fat formation) (*See also* terms beginning with LIPO-).

adipocyte (ăd′ə-pō-sīt′) N. fat cell that makes up fatty tissue of the body.

adiponecrosis (ăd′ə-pō-nə-krō′sĭs) N. death of fat cells or fatty tissue in the body.

adipose (ăd′ə-pōs′) ADJ. fatty, composed of fat.

adipose tissue N. type of connective tissue containing many fat cells. It forms a layer under the skin and serves as an insulating layer and as an energy reserve.

adipose tumor *See* LIPOMA.

adiposis (ăd′ə-pō′sĭs) N.
1. condition in which there is an abnormal amount of fat present in the body because of overeating, a metabolic disorder, or glandular malfunction.
2. corpulence, obesity.

adiposuria (ăd′ə-pō-soŏr′ē-ə) N. passing of fat in the urine. This condition is almost always abnormal and may be due to a variety of conditions, including elevated blood fats (hypercholesterolemia, hypertriglyceridemia) and kidney disease (nephrotic syndrome). Also called lipuria.

adipsia N. absence of thirst; lack of desire to drink fluids.

adjunct N. something that is added, as an accessory agent or procedure. ADJ. adjunctive

adjustment (ə-jŭst′mənt) N.
1. change to a more satisfactory condition, as in overcoming emotional problems.
2. in chiropractic, correction of a displaced vertebra.

adjuvant (ăj′ə-vənt) N. something that helps or reinforces a process, as in enhancing an immune response (*see also* ADJUNCT; BUFFER; CATALYST).

adnexa N., *pl.,* accessory parts that enable an organ to function; for example, the adnexa of the eye are the eyelids, tear glands, and tear ducts, and the fallopian tubes are adnexa of the uterus. ADJ. adnexal

adolescence (ăd′l-ĕs′əns) N. period between puberty and adulthood (*see also* AGE), marked by extensive physical, psychological, and emotional changes.

adrenal (ə-drē′nəl) ADJ.
1. pert. to the adrenal gland.
2. near the kidney(s).

adrenal gland N. either of a pair of triangular endocrine, or ductless, hormone-secreting glands situated atop a kidney.

ADRENAL GLAND

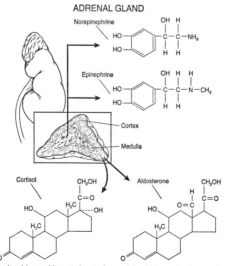

The adrenal gland in position at the surface of the kidney, the two main regions of the adrenal gland, and representative hormones from each region.

There are two functional portions—the adrenal cortex manufactures and secretes sex hormones (estrogen), glucocorticoids (cortisone), essential to the function of many body systems, and mineralocorticoids (aldosterone), essential for the maintenance of water and salt balance in the body. The medulla manufactures and secretes catecholamines (epinephrine and norepinephrine) into the circulation. These are essential in the maintenance of numerous body functions, including normal blood pressure and heart function, as well as the response to stress (fight or flight response). *See also* FIGHT OR FLIGHT RESPONSE.

adrenalectomize v. destroy or eliminate adrenal gland function either by removal of both glands, total destruction of the blood supply, or experimentally, by toxic drugs.

adrenaline (ə-drĕn′ə-lĭn) *See* EPINEPHRINE.

adrenergic (ăd′rə-nûr′jĭk) ADJ. indicating a relationship to either epinephrine or norepinephrine, their release, or their actions, esp. in association with the sympathetic nervous system; also called sympathomimetic (*compare* CHOLINERGIC).

adreno- comb. form indicating an association with the adrenal glands (e.g., adrenomegaly, enlargement of one or both of the adrenal glands; adrenocortical, pert. to the cortex of the adrenal gland).

adrenocorticotropic hormone (ACTH) (ə-drē′nō-kôr′tĭ-kō-trŏp′ĭk) N. hormone secreted by the anterior pituitary gland that is essential for the development of the cortex of the adrenal gland and for its secre-

tion of corticosteroids (mineralocorticoids and glucocorticoids). Stress, trauma, major surgery, fever, and other conditions stimulate ACTH secretion. Also called corticotropin.

adsorption (ăd-sôrp′shən) N. adherence of a thin layer of a gas, liquid, or dissolved substance to the surface of another. For example, in some gas masks, activated charcoal acts as an adsorbent, picking up gases on its surface. (*Compare* ABSORPTION.) ADJ. adsorbent

adult (ə-dŭlt′) N. fully grown and developed organism.

adulterant (ə-dŭl′tər-ənt) N. added matter that lessens the purity, effectiveness, or reliability of a substance.

advance directive N. any of a number of means (e.g., conversations, written directives, living wills, and durable power of attorney) by which a mentally competent patient indicates what interventions he or she would refuse or accept after losing the capacity to make decisions. Federal legislation now requires that all hospitalized patients have a form on file indicating their desires; in many cases, failure to follow a patient's requests on an advanced directive is considered unethical and may result in legal action.

advanced life support *See* EMERGENCY MEDICAL TECHNICIAN.

advancement (ăd-văns′mənt) N. act of freeing a part (e.g., a tendon) and reattaching it surgically at another (advanced) place.

adventitia (ăd′vĕn-tĭsh′ə) *See* TUNICA. ADJ. adventitial

adventitious (ăd'věn-tĭsh'əs) ADJ. not inherited; accidental; acquired from outside the organism (e.g., a scar on the arm).

Advil N. trade name for over-the-counter ibuprofen tablets.

aer-, aero- comb. forms indicating an association with air, oxygen, or other gas (e.g., aerocele, air-filled swelling). *See also* PNEUMO-.

aerate V. to charge with air or oxygen.

aerobe N. organism that thrives in air or more particularly oxygen (compare anaerobe). ADJ. aerobic

aerobic exercise N. exercise system based on continuous action movements, as in swimming, dancing, bicycling, running, or walking. Designed to increase oxygen consumption and improve functioning of the lungs and cardiovascular system (*compare* CALISTHENICS).

Aerobid N. trade name for the inhaled steroid flunisolide.

aerodontalgia (âr'ə-dŏnt-ăl'gĭ-ă) N. pain in the teeth resulting from change in air pressure, as in flying or climbing a mountain.

aeroembolism (âr'ə-em'bō-lizm) *See* AIR EMBOLISM.

aerophagia (âr'əfā'jə) N. swallowing of air, usually followed by belching, flatulence, and discomfort; also called aerophagy.

afebrile (ā-fĕb'rəl, ā-fē'brəl) ADJ. having no fever.

affect (ə'-fĕkt) N.
1. emotional reactions associated with an experience.

2. in psychiatry, emotional tone behind an expressed emotion or behavior (e.g., some schizophrenics have flattened affect).

affective disorder N. mood disturbance accompanied by manic or depressive symptoms not caused by any other organic or mental disorder.

afferent (ăf'ər-ənt) ADJ. carrying inward, toward the center, as a nerve carrying a sensory impulse (e.g., cold, texture) to the brain (*compare* EFFERENT).

affinity (ə-fĭn'ĭ-tē) N. attraction to, attracting force causing certain atoms to combine with others to form molecules. Certain antibiotics exhibit an affinity for particular microorganism (e.g., penicillin for streptococcus). Oil layers in water because the two substances lack affinity for each other.

aflatoxin (ăf'lə-tŏk'sĭn) N. toxin produced by various fungi that may contaminate food; thought to predispose to development of hepatoma (primary liver cancer).

AFP *See* ALPHA FETOPROTEIN.

Afrin N. trade name for the over-the-counter decongestant nasal spray, oxymetazoline hydrochloride.

afterbirth N. fetus-supporting material (placenta and fetal membranes) expelled from the mother's uterus after a baby is born.

aftercare N. care of a convalescent, chronically ill, or handicapped person after formal acute medical care has ended; may include the provision of special aids or facilities (e.g., handrails, ramp) necessary for living at home.

afterhearing N. continuing sensation of hearing a sound that has actually stopped.

afterimage N. continuing sensation of seeing an image that is no longer visible.

afterpains N. pains from uterine contractions felt by a woman after her baby is born.

aftertaste N. persistence of a taste sensation after the stimulus is gone.

agalactia (ă-gə-lăk′tē-ə) N. condition in which milk is not secreted or is not contained in a mother's breasts after she has delivered a child; also called agalactosis.

agalorrhea (ă-gal′ō-rē′ă) N. stopping or limiting of milk flow from the breasts.

agammaglobulinemia (ā-găm′ə-glŏb′yə-lə-nē′mē-ə) N. rare immunological disorder characterized by the virtual absence of gamma globulins (immunoglobulins) from the blood serum and resultant heightened susceptibility to infection. It may be congenital (sex-linked and persistent or transient during the first few weeks of life) or acquired (often as the result of a cancer and/or its treatment). (*Compare* HYPOGAMMAGLOBULINEMIA.)

agastria (ā-gas′trē-ă) N. absence of the stomach, usually as a result of surgical removal.

age N. lifetime, from birth to the present (or to death), generally given in calendar years for these common groups: neonate—birth to 4 weeks; infant—birth to 1 year; child—birth to puberty; adolescent—puberty to adulthood; adult—maturity onward; aged—a nonspecific term, generally meaning of retirement age and beyond. *See also* BONE AGE; CHRONOLOGICAL AGE; DEVELOPMENTAL AGE; MENTAL AGE.

agenesis (ā-jĕn′ĭ-sĭs) N. nondevelopment of a part or an organ; also called agenesia.

Agent Orange N. chemical defoliant mixture containing the toxic substance dioxin, used during the Vietnam War as a means of removing underbrush, and containing a poison that can adversely affect the skin, liver, kidneys, and nervous system. Since the war ended, thousands of veterans have filed lawsuits against the U.S. government and the manufacturers of Agent Orange, seeking compensation for both illnesses of their own and birth defects in their offspring that were allegedly caused by exposure to dioxin.

agerasia (ā-jĕr-ā′sĭ-ă) N. appearance of youthfulness in an old person.

agglutination (ə-gloōt′n-ā′shən) N. clumping together of antigen-carrying cells or microorganisms as a result of their interaction with specific antibodies.

agglutination test N. blood test used to identify unknown antigens. A sample with the unknown antigen is mixed with a known antibody; whether or not agglutination occurs helps in identifying the unknown antigen. The test is useful in determining susceptibility to certain diseases, in blood typing, and in tissue matching (e.g., for transplants).

agglutinin (ə-glo͞ot′n-ĭn) N. substance in an antibody that causes clumping of a specific antigen (e.g., the Rh factor).

agglutinogen (ăg′lo͞o-tĭn′ə-jən) N. substance that causes agglutinin production.

aggregation (ăg′rĭ-gā′shən) N. assembly, clumping, or clustering of cells, molecules, or substances. For example, platelets aggregate to help form a blood clot; white blood cells form an aggregation around foreign bodies (such as viruses) to try and destroy them.

aggression (ə-grĕsh′ən) N. hostile behavior directed against oneself or others, arising from frustration or inner drives.

aging N. process of growing old. Generally during aging a person's height decreases, bone tissue diminishes, hair becomes gray and/or is thinned or lost, nose and ears lengthen, eye lenses become more rigid, and other physical changes occur. The process seems to relate to an internal clock that is specific for each type of organism, the human maximum being about 105 years. Aging is believed to be influenced by genetics and lifestyle and possibly inhibited by exercise and mental activity, a positive attitude, and a balanced and restricted diet.

aging pigment *See* LIPOFUSCIN.

agnosia (ăg-nō′zhə) N. inability to recognize things because of loss in sensory perception.

agonadal ADJ. lacking gonads, or sex glands.

agonist (ăg′ə-nĭst) N.
1. one of a pair of muscles (e.g., the triceps) that contracts during the relaxing phase of the other, the antagonist.

2. drug or other substance that aids another drug or a bodily process.

agoraphobia (ăg′ər-ə-fō′bē-ə) N. abnormal fear of open or public places.

-agra suffix indicating sharp pain or seizure (e.g., melagra, muscle pain in the arms or legs).

agranulocyte (ā-grăn′yə-lō-sīt′) N. type of white blood cell (leukocyte) that lacks intracellular granules when observed under the microscope; includes lymphocytes and monocytes. Note the term agranulocytosis, however, refers to the absence of granulocytes ("a" = without + granulocytosis).

agranulocytosis (ā-grăn′yə-lō-sī-tō′sĭs) N. acute blood disorder, often resulting from radiation or drug therapy, characterized by a severe decrease in granulocytes (a type of white blood cell). Rarely asymptomatic, agranulocytosis is usually accompanied by fever, prostration, and ulcers of the mucous membranes of the mouth, rectum, and vagina. Also called agranulosis; granulocytopenia. ADJ. agranulocytic

agraphia (ā-grăf′ē-ə) N. loss of ability to write one's thoughts, caused by a lesion in the cerebral cortex of the brain. ADJ. agraphic

agromania N. strong desire to be alone or out in open space.

ague (ā′gyo͞o) N. old term for chill or fever, esp. during malaria.

AI *See* ARTIFICIAL INSEMINATION.

AID abbreviation for artificial insemination by a donor.

AIDS *See* ACQUIRED IMMUNE DEFICIENCY SYNDROME.

ailment (āl′mənt) N. slight but often persistent bodily disorder or disease.

air bed N. bed (used for patients with extensive burns or decubitus ulcers) having a special mattress in which air is forced under pressure through thousands of holes on the upper surface, so that the patient floats on a cushion of air.

air embolism N. blockage of a blood vessel by an air bubble that has moved through the bloodstream. It can occur accidentally during surgery, hypodermic injection, intravenous fluid or drug administration, or puncture injury, or as a complication from scuba diving. *Compare* DECOMPRESSION SICKNESS, BENDS.

air sickness N. nausea, vomiting, and headache caused by airplane motion and the changes in gravity experienced during flight, esp. in turbulence. Symptomatic relief is provided by antihistamines and motion sickness bands. *Compare* CAR SICKNESS; MOTION SICKNESS; SEASICKNESS.

airway obstruction N. blockage of any portion of the respiratory tract; usually with reference to the upper tract. When complete, airway obstruction may be life-threatening and is treated with the Heimlich maneuver.

akaryocyte (ā-kăr′ē-ə-sīt′) N. cell without a nucleus, such as an erythrocyte (red blood cell).

akinesia (ā′kĭ-nē′zhə) N. motionlessness; temporary paralysis; also called akinesis.

Al symbol for the element aluminum.

ala N., *pl.* alae, structure that resembles a bird's wing (e.g., ala nasi, flared walls of the nose). ADJ. alar, alate.

alalia (ə-lā′lē-ə) N. inability to speak, e.g., in paralysis of the vocal cords. ADJ. alalic.

alanine (ăl′ə-nēn′) N. nonessential (produced by the body, not required in the diet) amino acid.

Al-Anon N. group that provides support services to relatives of alcoholics or to those who have friends with alcohol-related problems.

alba ADJ. general term meaning white, for some structures, tissues, or diseases (e.g., linea alba, white line of the front of the abdomen, between two muscles); also called albicans.

albedo retinae N. fluid swelling of the retina.

Albers-Schonberg disease (ăl-bärs-shĕn′bärg) *See* OSTEOPETROSIS.

albinism (ăl′bə-nĭz′əm) N. abnormal congenital condition characterized by lack of normal pigment in the skin, eyes, and hair. An albino has pale skin, white hair, and pink eyes and is susceptible to eye and skin disorders.

albino (ăl-bī′nō) N. person with albinism.

Albright's disease N. disorder of bone and cartilage that causes skeletal lesions, sometimes skin lesions, and, in girls, precocious puberty; also called polyostotic fibrous dysplasia.

albuginea (ăl-bū-jĭn'ĭ-ă) N. whitish cover, as of the testicle (also: tunica albuginea testes) or of the eyeball. *See also* SCLERA.

albumin (ăl-byoo'mĭn) N. water-soluble protein found in most animal tissues. Determination of the types and levels of albumin in blood, urine, and other body tissues and fluids is the basis of many diagnostic tests. The constant presence of albumin in the urine (albuminuria) usually indicates kidney disease.

albuminemia N. presence of albumin in the blood, specifically in the serum or plasma.

albuminuria (ăl-byoo mə-noor' ē-ə) N. presence of excessive albumin in the urine, usually indicative of kidney impairment but sometimes due to vigorous exercise. *See also* PROTEINURIA.

albuterol (ăl-byoo'tə-rôl') N. bronchodilator (trade names Ventolin and Proventil) available in oral and inhalant forms. It is used in asthma, emphysema, and other lung conditions. Adverse effects include tachycardia and shakiness. *See* TABLE OF COMMONLY PRESCRIBED DRUGS—GENERIC NAMES.

alcohol (ăl'kə-hôl') N. general term for liquids that are volatile organic compounds made from hydrocarbons by distillation; most often refers to ethyl alcohol (C_2H_5OH), which is used as a rubbing compound and topical antiseptic and as a solvent and preservative in many drugs and biological preparations, and is drunk in alcoholic beverages. When ingested, alcohol acts as a central nervous system depressant and has many other physiological effects. *See also* ALCOHOLISM.

alcohol withdrawal syndrome N. specific set of signs and symptoms that occur from abrupt cessation of drinking alcohol. Typically divided into three phases: 1) the "shakes"—occur within 24 hours of the last drink; consist of tachycardia, tremors, red eyes; 2) alcohol withdrawal seizures—occur within 24–72 hours of the last drink and are generalized (grand mal) in nature; 3) delirium tremens (DTs)—occur approx. 72 hours after last drink; consist of hallucinations, potentially violent behavior, and may be fatal. *See* WITHDRAWAL SYMPTOMS.

alcoholic (ăl'kə-hô'lĭk) N. person with alcoholism; one who uses alcohol to such an extent or in such a way as to interfere with his/her health or efficient functioning.

Alcoholics Anonymous (AA) N. international organization established in 1935 as a support group for persons who want to free themselves, by means of self-help and other programs, from their dependence on, or addiction, to alcohol. A member is expected to acknowledge his/her drinking problem, to attend meetings regularly, to share experiences and difficulties, and to try to maintain sobriety one day at a time. Even after prolonged abstinence, members do not consider themselves cured; rather, they refer to themselves as recovering alcoholics.

alcoholism N. chronic condition in which alcoholic drinks are taken to excess, leading to a breakdown in health and inability to function properly; dependence on, or addiction to, alcoholic beverages such that abrupt deprivation leads to withdrawal symptoms. Alcoholism may occur at any age; its cause is unknown, but hereditary and biochemical as well as cultural and psychosocial factors are believed to play important roles. The consequences of alcoholism include impaired intellectual functioning, physical skills, memory, and judgment; peripheral abnormalities in nerve function; esophageal and gastrointestinal problems, impaired liver function, sometimes leading to cirrhosis of the liver, and damage to the heart muscle. Impaired emotional, social, and often economic/professional functioning also affects the self, family, and community. Alcoholism in pregnant women is also thought to damage the growth and development of the fetus (fetal alcohol syndrome). Acute withdrawal symptoms include tremor, anxiety, hallucinations, and in severe cases delirium tremens. Treatment includes psychotherapy, often in groups such as Alcoholics Anonymous, and the use of certain drugs like Antabuse that cause vomiting if alcohol is ingested. ADJ. alcoholic

Aldactone N. trade name for the diuretic, anti-hypertensive agent, spironolactone.

aldosterone (ăl-dŏs′tə-rōn′) N. hormone (one of the mineralocorticoids) released by the cortex of the adrenal gland; it regulates salt (sodium and potassium) and water balance in the body. Along with antidiuretic hormone (ADH), aldosterone plays a crucial role in the body's water regulation.

ALDOSTERONE

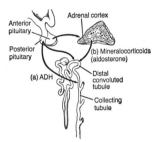

The two hormones that control water reabsorption in the nephron. (a) Antidiuretic hormone (ADH) from the hypothalamus and posterior pituitary gland. (b) Aldosterone from the adrenal cortex.

aldosteronism (ăl-dŏs′tə-rō-nĭz′əm) N. condition characterized by an overproduction of aldosterone from the adrenal cortex. It may result from disease of the adrenal cortex (Conn's syndrome) or secondarily as a result of kidney or liver disease or other disorders. Symptoms include sodium retention, increased blood pressure, alkalosis, muscular weakness, and cardiac abnormalities. Also called hyperaldosteronism.

alendronate N. *See* TABLE OF COMMONLY PRESCRIBED DRUGS —GENERIC NAMES.

aleppo boil (ə-lĕp′ō) *See* ORIENTAL SORE.

alexia (ə-lĕk′sē-ə) N. loss of reading ability; also called word blindness. ADJ. alexic

alexithymia (ə-lĕk′sə-thī′mē-ə) N. inability to express one's feelings; inability to identify particular bodily reactions (e.g., sweating, fast heartbeat) occurring with emotional excitement.

alge-, algesi-, algo- comb. forms indicating an association with pain (e.g., algesia, sensitivity to pain).

-algia suffix indicating an association with pain (e.g., neuralgia).

alimentary canal (ăl′ə-měn′tə-rē) N. digestive tube through which food passes and is digested and absorbed. It extends from the mouth to the anus. Also called alimentary tract. *See also* DIGESTIVE SYSTEM.

alimentation (ăl′ə-měn-tā′shən) N. act or process of providing or receiving nourishment.

aliquot N. portion of the total amount of a liquid, solid, or gaseous substance; often, but not always, an equal fraction of the whole amount (such as one-half, 50 cc).

alkalemia (ăl′kă-lē′mĭ-ă) N. state of higher than normal alkalinity in the blood (representing a lower concentration of hydrogen ions), state in which the pH of the blood is higher than the normal range (7.35–7.45).

alkali (ăl′kə-lī′) N. general term for a compound (e.g., potassium hydroxide) that has the properties of a base (vs. acid), it contains the hydroxyl ion (OH), forms a salt when combined with an acid, and forms a soap when combined with a fatty acid. ADJ. alkaline

alkali poisoning N. poisoning resulting from the ingestion of an alkali compound (e.g., ammonia, lye); for emergency treatment, contact a local poison control center for advice.

alkalinuria N. condition in which the normally slightly acid urine is alkaline.

alkaloid (ăl′kə-loid′) N. natural nitrogen-containing base found in plants.

alkalosis (ăl′kə-lō′sĭs) N. disturbance in the normal acid-base balance of the body in which the blood and body tissues are more alkaline than normal; it may result from hyperventilation, vomiting, or other conditions that cause an increase in base ions or a decrease in acid ions (*compare* ACIDOSIS). ADJ. alkalotic

alkylating agent (al′kĭ-lāt-ing) N. any of a group of drugs used in the chemotherapeutic treatment of cancer. Antineoplastic drugs that are alkylating agents interfere with the proliferation of cells.

ALL *See* ACUTE LYMPHOCYTIC LEUKEMIA.

allantois (ə-lăn′tō-ĭs) N. one of the extraembryonic membranes surrounding the developing fetus. Lying between the inner amnion and outer chorion, it carries blood from the fetus to the placenta and forms umbilical blood vessels.

Allegra N. *See* TABLE OF COMMONLY PRESCRIBED DRUGS—TRADE NAMES.

allele (ə-lēl′) N. one of two or more alternative forms of a hereditary unit (gene) situated in the same site on paired (homologous) chromosomes and determining a given characteristic of an organism. For example, the gene for blue eye color and the gene for brown eye color are two alleles of the gene for eye color. Also called allelomorph. ADJ. allelic

allergen (ăl′ər-jən) N. substance (e.g., ragweed pollen or the proteins of milk, egg, or wheat) that can cause an allergy. ADJ. allergenic

allergist (ăl'ər-jĭst) N. physician who specializes in allergology.

allergology N. medical specialty dealing with allergies, their causes and treatment.

allergy (ăl'ər-jē) N. hypersensitivity reaction to the presence of an agent (allergen) that is intrinsically harmless, such as animal hairs, dust, pollen, or substances in certain foods. Symptoms vary widely but may include bronchial congestion, the appearance of a rash (often itchy), vomiting, edema, conjunctivitis, runny nose, or serious systemic reactions leading to anaphylactic shock and possibly death. Allergies are very common, affecting probably more than 15% of the U.S. population. Allergies are diagnosed through skin tests (patch test, scratch test) and other laboratory procedures. Treatment is avoidance of the allergen, if possible; the use of antihistamine drugs to relieve the symptoms, desensitizing injections in some cases (e.g., hay fever), and other measures. (*See also* HAY FEVER; URTICARIA.) ADJ. allergic

allo- comb. form indicating an association with another or a condition of abnormality or reversal (e.g., alloploidy, condition of having inherited two or more sets of chromosomes from different species).

allodynia (ăl'ə-dĭn-ē-ə) N. pain from stimuli that are not normally painful. The pain may occur other than in the area stimulated. Various diseases can cause hypersensitivity to pain, such as trigeminal neuralgia and complex regional pain syndrome (reflex sympathetic dystrophy). *See also* TRIGEMINAL NEURALGIA; COMPLEX REGIONAL PAIN SYNDROME.

allograft (ăl'ə-grăft') N. tissue segment from one member to be applied as a graft to another member of the same species but of a different genetic makeup.

allopathy (ə-lŏp'ə-thē) N. system of medicine that aims to produce (e.g., through drugs, compresses) a condition opposite to or antagonistic to that affecting the ill person (e.g. applying cold for a fever) (*compare* HOMEOPATHY). ADJ. allopathic

allopurinol N. drug (trade name Zyloprim) used to treat gout and other conditions in which there is a buildup of uric acid. Adverse effects include blood abnormalities, gastrointestinal upsets, and allergic reactions.

all-or-none law N. principle describing the characteristic response of a nerve fiber or a muscle, esp. the heart muscle, whereby any stimulus above threshold level causes the nerve or muscle to respond to its fullest extent or not at all.

alogia (ə-lō'jē-ə) N. loss of speaking ability, resulting from brain defect or injury.

alopecia (ăl'ə-pē'shə, -shē-ə) N. loss of hair; baldness. It may be partial or complete, permanent or temporary. It can result from hereditary factors, hormonal imbalances, certain diseases, drugs and treatments (e.g., chemotherapy for cancer), and sometimes normal aging. Treatment is limited; the Food and Drug Administration has approved the drug minoxidil, marketed in a liquid form called Rogaine, for use in male-pattern baldness (loss of hair on the crown of the head). Human hair transplants have worked well in selected cases.

alpha fetoprotein (AFP) N. protein normally synthesized by a fetus. Determination of the AFP levels in amniotic fluid (through amniocentesis) or in the blood of pregnant women during a certain time in pregnancy can be used to detect the presence of neural tube defects such as spina bifida and anencephaly in the fetus. Elevated AFP levels in the serum of adults may indicate certain cancers and other diseases.

alpha rhythm N. brainwave frequency of moderate voltage that is characteristic of a person who is awake but relaxed; also called alpha wave. It is one of four brain wave patterns (*compare* BETA RHYTHM; DELTA RHYTHM; THETA RHYTHM).

alprazolam (ăl-prā′zə-lăm′) N. antianxiety agent (trade name Xanax) of the benzodiazepine class. Adverse effects include fatigue, dry mouth, confusion, and nasal congestion. *See* TABLE OF COMMONLY PRESCRIBED DRUGS—GENERIC NAMES.

ALS *See* AMYOTROPHIC LATERAL SCLEROSIS.

Altace N. trade name for the antihypertensive agent ramipril. *See* TABLE OF COMMONLY PRESCRIBED DRUGS—TRADE NAMES.

alternative medical systems *See* TABLE OF ALTERNATIVE MEDICINE TERMS.

alternative medicine *See* TABLE OF ALTERNATIVE MEDICINE TERMS.

altitude sickness N. syndrome caused by low oxygen concentration at high altitudes associated with mountain climbing or air travel in unpressurized aircraft. Symptoms include rapid breathing, headache, dizziness, anxiety, or euphoria. Also sometimes called mountain sickness.

aluminum N. common metallic element. Aluminum preparations are widely used in astringents, deodorants, antiperspirants, antiseptics, and antacids. *See also* TABLE OF IMPORTANT ELEMENTS.

Alupent N. trade name for the inhaled bronchodilator metaproterenol.

alveoli N., *pl.* of alveolus.

alveolitis (ăl′vē-ə-lī′tĭs) N.
1. inflammation of the small saclike structures (alveoli) in the lungs, caused by inhaling dusts and marked by shortness of breath, cough, fever, and joint pain. With repeated exposure to the source of irritation, the condition may become chronic. *See also* BAGASSOSIS AND FARMER'S LUNG.
2. inflammation of the socket of a tooth, sometimes occurring after tooth extraction. *See also* DRY SOCKET.

alveolo- comb. form indicating an association with an alveolus or alveoli (e.g., alveolocapillary, pert. to the alveoli and capillaries of the lungs).

alveolus (ăl-vē′ə-ləs) N., *pl.* alveoli
1. any tiny saclike structure, esp. the tiny air sacs of the lungs where the exchange of oxygen and carbon dioxide takes place.
2. socket in the jaw that retains the root of a tooth.
3. small depression or pit. ADJ. alveolar

GAS EXCHANGE IN THE ALVEOLUS

Alveolus

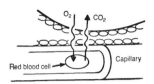

Oxygen (O_2) taken into the lungs during breathing passes through the thin walls of the alveolus to a capillary and then into red blood cells. Simultaneously, carbon dioxide (CO_2) waste products pass from red blood cells to the alveolus, where they are exhaled into the atmosphere.

Alzheimer's disease N. progressive loss of mental ability and function, often accompanied by personality changes and emotional instability. A common disorder affecting both men and women, it usually starts between ages 50 and 60, often with memory lapses and changes in behavior; it progresses to include symptoms of confusion, restlessness, inability to plan and carry out activities and sometimes hallucinations and loss of sphincter (i.e., bladder) control. The cause is unknown but plaques and neurofibrillary tangles are commonly found in the brain tissue. There is no cure, with treatment aimed at alleviating the symptoms. Also called presenile dementia.

Amaryl N. See TABLE OF COMMONLY PRESCRIBED DRUGS—TRADE NAMES.

amastia (ā-măs'tē-ə) N. absence of one or both breasts, from either developmental fault or surgery.

amaurosis (ăm'ô-rō'sĭs) N. blindness, esp. in the absence of an obvious eye lesion (e.g., that due to disease of the spine or brain). ADJ. amaurotic

amaurotic family idiocy See TAY-SACHS DISEASE.

amb-, ambi- comb. forms indicating an association with both sides (e.g., ambidexterity, ability to use both hands with equal skill, as in writing).

Ambien N. See TABLE OF COMMONLY PRESCRIBED DRUGS—TRADE NAMES.

ambient (ăm'bē-ənt) ADJ. pert. to a surrounding or environmental quality (e.g., ambient air).

amblyopia (ăm'blē-ō'pē-ə) N. dimness of vision without detectable organic lesion of the eye.

ambulation N. act of walking or moving about.

ambulatory (ăm'byə-lə-tôr'ē) ADJ. able to walk, thus descriptive of a patient not confined to bed.

ameba (ə-mē'bə) N. one-celled jellylike organism whose shape changes. Some amebas cause disease in humans. See also AMEBIASIS.

amebiasis (ăm'ə-bī'ə-sĭs) N. infection with a disease-causing ameba, esp. *Entamoeba histolytica,* the cause of amebic dysentery; also called amebiosis, amebosis.

amebic (ə-mē'bĭk) ADJ. pert. to or caused by an ameba (e.g., amebic dysentery).

amebic dysentery N. inflammation of the intestine caused by *Entamoeba histolytica,* usually acquired through feces-contaminated food or water, and characterized by frequent, loose, usually blood-tinged stools and sometimes liver involvement.

Treatment usually includes metronidazole.

amelia (ə-mĕl′ē-ə, ə-mē′lē-ə) N. congenital absence of an arm or leg (*compare* PHOCOMELIA).

ameloblast (ăm′ə-lō-blast′) N. enamel-forming cell (of teeth).

amenorrhea (ā-mĕn′ə-rē′ə) N. abnormal stoppage or absence of the menstrual flow. It may be caused by congenital abnormality of the reproductive tract or by endocrine (hormonal) dysfunction, malnutrition, marked change in the amount of body fat (as occurs in strenuous exercise programs), severe trauma, or emotional upset. Primary amenorrhea is arbitrarily defined as delay of onset of the menstrual flow (menarche) beyond age 18. Secondary amenorrhea refers to cessation of menstruation in a woman who has previously menstruated. Treatment involves correction of the underlying cause and hormone therapy if necessary. Also called amenia. ADJ. amenorrheal

Americans with Disabilities Act (ADA) N. Federal statute signed into law on July 26, 1990. The ADA prohibits discrimination on the basis of disability in employment, programs, and services provided by state and local governments, goods and services provided by private companies, and in commercial facilities. It contains requirements for new construction, for alterations or renovations to buildings and facilities, and for improving access to existing facilities of private companies providing goods or services to the public. It also requires that state and local governments provide access to programs offered to the public.

The ADA also covers effective communication with people with disabilities, eligibility criteria that may restrict or prevent access, and requires reasonable modifications of policies and practices that may be discriminatory.

ametria (ə-mē′trē-ə) N. congenital absence of the uterus.

ametropia (ăm′ĭ-trō′pē-ə) N. abnormal eye condition marked by failure of the image to focus properly on the retina; common types of ametropia are astigmatism, myopia (nearsightedness), and hyperopia (farsightedness). ADJ. ametropic

amine (ə-mēn′, ăm′ēn) N. organic compound that contains nitrogen.

amino acid N. organic compound, containing an amino group (NH_2) and a carboxyl group (COOH), that is the end product of protein digestion and the basic building block from which proteins are synthesized in the cell. During protein synthesis, amino acids are linked together by peptide bonds. These are broken down during digestion. Ten amino acids, termed essential amino acids, cannot be synthesized in adequate amounts and at the necessary rate by the body and must be supplied in foods; they are isoleucine, leucine, lysine, methionine, phenylalanine, threonine, tryptophan, valine, histidine (essential for children), and arginine (essential in early life). Other amino acids necessary for growth and metabolism of the body, including alanine, glycine, cystine, tyrosine, glutamic acid, and serine, can be synthesized in the body. Protein-rich foods (e.g., milk, meat, cheese, eggs) supply the body with essential amino acids. *See also* PEPTIDE BOND.

aminoaciduria (ə-mē'nō-ăs'ĭ-dŏŏr'ē-ə) N. abnormal presence of amino acids in the urine, usually a result of a metabolic defect.

aminophylline (ăm-ĭ-nŏf'ĭ-lĭn) N. bronchodilator used to treat asthma, bronchitis, and emphysema. Adverse effects include gastrointestinal upset and central nervous system stimulation.

amiodarone N. oral parenteral antiarrhythmic (trade name Cordarone) useful in the treatment of arrhythmias that are difficult to control. Since this agent is associated with potentially fatal toxic side effects, including interstitial pneumonia, its use is limited to patients for whom no safer agent has been effective, and who still have life-threatening heart rhythm problems.

amitriptyline (ăm'ĭ-trĭp'tə-lēn') N. drug (trade name Elavil) used to treat depression. Adverse effects include sedation and various cardiovascular, neurologic, and gastrointestinal problems; it also interacts with many other drugs and is used with caution in combination with any other agents. *See* TABLE OF COMMONLY PRESCRIBED DRUGS—GENERIC NAMES.

AML *See* ACUTE MYELOCYTIC LEUKEMIA.

amlodipine besylate N. oral calcium blocker (trade name Norvasc) indicated for once-daily administration in the treatment of hypertension and of angina; side effects include edema, dizziness, flushing, and palpitations. *See* TABLE OF COMMONLY PRESCRIBED DRUGS—GENERIC NAMES.

amlodipine/benazepril N. *See* TABLE OF COMMONLY PRESCRIBED DRUGS—GENERIC NAMES.

ammoniuria (ə-mō'nē-yŏŏr'ē-ə) N. presence of excessive ammonia in the urine.

amnesia (ăm-nē'zhə) N. loss of memory, due to injury to the brain or severe emotional trauma. There are several kinds of amnesia, including anterograde amnesia, retrograde amnesia, and transient global amnesia. ADJ. amnesic

amniocentesis (ăm'nē-ō-sěn-tē'sĭs) N. extraction of amniotic fluid by needle puncture through the abdominal wall of a pregnant woman to aid in the diagnosis of fetal abnormalities (e.g., Down's syndrome, Tay-Sachs disease). The test cannot be performed until about the 15th or 16th week of pregnancy and is recommended when a hereditary pattern in the family or the mother's age (over 35) increases the chance of fetal defects.

amnion (ăm'nē-ən) N. inner membrane sac around the developing fetus (the outer membrane sac being the chorion) (*compare* PLACENTA). ADJ. amnionic, amniotic

amniotic fluid N. liquid that surrounds the fetus during pregnancy, serving as protection for the developing fetus, as a shock absorber, and as medium for the exchange of materials between fetus and mother.

amniotic sac N. thin-walled bag that contains the fetus and amniotic fluid during pregnancy.

amniotomy (ăm'nē-ŏt'ə-mē) N. deliberate surgical breakage of

AMNIOCENTESIS

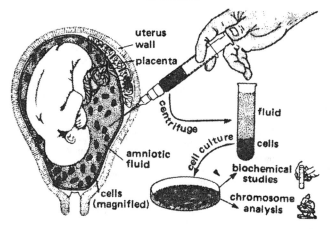

uterus
wall
placenta
centrifuge
fluid
cells
amniotic
fluid
cell culture
biochemical
studies
cells
(magnified)
chromosome
analysis

the fetal membranes; used to induce labor.

amobarbital (ăm′ō-bär′bĭ-tăl′) N. barbiturate drug with sedative-hypnotic effects used for the relief of insomnia and as an anticonvulsant; commonly known as truth serum.

amoeba (ə-mē′bə) N. animal composed of only one cell that has no fixed shape. It is the best known of the single-celled animals, or protozoa. *Also spelled* AMEBA.

amorphous (ə-môr′fəs) ADJ. lacking a specific shape or form (e.g., an ameba).

amoxicillin (ə-mŏk′sĭ-sĭl′ĭn) N. antibiotic, specifically a semi-synthetic oral penicillin, used in the treatment of several bacterial infections. *See* TABLE OF COMMONLY PRESCRIBED DRUGS—GENERIC NAMES.

amoxicillin/clavulanate N. *See* TABLE OF COMMONLY PRESCRIBED DRUGS—GENERIC NAMES.

Amoxil N. trade name for amoxicillin. *See* TABLE OF COMMONLY PRESCRIBED DRUGS—TRADE NAMES.

AMP *See* ADENOSINE MONOPHOSPHATE.

amphetamine (ăm-fĕt′ə-mēn′, mĭn) N. central nervous system stimulant used to treat narcolepsy and some forms of depression and attention-deficit disorders. It alleviates fatigue, promotes alertness, and decreases appetite. Overdosage causes gastrointestinal complaints, rapid heart rate, restlessness, sleeplessness, and in very high doses hallucinations and feelings of panic. It has a high potential for abuse, resulting in tolerance and dependence. Slang: speed. *See* TABLE OF COMMONLY PRESCRIBED DRUGS—GENERIC NAMES.

amphi- comb. form indicating a doubling, affecting both sides, of both kinds (e.g., amphigonadism, state of having tissues for both ovaries and testes; true hermaphroditism).

amphiarthrosis (ăm′fē-är-thrō′sĭs) N. type of joint in which the bones are connected by cartilage allowing only slight motion, but in all directions. The joints between the spinal vertebrae are prime examples.

amphoric breath sound N. abnormal hollow sound heard with a stethoscope that indicates a cavity in the lung.

Amphotericin B (ăm′fə-tĕr′ĭ-sĭn) N. drug, used topically and systemically, to treat certain fungal infections. Adverse effects with systemic use include thrombophlebitis, nausea, and fever; with topical use, local hypersensitivity reactions.

ampicillin (ăm′pĭ-sĭl′ĭn) N. antibiotic (semisynthetic penicillin) used to treat a wide variety of infections. Adverse effects include nausea, diarrhea, skin rash, and anaphylaxis.

amplitude (ăm′plĭ-to͞od) N. size, magnitude, extent of anything; in medicine, often refers to the height of a wave, such as on an electrocardiogram.

ampule (ăm′po͞ol, -pyo͞ol) N. sealable sterile glass tube used to contain medicines, usually for injection by needle. Also called ampul.

ampulla (ăm-po͞ol′ə, -pŭl′ə) N., *pl.* ampullae dilated, flasklike part or structure, esp. the widened portion of a tube. ADJ. ampullar, ampullary

amputation (ăm′pyo͞o-tā′shən) N. surgical removal of a limb, part of a limb, or other body part by surgery (e.g., to treat gangrene or recurrent infection,

severe trauma, or malignancy) or by trauma.

amputee (ăm′pyo͞o-tē′) N. person who has had a limb removed through surgery, trauma, or congenital malformation.

amrinone (ăm′rə-nōn′) N. drug (trade name Inocor) used intravenously in heart failure; it increases the strength of contraction of the myocardium via a mechanism independent of other agents such as digitalis or nitroglycerin. Adverse effects include reduction in the platelet count, which is reversible. *See* MILRINONE.

amygdala (ə-mĭg′də-lə) N. almond-shaped part or structure, specifically the two rounded bulges on the bottom sides of the cerebellum, part of the brain's limbic system. Destruction of the amygdala can result in rage and peculiar sexual behavior.

amyl nitrate N. vasodilator sometimes used to treat angina pectoris. Adverse effects include hypotension, nausea, headache, dizziness, and allergic reactions.

amylase (ăm′ə-lās′, lāz′) N. enzyme that catalyzes part of the reactions by which starch is broken down into simpler carbohydrates. It is present in saliva, pancreatic juices, certain microorganisms, and certain foods.

amyloidosis (ăm′ə-loi-dō′sĭs) N. disorder in which starchlike proteins, called amyloids, accumulate in body tissues, impairing their function. The condition usually results from chronic infections or inflammatory diseases or from certain malignancies.

amyoplasia (ă-mī′ō-plā′zē-ə) N. deficiency in muscular development.

amyotonia (ā′mī-ə-tō′nē-ə) N. lack of muscle tone, weakness.

amyotrophia (ă-mī′ə-trŏf′ē-ə) N. progressive wasting of a muscle or group of muscles; also called amyotrophy.

amyotrophic lateral sclerosis (ALS) (ă-mī′ə-trŏf′ĭk, -trō′fĭk) N. degenerative disease of the central nervous system characterized by progressive muscle atrophy starting in the limbs and spreading to the rest of the body, often accompanied by hyperreflexia (overactive reflexes). Of unknown cause, it usually manifests itself after age 40, affecting more men than women, and progresses rapidly. There is no known treatment. Also called Lou Gehrig's disease.

amyxia (ă-mĭks′ĭ-ă) N. condition in which no mucus is produced.

an-, ana-
1. prefixes meaning upward, backward, duplicate (e.g., anastalsis, reversed muscular action of the intestine, opposite to peristalsis).
2. prefix meaning not (e.g., anaerobe, an organism not needing air or oxygen).

anabolic steroid N. any of a group of compounds, derived from testosterone or prepared synthetically, which aid in constructive metabolism, including the building of cell components such as proteins and fats. They are used to treat certain anemias and malignancies, to promote body growth and weight gain, to strengthen bones in osteoporosis, to counter the effects of estrogen, or to promote masculinizing characteristics. Anabolic steroids are sometimes used illegally by athletes in an attempt to improve their strength and performance.

anabolism (ə-năb′ə-lĭz′əm) N. phase of metabolism involving the conversion, in cells, of simple structures into the complex molecular forms of living material (*compare* CATABOLISM).

anaclisis (ăn′ə-klī′sĭs) N. in psychoanalysis, state of needing someone for support, as an infant's dependence on the mother.

anaerobe (ăn′ə-rōb′, ăn-âr′ōb′) N. organism that thrives without oxygen (*compare* AEROBE). ADJ. anaerobic

anal (ā′nəl) ADJ. pert. to the anus.

anal phase N. in psychoanalytic theory, the second stage in a person's development. The phase occurs in early childhood (1–3 years) and involves conflicts of autonomy with shame and doubt (*compare* ORAL PHASE; PHALLIC PHASE; LATENCY PHASE; GENITAL PHASE).

analbuminemia (ăn′ăl-byōō′mə-nē′mē-ə) N. abnormally low level of albumin in the blood serum.

analeptic (ăn′ə-lĕp′tĭk) N. drug that stimulates (e.g., caffeine) the central nervous system or strengthens or invigorates the body.

analgesia (ăn′əl-jē′zē-ə) N. absence of sensitivity to pain, while remaining conscious, due to nerve damage (as in leprosy), hypnosis, acupuncture, the use of pain-relieving drugs (analgesics), or anything that activates the body's natural pain-relieving system (endorphins). (*Compare* ANESTHESIA.) ADJ. analgesic

analgesic (ăn'əl-jē'zĭk, sĭk) N. pain-relieving substance (e.g., aspirin, acetaminophen).

analogue (ăn'ə-lôg') N. part having a function like that of another but of a different source or species (e.g., the crop of an earthworm is analogous to the human stomach); also called analog.

analysis (ə-năl'ĭ-sĭs) N., pl. analyses
1. division of a thing into its elements (as a chemical) or fundamental parts (as in a procedure).
2. shortened form for psychoanalysis. ADJ. analytic

anamnesis (ăn'ăm-nē'sĭs) N.
1. memory, the faculty of remembering, of recollecting.
2. detailed data collected about a patient and used in analyzing the case.

anamnestic (ăn'ăm-nĕs'tĭk) ADJ. pert. to the antibody production that occurs rapidly the second time a given substance (antigen) is put into the body.

anaphase (ăn'ə-fāz') N. stage in cell division in which the chromosomes move from the center plane of the cell toward the poles. See MITOSIS.

anaphoresis N. condition marked by lack of function of the sweat glands.

anaphrodisia (ăn-ăf'rə-dĭz'ē-ə) N. loss or absence of sexual feeling. ADJ. anaphrodisiac

anaphylactic shock (ăn'ə-fə-lăk'tĭk) N. severe and sometimes fatal hypersensitivity reaction to the injection or ingestion of a substance (e.g., penicillin, shellfish, insect venom, vaccine) to which the organism has become sensitized by a previous exposure. Symp-toms, including anxiety, weakness, shortness of breath, laryngeal edema, cardiac and respiratory abnormalities, hypotension, and shock, may occur within minutes of exposure. Treatment must be prompt and usually involves use of epinephrine, the maintenance of an open airway, and the treatment of cardiac and other problems. Persons with known hypersensitivity reactions are advised to avoid the offending agent and, if that is not always possible (e.g., insect venom), to carry an emergency kit with epinephrine and other necessary first-aid items.

anaphylaxis (ăn'ə-fə-lăk'sĭs) N. strong hypersensitivity reaction to the ingestion or injection of a substance (e.g., penicillin, shellfish) to which the organism has become sensitized by a previous exposure. Symptoms may include localized wheal, itching and swelling, or, in severe cases, anaphylactic shock and even death. ADJ. anaphylactic

anaplasia (ăn'ə-plā'zhə) N. regression of fully developed cells into a more primitive (embryonic) form, occurring in some tumors.

Anaprox N. See TABLE OF COMMONLY PRESCRIBED DRUGS—TRADE NAMES.

anastomosis (ə-năs'tə-mō'sĭs) N., pl. anastomoses
1. communication between two blood vessels, lymph vessels, or nerves.
2. opening or passage, made by surgery, trauma, or pathology, between two normally separate tubular and hollow parts (e.g., two parts of the intestine) (compare FISTULA). ADJ. anastomotic

anatomy (ə-năt′ə-mē) N. study and science of the structure of an organism and its parts (*compare* PHYSIOLOGY) (*see also* GROSS ANATOMY; MICROSCOPIC ANATOMY). ADJ. anatomic, anatomical

andr-, andro- comb. forms indicating an association with the male sex (e.g., androglossia, male-quality voice in a woman).

androgen (ăn′drə-jən) N. general term for substances that produce secondary masculine characteristics (e.g., deep voice, facial hair); a male hormone (e.g., testosterone). Androgens are also chemical precursors to the female hormones (e.g., estrogen) and are present in females as well. ADJ. androgenous, androgenic

androgyne N. person with both ovaries and testes and underdeveloped external male and female sex organs but a predominantly female aspect (*compare* PSEUDOHERMAPHRODITISM). ADJ. androgynous

androsterone (ăn-drŏs′tə-rōn′) N. male sex hormone.

anecdotal ADJ. not based upon systematic collection of scientific data; based upon experience or hearsay evidence. Certain medical practices are said to be based on anecdotal evidence only.

anemia (ə-nē′mē-ə) N. condition in which the hemoglobin content of the blood is below normal limits. It may be hereditary, congenital, or acquired. Basically, anemia results from a defect in the production of hemoglobin and its carrier, the red blood cell (e.g., production of abnormal hemoglobin, misshapen red blood cells, or inadequate levels of hemoglobin), increased destruction of red blood cells, or blood loss (e.g., in hemorrhage after injury or in excessive menstrual flow). The most common cause is a deficiency in iron, an element necessary for the formation of hemoglobin. Symptoms vary with the severity and cause of the anemia but may include fatigue, weakness, pallor, headache, dizziness, and anorexia. Treatment also depends on the cause and severity and may include an iron-rich diet, iron supplements, blood transfusions, and the correction or elimination of any pathological conditions causing the anemia. There are several types of anemia, including aplastic anemia, pernicious anemia, sickle-cell anemia, and thalassemia. ADJ. anemic

anencephaly (ăn′ən-sĕf′ə-lē) N. defect in the development of the brain and skull, resulting in small or missing brain hemispheres; also called anencephalia. ADJ. anencephalic, anencephalous

anergic ADJ.
1. characterized by inactivity, lack of energy.
2. pert. to anergy.

anergy (ăn′ər-jē) N. lack or reduction of immune response to a specific antigen; also called anergia.

anesthesia (ăn′ĭs-thē′zhə) N. absence of sensation, esp. pain. In general anesthesia, which is administered before a major operation (e.g., removal of a lung), total unconsciousness results from injection or inhalation of anesthetic drugs. In local anesthesia loss of sensation is confined to a given small part or area of the body (e.g., the tissues surrounding a tooth to be extracted). In regional anesthesia loss of sensation is produced in a specific area of the body (e.g., in the pelvic area during childbirth by an epidural anesthetic). In topical anesthesia loss of sensation is confined to the surface skin or mucous membranes (e.g., benzocaine solution sprayed on the skin). Hypnosis, acupuncture, and nerve damage, as in leprosy, may also produce anesthesia. (*Compare* ANALGESIA.) ADJ. anesthetic

anesthesiologist (ăn′ĭs-thē′zē-ol′ə-jĭst) N. physician who specializes in anesthesiology.

anesthesiology (ăn′ĭs-thē′zē-ŏl′ə-jē) N.
1. science and study of the use of anesthesia and of anesthetic drugs;
2. medical specialty in the use of drugs and other means to avert or reduce pain in patients, esp. during surgery.

anesthetic (ăn′ĭs-thĕt′ĭk) N. drug (e.g., procaine hydrochloride, Novocain) that causes temporary loss of sensation.

aneuploidy (ăn′yə-ploĭ′dē) N. condition in which the number of chromosomes is either more or fewer than normal. ADJ. aneuploid

aneurysm (ăn′yə-rĭz′əm) N. saclike widening in a blood vessel; it occurs most often in the aorta but can also occur in other blood vessels. Aneurysms are usually caused by atherosclerosis or hypertension, sometimes by trauma, infection, or other factors. An aneurysm may rupture, causing hemorrhage, or it may lead to the formation of thrombi and/or emboli that may block an important blood vessel. Common types of aneurysms include aortic aneurysm

(aneurysm of the aorta) and cerebral aneurysm (aneurysm of any of the major arteries within the brain). Treatment includes use of drugs to reduce the force of cardiac contraction, analgesic and antihypertensive drugs if indicated, and, in some cases, surgical resection of the aorta or affected artery. ADJ. aneurysmal

ANEURYSM OF THE
ABDOMINAL AORTA

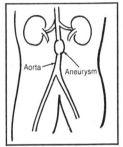

angel dust N. street term for phencyclide hydrochloride; also known as PCP.

angi-, angio- comb. forms indicating an association with blood vessels or lymph vessels (e.g., angiectasis, abnormal widening and sometimes lengthening of an artery or vein).

angiitis (ăn′jē-ī′tĭs) N. inflammation of a blood or lymph vessel.

angina (ăn-jī′nə) N. severe pain, often spasmodic and accompanied by a choking feeling, esp. choking pain in the chest (angina pectoris).

angina pectoris (pĕk′tər-ĭs) N. chest pain, often accompanied by a feeling of choking or impending death; the pain typically radiates down the left arm. It is usually caused by lack of oxygen to the heart muscle, resulting from atherosclerosis of the coronary arteries; attacks are precipitated by exertion, exposure to cold, or stress. Rest and use of drugs (e.g., nitroglycerine) to dilate the coronary arteries relieve pain.

angiocardiogram N. X ray of the heart obtained by following with a rapid series of X-ray films the passage of a contrast medium through the heart and its associated vessels. It is useful in diagnosing heart defects and disorders.

angiogram (ăn′jē-ə-grăm′) N. serial set of X rays taken of an artery or arteries following the injection of a radiopaque contrast medium; used to define the location and condition of an artery, such as the presence of atherosclerosis.

angiography (ăn′jē-ŏg′rə-fē) N. the process of obtaining an angiogram.

angiologist N. physician who specializes in angiology.

angiology N. medical specialty dealing with diseases of the blood and lymph vessels and their treatment; the science of vessels.

angioma (ăn′jē-ō′mə) N. benign tumor made up primarily of blood vessels (hemangioma) or lymph vessels (lymphangioma).

angiopathy (ăn′jē-op′ə-thē) N. any abnormality affecting the blood vessels.

angioplasty (ăn′jē-ə-plăs′tē) N. surgery done on arteries, veins, or capillaries; a technique in which a balloon is inflated inside a blood vessels to flatten any plaque (patch) that obstructs it and causes it to become narrowed (used esp. to open coronary arteries).

PERCUTANEOUS TRANSLUMINAL ANGIOPLASTY

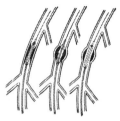

Inflation of the balloon dilates the artery by breaking apart the atherosclerotic plaque.

angiospasm (ăn′jē-ō-spăz′əm) N. involuntary and abnormal contraction of the muscular layer of a blood vessel, leading to decreased blood flow. Depending on the location, such spasms may lead to lack of oxygen (ischemia) to tissues, causing heart pains (angina) or leg cramps (claudication). Some evidence suggests that smoking crack cocaine leads to either heart attack or stroke because it provokes spasm in either the coronary (heart) or cerebral (brain) arteries.

angiotelectasia (ăn′jē-ō-tĕl′ĭk-tā′zē-ə) N. condition characterized by dilation and enlargement of arterioles.

angiotensin (ăn′jē-ō-tĕn′sĭn) N. chemical in the blood that causes blood vessels to become narrowed; also called angiotonin. *See* ANGIOTENSIN CONVERTING ENZYME INHIBITORS. Renin catalyzes the formation of angiotensin I from angiotensinogen. Angiotensin I is converted by angiotensin converting enzyme in the lung to angiotensin II which is then further metabolized to angiotensin III. Angiotensin II is a potent vasoconstrictor and stimulant of sodium and water retention. Angiotensin III is the final metabolically active product and is a strong stimulant of aldosterone secretion.

ANGIOTENSIN METABOLISM

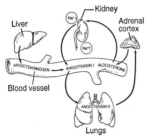

angiotensin converting enzyme inhibitors N. class of drugs that inhibit the angiotensin converting enzyme that converts angiotensin I to the vasoconstrictor, angiotensin II. By blocking this conversion, the blood vessels dilate and the result is improved blood flow. Used in the treatment of hypertension, congestive heart failure, and myocardial infarction. Side effects include orthostatic hypotension, cough, and rarely, life-threatening edema.

angle (ăng′gəl) N., *pl.* anguli, shape formed by the joining of two lines or parts (e.g., costovertebral angle, formed by the attachment of the lowest rib to the spinal column at the lumbar region); also called angulus. ADJ. angular

angstrom N. unit of measure of wavelength (as of ultraviolet radiation or X rays) equal to 1 ten-millionth of a meter, or 0.1 nanometer.

anhidrosis (ăn′hĭ-drō′sĭs) N. failure of sweat gland function.

anhydrous ADJ. having no water (e.g., the waterless form of a chemical compound, as anhydrous ammonia).

anicteric ADJ. without jaundice.

anile ADJ. imbecilic; acting like a feeble, trembling person.

anima (ăn′ə-mə) N. inner self (compare persona).

anion (ăn′ī′ən) N. negatively charged atom.

aniridia (ăn′ī-rĭd′ē-ə) N. congenital absence of all or part of the iris of the eye.

ankle N. joint at which the foot attaches to the leg, formed by the ends of the lower leg bones (tibia and fibula) and the talus, the topmost bone in the foot.

THE ANKLE BONES

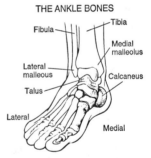

ankle bone *See* ANKLE.

ankyloglossia N. condition in which the band of tissue (frenum) connecting the lower surface of the tongue to the floor of the mouth is abnormally short, limiting the normal movement of the tongue; also called tongue-tied.

ankylosing spondylitis (spŏn′dl-ī′tĭs) N. chronic disease, affecting primarily males under the age of 30, characterized by inflammation and stiffening of the spine and joints, sometimes leading to ankylosis, or fusion, of the involved joints. Treatment includes anti-inflammatory agents and pain relievers. Also called Marie-Strumpell disease. (*Compare* RHEUMATOID ARTHRITIS.)

ankylosis (ăn′kə-lō′sĭs) N., *pl.* ankyloses, rigidity of a joint, often in an abnormal position, resulting from disease (e.g., rheumatoid arthritis) or injury, or produced intentionally as a surgical treatment.

anlage (än′lä-gə) N. in the developing embryo, a structure or part on which some later development depends; rudiment; primordium.

anodyne (ăn′ə-dīn′) N. pain-relieving drug.

anomaly (ə-nŏm′ə-lē) N. marked abnormality, as of an organ or part, esp. a congenital or inherited defect. ADJ. anomalous

anomie N. feeling of isolation, anxiety, or disorientation from any norms (considered by some as a major cause of suicide).

anoperineal ADJ. pert. to the anus and surrounding area (perineum).

anorchism (ă-nôr′kĭz′əm) N. absence of one testis or both testes; also called anorchia, anorchidism. ADJ. anorchidic

anorectal ADJ. pert. to the anus and rectum or to the junction region between the two.

anorexia (ăn′ə-rĕk′sē-ə) N. lack or loss of appetite; possible causes include depression, alcoholism or other drug dependence, fever, and disorders of the alimentary canal (e.g., liver cancer) (*See also* ANOREXIA NERVOSA). ADJ. anorectic, anorexic

anorexia athletica N. use of excessive exercise to lose weight, normally associated with anorexia nervosa. Athletes often restrict calories and/or overexercise to achieve or maintain low body and fat masses. Even though exercise provides many health benefits, there appears to be a unique set of risks associated with intense exercise, especially for the female athlete. Female athletes with eating disorders (ED) significantly outnumber male athletes with the same conditions. However, ED in male athletes are still significantly more frequent than in the general population. *See also* EATING DISORDERS.

anorexia nervosa N. emotional disorder, occurring most commonly in adolescent females, characterized by abnormal body image, fear of obesity, and prolonged refusal to eat, and leading to emaciation, amenorrhea, and other symptoms, and sometimes resulting in death. Treatment includes psychotherapy and nourishment. *See also* BULIMIA.

anorgasmia (ăn′ôr-găz′mē-ə) N. absence of a climax (orgasm) in sexual relations.

anosmia (ăn-ŏz′mē-ə) N. absence of the sense of smell. It may be temporary, as from a cold or respiratory infection, or permanent, resulting from damage to olfactory nasal tissue or the olfactory nerve. ADJ. anosmatic, anosmic

anovulation (ăn-ō′vyə-lā′shən) N. absence of egg production or release from the ovary. It may be caused by ovarian immaturity or postmaturity, pregnancy or lactation, dysfunction of the ovary, hormonal imbalance, or oral contraceptive pills; or be a side effect of other medication.

Also called anovulia. ADJ. anovular, anovulatory

anovulatory ADJ. not associated with ovulation, the development and release of a mature ovum (egg) from the ovary, as in anovulatory menstruation.

anovulatory drug N. drug that inhibits ovulation, as an oral contraceptive pill.

anoxia (ăn-ŏk′sē-ə) N. absence or abnormally low amount of oxygen in the body; can occur in certain abnormal states (e.g., cardiac arrest, anemia, heart failure, impaired respiration) and at high altitudes. ADJ. anoxic

Ansaid N. trade name for the nonsteroidal anti-inflammatory agent flurbiprofen.

Antabuse N. trade name for disulfiram, drug used in the treatment of alcoholism. Reactions can be severe and life-threatening if a patient on this drug ingests alcohol.

antacid (ănt-ăs′ĭd) N. chemical that reduces acidity (e.g., sodium bicarbonate), esp. one taken to relieve upset stomach.

antagonist (ăn-tăg′ə-nĭst) N.
1. one of a pair of muscles (e.g., the biceps) that relaxes during the contraction of the other muscle (the agonist, e.g., the triceps).
2. any chemical that works against the action of another.

ante- comb. form referring to a preceding time, place, or condition (e.g., antenatal, before birth).

antecubital ADJ. pert. to the region of the arm in front of the elbow; it is the site often used for drawing blood for examination.

antemortem ADJ. before death.

antenatal See PRENATAL.

antepartum ADJ. occurring during pregnancy, before childbirth.

anterior (ăn-tēr′ē-ər) ADJ. at or toward the front of a part, organ, or structure, or toward the head in four-legged animals (*compare* POSTERIOR).

anterior crural nerve See FEMORAL NERVE.

anterior nares See NARES.

anterior pituitary gland N. anterior lobe of the pituitary gland, the endocrine gland situated at the base of the brain. Under the control of the hypothalamus, it secretes hormones that control other endocrine glands throughout the body as well as hormones that have a direct effect on body growth and metabolism. Important anterior pituitary hormones are growth hormone (GH), follicle-stimulating hormone (FSH), thyroid-stimulating hormone (TSH), adrenocorticotropic hormone (ACTH), luteinizing hormone (LH), and prolactin, also called adenohypophysis.

ANTERIOR PITUITARY HORMONES

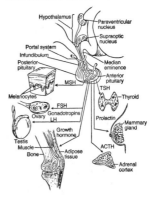

The anterior pituitary gland, its hormones, and their target organs.

antero- comb. form indicating a position to the front of, or placement before, a part or reference point (e.g., anteroinferior, at or toward the front and below) (*compare* RETRO-; POSTERO-). *See* TABLE OF POSITIONAL AND DIRECTIONAL TERMS.

anterograde (ăn'tə-rō-grād') N. in a forward direction, advancing. Often used to refer to the movement of blood or nerve impulses in the normal physiological direction. Compare to retrograde (moving backwards or opposite from the normal physiological direction).

anterograde amnesia N. inability to recall long-ago events but with normal recall of recent happenings (*compare* ANTEROGRADE MEMORY).

anterograde memory N. ability to recall events long past but not recent happenings; also called senile memory (*compare* ANTEROGRADE AMNESIA).

anthelmintic (ănt'hĕl-mĭn'tĭk) N. drug (e.g., piperazine) or chemical that kills intestinal worms.

anthracosis (ăn'thrə-kō'sĭs) N. chronic lung disease, occurring in coal miners and others exposed to coal dust and soot characterized by black deposits on the lungs and bronchi and impaired lung function. *See also* BLACK LUNG DISEASE; PNEUMOCONIOSIS.

anthracycline (ăn'thrə-sĭ-klēn) N. type of antibiotic that comes from the fungus *Streptococcus peucetius*. Anthracyclines are used as treatments for cancer. Examples include daunorubicin (Daunomycin), doxorubicin (Adriamycin), and epirubicin (Ellence). All drugs of this class can cause severe heart damage, even months or years after the patient has stopped taking them.

anthrax (ăn'thrăks') N. bacterial (*Bacillus anthracis*) disease of cattle and other farm animals that can be transmitted to humans from infected animals and animal products. The disease causes skin lesions, fever, muscle pain, nausea, and internal hemorrhage; in a serious, often fatal form, it also attacks the lungs. Treatment is by penicillin or tetracycline. ADJ. anthracic

anti- prefix meaning counter, against, opposite (e.g., antibacterial, pert. to a substance that destroys bacteria).

antiadrenergic ADJ. pert. to blocking or countering the effects of impulses conveyed by the adrenergic postganglionic fibers of the sympathetic nervous system.

antiarrhythmic N. drug used in the treatment of an abnormal heart rhythm.

antiberiberi factor See THIAMINE.

antibiotic (ăn'tĭ-bī-ŏt'ĭk) N. drug (e.g., penicillin), derived from a microorganism or produced synthetically, that destroys or limits the growth of a living organism, esp. a disease-producing bacterium (e.g., *Streptococcus*) or fungus.

antibody N. complex molecule (immunoglobulin), produced by lymph tissue in response to the presence of an antigen (such as a protein of bacteria or other infecting organism), that neutralizes the effect of the foreign substance (*see also* MONOCLONAL ANTIBODY).

anticancer ADJ. used in the treatment of cancer, esp. anticancer drugs (e.g., vincristine sulfate).

THE FIVE TYPES OF ANTIBODIES

Antibody Designation	Percentage of Antibody in Serum	Location in Body	Molecular Weight (daltons)	Number of Four Chain Units	Crosses Placenta	Functions
IgM	5–10	Blood, lymph	900,000	5	No	Principal antibody
IgG	80	Blood, lymph	150,000	1	Yes	Principal component of secondary response
IgA	10	Body secretion, body cavities	400,000	2	No	Protection in body cavities
IgE	~1	Blood, lymph	200,000	1	No	Role in allergic reactions
IgE	0.05	Blood, lymph	180,000	1	No	Receptor site on B-lymphocyte

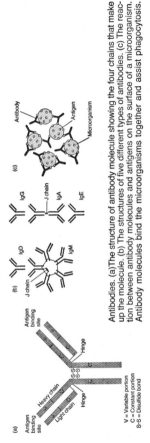

ANTIBODIES

Antibodies. (a) The structure of antibody molecule showing the four chains that make up the molecule. (b) The structures of five different types of antibodies. (c) The reaction between antibody molecules and antigens on the surface of a microorganism. Antibody molecules bind the microorganisms together and assist phagocytosis.

(a) Antigen binding site, Hinge, Heavy chain, Light chain, Hinge, Antigen binding site
V = Variable portion
C = Constant portion
S-S = Disulfide bond

(b) IgD, J chain, IgM, J chain, IgG, IgA, IgE

(c) Antibody, Antigen, Microorganism

anticholinergic (ăn′tē-kō′lə-nûr′jĭk) ADJ. pert. to the blocking of acetylcholine receptors; this results in the inhibition of nerve impulse transmission in the parasympathetic nervous system.

anticoagulant (ăn′tē-kō-ăg′yə-lənt) N. substance that delays blood clotting coagulation (e.g., coumarin, heparin). Anticoagulants are used to prevent clotting in blood used for transfusions and in blood vessels (e.g., in patients with phlebitis). Also called decoagulant. ADJ. anticoagulative

anticonvulsant (ăn′tē-kən-vŭl′sənt) N. drug (e.g., Dilantin) effective in preventing or treating convulsions (e.g., in epilepsy).

antidepressant (ăn′tē-dĭ-prĕs′ənt) N. drug used to treat depression.

antidiabetic N. drug used to treat diabetes mellitus.

antidiarrheal (ăn′tē-dī′ə-rē′əl) N. drug or other substance used to control or stop diarrhea (e.g., Lomotil).

antidiuretic N. drug that limits the formation of urine.

antidiuretic hormone (ADH) (ăn′tē-dī′ə-rĕt′ĭk) N. hormone that inhibits the production of urine by increasing the reabsorption of water in the kidney; it also constricts blood vessels. It is secreted by the hypothalamus and stored and released by the posterior pituitary gland in response to stress, pain, and certain changes in electrolyte balance and blood volume. Along with aldosterone, ADH plays a major role in the body's regulation of water. Also called vasopressin.

antidote (ăn′tĭ-dōt′) N. drug that neutralizes or minimizes the effects of a poison (e.g., pralidoxime chloride, an antidote against poisoning by intake of an organophosphate pesticide) (*compare* ANTITOXIN).

Anti-dumping law of 1985 N. law to prevent hospital emergency departments from refusing to treat patients with an emergency condition, regardless of their ability to pay. Commonly known as COBRA, this law originally passed as part of the Medicare Legislation of 1985 and subsequently was revised several times. It mandates that any person who presents at the Emergency Department of a hospital that receives Medicare funds must get a medical screening examination to rule out the existence of an emergency medical condition or of active labor. If either of these conditions is present, the hospital must, within its resources, do everything possible to stabilize the patient before transferring him to another facility. The patient does not need to be a Medicare recipient for the law to apply; all persons who come to the Emergency Department are covered. Failure of the hospital to comply with COBRA regulations subjects it to a $50,000 fine and loss of Medicare benefits. Also called Emergency Medical Treatment and Active Labor Act (EMTALA).

antiemetic (ăn′tē-ĭ-mĕt′ĭk) N. drug or other substance that prevents or alleviates vomiting and nausea or limits their effects, sometimes used to treat motion sickness (e.g., Emetrol, a mint-flavored solution of glucose, fructose, and orthophosphoric acid).

antiepileptic *See* ANTICONVULSANT.

antiflatulent N. agent that reduces intestinal gas (flatus).

antifungal (ăn′tē-fŭng′gəl) N. agent that destroys or prevents the growth of fungi (e.g., Griseofulvin).

antigen (ăn′tĭ-jən) N. substance (e.g., a toxin) or organism (e.g., an ameba) that, when entering the body, causes the production of an antibody that reacts specifically with the antigen to neutralize, destroy, or weaken it. The presence of certain antigens is the criterion for typing in the ABO blood group system and is important in tissue crossmatching for transplants (e.g., the HLA antigen in kidney transplants). ADJ. antigenic

antigen-antibody reaction N. process by which the immune system recognizes an antigen and causes the production of antibodies specific against that antigen.

antihistamine (ăn′tē-hĭs′tə-mēn′) N. drug, used to treat allergies, hypersensitivity reactions, and colds, that works to reduce the effects of histamine (e.g., chlorpheniramine maleate, Teldrin). ADJ. antihistaminic

antihypertensive (ăn′tē-hī′pər-tĕn′sĭv) N. drug that reduces hypertension (high blood pressure).

anti-inflammatory N. drug (e.g., aspirin, ibuprofen) that counteracts or reduces inflammation. These agents are thought to act by reducing the production of prostaglandins, which contribute to inflammatory processes.

antimalarial (ăn′tē-mə-lâr′ē-əl) ADJ. pert. to destruction or suppression of the causes and carriers of malaria. N. drug used to prevent and treat malaria.

antimicrobial (ăn′tē-mī-krō′bē-əl) N. agent that destroys or limits the growth of a microscopic organism.

antimony (ăn′tə-mō′nē) N. metallic element, also known as stibium (symbol, Sb) used in formation of metallic alloys and in several types of medications.

antimycotic N. agent that destroys or limits the growth of a fungus.

antineoplastic (ăn′tē-nē′ə-plăs′tĭk) N. drug that controls or kills cancer cells, used in the treatment of cancer by chemotherapy. There are several types of antineoplastic drugs, including alkylating agents (e.g., chlorambucil), antimetabolites (e.g., fluorouracil), periwinkle plant derivatives (e.g., vinblastine, vincristine), and antineoplastic antibiotics (e.g., adramycin, actinomycin-D, mithramycin). All are associated with unpleasant and sometimes serious side effects, which may include nausea and vomiting, hair loss, and suppression of bone marrow function.

antioxidant N. type of drug or other substance that absorbs, blocks, or prevents the formation of free radicals, highly reactive compounds that are felt to be potentially responsible for a wide number of conditions, including aging (e.g., vitamin E).

antipernicious anemia factor (ăn′tē-pər-nĭsh′əs) *See* CYANOCOBALAMIN.

antipruritic (ăn′tē-prōō-rĭt′ĭk) N. substance that prevents or relieves itching (e.g., topical anesthetic).

antipsychotic (ăn′tē-sī-kŏt′ĭk) N. drug used to treat a psychosis (e.g., schizophrenia).

antipyretic (ăn′tē-pī-rĕt′ĭk) N. drug that reduces fever (e.g., aspirin).

antisepsis (ăn′tĭ-sĕp′sĭs) N. destruction or inhibition of infection-producing microorganisms, thus preventing infection.

antiseptic (ăn′tĭ-sĕp′tĭk) N. agent (e.g., soap) that slows or stops the continuing growth of microorganisms but may not actually kill them. ADJ. antiseptic

antiserum (ăn′tĭ-sēr′əm) N. serum that contains antibodies against a specific disease; it is used to confer passive immunity (*compare* VACCINE).

antispasmodic (ăn′tē-spăz-mŏd′ĭk) N. agent that relieves or prevents spasm.

antitoxin (ăn′tē-tŏk′sĭn) N. drugs or other agent (e.g., antivenin) that prevents or limits the effect of a microorganism's poison (toxin) (*compare* ANTIDOTE). ADJ. antitoxic

antitussive (ăn′tē-tŭs′ĭv) N. substance (e.g., codeine) that relieves coughing.

antivenin (ăn′tē-vĕn′ĭn) N. drug (antitoxin) used to counteract the effects of venom from the bite of an insect, a snake, or other animal.

Antivert N. trade name for the antihistamine meclizine hydrochloride, used to prevent and treat motion sickness.

antiviral (ăn′tē-vī′rəl) N. drug (e.g., interferon) that destroys viruses.

antrum (ăn′trəm) N., *pl.* antra, in anatomy, cavity or cavelike structure. ADJ. antral

anulus N., *pl.* anuli, ringlike part; also called annulus.

anuria (ə-nōōr′ē-ə) N. inability to urinate, cessation of urine production and excretion. It can be caused by disease of the kidney and bladder or by serious decline of blood pressure. Untreated, it leads to uremia and death. Also called anuresis. ADJ. anuretic

anus N. opening of the rectum, at which the passing of feces is controlled by a circular muscle system (sphincter ani). ADJ. anal

anvil *See* INCUS.

anxiety N. state of mild to severe apprehension, often without specific cause, resulting in body changes such as quickened heartbeat and sweat. Natural body chemicals (e.g., inosine) help to reduce anxiety and its effects.

anxiety attack N. acute episode of intense anxiety and feelings of panic, accompanied by symptoms such as palpitations, breathlessness, sweating, gastrointestinal complaints, and feelings of imminent disaster. The attacks usually occur suddenly, may last from a few seconds to an hour or more, and may occur infrequently or several times a day. Treatment includes reassurance; the use of anxiolytic and ataraxic drugs, sedation, if necessary; and often psychotherapy to alleviate the underlying causes.

anxiolytic (ăng′zē-ō-lĭt′ĭk) N. drug that relieves anxiety. ADJ. anxiety-relieving

aorta (ā-ôr′tə) N. main trunk of the arterial blood circulatory system from which all other arteries (except the pulmonary) branch. This large artery stems from the heart at the left ventricle, passes upward (ascending aorta) toward the neck, arches (aortic arch) and loops, and descends downward (descending aorta) along the left side of the vertebral column through the chest region (thoracic aorta), through the diaphragm to the abdomen (abdominal aorta), where it divides into two iliac arteries. Major arteries (e.g., carotid, coronary) branch from the aorta, transporting the aorta's freshly oxygenated blood to the various organs of the body. The aortic valve, situated between the left ventricle and the aorta, prevents blood from flowing back from the aorta into the heart. ADJ. aortal, aortic

aortic aneurysm See ANEURYSM.

aortic arch See AORTA.

aortic stenosis N. narrowing or stricture of the aortic valve, due to congenital malformation or the result of disease (e.g., rheumatic fever), that obstructs the flow of blood from the heart's left ventricle into the aorta, leading to decreased cardiac output. Symptoms include faint pulse in the extremities, systolic murmur, and exercise intolerance. Children with aortic stenosis are usually restricted from strenuous sports activities (e.g., football). Treatment involves surgical repair of the valve.

aortic valve N. valve in the heart, between the left ventricle and the aorta, that prevents blood from flowing from the aorta back into the heart.

aortitis (ā′ôr-tī′tĭs) N. inflammation of the aorta, usually due to advanced syphilis, sometimes to rheumatic fever.

apathy (ăp′ə-thē) N. absence or suppression of feeling, concern, passion; indifference to things generally found exciting. ADJ. apathetic

APC abbreviation for aspirin, phenacetin, and caffeine, a drug combination found in some over-the-counter remedies for headache and other mild pain.

aperture (ăp′ər-chər) N. hole or opening. See also ORIFICE; PUPIL.

apex N., *pl.* apices, top or pointed end of a structure, as the apex, or tip, of the tongue. ADJ. apical

Apgar score (ăp′gär) N. evaluation of the infant's physical condition usually made one minute after birth and then repeated five minutes after birth. Five factors—heart rate, muscle tone, respiratory effort, color, and reflex irritability—are scored from a low of 0 to a normal of 2 and the five scores combined to give a total score of 0 to 10. In general, a total score below 7 indicates distress.

aphagia (ə-fā′jē-ə) N. inability to swallow, due to pain or paralysis, as in myasthenia gravis.

aphakia (ə-fā′kē-ə) N. absence of the natural lens of the eye, as when a cataract has been surgically removed. ADJ. aphakic

aphasia (ə-kā′zhə) N. inability to speak or express oneself in writing or to comprehend spoken or written language because of a brain lesion (e.g., the result of a cerebrovascular accident stroke). ADJ. aphasic

apheresis (ăf'ə-rē'sĭs) N. procedure, similar to dialysis, for cleansing the blood through filters; used experimentally to treat persons with certain disorders. *See also* PLASMAPHORESIS.

aphrodisia N. sexual desire, esp. if extreme.

aphrodisiac (ăf'rə-dĭz'ē-ăk') N. any substance (e.g., plant, food, or drug) that may stimulate sexual desire.

apical (ā'pĭ-kəl) ADJ. pertaining to the point (apex) of a cone-shaped structure. Typically refers to the tip of the heart as it lies in the chest. This location is commonly used to listen to and count the apical pulse or heart rate.

aplasia (ə-plā'zē-ə) N. failure of an organ or part to develop (*compare* HYPERPLASIA; HYPOPLASIA; PHOCOMELIA, *see also* APLASTIC ANEMIA). ADJ. aplastic

aplastic anemia (ā-plăs'tĭk) N. deficiency of the formed elements (e.g., red blood cells, white blood cells) of the blood due to a failure of the cell-producing machinery of the bone marrow, caused by a neoplasm or, most commonly, by exposure to toxic chemicals, radiation, or certain drugs.

apnea (ăp'nē-ə) N. state of not breathing; arrest of respiration. Attacks of temporary apnea occur in some people during sleep (sleep apnea) and in some newborn babies. *See also* PERIODIC APNEA OF THE NEWBORN. ADJ. apneic

apocrine gland (ăp'ə-krĭn) N. any of several large, deep exocrine glands found in the axillary (armpit), genital, anal, and mammary regions, that secrete a strong sweat with a characteristic odor.

apoenzyme (ăp'ō-ĕn'zīm) N. protein that combines with a coenzyme (non-protein, e.g., some vitamins) to form an active enzyme.

aponeurosis (ăp'ə-nŏŏ-rō'sĭs) N., *pl.* aponeuroses, tendon-like expansion with which a flat muscle attaches to other parts. ADJ. aponeurotic

apoplexy (ăp'ə-plĕk'sē) N. long-used (now obsolete) term for a cerebrovascular accident stroke in which the brain's blood system becomes impaired and muscle control and other nerve function may be affected. ADJ. apoplectic

apoptosis N. programmed death of cells that is under genetic control; the cell's own genes play an active role in its demise. Apoptosis is different from cell necrosis where healthy cells are destroyed by external processes, such as inflammation. This is a common process during development (e.g., formation of the central nervous system) as well as in adulthood (e.g., cyclic breakdown of the endometrial lining of the uterus that leads to menstruation). Certain cancer patients lack the p53 tumor suppressor gene that helps prevent cancer by making a protein that triggers apoptosis in abnormal cells. Absence or abnormality of p53 permits cancer cells to continue to grow.

apparatus (ăp'ə-rā'təs) N., *pl.* apparatuses, in anatomy, group of parts that work together in performing a given function (e.g., auditory apparatus, all the components of the organ of hearing—the ear, including outer, inner, and middle parts).

appendage (ə-pĕn′dĭj) N. something attached or appended. The cecal appendage is the vermiform appendix, commonly called simply the appendix. *See also* ADNEXA.

appendectomy (ăp′ən-dĕk′tə-me) N. surgical removal of the appendix. When a patient has appendicitis, the operation is performed to prevent the appendix from rupturing.

appendicitis (ə-pĕn′dĭ-sī′tĭs) N. inflammation of the vermiform appendix. Symptoms are pain in the abdomen, generally but not exclusively on the right side, nausea, vomiting, low-grade fever, and elevated white blood cell counts. Treatment is appendectomy.

appendix (ə-pĕn′dĭks) N. appendage, esp. the vermiform appendix, the apparently functionless wormlike (vermiform) or fingerlike attachment to the first part of the large intestine (cecum) in the lower right abdomen. *See also* APPENDICITIS.

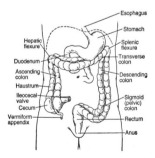

Esophagus
Stomach
Hepatic flexure
Splenic flexure
Duodenum
Transverse colon
Ascending colon
Descending colon
Haustrum
Ileocecal valve
Sigmoid (pelvic) colon
Cecum
Vermiform appendix
Rectum
Anus

Anatomical location of the appendix.

apperception (ăp′ər-sĕp′shən) N. whole perception process: receiving, recognizing, appreciating, assimilating, and interpreting stimuli taken in by the senses (e.g., hearing the roar of a wave on the beach and appreciating the contribution of the separate drops of water that cause the roar) (*compare* GESTALTISM). ADJ. apperceptive

appetite (ăp′ĭ-tīt′) N. normal desire, esp. for food, but also for other needs, including sex.

apraxia (ā-prăk′sē-ə) N. loss or impairment of the ability to make purposeful movements, usually caused by a neurological disorder. ADJ. apraxic

APSAC N. intravenous thrombolytic drug (trade name Eminase) used in the treatment of acute myocardial infarction; side effects include bleeding and stroke.

aqueduct (ăk′wĭ-dŭkt′) N. canal or channel; medically, refers to any of several normal round anatomical pathways for the flow of various body fluids. For example, the cerebral aqueduct connects the third and fourth ventricles in the brain and allows cerebrospinal fluid to flow freely. Obstruction of this duct may lead to swelling and hydrocephalus.

aqueous (ā′kwē-əs) ADJ.
1. made with water (e.g., a chemical compound).
2. like water (e.g., the aqueous humor of the eye).

aqueous humor N. clear, watery fluid circulating in the anterior and posterior chambers of the eye.

arachnodactyly (ə-răk′nō-dăk′tə-lē) N. congenital condition in which the fingers and/or toes are long, thin, and spiderlike.

arachnoid membrane N. thin, delicate membrane that is the middle of the three membranes (meninges) enclosing the brain and spinal cord; the outer membrane is the dura mater, the inner the pia mater. *See* SUB-ARACHNOID SPACE.

ARACHNOID MEMBRANE

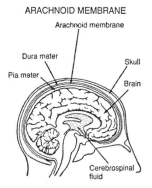

arbovirus (är′bə-vī′rəs) N. large group of viruses that grow in both mammals and in insects such as mosquitos and ticks. Cause viral encephalitis and yellow fever.

arc N. structure or pathway shaped like a bow or loop. *See also* ARCH. Also called arcus.

arch N. bowlike structure or part (e.g., maxillary arch, structure that forms the palate).

arch support N. artificial support for the arch of the foot, generally inserted in shoes, helping, in some cases, to relieve back pain.

area N. general anatomical region (e.g., aortic area, that portion of the chest surface over the cartilage of the right second rib where it attaches to the breastbone, the site at which aortic sounds are best heard through a stethoscope).

areata ADJ. developing or showing as patches (e.g., alopecia

areata, patchy baldness). Also called areatus.

areflexia (ā′rĭ-flĕk′sē-ə) N. absence or loss of reflexes, a sign of possible nerve damage.

areola (ə-rē′ə-lə) N., *pl.* areolae
1. small space as that in tissue (interstice).
2. circle around a pimple, the iris, or the nipple. ADJ. areolar.

arginine (är′jə-nēn′) N. nonessential (produced by the body, not required in the diet) amino acid.

Aristocort N. trade name for the glucocorticoid triamcinolone.

arm N. upper extremity or limb, esp. from the shoulder to the hand and including the upper arm (humerus), forearm (ulna and radius), and wrist (carpus).

MAJOR MUSCLES OF THE UPPER EXTREMITY

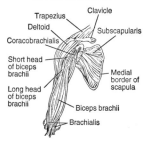

aromatherapy (ə-rō′mə-thĕr′ə-pē) *See* TABLE OF ALTERNATIVE MEDICINE TERMS.

arousal N. increased responsiveness to stimulation; increased desire for sexual activity.

arrector pili (ə-rĕk′tər) N. small muscle of a hair follicle that, when contracted, causes a goose bump.

arrest N. stopping, as of a rhythm or muscle function (e.g., cardiac arrest, sudden stopping of the heart).

arrhythmia (ə-rǐth′mē-ə) N. abnormal heartbeat rhythm, caused by drugs, disease, the body's physiology, or a combination of factors. ADJ. arrhythmic

arsenic (är′sə-nǐk) N. metallic, highly poisonous element. *See also* TABLE OF IMPORTANT ELEMENTS.

arsenic poisoning N. poisoning caused by the ingestion or inhalation of arsenic, an ingredient in some pesticides, dyes, and medicinal products. Small amounts absorbed over a long period may cause headache, nausea, coloring of the skin, and the appearance of white lines on the nails. Ingestion of large amounts leads to severe gastrointestinal problems, swelling of the arms and legs, and possibly renal failure, shock, and death.

arterial bleeding (är-tîr′ē-əl) N. bleeding from an artery, with the blood bright red and coming in spurts. Applying pressure to the artery between the wound and the heart can stop it.

arterial blood N. blood found in the arteries. Except in the pulmonary artery, arterial blood is rich in oxygen transported to the tissues of the body.

arterial blood gases N. laboratory measurement of the pH level and the oxygen and carbon dioxide concentrations in arterial blood. Determination of these parameters is important in the diagnosis and treatment of many diseases (e.g., emphysema, chronic obstructive pulmonary disease, polycythemia).

arterial pressure N. stress exerted by the circulating blood on the arteries. It is a result of the product of cardiac output and vascular resistance. *See also* BLOOD PRESSURE.

arteriectasis (är-tēr′ē-ĕk′tə-sĭs) N. abnormal distension of an artery; also called arteriectasia.

arterio- comb. form indicating an association with an artery or arteries (e.g., arteriocapillary, pert. to arteries and capillaries; arteriovenous, pert. to arteries and veins).

arteriogram (är-tēr′ē-ə-grăm′) N. X ray of an artery filled with a contrast medium.

arteriole (är-tîr′ē-ōl′) N. smallest branch of an artery, leading to a capillary network. ADJ. arteriolar

arteriosclerosis (är-tēr′ē-ō′sklə-rō′sĭs) N. disorder of the arteries, common with advancing age and in certain diseases (e.g., hypertension), characterized by calcification, loss of elasticity and hardening of the walls of the arteries, and resulting in decreased blood flow, especially to the brain and extremities. Symptoms include intermittent limping, memory deficits, headache, and dizziness. There is no specific treatment, but moderate exercise, a low-fat diet, and avoidance of stress are generally recommended. Also called hardening of the arteries.

arteritis (är′tə-rī′tĭs) N. inflammation of an artery or arteries, occurring alone or accompanying another disorder (e.g., rheumatic fever).

artery (är′tə-rē) N. vessel that carries blood away from the heart to the other tissues throughout the body. Except for the pulmonary artery (which carries blood to the lungs), arteries carry oxygen-rich blood. Most arteries are named for the body part they traverse or reach (e.g., the femoral artery courses along the femur). (*Compare* VEIN; *see also* AORTA.) ADJ. arterial. *See* MAJOR ARTERIES AND VEINS OF THE BODY, in Appendix.

arth-, arthro- comb. forms indicating an association with a joint or joints (e.g., arthrodysplasia, joint abnormality or deformity).

arthralgia (är-thrăl′jə) N. pain in a joint or joints.

arthritis (är-thrī′tĭs) N. inflammation of a joint that may cause swelling, redness, and pain. There are several types of arthritis, the most common of which are gout (gouty arthritis), osteoarthritis, and rheumatoid arthritis. ADJ. arthritic

arthrocentesis (är′thrō-sĕn-tē′sĭs) N. introduction of a needle into a joint and the removal of fluid from it (e.g., to determine what chemicals or microorganisms may be present).

arthrography (är-thrŏg′rə-fē) N. X ray of a joint.

arthroplasty (är′thrə-plăs′tē) N. surgical reconstruction or replacement of a joint that is congenitally malformed or that has degenerated as a result of injury or disease (e.g., osteorarthritis).

articulation (är-tĭk′yə-lā′shən) N. *See* JOINT. ADJ. articular

artifact (är′tə-făkt′) N. synthetic object found in a body part, esp. something (as a clip or thread) seen on an X-ray film or in a microscopic field, that does not normally belong there.

artificial blood N. fluid that can carry large amounts of oxygen and is being used as a temporary substitute for blood. The most common is known as Fluosol-DA; it is similar to Teflon and made up of inert perfluorochemicals. Most clinical studies have involved persons who are seriously in need of blood but refuse blood transfusions (e.g., on religious grounds, such as Jehovah's Witnesses).

artificial heart N. device designed to replace the heart and to pump blood throughout the body. An artificial heart (the Jarvik heart) was implanted in a human for the first time in late 1982 and worked in the patient for over 110 days, before he died of complications. Work on these devices is continuing.

artificial insemination (AI) N. introduction of spermatozoa into the female birth canal by means of an instrument (e.g., a slender tube and syringe) to increase the likelihood of conception. The sperm specimen may be provided by the woman's husband (AIH) or partner or by an anonymous donor (AID).

artificial organ N. synthetic device to replace a natural organ or to assist its function (e.g., artificial heart, artificial kidney, artificial pancreas).

artificial respiration N. emergency procedure for maintaining a flow of air through the pulmonary system by using mechanical means or hand pressure to aid a person whose breathing has stopped (e.g., because of drowning, injury, or drugs) or is otherwise not controlled. *See also* CARDIOPULMONARY RESUSCITATION; IRON LUNG.

artificial skin N. synthetic (e.g., plastic, cowhide collagen, shark cartilage) two-layer covering used experimentally to treat burn victims.

As symbol for the element arsenic.

asbestos (ăs-bĕs′təs) N. fiberlike, fire-resistant mineral commonly used as an insulator and roofing material; now implicated in causing lung disease (asbestosis) (even when inhaled in small amounts and for a limited time) and as a carcinogen.

asbestosis (ăs′bĕs-tō′sĭs) N. chronic, progressive lung disease, resulting from breathing in the mineral asbestos and common among asbestos miners and roofers; it is marked by fibrosis of lung tissue. Symptoms include shortness of breath and cough, often leading to respiratory failure; lung cancer is a frequent complication. *See also* PNEUMONOCONIOSIS.

ascariasis (ăs′kə-rī′ə-sĭs) N. infection with ascaris worms, acquired through feces-contaminated water or food. Symptoms may involve cough, wheezing, and fever or gastrointestinal complaints. Treatment is by piperazine and other drugs.

ascites (ə-sī′tēz) N. abnormal accumulation of protein and electrolyte-rich fluid in the abdomen (peritoneal cavity), often a complication of another serious disease (e.g., cirrhosis, nephrosis, congestive heart failure). ADJ. ascitic

ascorbic acid (ə-skôr′bĭk) N. water-soluble vitamin C (*See also* TABLE OF VITAMINS), essential for normal connective tissue, bone and skin development, for fighting bacterial infection, and for preventing scurvy; found esp. in citrus fruits, potatoes, and leafy vegetables.

-ase suffix that identifies an enzyme (e.g., cholinesterase, an enzyme found esp. in blood plasma).

asepsis (ə-sĕp′sĭs) N. state of being without infection or contamination; sterile. ADJ. aseptic

asexual (ā-sĕk′shoō-əl) ADJ. lacking sexual involvement; having no sex.

Asiatic flu N. influenza caused by the Asian virus, first isolated in 1957.

-asis comb. form denoting a condition (e.g., elephantiasis) (*compare* -OSIS).

asparagine (ə-spăr′ə-jēn′) N. nonessential (produced by the body, not required in the diet) amino acid.

aspartame (ăs′pər-tām′) N. artificial sweetener made from the amino acids aspartic acid and phenylalanine. Nearly 200 times as sweet as sugar, aspartame should be avoided by persons with phenylketonuria (PKU).

aspergillosis (ăs′pər-jə-lō′sĭs) N. uncommon and serious infection with a fungus of the genus Aspergillus, most often occurring in persons weakened by another disease or having impaired immunological responses (e.g., those undergoing chemotherapy, receiving immunosuppressive drugs following a transplant, or having acquired immune deficiency syndrome (AIDS)) and characterized by inflammation and lesions of the ear and other organs.

asphyxia (ăs-fĭk′sē-ə) N. condition in which insufficient or no oxygen reaches the tissues, thereby threatening the life of the organism. Common causes are drowning, electric shock, inhaling poison gas, and choking. v. asphyxiate, ADJ. asphyxiated

aspiration (ăs′pə-rā′shən) N.
1. action of breathing in, esp. inhaling an unwanted substance or foreign object.
2. use of suction to take liquids or gases from a body cavity or area, as in aspiration biopsy.

aspiration pneumonia N. inflammation of the lungs and bronchi caused by inhaling or choking on vomit; may occur during anesthesia or recovery from anesthesia, or during an acute episode of alcoholism, seizure, loss of consciousness, or cardiac arrest. Treatment includes suctioning and the administration of oxygen and, in some cases, drugs to reduce inflammation.

aspirin (ăs′pər-ĭn) N. acetylsalicylic acid, a drug commonly used to relieve pain (analgesic) and reduce fever (antipyretic) and inflammation (anti-inflammatory); it may also (in prescribed amounts) prevent blood clotting and help prevent cardiovascular accidents (strokes), heart attacks, and cataracts. Side effects include stomach discomfort and gastrointestinal bleeding (which may be small in amount and occult), for these reasons buffered aspirins are available. *See also* BUFFERED ASPIRIN. Accidental overdosage of aspirin is a common form of poisoning, esp. among children. *See also* SALICYLATE POISONING.

Assam fever *See* KALA-AZAR.

assay (ăs′ā) N. test to determine the amount of a given chemical in a mixture, the potency of a drug, or the purity of a compound. v. to analyze a substance.

assertiveness training N. method used in psychotherapy in which

one is taught to state negative and positive feelings directly and frankly.

assimilation (ə-sĭm′ə-lā′shən) N. portion of the digestive process where food breakdown products are absorbed into the body and metabolized to living tissue. Also called anabolic (building-up) metabolism.

association (ə-sō′sē-ā′shən) N. connection of two or more things or events. *See also* FREE ASSOCIATION.

astemizole N. antihistamine drug (trade name Hismanal) used in the treatment of allergy and rhinitis. Side effects include drowsiness; overdoses of this drug may result in severe cardiac arrhythmias.

asthenia N. weakened state; lack or loss of physical strength (*see also* NEURESTHENIA). ADJ. asthenic

asthenopia *See* EYE STRAIN.

asthma (ăz′mə) N. respiratory disorder characterized by recurrent episodes of difficulty in breathing, wheezing (esp. on expiration), cough, and thick mucus production, caused by spasm or inflammation of the bronchi. Most attacks are precipitated by infection, strenuous exercise, stress, or exposure to an allergen (e.g., pollen, dust, food). Treatment involves the use of bronchodilators, corticosteroids, and elimination, if possible, of causative agents. Between attacks, respiratory function is normal. (Also called bronchial asthma.) ADJ. asthmatic

astigmatism (ə-stĭg′mə-tĭz′əm) N. defect in vision in which the light rays cannot be focused properly on the retina because of abnormal curvature of the

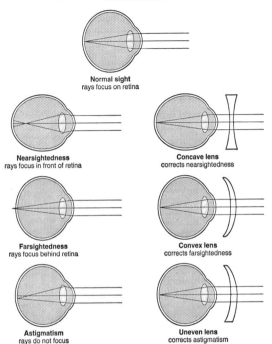

ASTIGMATISM

Normal sight
rays focus on retina

Nearsightedness
rays focus in front of retina

Concave lens
corrects nearsightedness

Farsightedness
rays focus behind retina

Convex lens
corrects farsightedness

Astigmatism
rays do not focus

Uneven lens
corrects astigmatism

Common disorders of the eye. During normal sight, the light rays focus on the retina. In the nearsighted and farsighted individual, the rays focus in front of and behind the retina, respectively. Concave and convex lenses correct these problems, as shown. In astigmatism, the rays do not focus, but uneven lenses correct this problem.

cornea or lens of the eye; corrective lenses improve vision. ADJ. astigmatic

astragalus (ə-străg′ə-ləs) N. *See* TALUS.

astringent (ə-strĭn′jənt) ADJ. causing the skin to draw tight; also styptic (as styptic pencil, containing the astringent alum, to stop bleeding in minor cuts from shaving). N. substance that when applied to the skin draws it tight.

astrocyte (ăs′trə-sīt′) N. star-shaped nerve cell with many branching processes. These processes cover the surfaces of the blood vesselss, neurons, and the pia mater, providing a nonrigid supportive matrix. The matrix helps to regulate the composition of the fluid which surrounds nerve cells (extracellular fluid).

asymmetry (ā-sĭm′ĭ-trē) N. lack of mirror-image correspondence between paired parts or normally similar sides of a body or organ (e.g., having one hand or a side of the face that is not the mirror image of the other). ADJ. asymmetrical

asymptomatic (ā'sĭmp-tə-măt'ĭk) ADJ. without symptoms.

asynclitism (ā-sĭn'klĭ-tĭz'əm) N. in labor, presentation of the head of the fetus at an abnormal angle.

asynergy (ā-sĭn'ər-jē) N. discoordination of body parts or organs that normally work together harmoniously. Also called asynergia. ADJ. asynergic

asystole (ā-sĭs'tə-lē) N. absence of heart beat; failure of the ventricles of the heart to contract, cardiac arrest. ADJ. asystolic

Atabrine (ăt'ə-brĭn, -brēn') N. trade name for the antimalarial drug quinacrine hydrochloride.

Atarax N. trade name for the minor tranquilizer hydroxyzine hydrochloride.

ataraxic drug N. tranquilizer; sedative drug that does not produce sleep. *See also* NEUROLEPTIC.

ataraxis N. mental calm esp. when consciousness is unimpaired. ADJ. ataractic, ataraxic

atavism (ăt'ə-vĭz'əm) N. throwback, development of a characteristic or disease known to have occurred in an earlier ancestor rather than in the parents. ADJ. atavistic

ataxia N. lack of coordination in muscle action, manifested as unsteady movements and staggering gait and caused by brain or spinal cord lesion. *See also* DEGENERATIVE DISORDER. ADJ. ataxic

atelectasis N. incomplete expansion of all or part of the lung in a newborn or collapse of lung tissue in the adult. Collapse, caused by obstruction of the airways or compression on the lung (e.g., by tumor or enlarged lymph glands), produces increasing difficulty in breathing and fever, and often leads to pneumonia and serious complications. ADJ. atelectatic

atenolol N. oral beta blocker (trade name Tenormin) used in the treatment of hypertension and angina. Adverse effects include depression, exacerbation of congestive heart failure or asthma, and acrocyanosis. *See* TABLE OF COMMONLY PRESCRIBED DRUGS—GENERIC NAMES.

atherectomy N. procedure used to treat coronary artery disease in which a small catheter is passed into the involved artery by way of a percutaneous incision. The catheter contains a small blade that rotates and shaves away a portion of the obstructive atherosclerotic debris, which is collected in a chamber and discarded. Although used in several larger medical centers, this technique is not widely available.

atherogenesis (ăth'ər-ō-jĕn'ĭ-sĭs) N. formation of fatty (lipid) deposits (atheromas), on the walls of the arteries, as in atherosclerosis.

atheroma (ăth'ə-rō'mə) N. clump of material, a fatty deposit, from the lining (intima) of an artery.

atherosclerosis (ăth'ə-rō-sklə-rō'sĭs) N. common disorder of the arteries in which plaques consisting mostly of cholesterol and lipids form on the inner arterial wall. As a result the vessels become nonelastic and the lumen is narrowed, leading to decreased blood flow. Atherosclerosis is also associated with hypertension, obesity, diabetes, and some hereditary metabolic disorders. In some cases, segments of occluded arteries may be surgically bypassed (as in coronary bypass surgery). Preventive measures include cessation of smoking, a low-fat diet, exercise, and avoidance of stress. Also called coronary artery disease. ADJ. atherosclerotic

ATHEROSCLEROSIS

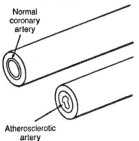

Normal coronary artery

Atherosclerotic artery

athetosis N. condition characterized by slow, continuous involuntary position changes of the hands and feet and other parts of the body, as sometimes seen in cerebral palsy.

athlete's foot N. fungal infection (ringworm) of the foot, generally starting between the toes, causing itching. Later, a bacterium may replace the fungus and cause the skin between the toes to turn white, crack, and peel off. Treatment is by antifungal preparations.

athlete's heart N. oversized heart commonly found in professional athletes and those trained for endurance; it is believed to result from overexertion for an extended period. The heart's increased pumping capacity delivers more oxygen to the skeletal muscles.

Ativan N. trade name for the benzodiazepine, lorazepam. *See* TABLE OF COMMONLY PRESCRIBED DRUGS—TRADE NAMES.

atlas N. first cervical vertebra; the first verebra in the neck, hinging with the skull at the occipital bone (*compare* AXIS).

atom N. the smallest part of an element consisting of a nucleus (contains protons and neutrons) and surrounding electrons. Physics studies suggest that protons and neutrons are made up of even smaller particles, called quarks. Hundreds of other very small particles are thought to exist, even if only momentarily. The latest theory, The Standard Model, explains all the hundreds of particles and complex interactions with only six types of quarks and six types of leptons, of which the best known is the electron. According to this model, all the known matter particles are composites of quarks and leptons, and they interact by exchanging force carrier particles. The study of these particles is known as particle physics. Particle physicists

THE ATOM

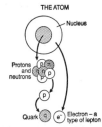

Nucleus

Protons and neutrons

Quark

Electron – a type of lepton

All the known matter particles are composites of quarks and leptons. The atom consists of a nucleus, which contains quarks that interact to form protons and neutrons. Electrons, the most common type of lepton, surround the nucleus.

study the fundamental particles that make up all of matter and how they interact with each other. *See also* FORCE-CARRYING PARTICLES; LEPTONS; PARTICLE PHYSICS; QUARKS.

atomic mass N. the mass of an atom, measured in atomic mass units.

atomic number N. number indicating the number of protons in the nucleus or the number of electrons in an uncharged atom.

atony (ăt′ə-nē, ăt′n-ē) N. lack of normal tone, usually of a muscle, muscle system, or the bladder, also: atonia, atonicity. ADJ. atonic

atopognosia (ă-tŏp′ŏg-nō′zē-ə) N. inability to locate correctly a pinprick point of touch, or other sensation; also called atopognosis.

atopy (ăt′ə-pē) N. allergy to which one has an inherited tendency.

atorvastatin N. *See* TABLE OF COMMONLY PRESCRIBED DRUGS —GENERIC NAMES.

atovaquone N. antibiotic specifically designed for the treatment of pneumocystosis, especially when sulfonamides have failed; possible side effects include rash, nausea, and diarrhea.

atoxic ADJ. not producing or resulting from poison; also called nontoxic.

ATP *See* ADENOSINE TRIPHOSPHATE.

ATP synthetase (sin-thə-tāz) N. enzyme that catalyzes the synthesis of adenosine triphosphate (ATP) from adenosine diphosphate (ADP) and phosphate by utilizing some form of energy. *See also* ELECTRON TRANSPORT SYSTEM.

atresia (ə-trē′zhə) N. condition in which a normal opening or

tube in the body (e.g., the urethra) is closed or absent. ADJ. atresic

atrial fibrillation (ā′trē-əl) N. condition characterized by rapid and random contraction of the atria of the heart causing irregular beats of the ventricles and resulting in decreased heart output and frequently clot formation in the atria. A type of cardiac arrhythmia, atrial fibrillation occurs in rheumatic heart disease, mitral valve stenosis, and other heart disorders. Treatment is by drugs (e.g., digitalis) or electroshock to restore normal heart rhythm.

atrial septal defect (ASD) N. common congenital heart defect, characterized by an abnormal opening in the septum dividing the atria, which allows blood to pass from the left to the right atrium. Small openings may cause no symptoms and may heal spontaneously during childhood. Larger openings may cause symptoms of congestive heart failure and usually require surgical repair of the defect. *Compare* VENTRICULAR SEPTAL DEFECT.

atrio- comb. form indicating an association with the atrium of the heart (e.g., atrioventricular, pert. to an atrium and ventricle of the heart, considered together).

atrioventricular (AV) node (ā′trē-ō-vĕn-trĭk′-yə-lər) N. area of specialized heart muscle, located in the septal wall of the right atrium that receives impulses from the sinoatrial node (pacemaker) and transmits them to the bundle of His and thus to the walls of the ventricles, causing them to contract.

atrioventricular bundle *See* BUNDLE OF HIS.

atrioventricular valve N. either of two valves in the heart through which blood flows from the atria to the ventricles. The left atrioventricular valve is the mitral valve; the right, the tricuspid valve. (*Compare* SINOATRIAL NODES.)

atrium (ā'trē-əm) N., *pl.* atria 1. either of the two upper chambers of the heart. The right atrium receives deoxygenated blood from the vena cava and then passes it into the right ventricle, which pumps it to the lungs, where it gives off waste products and receives oxygen. The freshly oxygenated blood then passes through the pulmonary vein to the left atrium and from there to the left ventricle and then the rest of the body.
2. main section of the middle ear.
3. chamber serving as the entrance to another organ (e.g., atrium of the larynx). ADJ. atrial

Atromid-S N. trade name for the drug clofibrate, which reduces lipids in the blood serum and is used to treat some cardiovascular diseases.

atrophy (ăt'rə-fē) N. decrease in size of a part or organ, resulting from a wasting away of tissue, as may occur in disease or from lack of use (*compare* HYPERTROPHY). ADJ. atrophic

atropine (ăt'rə-pēn', -pǐn) N. antispasmodic drug commonly obtained from belladonna and related plants and used in various forms to calm gastrointestinal motility, treat certain abnormalities of the heart rhythm, and dilate the pupil of the eye. In an inhaled form, atropine has been used to treat asthma and emphysema.

Atrovent N. trade name for the inhaled bronchodilator ipratropium bromide. *See* TABLE OF COMMONLY PRESCRIBED DRUGS—TRADE NAMES.

attachment N. dependence of a person on an object or another human being. Personality problems can result if the relationship is broken, as by separation, before the person is fully mature.

attention deficit disorder N. syndrome, affecting mostly males, characterized by learning and behavioral problems. These include short attention span, impulsivity, hyperactivity, and impairments in perceptual, language, and motor skills. The cause is unknown; originally thought to just affect children, an adult form is now recognized.

attention span N. length of time that one can concentrate on a given object or activity (*compare* AUTISM). Some disturbed patients have extremely short attention spans (i.e., less than a few minutes).

attenuation (ə-tĕn'yoo-ā'shən) N. process of weakening, esp. of the potency of a drug or other agent or of the virulence of a disease-causing germ. V. attenuate; ADJ. attenuated.

atypical antipsychotics N. class of prescription medications (also known as second-generation antipsychotics) used to treat psychiatric conditions, especially schizophrenia. Some are also used for bipolar disease. Hyperglycemia (elevated blood sugar), in some cases extreme, has been reported in patients treated with atypical antipsychotics. *See also* BIPOLAR DISEASE; HYPERGLYCEMIA; SCHIZOPHRENIA.

Au N. symbol for the element gold. Various drug preparations containing gold are used in the treatment of rheumatoid arthritis.

audio- comb. form indicating an association with sound or hearing (e.g., audiovisual, pert. to sound and sight).

audiogram (ô′dē-ə-grăm′) N. record of an individual's hearing sensitivity.

audiometry N. measurement of the sense of hearing. Originally it included only measures of pure-tone thresholds but now the hearing of different speech sounds and the processing of sound stimuli in the brain are also measured.

audition (ô-dĭsh′ən) N. act of hearing; the ability to hear. *See also* EAR. ADJ. auditory

auditory canal (ô′dĭ-tôr′ē) N. tubelike structure that leads from the outside of the ear to the tympanic membrane. Also called auditory meatus.

auditory center N. part of the brain that receives impulses from the ear by way of the auditory nerve for interpretation as hearing. The center is at the side of each brain hemisphere (temporal lobe) in a fold of the cerebral cortex.

auditory nerve N. one of a pair of major sensory nerves, the eighth cranial nerves, that carry impulses from the inner ear to the brain for interpretation as hearing, position sense, and balance. Also called auditory vestibular nerve or, less commonly now, acoustic nerve.

auditory tube *See* EUSTACHIAN TUBE.

Augmentin N. trade name for a fixed-combination oral antibiotic consisting of amoxicillin and clavulanic acid, and used in the treatment of mild to moderate infections involving the ears, throat, skin, and lungs. *See* TABLE OF COMMONLY PRESCRIBED DRUGS—TRADE NAMES.

aura (ôr′ə) N., *pl.* aurae, sensation (e.g., flickering light, halos, or warmth) that may signal the start of a migraine or an epileptic seizure. ADJ. aural

aural (ôr′əl) ADJ. pert. to the ear.

auranofin (ô-răn′ə-fĭn) N. oral preparation of the metal gold (trade name Ridaura) that is taken, in a chemically ingestable form (as a salt), for the treatment of rheumatoid arthritis. Side effects include leukopenia, thrombocytopenia, rash, mouth sores (stomatitis), and kidney dysfunction.

auricle (ôr′ĭ-kəl) N.
1. outer visible part of the ear, also called pinna.
2. atrial auricle is a small conical pouch projecting from the upper anterior portion of each atrium of the heart. ADJ. auricular

auscultation (ô′skəl-tā′shən) N. act of listening to body sounds, including those of the lungs, heart, and abdomen, as an aid to diagnosis. *See also* STETHOSCOPE. ADJ. auscultatory

aut-, auto- comb. forms meaning self (e.g., autoagglutination, clumping of blood cells caused by factors in one's own blood serum).

autism (ô′tĭz′əm) N. abnormal withdrawal into oneself, marked by severe communication problems, short attention span, inability to interact socially, and extreme resistance to change. Children with autism are extremely difficult to teach. Treatment involves specialized education and the use of drugs (e.g., phenothiazines) to control behavior problems and anxiety. ADJ. autistic

autoclave (ô′tō-klāv′) N. tanklike device that securely seals itself (hence the name) and can withstand high internal temperatures and pressures, used in sterilizing with steam, surgical instruments and research materials.

autoeroticism (ô′tō-ĭ-rŏt′ĭ-sīz′əm) N. sexual gratification through self-stimulation, without regard for another person; sensual gratification through masturbation, fantasy, or visual experience.

autograft (ô′tō-grăft′) N. tissue that is removed from one site and then attached to another site on the same person (e.g., skin from the thigh to replace burned skin on the arm).

autoimmune disease (ô′tō-ĭ-myōōn′) N. any of a large group of diseases marked by an abnormality of the functioning of the immune system that causes the production of antibodies against one's own tissues and other body materials. Autoimmune diseases include systemic lupus erythematosus, rheumatoid arthritis, and other collagen diseases; and idiopathic thrombocytopenic purpura, autoimmune leukopenia, and other hemolytic disorders.

autoimmunity N. production of antibodies against the tissues of one's own body, producing autoimmune disease or hypersensitivity reactions.

automated implantable cardioverter-defibrillator (AICD) N. medical device implanted in the chest wall for the treatment of life-threatening cardiac arrhythmias. Wires, called leads, run from the device directly to the heart. These continuously monitor the cardiac rhythm. If a dangerous arrhythmia develops, an electric shock is delivered to the heart muscle via the lead wires, terminating the arrhythmia. AICDs have been life saving in a wide variety of patients, including those with life-threatening arrhythmias following heart attack and severe mitral valve prolapse. *See also* ARRHYTHMIA; MITRAL VALVE PROLAPSE.

autonomic (ô′tə-nŏm′ĭk) ADJ. regulated or controlled by the mechanisms within oneself, specifically referring to the autonomic nervous system, which maintains many of the body's involuntary functions (e.g., breathing, digestion).

autonomic nervous system N. that part of the nervous system that regulates involuntary vital functions, such as the activity of the heart and smooth muscle. It is divided into two parts: the sympathetic nervous system, which, when stimulated, constricts blood vessels, raises blood pressure, and increases heart rate; and the parasympathetic nervous system, which, when stimulated, increases intestinal and gland activity, slows heart rate, and relaxes sphincter muscles.

autonomic reflex N. any of a number of reflexes that control the activity of body parts (e.g., urination, sweating, heart rate).

autopsy (ô′tŏp′sē) N. examination, using dissection and other methods, of a body after death to determine the cause of death, the extent of injuries, or other factors.

autoregulation (ô′tō-rĕg′yə-lā′shən) N. process of maintaining

THE AUTONOMIC NERVOUS SYSTEM

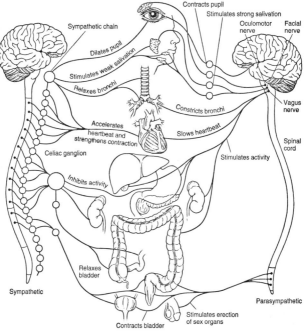

a generally constant physiological state of a cell or organism.

autosomal dominant disease N. disorder (e.g., Huntington's chorea) caused by a dominant mutant (abnormal) gene on an autosome (nonsex chromosome). Evidence of the disorder may not occur for several decades. The mutant gene is inherited from one or both parents or is the result of a fresh mutation. If both parents have the mutant dominant gene, all offspring will be affected; if one parent is affected, 50% of the offspring will be affected; the normal children of an affected parent do not carry the trait.

autosomal recessive disease N. disorder caused by the presence of two recessive (homozygous) mutant (abnormal) genes on an autosome. If only one mutant recessive (heterozygous) gene is present the person is not affected with the disease but is a carrier of it. One fourth of the children of two heterozygous (carrier) parents will be affected and another one half will be carriers. All of the children of two homozygous affected persons will be affected. The children of one normal and one affected with the disease will all be carriers. When close relatives (e.g., first cousins) marry, the chance that an offspring will inherit an abnormal recessive gene from

A COMPARISON OF THE SYMPATHETIC AND PARASYMPATHETIC NERVOUS SYSTEMS

Characteristic	Sympathetic System	Parasympathetic System
General Effect	Prepares body to cope with stressful situations; mediatesabnormal configuration of bodyfunctions	Restores body to resting state after stressful situation; actively maintains normal configuration of bodyfunctions
Extent of effect	Widespread throughout the body	Localized in tissues
Neuro-transmitter released at synapse	Norepinephrine (usually)	Acetylcholine
Duration of effect	Lasting	Brief
Outflow from CNS	Thoracolumbar levels of spinal cord	Craniosacral levels (from brain and spinal cord)
Location of ganglia	Chain and collateral ganglia	Terminal ganglia
Number of postgangli-onic fibers	Many	Few

both parents is increased, as it is among persons marrying within certain ethnic groups (e.g., Tay-Sachs disease among Ashken-azic Jews).

autosome (ô'tə-sōm') N. chromosome (other than a sex chromosome), usually appearing in pairs in body cells but as single chromosomes in spermatazoa or ova (gametes, or sex cells); also called somatic chromosome.

avascular (ā-văs'kyə-lər) N. ADJ. without blood vessels.

avascular necrosis N. death of any tissue due to loss of blood supply, usually due to trauma or congenital blood vessel abnormalities. For example, fractures of the navicular bone of the wrist are at a high risk for avascular necrosis because of a perilous blood supply.

aversion (ə-vûr'zhən, -shən) N. extreme dislike and desire to move away from the source of antagonism (e.g., wanting to run away from a snake).

aversion therapy N. process in which undesirable behavior is treated by accompanying the behavior with a disagreeable experience, such as extreme nausea (the treatment has been used to help persons stop smoking cigarettes or drinking alcohol).

aversive N. ADJ. repelling; noxious, as a stimulus used in avoidance training or aversion therapy.

avian influenza N. infection caused by avian influenza (bird flu) viruses; also called bird flu. These viruses occur naturally among birds. Wild birds worldwide carry the viruses in their intestines, but usually do not get sick from them. However, bird flu is very contagious among birds and can make some domesticated birds, including chickens, ducks, and turkeys, very sick and kill them. Bird flu viruses do not usually infect humans, but several cases of human infection with bird flu viruses have occurred since 1997. The risk from bird flu is generally low to most people because the viruses occur mainly among birds and do not usually infect humans. However, during an outbreak of bird flu among poultry (domesticated chicken, ducks, turkeys), there is a possible risk to people who have contact with infected birds or surfaces that have been contaminated with excretions from infected birds. An outbreak of avian influenza A (strain H5N1) among poultry in Asia (October 2005) is an example of a bird flu outbreak that caused human infections and deaths. In such situations, people should avoid contact with infected birds or contaminated surfaces and should be careful when handling and cooking poultry. Symptoms of bird flu in humans have ranged from typical flu-like symptoms (fever, cough, sore throat, and muscle aches) to eye infections, pneumonia, severe respiratory diseases (such as acute respiratory distress), and other severe and life-threatening complications. Laboratory testing to confirm human infection with H5N1 avian influenza is technically difficult; some tests produce inconclusive or unreliable results. Currently, World Health Organization (WHO) reference laboratories must be used for diagnostic confirmation. The H5N1 virus currently infecting birds in Asia that has caused human illness and death is resistant to amantadine (Symmetrel) and rimantadine (Flumadine), two antiviral medications commonly used for influenza. Two other antiviral medications, oseltamivir (Tamiflu) and zanamavir (Relenza), can be used for treatment and prophylaxis. There currently is no vaccine to protect humans against the H5N1 virus that is being seen in Asia. However, vaccine development efforts are under way. Research studies to test a vaccine to protect humans against H5N1 virus began in April 2005. *See also* INFLUENZA; TABLE OF COMMONLY PRESCRIBED DRUGS—TRADE NAMES.

avirulent ADJ. unable to produce disease or its effects.

avitaminosis (ā-vī′tə-mĭ-nō′sĭs) N. vitamin deficiency; also called hypovitaminosis (*compare* HYPERVITAMINOSIS).

avoidance N. noninvolvement, as a psychological defense to free oneself from fear, anxiety, or other adverse feelings.

avulsion (ə-vŭl′shən) N. tearing or forcible separation of one body part from another.

Axid N. trade name for the histamine blocker, nizatidine. *See* TABLE OF COMMONLY PRESCRIBED DRUGS—TRADE NAMES.

axilla (ăk-sĭl′ə) N., *pl.* axillae, armpit. ADJ. axillary

axillary node (ăk′sə-lĕr′ē) N. any of the lymph glands of the armpit that help to fight infection in the neck, chest, and arm area.

axis (ăk′sĭs) N., *pl.* axes
1. second cervical vertebra; the second bone of the vertebral column, located in the neck region (*compare* ATLAS).
2. imaginary line used as a reference for the relationship of parts or actions (e.g., the body axis being the imaginary line from the head to the feet). ADJ. axial

axolemma (ăk′sō-lĕm′ə) N. outer membrane cover of an axon.

axon (ăk′sŏn′) N. nerve cell process that carries the impulse away from the cell body to the site of action or response, the effector (e.g., muscle); some axons have a myelin sheath (*compare* DENDRITE). ADJ. axonal

THE NERVE CELL

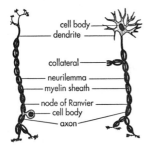

cell body
dendrite

collateral

neurilemma
myelin sheath

node of Ranvier
cell body
axon

ayurveda *See* TABLE OF ALTERNATIVE MEDICINE TERMS

azathioprine (ăz′ə-thī′ə-prēn′) N. immunosuppressive drug (trade name Imuran) used to prevent rejection following organ transplants and to treat certain inflammatory conditions.

azidothymidine (AZT) (ăz′ĭ-dō-thī′mĭ-dēn′) N. drug authorized by the Food and Drug Administration for the treatment of acquired immune deficiency syndrome (AIDS). Adverse effects include liver damage and bone marrow suppression.

azithromycin N. once-daily antibiotic agent (trade name Zithromax) used in respiratory infections and in skin infections; similar to erythromycin. *See* TABLE OF COMMONLY PRESCRIBED DRUGS—GENERIC NAMES.

Azmacort N. trade name for an inhaled form of the corticosteroid, triamcinolone; used in asthma. *See* TABLE OF COMMONLY PRESCRIBED DRUGS—TRADE NAMES.

azotemia (ăz′ə-tē′mē-ə) N. presence of an abnormally high level of nitrogen-bearing materials (e.g., urea) in the blood. ADJ. azotemic

azoturia (ăz′ə-toōr′ē-ə) N. excess of urea or other nitrogen-containing compounds in the urine. ADJ. azoturic

AZT N. abbrev. for the drug azidothymidine, used in the treatment of acquired immune deficiency syndrome (AIDS).

aztreonam (ăz-trē′ə-năm′) N. parenteral antibiotic (trade name Azactam) that is particularly useful against severe infections and produces minimal side effects.

azygous ADJ. not paired, as some organs (e.g., the heart).

azymia N. absence of an enzyme.

B

B symbol for the element boron.

B blood type N. one of the four blood groups (the others being A, AB, and O) in the ABO blood group system for classifying human blood based on the presence or absence of two antigens A and B on the surface of red blood cells (erythrocytes). A person with type B blood produces antibodies against A antigens that cause the blood cells to agglutinate, or clump together. A person with type B blood must receive blood transfusions only from others with type B or type O blood. *See also* BLOOD TYPING.

B cell N. a lymphocyte (a type of white blood cell) important in the body's immune system and response to infection, esp. by bacteria, or to invasion by other foreign substance (antigen). B cells develop in the bone marrow and circulate through the body until, when confronted by an antigen, they greatly increase in number and produce antibodies specific against that antigen.

B vitamins N. series of water-soluble vitamins (e.g., thiamine, riboflavin, niacin, pyridoxine, folic acid, cyanocobalamin) essential for normal metabolism and first believed to be a single vitamin. *See also* VITAMIN; TABLE OF VITAMINS.

Ba symbol for the element barium.

babesiosis (bə-bē′zē-ō′sĭs) N. infection caused by a protozoan (*Babesia*), transmitted by the bite of certain ticks; it is characterized by headache, fever, muscle pain, and nausea; also called babesiasis.

Babinski's reflex (bə-bĭn′skēz) N. extension or moving of the big toe upward or toward the head, with the other toes fanned out and extended, when the sole of the foot is stroked from below the heel toward the toes on its lateral side (outside). The reflex is normal in infants, but in others usually indicates brain or spinal cord disease. Also called Babinski sign.

baby N. infant; child under 1 year of age, or not yet able to walk.

bacillary (băs′ə-lĕr′ē) (bə-sĭl′ə-rē) ADJ.
1. pert. to or caused by a bacillus.
2. rod-shaped, like a bacillus; also called bacillar, bacilliform

bacillary dysentery *See* SHIGELLOSIS.

bacillemia (băs′ə-lē′mē-ə) N. presence of bacilli in the blood.

bacilli N., *pl.* of bacillus.

bacilluria (băs′ə-loor′ē-ə) N. presence of bacilli in the urine, usually due to bladder or kidney infection.

bacillus (bə-sĭl′əs) N. *pl.* bacilli, common rodshaped bacterium (genus *Bacillus*) that normally lives in soil, water, and organic materials and helps in the process of decay. Only a few species (e.g., *Bacillus anthracis*, the cause of anthrax) cause human disease.

bacitracin (băs′ĭ-trā′sĭn) N. antibiotic used to treat many bacterial infections, esp. those involving the skin.

back N. posterior part of the body trunk from the nape of the neck to the buttocks.

backache (băk'āk') N. pain in the back. Backache is a common complaint; it may be caused by muscle strain or other muscle injury or disorder, or by pressure on a nerve, resulting from vertebral disk injury or other injury, or as a symptom of many other disorders. Treatment depends on the cause; it may include bed rest, heat or ice, and the use of drugs to relieve pain and muscle spasms.

backbone (băk'bōn') *See* VERTEBRAL COLUMN.

bacteremia (băk'tə-rē'mē-ə) N. presence of bacteria in the blood.

bacteria N., *pl.* of bacterium.

bacterial ADJ. pert. to or caused by bacteria, as in bacterial endocarditis.

bacterial resistance N. development of resistance to a drug (e.g., penicillin) by bacteria previously susceptible to its destructive effects.

bactericide N. drug or other chemical that kills bacteria (*compare* BACTERIOSTASIS). ADJ. bactericidal

bacteriogenic (băk-tēr'ē-ə-jĕn'ĭk) ADJ. caused by, or producing, bacteria.

bacteriology (băk-tîr'ē-ŏl'ə-jē) N. science and study of bacteria, their development, and their effects on human tissue; today generally included in microbiology. ADJ. bacteriologic, bacteriological

bacteriolysin (băk-tēr'ē-ŏl'ĭ-sĭn) N. antibody, produced against bacteria, that causes the microorganisms to break down (lyse).

bacteriolysis (băk-tēr'ē-ŏl'ĭ-sĭs) N. the breakdown of microorganisms, specifically bacteria. ADJ. bacteriolytic

bacteriophage (băk-tēr'ē-ə-fāj') N. a virus, sometimes called a bacterial virus but more generally simply phage, that causes bacteria to break down (lyse).

bacteriostasis N. condition in which the growth and multiplication of bacteria are inhibited, but the bacteria are not killed, by the use of biological or chemical agents (*compare* BACTERICIDE). ADJ. bacteriostatic

bacteriotoxic ADJ.
1. having the effect of poison (toxin) on bacteria.
2. caused by poisons produced by bacteria.

bacterium (băk-tēr'ē-əm) N., *pl.* bacteria, any of a large group of small, unicellular microorganisms (class Schizomycetes)

BACTERIA

cocci

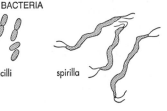

bacilli

spirilla

found in the soil, water, and air, some of which cause disease in humans and other animals. Bacteria are generally classified as rod-shaped (bacillus), spherical (coccus), comma-shaped (vibrio), or spiral (spirochete). ADJ. bacterial

Bactoban N. trade name for the antibiotic ointment, mupirocin. *See* TABLE OF COMMONLY PRESCRIBED DRUGS—TRADE NAMES.

Bactrim N. *See* TABLE OF COMMONLY PRESCRIBED DRUGS—TRADE NAMES.

bag N. pocketlike container for fluids or other substances, esp. a plastic or rubber container attached to the body to receive the contents (urine or feces) emitted from an artificial opening created in an ileostomy or other operation.

bag of waters N. colloq. for the sac of amniotic fluid surrounding the fetus during pregnancy.

bagassosis (băg'ə-sō'sĭs) N. lung disease caused by inhaling bagasse (sugarcane dust) and marked by fever, malaise, and difficulty in breathing; also called bagasscosis.

balance (băl'əns) N.
1. coordinated, harmonious working of parts or systems. *See also* ACID-BASE BALANCE.
2. instrument for weighing.

balanced diet N. diet containing adequate amounts of all essential nutrients (vitamins and minerals, proteins, fats, and carbohydrates) needed for growth and the maintenance of normal health and energy levels.

balanitis (băl'ə-nī'tĭs) N. inflammation of the head (glans) of the penis, usually accompanied by a discharge and tightening of the foreskin.

balanoposthitis (băl'ə-nō-pŏs-thī'tĭs) N. inflammation of the head (glans) of the penis and of the foreskin, often the result of bacterial or fungal (frequently venereal) infection; it is characterized by soreness and discharge.

baldness (bôld'nĭs) N. loss or absence of hair, commonly of the scalp. In male-pattern baldness the hairline recedes at the forehead and hair is lost at the back and top of the head. *See also* ALOPECIA.

ball-and-socket joint N. joint in which the globular head of an articulating bone fits into a cuplike cavity of another to allow the distal bone to rotate, as in the shoulder joint and hip joint.

ballistics N. science of the movement and path of projectiles, such as bullets and missiles. Medically important in the treatment of victims of gunshot and shrapnel wounds. For example, bullets typically tumble as they pass through tissue, causing far more damage than the exterior wound might suggest.

ballottement (bə-lŏt'mənt) N. checking for the correctness of position or the size of a floating part or organ or a fetus by gently flicking or bouncing it with the hand or finger(s) and feeling its response (e.g., an unborn child felt through the birth canal or the abdominal wall).

balneotherapy N. use of baths to treat disease, esp. to relieve pain and improve circulation.

bandage (băn'dĭj) N., V. piece of soft material that protects an injured part of the body; wrap around with something so as to cover or enclose. There are numerous types of bandages. Typically the wound is covered first by a dressing, which is held in place by a bandage.

bandy leg See BOWLEG.

bank N. in medicine, storage of human materials for later use, usually by other persons (e.g., blood bank, eye bank, sperm bank).

Banti's syndrome N. progressive disorder characterized by enlargement of the spleen, anemia, gastrointestinal bleeding, and other symptoms and often occurring as a complication of alcoholic cirrhosis of the liver; also called Banti's disease.

baragnosis (băr'ăg-nō'sĭs) N. inability to determine weight differences.

barber's itch (bär'bərz) N. inflammation of the hair follicles of the face, caused by bacterial or fungal infection.

barbiturate (bär-bĭch'ər-ĭt, bär' bĭ-tŏor'ĭt) N. drug (e.g., phenobarbital) that depresses brain and spinal cord activity. These agents are used to treat convulsions and, less commonly, to produce sedation. Barbiturates are potentially habit-forming.

barbiturism (bär-bĭch'ə-rĭz'əm) (bär'bĭ-tŏor'ĭz'əm) N. poisoning resulting from the use of barbiturates, marked by slurred speech, sleepiness, loss of memory, disorientation, and in serious cases, depressed respiration, coma, and death.

bariatrics (băr'ē-ăt'rĭks) N.
1. study of body weight, esp. the causes and treatment of obesity.
2. medical specialty for treatment of overweight.

barium (bâr'ē-əm) N. element, compounds of which (particularly barium sulfate) are used for diagnostic purposes in medicine. When swallowed or introduced via enema into the gastrointestinal tract, barium compounds present a contrast on X-ray film, thus outlining various anatomic structures. See also TABLE OF IMPORTANT ELEMENTS.

baroreceptor (băr'ō-rĭ-sĕp'tər) N. nerve ending that senses changes in pressure.

Barr body (bär) N. mass of chromosomal material normally seen within female body cells. Though females have two X-chromosomes, one is normally inactivated during development. The Barr body represents the inactivated X-chromosome.

barrel chest (băr'əl) N. large, rounded chest that is normal in some stocky persons and in some persons living in high-altitude areas where the oxygen content of the air is low, but is abnormal in others; often a sign of emphysema.

barren (băr'ən) ADJ. unable to produce young; sterile.

barrier (băr'ē-ər) N. object or structure that blocks an action or flow or separates parts from one another. See BLOOD-BRAIN BARRIER.

bartholinitis (bär'tə-lə-nī'tĭs) N. inflammation of one or both Bartholin's glands, usually caused by bacteria, and characterized by swelling, pain, and abscess formation.

Bartholin's gland N. either of two small, mucus-secreting glands located on the posterior and lateral parts of the vestibule of the vagina.

basal (bā'səl, zəl) ADJ. pert. to the fundamental, basic, or lowest (e.g., basal anesthesia, the first stage of unconsciousness).

basal body temperature N. temperature of the body taken in the morning before rising or moving about or eating or drinking anything; changes in the basal body temperature are used in the basal body temperature method of family planning to determine the fertile time in a woman's menstrual cycle.

basal body temperature method of family planning N. method of family planning based on the identification of the fertile period (the time when conception is most likely to occur) in a woman's menstrual cycle, obtained by noting the rise in basal body temperature that typically occurs with ovulation. The fertile period is calculated to start 6 days before ovulation is expected (from the data of previous cycles) and to continue until the temperature is elevated for 5 days. (*Compare* CALENDAR METHOD OF FAMILY PLANNING, OVULATION METHOD OF FAMILY PLANNING.) *See also* CONTRACEPTION.

basal ganglia N. masses of gray matter lying in the brain's cerebral cortex and involved in the control of body movements.

basal metabolism N. basic rate of energy flow needed to maintain the body.

basal metabolism test N. measurement of oxygen intake by a person about 14 hours after eating as an indication of the amount of energy required to maintain vital body functions (e.g., circulation, respiration, digestion). Breathing into a tube that leads to a measuring apparatus, the person remains at rest (but does not sleep) during the test. For each interval of time, the more oxygen consumed, the more oxidation is occurring and the higher is the basal metabolic rate (BMR). The test has largely been replaced by newer techniques.

base N.
1. bottom or supporting structure.
2. main part of a chemical compound.
3. substance that has a hydroxyl (OH) ion, tastes bitter, turns litmus paper blue, and, when combined with an acid, forms a salt. ADJ. basic, basilar

bashfulness N. chronic behavior response of self-consciousness, timidity, and avoidance of personal attention in public; a withdrawing, self-conscious temperament.

basi-, basio-, baso- comb. forms indicating an association with a chemical base (e.g., basophilic, easily stained with dyes that are chemical bases) or with a structural base (e.g., basicranial, pert. to the base of the skull).

basic life support *See* EMERGENCY MEDICAL TECHNICIAN.

basilar membrane (băs′ə-lər) N. cellular structure in the ear that forms a floor of the cochlear duct and provides a base for the organ of Corti, the main organ of hearing.

basophil (bā′sə-fĭl) N. type of white blood cell (leukocyte), with coarse granules that stain blue when exposed to a basic dye. Basophils normally constitute 1% or less of the total white blood cell count but may increase or decrease in certain diseases.

batho-, bathy- comb. forms indicating an association with depth (e.g., bathypnea, deep breathing).

bathycardia N. unusually low placement of the heart, not caused by disease.

bathyesthesia (băth′ē-ĭs-thē′zhə) N. sensation in the deeper parts of the body (e.g., the muscles and joints), as opposed to the skin.

battered child N. infant, child, or adolescent who has been seriously injured, generally many times, by one or more adults, frequently the parent(s), whose mistreatment of the victim shows a pattern of abnormal, abusive behavior. *See also* CHILD ABUSE.

battered elderly N. older adult victim of physical and emotional violence inflicted by another adult, often a relative. The injury may occur under circumstances that make it appear accidental when, in reality, this is not the case. Frequently the victim is afraid or reluctant (particularly when the abuser is a son or daughter) to report the violence.

battered spouse N. man or (more often) woman who is the victim of repeated episodes of physical violence, usually accompanied by verbal abuse. This often leads to serious physical and psychological damage being inflicted by the marriage partner. For a variety of reasons including physical, cultural, and personality factors, women are far more likely than men to suffer such abuse, and in some communities shelters have been made available for them and their children.

BCG vaccine N. immunizing agent, prepared from Calmette-Guérin bacillus, against tuberculosis.

bearing down N. sensation and effort by a pregnant woman to expel the fetus; it is characteristic of the second stage of labor.

beat N. single pulse or throb, esp. of the heart; the apical (apex) beat is heard over the left side of the chest, between the fourth and fifth ribs.

beclomethasone N. inhaled corticosteroid anti-inflammatory agent (trade name Beconase, Vancenase) used in the treatment of asthma and in allergies. *See* TABLE OF COMMONLY PRESCRIBED DRUGS—GENERIC NAMES.

Beconase N. trade name for the inhaled corticosteroid drug beclomethasone.

bed N.
1. in anatomy, general term for a structure or tissue that provides support, as a nail bed, the skin over which a nail extends as the fingernail or toenail grows.
2. special type of bed used to avert bedsores (decubitus ulcers). *See also* AIR BED; WATER BED.

bedbug N. arthropod (*Cimex lectularius*) that feeds on humans and other animals, sucking blood and causing redness, pain, and itching at the site of the bite. Bedbugs can be removed when covered with a jellylike preparation and the bite site treated with topical anti-inflammatory and analgesic preparations.

bedridden ADJ. unable to leave one's bed; not ambulatory.

bedsore *See* DECUBITUS ULCER.

bedwetting *See* ENURESIS.

bee sting N. injury caused by the venom of a bee, marked by pain and swelling at the site of the bite and often by the presence of a bee stinger, which should be removed. Ice or cold applications relieve pain. Multiple stings or stings to certain parts of the body can cause serious reactions. A single sting can cause anaphylactic shock and even death in a person hypersensitive to bee venom; such persons should carry emergency medical supplies if they expect to be exposed to the possibility of bee stings.

behavior modification N. technique for changing undesirable behavior into acceptable behavior generally by rewarding (*see also* REINFORCEMENT) appropriate responses and ignoring or punishing inappropriate behavior (*compare* BIOFEEDBACK).

behaviorism (bĭ-hāv′yə-rĭz′əm) N. branch of psychology concerned with objective observations of behavior, as evidence of such processes as intent and drive, without influence from personally biased (subjective) statements.

bejel N. chronic, nonvenereal form of syphilis, caused by the spirochete *Treponema pallidum,* widespread in the Middle East and northern Africa, most commonly among children and their family members. Lesions in the mouth region spread to other areas of the body. Treatment is by penicillin.

belching *See* ERUCTATION.

belladonna N. plant (*Atopa belladonna*) from which certain medicines (alkaloids, e.g., atropine) are derived.

belly N.
1. common term for the abdomen.
2. general term for the full and rounded part of a structure, as of a voluntary muscle (e.g., the biceps).

belly button N. colloquial term for umbilicus.

Bell's palsy N. feature-distorting paralysis of one side (or infrequently both sides) of the face, often affecting the eye or mouth and resulting from injury, disease of the facial nerve, or an unknown cause. If permanent deformity occurs, cosmetic surgery may be helpful.

Benadryl N. trade name for the antihistamine diphenhydramine hydrochloride.

benazepril N. *See* TABLE OF COMMONLY PRESCRIBED DRUGS—GENERIC NAMES.

bends N. painful, sometimes fatal condition in which, because of a rapid drop in outside pressure, nitrogen bubbles form in the body and cause pain, disorientation, and faintness, as when a diver ascends too quickly. Treatment is by return to a higher pressure environment and gradual decompression in a special chamber. Also called caisson disease, decompression sickness. *Compare* AIR EMBOLISM.

Benedict's solution N. copper sulfate dissolved in water containing sodium citrate and sodium carbonate; it is used to test for sugar (glucose) in the urine.

benign (bĭ-nīn′) ADJ. mild, noncancerous, and/or not spreading (*compare* MALIGNANT), as of a disease or growth, esp. a benign tumor.

Benzedrine (běn′zĭ-drēn′) N. trade name for the central nervous system stimulant amphetamine.

benzene (běn′zēn′, běn-zēn′) N. volatile liquid hydrocarbon chemical commonly used in the synthesis of dyes and various drugs.

benzocaine (běn′zə-kān′) N. local anesthetic agent found in many over-the-counter preparations for pain and itching. Frequent use of such preparations can lead to hypersensitivity reactions.

benzodiazepine (běn′zō-dī-ăz′ə-pēn′) N. class of psychoactive drugs; included are the tranquilizers diazepam (Valium) and chlordiazepoxide (Librium) and the sedative hypnotic flurazepam (Dalmane). Tolerance and dependence can occur with prolonged use of benzodiazepines.

beriberi (běr′ē-běr′ē) N. disease, resulting from a deficiency of vitamin B1 (thiamine), characterized by appetite and weight loss, disturbed nerve function, fluid retention, and heart failure. The disease is common in parts of Asia, particularly in areas where the diet is limited to highly milled rice, but is rare in the United States. Also called in endemic forms, kakke disease.

berylliosis (bə-rĭl′ē-ō′sĭs) N. poisoning, resulting from the inhalation of beryllium, marked by cough, chest pain, shortness of breath, and damage to lung tissue.

bestiality (běs′chē-ăl′ĭ-tē) N. sexual involvement of a human with an animal.

beta blocker N. any of a group of drugs (e.g., propranolol, naldolol, atenolol, metoprolol) widely used in the treatment of some forms of hypertension and arrhythmia. The drugs decrease the rate and force of heart contraction by blocking the beta-adrenergic receptors of the sympathetic nervous system.

beta cells N. insulin-producing cells found in the islands of Langerhans of the pancreas.

beta rhythm N. brain-wave frequency of low voltage, the busy waves of the brain, characteristic of a person who is awake and alert; also called beta wave. It is one of four brain-wave patterns (*compare* ALPHA RHYTHM; DELTA RHYTHM; THETA RHYTHM).

Betapace N. trade name for the antiarrhythmic drug, sotalol.

bi- prefix meaning two, twice, using both (e.g., bicapsular, pert. to two capsules).

Biaxin N. trade name for the antibiotic clarithromycin. *See* TABLE OF COMMONLY PRESCRIBED DRUGS—TRADE NAMES.

biceps (bī′sěps′) N. muscle having two heads, esp. the one at the front of the upper part of the arm, which flexes the arm and draws the hand toward the shoulder (*compare* TRICEPS).

bicuspid (bī-kŭs′pĭd) N. tooth (or other part) having two blunt points on its top. *See also* PREMOLAR.

bicuspid valve *See* MITRAL VALVE.

bid in prescriptions, abbreviation meaning twice a day.

bidet N. toilet-like basin designed to clean the genital and perineal areas by way of hand-controlled, small jets of water.

bifid (bī′fĭd) ADJ. consisting of two connecting parts.

bifocal glasses N. lenses that include curvatures of two focal lengths, to improve both near vision and distant vision (*compare* TRIFOCAL GLASSES).

bifurcation (bī'fər-kā'shən) N. split or branch point, often of either a nerve or a blood vessels (e.g., the bifurcation of the aorta into the iliac arteries).

bilateral (bī-lăt'ər-əl) ADJ. having or occurring on two sides, as in bilateral hearing loss; having two layers.

bile (bīl) N. thick, yellow-green-brown fluid made by the liver, stored in the gallbladder, and discharged into the upper part of the digestive tract (duodenum), where it breaks down fats, preparing them for further digestion; also called gall.

bilharziasis See SCHISTOSOMIASIS.

biliary (bĭl'ē-ĕr'ē) ADJ. pert. to bile or the gallbladder and its ducts.

biliary tract N. gallbladder and its ducts, which transport bile; also called biliary system.

bilious (bĭl'yəs) ADJ.
1. pert. to bile.
2. having the feeling of general irritability, loss of appetite, indigestion, constipation, and vomiting that can result from a liver disorder.

bilirubin (bĭl'ĭ-rōō'bĭn) N. orange-yellow pigment in bile. The abnormal accumulation of bilirubin in the blood and skin causes jaundice, and testing for bilirubin levels in the blood helps in the diagnosis of several diseases.

biliverdin (bĭl'ĭ-vûr'dĭn) N. early breakdown product of hemoglobin as part of the normal life-death cycle of red blood cells. After 120 days, these cells die and hemoglobin is metabolized in the spleen and other related tissues. The globin protein is recycled, while the heme portion is excreted. For this to occur, it must be chemically converted to biliverdin, then to bilirubin.

binge eating disorder N. disorder that resembles bulimia and is characterized by episodes of uncontrolled eating (or binging). It differs from bulimia, however, because its sufferers do not purge their bodies of the excess food, via vomiting, laxative abuse, or diuretic abuse. (*Compare* BULIMIA).

binocular ADJ. pert. to both eyes; using both eyes; made for use by both eyes (e.g., a binocular microscope).

bio- comb. form indicating an association with life (e.g., biometrics, application of statistical methods to data on living organisms).

bioassay N. test, usually involving living organisms, of the effect or potency of a drug.

biochemistry (bī'ŏ-kĕm'ĭ-strē) N. study of chemical processes in living organisms.

biocompatible ADJ. agreeable to or with the essential life processes of a cell, tissue, or organism.

biodegradable ADJ. able to be broken down by living organisms, esp. with reference to the action of microorganisms on organic wastes and refuse.

bioelectromagnetics N. unconventional use of electromagnetic fields for medical purposes.

bioengineering N. branch of biology dealing with (1) processing or artificial production of plant and animal materials, esp. in the fermentation of organic products; and (2) application of engineering principles to medical problems (e.g., manufacture of artificial limbs and other organs).

biofeedback (bī'ō-fēd'băk') N. learnable technique that enables a person to manipulate ordinarily involuntary processes, such as heartbeat and blood pressure, through concentration and knowledge (feedback) of bodily effects or responses as they occur.

biofield medicine *See* TABLE OF ALTERNATIVE MEDICINE TERMS.

biohazard (bī'ō-hăz'ərd) N. something that endangers life or living things (e.g., a radiation overdose, an oil spill, insecticide overuse).

biological (bī'ə-lŏj'ĭ-kəl) N. medicinal preparation made from living organisms and their products, as serums, vaccines, antitoxins.

biological clock *See* CIRCADIAN RHYTHM.

biology (bī-ŏl'ə-je) N. science of life and living things, including the study of microorganisms (microbiology), plants (botany) and animals (zoology). ADJ. biological, biologic

biomechanics (bī'ō-mĭ-kăn'ĭks) N. study of the effects of mechanical forces on the body; includes forces arising from both within and outside of the body.

biomedical (bī'ō-mĕd'ĭ-kəl) ADJ. pert. to the activities and applications of the basic sciences (e.g., biochemistry, anatomy) to the diagnosis and treatment of patients (clinical medicine).

biomedicine (bī'ō-mĕd'ĭ-sĭn) N. formal name for the health care

system in which the primary practitioner is a medical doctor (M.D.). Also called allopathic, Western, modern, orthodox, or conventional medicine.

biometry (bī-ŏm'ĭ-trē) N. use of mathematics and statistics in biological problem-solving.

bionics (bī-ŏn'ĭks) N. study of the applicability of machines and devices to resolving medical problems, as in the replacement of natural parts (e.g., the bionic arm).

biophysics N. science that applies physics to biological problems (e.g., applying the laws of hydraulics to development of an artificial heart).

biopsy (bī'ŏp'sē) N. removal of a small amount of tissue and/or fluid from a living body and its examination by microscopic and/or other analytical methods to establish or confirm the presence of a disease, to follow its course, and/or to estimate its outcome. The specimen is usually obtained by suction through a needle, but other methods and instruments, including surgery, are also used.

biorhythm (bī'ō-rĭth'əm) N. supposed regular pattern of changes in a person's energy level, responsiveness, and attitude, as determined by genetic, physiologic, or other internal individual factors, or by external factors such as atmospheric pressure, ion content of the air, or amount of stress accumulated. *See also* CIRCADIAN RHYTHM.

biosynthesis (bī'ō-sĭn'thĭ-sĭs) N. manufacture of chemical compounds by a living organism.

biotin (bī'ə-tĭn) N. B-complex vitamin (*See also* TABLE OF

VITAMINS) that aids in body growth and helps fix carbon dioxide in microorganisms and humans; found in liver, egg yolk, and yeast; formerly called vitamin H.

bipolar disorder (bī-pō′lər) N. mental disorder characterized by episodes of mania and depression. One or the other phase may be dominant at a given time, the phases may alternate or aspects of both phases may be present at the same time. Treatment is by psychotherapy and the use of antidepressants and tranquilizers. Also called manic-depressive psychosis.

bird flu *See* AVIAN INFLUENZA.

birth N. act of being born; emergence of the fetus from the uterus, its separation from the mother, and the start of its independent life (usually after about 266 days of gestation); also called parturition.

birth canal N. passage (uterus and vagina) through which the fetus passes during vaginal birth.

birth control *See* CONTRACEPTION.

birth control pill *See* ORAL CONTRACEPTIVE.

birth defect *See* CONGENITAL ANOMALY.

birth injury N. harm to an infant's body or to his/her ability to function as a result of instruments used or actions taken during the birth process.

birth order N. sequence of births among siblings; one's position in the sequence is believed by some psychologists to affect learning ability, intelligence, and the development of personality.

birth rate N. number of live babies born during a given period for a stipulated population (e.g., the 1983 birth rate for the United States was 15.6 per 1,000 population).

birth weight N. weight of a baby at birth; in the United States average birth weight is about 7.5 pounds (3,500 grams). Babies weighing less than 5.5 pounds (2,500 grams) at term are considered small for gestational age; those over 10 pounds (4,500 grams) large for gestational age.

birthing chair N. chair specially designed to aid and provide comfort for a woman during labor and childbirth. It may be a stool with a straight back and hole in the center of the seat or a specially contoured chair. The woman's upright position is thought by many to allow gravity to help shorten labor and aid in the expulsion of the fetus. The chair cannot be used if the woman is anesthetized. *See also* NATURAL CHILDBIRTH.

birthing room N. room, usually in a hospital or other health facility, set aside for childbirth. The room is usually designed to be warm, friendly, and familial. *See also* NATURAL CHILDBIRTH.

birthmark N. discoloration or other blemish present at birth. *See also* NEVUS.

bisect V. to divide into two parts or to separate one part from another.

bisexual ADJ. having both male and female gonads (*see also* HERMAPHRODITE); having the drives and characteristics of both sexes. N. bisexuality

bisoprolol/hydrochlorothiazide N. *See* TABLE OF COMMONLY

PRESCRIBED DRUGS—GENERIC NAMES.

bisphosphonates (bĭs-fäs-fō-nāts) N. general name for a family of medicines that slow the action of osteoclasts, decrease bone resorption, and slow bone loss. They also decrease the risks for fracture in both men and women. Commonly used drugs include etidronate (Didronel), alendronate (Fosamax), and risedronate (Actonel). *See also* OSTEOCLAST; TABLE OF COMMONLY PRESCRIBED DRUGS.

bite N.
1. wound or puncture resulting from a bite, as from an insect or other animal.
2. position of the jaws and teeth when biting, referred to as occlusion, in a closed bite, the lower jaw protrudes, and in an open bite, some opposing teeth do not touch (*compare* MALOCCLUSION).

black death *See* BUBONIC PLAGUE.

black eye N. bluish discoloration around the eye resulting from damage to the tissues and clotting of blood under the skin; a bruise about the eye socket. *See also* HEMATOMA.

black lung disease N. condition marked by increasing loss of lung function (pneumoconiosis), resulting from continuous inhalation of coal dust or other substances; it is prevalent among coal miners. Evidence shows that smoking tobacco may seriously aggravate the condition. Also called coal miner's lung.

black tongue *See* HAIRY TONGUE.

blackhead *See* COMEDO.

blackout N.
1. temporary loss of consciousness.

2. lapse of memory of occurrences and the passage of time during a period of heavy alcohol consumption, sometimes occurring after bouts of heavy drinking.

bladder N.
1. urinary bladder, a muscular and membranous sac that stores urine. Urine produced in the kidneys passes through the ureters into the bladder; sphincters control the release of urine from the bladder through the urethra and out of the body.
2. any saclike, fibrous and membranous organ that holds liquids secreted into it for later passage to another part of the body or out of the body (e.g., the gallbladder, which stores bile).

bland diet N. diet that is chemically and mechanically nonirritating, often prescribed in cases of peptic ulcer, colitis, and other intestinal disorders and after abdominal surgery. Spicy and highly seasoned foods, raw fruits and vegetables, and carbonated beverages are usually avoided.

-blast suffix indicating a development (embryonic) stage that precedes the mature cell (e.g., erythroblast, stage before the mature erythrocyte).

blasto- prefix indicating an association with early embryonic development (e.g., blastomere, one of the two cells resulting from the cleavage of a fertilized ovum).

blastocele (blăs′tə-sēl′) N. liquid-filled cavity of the early ball-shaped embryo (blastula). By increasing the embryo's surface area, the blastocele assists in the absorption of oxygen and nutrients. Also called blastocoele, blastocoel.

blastocyst (blăs′tə-sĭst′) N. embryonic stage, following the morula stage in human development, characterized by a spherical ball of cells with a central fluid-filled cavity (blastocele); during this time, usually about the eighth day after fertilization, implantation in the wall of the uterus occurs.

blastomycosis (blăs′tō-mī-kō′sĭs) N. infection, caused by the fungus of *Blastomyces dermatitidis*, that produces lesions on the skin, especially in exposed areas, or the lungs and other internal organs. Treatment is by antifungal agents.

blastula (blăs′chə-lə) N. ball-like, one cell-layer-thick stage of development of an embryo.

BLASTULA

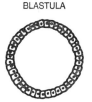

bleb N. blisterlike collection of fluid under the skin, varying from bean- to egg-sized.

bleeder (blē′dər) N.
1. common term for a person who has a tendency to bleed (e.g., a hemophiliac) because the ability of the blood to clot is deficient or absent.
2. bleeding blood vessels, as during surgery.

blenn-, blenno- comb. forms indicating an association with mucus (e.g., blennadenitis, mucous gland inflammation).

blennorrhagia N. excessive discharge of mucus.

blennuria (blĕ-nōōr′ē-ə) N. presence of mucus in the urine.

Blenoxane N. trade name for the antineoplastic bleomycin sulfate, used in the chemotherapeutic treatment of some cancers.

blephar-, blepharo- comb. forms indicating an association with an eyelid (e.g., blepharoplegia, paralysis of the eyelid).

blepharism N. condition in which the person blinks continuously (*compare* TIC).

blepharitis (blĕf′ə-rī′tĭs) N. inflammation of the eyelids, characterized by redness, swelling, and dried crusts of mucus and caused by infection, allergic reaction, or other factors.

blepharoplegia (blĕf′ə-rō-plē′jē-ə) N. paralysis of the movement of an eyelid.

blepharoptosis (blĕf′ə-rŏp-tō′sĭs) N. drooping of the upper eyelid due to paralysis.

blepharospasm N. eyelid muscle spasm, resulting in near closure of the eye, usually due to pain in the eye.

blind spot N. normal gap in the visual field, the result of a spot on the retina insensitive to light and located where the optic nerve enters the eye.

blindness N.
1. inability to see.
2. inability to perceive correctly information received by the eyes.

blister N. vesicle filled with serum; collection of fluid below the skin, usually resulting from a burn.

bloat N. swelling or filling with gas, as in abdominal distension.

block N.
1. anything that stops, interrupts, or obstructs a flow, as a nerve impulse, conscious ability, or blood passage. *See* BUNDLE-BRANCH BLOCK; MENTAL BLOCK.
2. anesthesia of a particular region of the body. *See also* CAUDAL; SADDLE-BLOCK ANESTHESIA.

blood N. fluid tissue that is pumped by the heart through arteries, capillaries, and veins carrying oxygen and nutrients to body cells and carbon dioxide and other waste products away from body cells. Human blood is composed of a pale yellow fluid called plasma in which red blood cells (erythrocytes), white blood cells (leukocytes), platelets, and a variety of chemicals, including hormones, proteins, carbohydrates, and fats are suspended. Adult males have about 70 ml/kg of body weight; women, about 65 ml/kg.

blood bank N. unit or department, usually associated with a hospital or laboratory, that collects, processes, and stores blood for use in blood transfusions and other purposes.

blood cell N. any of two types of cells—red blood cells (erythrocytes) and white blood cells (leukocytes) found in human blood. Platelets, though not true cells, are sometimes included. Also called blood corpuscles or formed elements of the blood. *See* ERYTHROCYTE, LEUKOCYTE, PLATELET.

blood clot N. gelatinous mass made up of red blood cells

COMPOSITION OF BLOOD

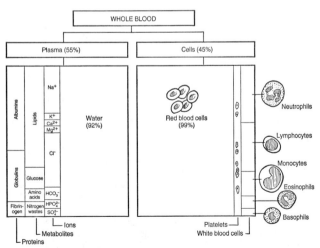

The composition of human blood. The two major components of whole blood are plasma and formed elements. The plasma contains water and numerous dissolved materials, including proteins, metabolites (nutrients and waste products), and ions. The great majority of formed elements are red blood cells.

CHARACTERISTICS OF THE FORMED ELEMENTS OF BLOOD

Cells	Number	Function	Role in Disease
Red blood cells (Erythrocytes)	Male: 5.4 million/mm^3 Female: 4.8 million/mm^3	Oxygen transport; carbon dioxide transport	Too few: anemia Too many: polycythemia
Platelets (Thrombo- cytes)	About 300,000/mm^3	Essential for clotting	Too few: clotting malfunctions; bleeding;easy bruising
White blood cells (Leukocytes, WBC)	About 700/mm^3 total		
Neutrophils	About 60% of WBC	Phago- cytosis	Too many; may be due to bacter- ial infection, inflammation, leukemia
Eosinophils	About 1% of WBC	Some role in allergic response	Too many may result from allergic reaction, parasite infections
Basophils	About 1% of WBC	Possible role in allergic response	
Lymphocytes	About 30% of WBC	Produce antibodies; destroy foreign cells	Atypical lymph- ocytes present in infectious mono- nucleosis; too many may result in leukemia
Monocytes	6 to 8% of WBC	Phago- cytosis; different- iate in tissues to form macro- phages	May increase in monocytic leukemia, tuber- culosis, fungal infections

OVERVIEW OF BLOOD COAGULATION

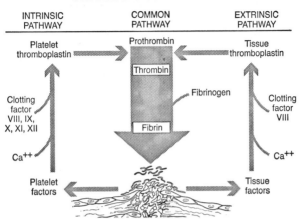

INTRINSIC PATHWAY	COMMON PATHWAY	EXTRINSIC PATHWAY

Platelet thromboplastin

Prothrombin

Tissue thromboplastin

Thrombin

Fibrinogen

Clotting factor VIII, IX, X, XI, XII

Clotting factor VIII

Fibrin

Ca⁺⁺

Ca⁺⁺

Platelet factors

Tissue factors

(erythrocytes), white blood cells (leukocytes), and platelets in a meshwork of the protein fibrin; it results from the process of blood coagulation.

TYPES OF BLOOD CELLS

Erythrocytes
Red blood cells

Leukocytes
White blood cells

Platelets

blood clotting *See* BLOOD COAGULATION, CLOTTING FACTORS.

blood coagulation N. process by which liquid blood is changed into a semisolid mass, a blood clot. It can occur in an intact blood vessel, but usually starts with an injury and the exposure of blood. Platelets clump at the wound site. A series of blood proteins, known as clotting factors, undergo chemical changes, leading to the formation of a fibrin meshwork and the trapping of blood cells into a clot.

Also called blood clotting. Absence of certain of these clotting factors leads to hemophilia.

blood corpuscle *See* BLOOD CELLS.

blood count N. enumeration of red blood cells (erythrocytes), white blood cells (leukocytes), and sometimes platelets found in an accurately diluted 1-cubic-millimeter sample of blood. Erythrocytes normally number 4.5 million (women) to 5 million (men), leukocytes 5,000 to 10,000, and platelets 150,000 to 450,000. Changes from the normal numbers usually indicate disease and are used as an aid to diagnosis. *See also* DIFFERENTIAL BLOOD COUNT.

blood crossmatching N. mixing of the red blood cells (erythrocytes) of a donor with the blood serum of a potential recipient to determine whether the blood is compatible and can be used for transfusion.

blood donor N. one who gives blood for transfusion purposes. Persons with type O blood are considered universal donors because their blood can be given not only to those with type O blood but also to those with type A, AB, or B blood.

blood gases *See* ARTERIAL BLOOD GASES.

blood group N. classification of blood, based on the presence or absence of certain antigens on the surface of red blood cells (erythrocytes), used to determine compatibility for transfusions. There are many systems for classifying blood; the most commonly used is the ABO blood group system.

blood plasma *See* PLASMA.

blood platelet *See* PLATELET.

blood poisoning *See* SEPTICEMIA.

blood pressure (BP) N. force of blood on the walls of the arteries resulting from the squeezing effect of the heart's left ventricle (systole), with residual maintenance (diastole) as the heart chambers relax and expand. Blood pressure is usually measured using a sphygmomanometer placed at the brachial artery in the arm, as the force needed to raise a column of mercury and expressed in millimeters (mm) of mercury (Hg) as a fraction, the upper number representing the systolic pressure, the lower number the diastolic pressure. Blood pressure varies with age, sex, condition of the arteries, force of the heart muscle contraction, emotional state, and general health of the arteries and heart. Adult blood pressure is usually considered normal at about 120/80 mm Hg; in children it is lower. High blood pressure is termed hypertension; low blood pressure, hypotension.

blood serum *See* SERUM.

blood substitute N. substance (e.g., plasma, packed blood cells) used to replace or expand the volume of blood. *See also* ARTIFICIAL BLOOD.

blood sugar *See* GLUCOSE.

blood test N.
1. any of several techniques used to determine whether the cellular makeup (e.g., blood count), chemical levels (e.g., amount of glucose), or other factors (e.g., capillary blood coagulation time) are within normal limits or to ascertain if disease-producing organisms or their products, alcohol, drugs, or poisons are present.
2. Informally, a test for syphilis (Wasserman test) required in many states before a marriage license can be obtained.

blood transfusion N. administration of whole blood or its components to replace blood lost through surgery, disease, or injury. Blood typing is the first step to ensure that donor and recipient's blood match in the transfusion of whole blood.

blood typing N. technique for determining a person's blood type or group. In typing for the commonly used ABO blood group system, blood cells are matched with serum known to be type A or type B, and whether or not agglutination (clumping) of the cells occurs determines the type.

blood urea nitrogen (BUN) N. amount of nitrogenous material present in the blood as urea; it is an indicator of kidney function. Higher-than-normal levels occur in kidney failure, shock, gastrointestinal bleeding, diabetes mellitus, and some other disorders; lower-than-normal values are found in malnutrition and liver disease.

A COMPARISON OF THE BODY'S BLOOD VESSELS

Vessel	Structure	Function
Artery	Thick, strong wall with three layers—endothelial lining, middle layer of smooth muscle and elastic tissue, and outer layer of connective tissue	Carries high-pressure blood from heart to arterioles
Arteriole	Thinner wall than artery, but with three layers; smaller arterioles have endothelial lining, some smooth muscle tissue, and small amount of connective tissue	Connects artery to capillary; helps to control blood flow into capillary by undergoing vasoconstriction of vasodilation
Capillary	Single layer of squamous epithelium	Provides semipermeable membrane through which nutrients, gases, and wastes are exchanged between blood and tissue cells; connects arteriole to venule
Venule	Thinner wall, less smooth muscle and elastic tissue than arteriole	Connects capillary to vein
Vein	Thinner wall than artery, but with similar layers; middle layer more poorly developed; some with flaplike valves	Carries low-pressure blood from venule to heart; valves prevent back flow of blood; serves as blood reservoir

blood vessel N. any of the network of tubes that transport blood throughout the body, including arteries, veins, arterioles, and venules. *See* MAJOR ARTERIES AND VEINS, in Appendix.

blood-brain barrier N. barrier that exists between circulating blood and brain tissue, due presumably to a property of the blood vessels or covering tissues of the brain, whereby large molecules in the blood (e.g., a virus) are prevented from entering the brain and its surrounding fluid. The barrier serves to protect the central nervous system.

blood-letting N. process of removing blood from the body. An ancient practice, generally discarded for centuries, it has recently become the object of renewed interest, esp. in the form of plasmapheresis, the removal of the fluid plasma from the blood.

bloody show N. colloq. for vaginal bleeding, often an early sign of labor.

blue baby N. infant born with a heart defect that limits blood flow to the lungs, causes arterial blood to mix with venous blood, and causes the skin to be bluish because of limited oxygen in the blood. Some of the heart defects can be corrected by surgery, usually performed in the first weeks or months of life. *See also* TETRALOGY OF FALLOT.

blush N. reddening of the face resulting from expansion and filling of the facial blood vessels, occurring in times of embarrassment, extreme self-consciousness, or heat exposure.

BMR N. abbr. for basal metabolic rate; determines the baseline rate of normal body metabolic functions. BMR has now been supplanted clinically by better tests, such as thyroid function tests.

board N. in medical specialties, a certifying body (e.g., the National Board of Medical Examiners, whose examinations must be passed for licensure in many states, or the American Board of Neurosurgery, whose examinations lead to certification in that specialty).

body N.
1. torso of an animal; the trunk.
2. cadaver.
3. specialized part within a larger structure (e.g., the polar bodies at the ends of certain microorganisms).

body image N. personal conception of one's own body, which may be realistic or unrealistic in terms of the way one is seen by others.

body language N. conveying of meaning, intent, or motive directly (e.g., making a fist) or subtly (e.g., changing stance or position) with the body, distinct from verbal communication.

body temperature N. level of heat produced and sustained by body

IONIC BONDING

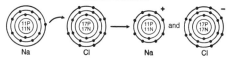

The formation of an ionic bond using sodium (Na) and chlorine (Cl) atoms. An electron moves from the Na to the Cl atom thereby creating ions whose electrical attractions form the ionic bond.

COVALENT BONDING

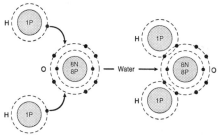

The formation of a covalent bond in a water molecule. The oxygen atom shares its electrons with two hydrogen atoms, thereby completing the outer electron shells of each.

processes. In adults, oral (taken by mouth) temperatures range from 96° to 99°F, with 98.6°F generally being regarded as normal; axillary (armpit) temperatures are typically lower, rectal temperatures higher. Body temperature normally varies during the day, depending on the level of activity, ambient temperature, and other factors; the normal range is greater for children than for adults. Marked changes in body temperature (e.g., fever) are generally indicative of disease.

boil *See* FURUNCLE.

bolus N. chewed mass of food in the mouth ready to be swallowed; also a concentrated mass of an injected drug.

bonding N.
1. attachment that occurs between infants and their parents, esp. the mother, considered significant for the child's psychological development and the child-parent relationship. With natural childbirth, the mother not anesthesized and the father often present, opportunities for bonding activities (e.g., eye-to-eye contact, fondling) immediately after birth, when the infant is in an alert and reactive state, are increased.
2. in chemistry, a chemical linkage. The most common kinds of chemical bonds are hydrogen bonds (weak bond involving the sharing of an electron with a hydrogen atom), ionic bonds (formed by electrical attraction between oppositely charged ions), and covalent bonds (formed by the sharing of a pair (single bond), two pairs (double bond), or three pairs of electrons (triple bond).

bone N.
1. hard, dense, specialized form of connective tissue that forms most of the skeleton. In addition to providing shape and structure to the body, bone stores mineral salts and aids in the formation of blood cells. Under an outer

BONE

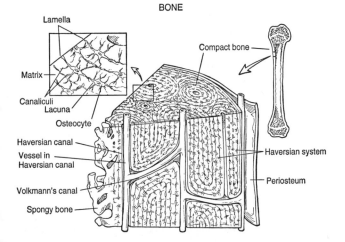

Lamella
Compact bone
Matrix
Canaliculi
Lacuna
Osteocyte
Haversian canal
Vessel in Haversian canal
Haversian system
Volkmann's canal
Periosteum
Spongy bone

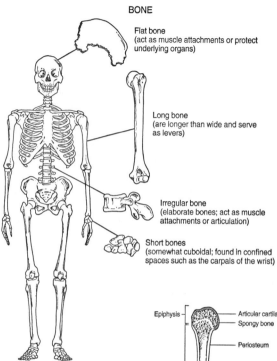

BONE

Flat bone
(act as muscle attachments or protect underlying organs)

Long bone
(are longer than wide and serve as levers)

Irregular bone
(elaborate bones; act as muscle attachments or articulation)

Short bones
(somewhat cuboidal; found in confined spaces such as the carpals of the wrist)

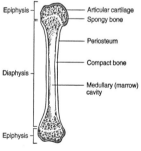

Epiphysis

Articular cartilage
Spongy bone

Periosteum

Compact bone

Diaphysis

Medullary (marrow) cavity

Epiphysis

periosteum layer, compact bone, a hard mass made up of layers of bone cell (osteocyte) tissue in concentric layers (Haversian system), forms the outer shell of most bones, surrounding inner spongy bone with its network of bony bars, bone marrow, blood vessels, and nerves. Bones are classified as long (e.g., femur), short (e.g., those in the wrist), flat (e.g., skull bones), or irregular (e.g., spinal column bones). 2. individual part of the skeleton, one of the 206 bones of the human body (e.g., rib, sternum, tibia). ADJ. bony. *See* MAJOR

BONES OF THE BODY, in Appendix.

bone age N. age determined by comparison of a person's bone development, as shown on X rays, with that of average persons of the same chronological age (*compare* CHRONOLOGICAL

AGE; DEVELOPMENTAL AGE; MENTAL AGE).

bone cancer N. malignant tumor of bone. Various types can occur. Symptoms include pain and spontaneous fractures; treatment involves surgery and sometimes chemotherapy or radiation therapy.

bone marrow N. specialized soft tissue found within bone. Red bone marrow, widespread in the bones of children and found in some adult bones (e.g., sternum, ribs), is essential for the formation of mature red blood cells. Fat-laden yellow bone marrow, more common in adults, is found primarily at the ends of long bones.

bone marrow aspiration N. withdrawal through a special needle of a sample of bone marrow tissue for examination, esp. in the diagnosis of certain blood disorders and malignancies.

bone marrow transplant N. procedure in which a section of bone marrow is taken from one person and transplanted into another; used to replace bone marrow that has been damaged or diseased, such as by leukemia or lymphoma. Autologous bone marrow transplant means that the patient's own bone marrow is used. In this case, the donor marrow is obtained prior to giving high doses of radiation or chemotherapy, usually for cancer, that essentially destroys the patient's own remaining bone marrow. An allogeneic bone marrow transplant uses marrow from a donor whose tissue type closely matches the patient's, usually a sibling.

bone powder N. bone tissue (usually from cadavers), which is reduced to a powder, treated with hydrochloric acid to remove minerals, dried, and sterilized, for implanting into areas where original bone has been injured and removed.

booster injection N. supplementary dose (booster shot) of a vaccine or other immunizing substance, given to raise or restore the presumably waning effectiveness of a previous dose.

border N. common term for the margin of a part (e.g., vermilion border, the deeper colored portion of the lip).

borderline personality disorder (BPD) N. serious mental illness characterized by pervasive instability in moods, interpersonal relationships, self-image, and behavior. A person with depression or bipolar disorder typically endures the same mood for weeks, but a person with BPD may experience intense bouts of anger, depression, and anxiety that may last only hours, or at most a day. These may be associated with episodes of impulsive aggression, self-injury, and drug or alcohol abuse. Patients have frequent changes in long-term goals, career plans, jobs, friendships, gender identity, and values. This instability often disrupts family and work life, long-term planning, and the individual's sense of self-identity. Patients often need extensive mental health services, and account for 20 percent of psychiatric hospitalizations. With help (e.g., dialectical behavioral therapy), many improve over time and are eventually able to lead productive lives. *See also* DIALECTICAL BEHAVIORAL THERAPY (*compare* BIPOLAR DISORDER; DEPRESSION).

borderline schizophrenia *See* LATENT SCHIZOPHRENIA.

boric acid N. white, odorless powder once commonly used as an eyewash and topical antiseptic.

boron N. nonmetallic chemical element used in antiseptics (e.g., boric acid). *See* TABLE OF IMPORTANT ELEMENTS.

botulism (bŏch′ə-lĭz′əm) N. severe and often fatal form of food poisoning that results from eating food (usually home-canned or otherwise preserved) containing the microorganism *Clostridium botulinum*. The microorganism produces a toxin (botulin) that causes fatigue followed by marked disturbances in vision, muscle weakness, and often fatal respiratory complications. Hospitalization and use of antitoxin are required. In infants, a recently reported form of botulism may be responsible for lethargy and failure to thrive. Its frequency is thought to be increased in infants who are fed honey.

bouton (bōō-tôn′) N. bulblike expansion at the tip of nerve axons that comes into contact with the cell bodies of other neurons at synapses; sometimes called the synaptic bouton.

bovine ADJ. pertaining to cattle; often used to indicate the source of a vaccine or serum (e.g., bovine serum).

bovine spongiform encephalopathy (BSE) N. chronic degenerative disease that affects the central nervous system of cattle. Commonly known as "mad cow disease," BSE belongs to a family of diseases known as the transmissible spongiform encephalopathies (TSEs). It is named because of the spongy appearance of the brain tissue of infected cattle when examined under a microscope. The only known bovine cases in the United States were confirmed in December 2003 and June 2005. No transmission to humans has occurred in the United States, but it has been reported in other parts of the world. The cause is a prion, an abnormal form of a normal protein known as a cellular prion protein. Animals become infected through consumption of feed contaminated with the infectious BSE agent. There is no scientific evidence to suggest that milk and dairy products carry the agent that causes BSE. There are strong data linking a rare, degenerative, fatal brain disorder in humans called variant Creutzfeldt-Jakob disease (vCJD) to the consumption of BSE-contaminated product. This type of disease begins primarily with psychiatric symptoms and affects younger patients (median age 28 years). Most cases have occurred outside of the United States. The Food and Drug Administration (FDA) has enacted numerous safety regulations to facilitate identification of potentially infected cattle and steps to prevent them from entering into the food cycle. *See also* CREUTZFELDT-JAKOB DISEASE; PRION.

bowel N. intestines, esp. the large intestine.

bowleg N. abnormal bending outward of the leg from the knee downward, with a gap between the knees; it is often the result of nutritional disorder or deficiency (e.g., insufficient vitamin D) but is sometimes caused by disease

THE BRAIN AND SPINAL CORD

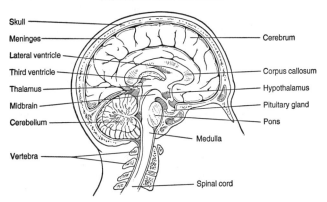

Skull
Meninges
Lateral ventricle
Third ventricle
Thalamus
Midbrain
Cerebellum
Vertebra
Cerebrum
Corpus callosum
Hypothalamus
Pituitary gland
Pons
Medulla
Spinal cord

(e.g., arthritis). It is also called bandy leg. *See also* RICKETS.

Bowman's capsule N. any of numerous cup-shaped structures in the kidney each of which contains a glomerulus that filters wastes from the blood.

BP *See* BLOOD PRESSURE.

BP cuff N. colloquial term for sphygmomanometer.

Br symbol for the element bromine.

brace N. device, usually of metal, plastic, wood, or leather, or a combination of these, used to support an injured or paralyzed part in the correct position.

brachi-, brachio- comb. forms indicating an association with the arm (e.g., brachiocrural, pert. to the arm and leg).

brachial (brā′kē-əl) ADJ. pert. to the arm.

brachial artery N. main artery of the upper arm. *See* MAJOR ARTERIES AND VEINS, in Appendix.

brachial plexus N. network of nerves arising from the spinal cord in the neck region and supplying the arm, hand, and parts of the shoulder.

brachialgia (brā′kē-ăl′jē-ə) N. pain in the arm.

brachy- comb. form meaning shortness (e.g., brachydactyly, shortness of the fingers and/or toes).

brachycephaly N. congenital malformation of the skull in which the skull is abnormally short and broad. Also called brachycephalia.

brachytherapy N. method of cancer treatment in which sealed radioactive sources are used to deliver radiation into or near the tumor. With this method of treatment, a high radiation dose can be delivered locally to the tumor with little effect to the surrounding normal tissue. This treatment may also be called internal radiation therapy. The most common uses of brachytherapy are radioactive seed implants for prostate cancer, cervical cancer, and certain head and

BRAIN

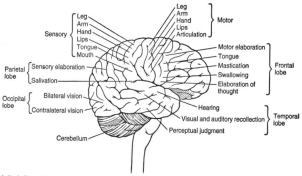

Well-defined areas of the brain control specific body functions.

neck cancers. In prostate cancer, radioactive seeds (iodine-125) are implanted into the prostate gland. The seeds remain in place permanently and become inactive after about 10 months. *See also* PROSTRATE CANCER.

Bradley method of childbirth N. method of psychophysical preparation for natural childbirth that includes education about the physiology of pregnancy, exercises and nutrition during pregnancy, and techniques of breathing and relaxation, with the assistance of the husband, for labor and childbirth (*compare* LAMAZE METHOD OF CHILDBIRTH; READ METHOD OF CHILDBIRTH).

brady- comb. form meaning slowness (e.g., bradyrhythmia, slowness of pulse or heart rate).

bradycardia (brăd′ĭ-kär′dē-ə) N. slow heartbeat (pulse rate lower than 60 in an adult). Some healthy people, esp. athletes, have normally low resting pulse rates, but bradycardia often indicates a disorder of either the cir-culatory or the central nervous system. Some medications (e.g., beta blockers) may also cause bradycardia. Symptoms of weakness or loss of consciousness (syncope) may be present. Treatment of the underlying disorder, removal of an offending drug, and a cardiac pacemaker are potential therapies.

bradykinesis N. abnormal slowness of all voluntary activity, including speech, caused by disease or sometimes tranquilizer use.

bradykinin N. one of a group of large protein molecules (kinins) that influence the contraction of smooth muscle. The result may be low blood pressure, pain, or changes in normal blood flow.

bradylalia N. extremely slow speech due to brain lesion.

bradypnea (brăd′ĭp-nē′ə, brăd′ē-nē′ə) N. abnormally slow breathing.

brain N. mass of nervous tissue in the skull (cranium); the main part of the central nervous system, the primary center for

BRAINSTEM

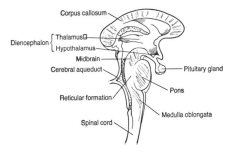

Corpus callosum

Diencephalon { Thalamus☐
Hypothalamus

Midbrain

Cerebral aqueduct

Reticular formation

Spinal cord

Pituitary gland

Pons

Medulla oblongata

The structures of the human brainstem. The major structures in descending order are the diencephalon, midbrain, pons, and medulla oblongata.

regulating body activities. The brain includes the two hemispheres of the cerebrum, the cerebellum, the pons, and the medulla oblongata, each part with specialized functions. The brain is covered by protective membranes (meninges) and contains cavities (ventricles) containing cerebrospinal fluid.

brain death N. irreversible unconsciousness with total loss of brain function, usually determined by loss of reflex activity and respiration and fixed, dilated pupils while the heart continues to beat. In the United States, legal definitions of brain death vary from state to state, but usually electrical activity of the brain must be shown to be absent on at least two electroencephalograms taken 12 to 14 hours apart. *See also* DEATH.

brain rhythm N. characteristic pattern of electrical activity (voltage) in the brain, recordable as a wave-form tracing (electroencephalogram). There are four basic brain rhythms: alpha rhythm, beta rhythm, delta rhythm, and theta rhythm.

brain scan N. painless diagnostic procedure using radioactive isotopes to examine the brain and localize and identify possible lesions or other abnormalities. *See also* COMPUTED TOMOGRAPHY; POSITRON EMISSION TOMOGRAPHY.

brain tumor N. tumor, often malignant, of brain tissue. Several types can occur. Symptoms include headache, visual disturbances, dizziness, loss of balance, nausea, and vomiting. Pain is not commonly present. Treatment involves surgery, chemotherapy, radiation therapy, or a combination.

brain wave *See* BRAIN RHYTHM.

brainstem N. portion of the brain that connects with the spinal cord and includes all parts of the brain (e.g., pons, medulla oblongata) except the cerebrum and cerebellum.

bran N. outer covering of a cereal grain that provides roughage when used as food. Bran is effective in promoting the elimination of solid wastes from the bowel and is recommended by some specialists as an aid to avoid certain diseases (e.g., diverticulosis).

Braxton-Hicks contractions (brăk′stən hĭks′) N. irregular contractions of the muscles of the pregnant uterus that increase in intensity and frequency as pregnancy progresses so that near term they may be hard to distinguish from true labor. Also called false labor.

breast N. front of the chest, esp. either of the two masses of tissue mammary glands that include and surround the nipples. In females the mammary glands produce milk after the birth of a baby. Each breast is made up of glandular lobules that secrete milk. The milk passes into ducts (lactiferous ducts), is stored in dilations of the ducts (ampullae), and is discharged through tiny openings in the nipple area. *See also* LACTATION.

BREAST

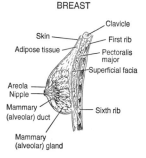

breast cancer N. one of the most common malignancies in women in the United States, with several known risk factors, including a family history of breast cancer, early menarche, late menopause, having no children or having them late in life, exposure to ionizing radi-

ation, obesity, hypertension, chronic cystic disease of breast, and possibly a high-fat diet. Early symptoms are usually detected by the woman during breast self-examination and include a small painless lump; thick or dimpled skin, or a change in the nipple; later symptoms include nipple discharge, pain, and swollen lymph glands in the armpit area. Diagnosis is made by physical examination, mammography, and laboratory examination of tumor cells obtained through biopsy. Treatment depends on the location and size of the tumor and whether or not it has spread to other areas, and may be lumpectomy or some type (e.g., radical or simple) of mastectomy, often followed by chemotherapy and/or radiotherapy. Since early diagnosis and treatment greatly improve the rate of cure, women are advised to practice regular breast self-examination.

breast feeding N. suckling (nursing) of an infant at a mother's breast (as contrasted with bottle feeding). Many authorities recommend breast feeding as a means for establishing a bond between mother and infant and giving the infant the natural benefits of mother's milk for nutrition and immunity.

breast milk N. milklike fluid secreted by female breasts after childbirth and used as food for newborns, providing all necessary nutrients and some level of immunity against certain diseases.

breast pump N. device for extracting milk from the breast of a woman who is nursing or has recently given birth.

How to examine your breasts

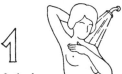

In the shower:

Examine your breasts during bath or shower; hands glide easier over wet skin. Fingers flat, move gently over every part of each breast. Use right hand to examine left breast, left hand for right breast. Check for any lump, hard knot or thickening.

Before a mirror:

Inspect your breasts with arms at your sides. Next, raise your arms high overhead. Look for any changes in contour of each breast, a swelling, dimpling of skin or changes in the nipple.

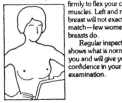

Then, rest palms on hips and press down firmly to flex your chest muscles. Left and right breast will not exactly match—few women's breasts do.

Regular inspection shows what is normal for you and will give you confidence in your examination.

American Cancer Society

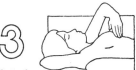

Lying down:

To examine your right breast, put a pillow or folded towel under your right shoulder. Place right hand behind your head—this distributes breast tissue more evenly on the chest. With left hand, fingers flat, press gently in small circular motions around an imaginary clock face. Begin at outermost top of your right breast for 12 o'clock, then move to 1 o'clock, and so on around the circle back to 12. A ridge of firm tissue in the lower curve of each breast is normal. Then move in an inch, toward the

nipple, keep circling to examine *every part of your breast*, including nipple. This requires at least three more circles. Now slowly repeat procedure on your left breast with a pillow under your left shoulder and left hand behind head. Notice how your breast structure feels.

Finally, squeeze the nipple of each breast gently between thumb and index finger. Any discharge, clear or bloody, should be reported to your doctor immediately.

breast self-examination N. process of observing (in front of a mirror) and palpating the breast and surrounding area to detect any lumps or other changes that may indicate disease (e.g., breast cyst or breast cancer); many authorities recommend that women examine their breasts monthly.

breastbone *See* STERNUM.

breath N. air that is taken into and let out from the lungs through the nose or mouth; one inhalation and one exhalation.

breathing N. action of taking air into the lungs and then letting it out, a process normally done without thinking and controlled by the autonomic nervous system (*compare* EXPIRATION; INHALATION; RESPIRATION).

breech presentation N. situation at birth in which the feet, knees, or buttocks of the infant appear first; occurs in about 3% of all births and is sometimes hazardous. Also called breech birth. *See also* FRANK BREECH.

bregma N. junction point at the top of the skull at which two bone seams (coronal and sagittal sutures) meet. ADJ. bregmatic

Brevibloc N. trade name for the intravenous beta blocker esmolol.

bridge N. narrow band of tissue, usually considered abnormal. For example, myocardial bridges in the heart represent growth of excess heart muscle that may interfere with coronary artery circulation or the transmission of electrical impulses through the heart's conduction system. In dentistry, an oral appliance that replaces missing teeth and is attached to adjacent normal teeth for support.

Bright's disease *See* NEPHRITIS.

Brill's disease N. mild form of typhus.

Broca's area N. area of the cerebral cortex involved in speech production.

Brodie's abscess N. form of osteomyelitis, with chronic abscess at the head of a bone. Treatment is by antibiotics and excision and drainage of the abscesses.

Brodmann areas N. numbered (1–47) areas of the cerebral cortex, each distinguished by different cellular components and each involved in a specific function (e.g., area 17 is involved in vision, area 4 in motor function).

bromhidrosis N. bad-smelling body odor resulting from bacterial action on sweat from armpits, groin, and/or feet.

bromide N. salt containing bromine, once formerly used as a sedative but now replaced by safer drugs.

bromide poisoning N. poisoning caused by excessive intake of bromides; symptoms include vomiting, confusion, hallucinations, irritability, a skin rash, and sometimes coma; also called brominism.

bromine (brō′mēn) N. liquid, nonmetallic element used in some medicinal compounds. *See also* TABLE OF IMPORTANT ELEMENTS.

brominism N. *See* BROMIDE POISONING.

bronchi N., *pl.* of bronchus.

bronchi-, broncho- comb. forms indicating an association with one (bronchus) or more (bronchi) passages leading to the lungs (e.g., bronchoesophageal, pert. to the bronchi and esophagus).

bronchial (brŏng′kē-əl) ADJ. pert. to a bronchus or the bronchi.

bronchial asthma *See* ASTHMA.

bronchiectasis (brŏng′kē-ĕk′tə-sĭs) N. persistent, abnormal widening of the bronchi, with an associated cough and the spitting up of pus-filled mucus. The condition may be congenital or may result from infection (e.g., whooping cough, pertussis) or obstruction due to a tumor or an inhaled foreign body. Treatment is by antibiotics, physiotherapy, or (less often) surgery.

bronchiole (brŏn′kē-ōl′) N. small branch in the bronchial system, leading toward and ending in the alveoli of the lung.

bronchiolitis (brŏn′kē-ō-lī′tĭs) N. viral infection of the lower respiratory tract, occurring most often in children under 1 or 2 years of age and characterized by respiratory distress, wheezing on expiration, low-grade fever, cough, and nasal discharge. The disease usually disappears within a week or 10 days. Antibiotics and bronchodilators are not generally used, treatment being mainly symptomatic (e.g., vaporizer, suctioning if necessary).

bronchitis (brŏn-kī′tĭs) N. inflammation of a bronchus or of the bronchi. Acute bronchitis, a common disorder often following an upper respiratory infection, is characterized by cough, fever, and chest pain. Treatment is by pain and fever reducers, steam inhalation and antibiotics, if indicated. Chronic bronchitis, bronchial inflammation that is persistent, often caused by cigarette smoking, exposure to other irritants or recurrent infections, is characterized by mucus secretions, cough, and frequently increasing difficulty in breathing.

bronchoconstrictor (brŏn′kō-kən-strĭk′tər) N. substance that causes contraction of the smooth muscle walls of bronchi, leading to constriction or narrowing of the opening (lumen). Symptoms (e.g., wheezing, shortness of breath) and abnormalities in lung function tests may result. A bronchodilator has the opposite effect (dilates the airways).

bronchodilator (brŏn′kō-dī-lā′tər) N. substance that causes relaxation of smooth muscle walls of bronchi, leading to dilation or widening of the opening (lumen). May result in improvement in a patient's symptoms (e.g., wheezing, shortness of breath) and lung function tests. A bronchoconstrictor has the opposite effect (constricts the airways).

bronchopneumonia (brŏn′kōnoŏ-mōn′yə) N. acute inflammation of the bronchi and of the alveoli of the lungs, characterized by fever, chills, shallow breathing, cough, and chest pain. It usually follows an earlier infection, starting at the smallest, most remote air channels (bronchioles) and resulting in the formation of pus and the clogging of those channels. Treatment is by bedrest, and antibiotics and oxygen, if necessary. (*Compare* INTESTINAL PNEUMONIA; LOBAR PNEUMONIA.)

bronchoscopy (brŏn-kŏs′kə-pē) N. examination of the bronchi through a special device (bronchoscope). Sometimes samples of tissue or fluid are taken for examination, and small foreign bodies can sometimes be removed. ADJ. bronchoscopic

bronchospasm (brŏn′kə-spăz′əm) N. spasm of the bronchi, causing them to narrow, making exhalation difficult and noisy; it is commonly associated with asthma and bronchitis.

bronchus (brŏn′kəs) N., *pl.* bronchi, one of the two large channels that lead from the trachea to smaller branches (bronchioles) and ultimately to the air sacs (alveoli) of the lung. ADJ. bronchial

Bronkosol N. trade name for the bronchodilator isoetharine hydrochloride, used in the treatment of asthma, emphysema, and bronchitis.

bronzed diabetes *See* HEMOCHROMATOSIS.

brucellosis (broo'sə-lo'sĭs) N. disease caused by infection with a bacterium (*Brucella* species), obtained by association with infected livestock or their products and causing chills, weakness, headache, and recurring fever. Treatment includes bedrest and tetracyclines. Also called Malta fever; Mediterranean fever; undulant fever.

bruise (brooz) N. injury that does not cause the skin to break or bleed but usually results in discoloration because of clotted blood below the skin's surface.

bruit (broo'ē) N. abnormal sound, heard on listening with a stethoscope, which indicates turbulent flow of blood in a vessel.

bruxism (brŭk'sĭz'əm) N. rhythmic or spasmodic grinding of the teeth, esp. during sleep; often caused by emotional tension.

bubo (boo'bō) N. lymph node, esp. in the armpit or groin, that is inflamed and enlarged because of tuberculosis, gonorrhea, plague, or other infection. ADJ. bubonic

bubonic plague (boo-bŏn'ĭk) N. serious, sometimes fatal infection, caused by toxin of the bacteria *Yersinia pestis* and transmitted by the bite of fleas from infected rats or squirrels; it is characterized by high fever, prostration, painful swollen lymph glands (buboes) in the groin and armpits, delirium, and bleeding from superficial blood vessels. Treatment is by antibiotics and drainage of buboes if necessary. Bubonic plague, the Black Death of the Middle Ages, can become epidemic in areas with large populations of infected rats.

bucca (bŭk'ə) N. cheek; fleshy portion of the side of the face below the eyes. ADJ. buccal

budesonide N. *See* TABLE OF COMMONLY PRESCRIBED DRUGS—GENERIC NAMES.

Buerger's disease N. disease of unknown cause, affecting primarily men who are heavy tobacco users, in which arteries, most often in the legs and feet, become inflamed and occluded, causing burning, numbness, tingling, and, if inadequate blood supply continues, phlebitis, tissue damage and possibly gangrene; also called thromboangiitis obliterans.

buffer N. chemical that is added to another to avert a radical change in concentration or pH in the second; a device or system that tends to prevent change, as in body temperature or blood pressure.

buffered aspirin N. aspirin that has been combined with one or more other chemicals to prevent change in the aspirin's composition under certain circumstances, as in passing through the stomach. Buffered aspirin was formulated to help persons who become ill as the result of the action of gastric juice on ordinary aspirin.

bulb (bŭlb) N., *pl.* bulbi.
  1. knoblike structure, mass, or part (e.g., bulbus pili; the bulb of a hair).
  2. old term for the medulla oblongata part of the brain. Also called bulbus. ADJ. bulbar

bulbourethral gland N. either of two small glands located on each side of the prostate and secreting a fluid component of semen.

bulimia (byoo-lǐm′ē-ə) N. potentially serious disorder, esp. common in adolescents and young women, marked by insatiable craving for food and leading to episodes of excessive overeating, often followed by self-induced vomiting, purging, or fasting. Treatment involves primarily psychotherapy. *See also* ANOREXIA NERVOSA. ADJ. bulimic

bulk N. that part of a food (e.g., fiber) that, when eaten, forms a mass that promotes intestinal movement (peristalsis). *See also* ROUGHAGE.

bulk cathartic N. laxative that acts by softening and increasing the mass of fecal matter.

bulla (boŏl′ə) N., *pl.* bullae, blister (vesicle); a large bleb in the skin that contains fluid (serum). ADJ. bullous

bumetanide (byoo-mĕt′ə-nīd′) N. oral/parenteral diuretic (trade name Bumex) used in the treatment of hypertension, edema, and congestive heart failure. Adverse effects include fluid and electrolyte imbalances.

BUN *See* BLOOD UREA NITROGEN.

bundle N. cluster (fascicle) of filaments or elongated parts, specifically muscle fibers or nerves (e.g., bundle of His).

bundle branch block N. defect in the electrical tissues of the heart that results in abnormal conduction of the cardiac depolarization wave. There may be no symptoms, or symptoms due to a reduced heart rate (bradycardia), or cardiac arrest. The most common cause is atherosclerosis, although myocardial infarction or other cardiac disease may also be responsible. A pacemaker may be required in severe cases.

bundle of His N. band of fibers in the heart through which the cardiac impulse is transmitted from the atrioventricular node to the ventricles; also called atrioventricular bundle.

bunion (bŭn′yən) N. swelling and thickening of the joint where the big toe joins the foot, displacing the big toe toward the other toes. Caused by chronic irritation from ill-fitting shoes, bunions may become painful and require surgery.

bupropion (byoo-prō′pē-ŏn′) N. *See* TABLE OF COMMONLY PRESCRIBED DRUGS—GENERIC NAMES.

Burkitt's lymphoma (bûr′kĭts) N. malignancy of the lymphatic system, seen mostly in central Africa, characterized by lesions of the jaw or abdomen (esp. in children) often followed by central nervous system involvement. The Epstein-Barr virus (EBV) is believed to be the cause; chemotherapy is usually effective treatment.

burn N. tissue injury resulting from exposure to excessive sun, heat, radiation (e.g., overexposure to X rays or radioactive elements), a caustic, or electricity. Tissue changes include reddening and pain (first degree), blistering (second degree), and destruction of tissue (third degree). Treatment involves alleviation of pain, careful cleaning of injuries, prevention of infection, maintenance of normal fluid and electrolyte balances in the body, care of wounds, and, in cases of severe burn, prevention or care of shock. In severe burns skin grafts and plastic surgery may be necessary.

burn center N. facility specially designed for the care of severely burned persons.

burnout N. condition marked by physical and emotional exhaustion, often described as having no energy, being apathetic, not caring anymore; it typically occurs in people who are overworked, frustrated by lack of accomplishments, and/or subject to continued job stress, particularly those in service professions (e.g., teacher, nurse, social worker).

bursa (bûr′sə) N., *pl.* bursae, fluid-filled, membrane-lined sac, usually in the vicinity of joints, which serves as a lubricating and protective system between various structures, including tendon and bone, tendon and ligament, or other structures.

ELBOW (OLECRANON) BURSA

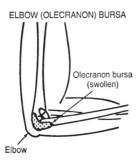

Olecranon bursa (swollen)

Elbow

bursitis (bər-sī′tĭs) N. inflammation of a bursa, often preci-

pitated by injury, infection, excessive trauma or effort, or arthritis or similar condition and characterized by pain and often limited mobility. Common locations include the shoulder, knee, and hip. Treatment is by analgesics, anti-inflammatory agents, immobilization of the affected area, and in some cases the use of corticosteroid injections at the affected site.

BuSpar N. trade name for the antianxiety agent buspirone HCl. *See* TABLE OF COMMONLY PRESCRIBED DRUGS—TRADE NAMES.

buspirone HCl (byo͞o-spī′rōn′) N. drug used in the treatment of anxiety (trade name BuSpar) with or without coexisting depression; side effects include dizziness, nausea, headache, and nervousness. *See* TABLE OF COMMONLY PRESCRIBED DRUGS—GENERIC NAMES.

butterfly rash N. red, scaly eruption on both cheeks with a narrow band across the nose, characteristic of certain diseases (e.g., lupus erythematosus, rosacea).

buttock N. external prominence posterior to the hips; consists of the gluteal muscles and underlying structures; *see* NATES.

bypass (bī′păs′) N. any surgically created, temporary or permanent channel or route around a part, esp. a part that has been damaged (e.g., a coronary bypass); a shunt.

byssinosis (bĭs′ĭ-nō′sĭs) N. lung disease caused by breathing in the dust of cotton, flax, or hemp. Symptoms, which are typically more pronounced when the patient returns to work after the weekend rest, are tightness of the chest, shortness of breath, and wheezing.

C

C
1. symbol for the element carbon.
2. abbreviation for the Celsius (centigrade) temperature scale.

C vitamin N. vitamin (ascorbic acid) essential for general metabolism, the health of capillary walls, and wound healing, and believed by some to help guard against certain infections. Rich sources are citrus fruits, tomatoes and potatoes. *See also* VITAMIN; TABLE OF VITAMINS.

Ca
1. symbol for the element calcium.
2. abbreviation for cancer.

cachexia (kə-kĕk′sē-ə) N. severe state of wasting, malnutrition, and poor health, as occurs, for example, in certain advanced cancers and advanced tuberculosis. Also called cachexy. ADJ. cachectic

cadaver (kə-dăv′ər) N. dead body, corpse, esp. one used for the study of anatomy. ADJ. cadaveric

caduceus (kə-doō′sē-əs) N. symbol often used to represent the medical profession consisting of two serpents entwined around a staff, topped by two wings.

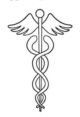

caesarean *See* CESAREAN SECTION.

caffeine (kă-fēn′, kăf′ēn′, kăf′ē-ĭn) N. central nervous system stimulant that is an alkaloid derived from the dried leaves of tea plants and the beans of coffee plants, found in coffee, tea, cola drinks, and some medicines. It is used to counter drowsiness and mental fatigue; it also acts as a diuretic. Excessive intake of caffeine frequently causes restlessness, insomnia, and gastrointestinal complaints. *See also* CAFFEINISM.

caffeinism N. poisoning from excessive intake of coffee or other caffeine-containing products, resulting in upset stomach, restlessness, nervousness, and increased heartbeat.

caisson disease (kā′sŏn′) *See* BENDS; AIR EMBOLISM.

calamine (kăl′ə-mīn′) N. chemical (zinc oxide with added iron oxide) used in the form of a pink powder or lotion to treat itching and mild skin irritations.

Calan N. trade name for the calcium-blocker verapamil. *See* TABLE OF COMMONLY PRESCRIBED DRUGS—TRADE NAMES.

calcaneus (kăl-kā′nē-əs) N. heelbone, the largest of the tarsals; also called calcaneum. ADJ. calcaneal

calcar (kăl′kär′) N. a spurlike projection, as that of the femur neck (calcar femorale).

calcareous (kăl-kâr′ē-əs) ADJ. chalky, containing calcium or lime.

calciferol (kăl-sĭf′ə-rôl′) N. one of the D vitamins, a chemical found in milk and fish liver oils and used to prevent and treat rickets, osteomalacia, and other disorders of calcium metabolism; also called vitamin D_2; ergocalciferol.

calcification (kăl′sə-fĭ-kā′shən) N. hardening of tissue resulting from the formation of calcium salts within it; the abnormal hardening (calcinosis) leads to impaired organ function (e.g., in the kidneys or arteries). The process can result from a disturbance in the normal balance of hormones, vitamin D, and calcium and other minerals in the body.

calcitonin (kăl′sĭ-tō′nĭn) N. hormone secreted by the thyroid gland that regulates the level of calcium in the blood and stimulates bone formation. *See* TABLE OF COMMONLY PRESCRIBED DRUGS—GENERIC NAMES.

calcium (kăl′sē-əm) N. element, the fifth most abundant in the human body, found primarily in bone but also present in body fluids and soft tissue cells. It is important for nerve impulse transmission, muscle function, blood coagulation, teeth and bone formation, and heart function. *See also* TABLE OF IMPORTANT ELEMENTS.

calcium channel blocker N. any of a class of drugs that block the flow of the electrolyte calcium either within the cells' electrical conduction system or in the contraction of smooth muscle. These agents are used in the treatment of hypertension, angina, arrhythmias, and migraine.

calculus (kăl′kyə-ləs) N., *pl.* calculi, stone that forms in the body, usually in hollow organs or ducts, where it may cause obstruction and inflammation. *See also* GALLSTONE; RENAL CALCULUS.

calefacient ADJ. producing warmth or the sensation of warmth (e.g., a hot-water bottle or a commercial ointment for muscle soreness).

calendar method of family planning N. method of family planning in which the fertile days (the days during which conception is most likely to occur) in a woman's menstrual cycle are determined by examining the timing of six or more consecutive menstrual cycles on a calendar, determining the average length of the menstrual cycle, and then applying the fact that ovulation typically occurs 14 days before the onset of a period and that sperm and ovum are each viable for a few days in the female reproductive tract. The fertile period therefore extends from a few days before ovulation to a few days after. If, for example, a woman has an average menstrual cycle of 28 days, she would be expected to ovulate on day 14 and her fertile days to extend from approximately day 10 through day 18 of her cycle. During these fertile, or unsafe, days, coitus should be avoided if pregnancy is not desired; should be practiced if pregnancy is desired. Since a woman's menstrual cycle is often not regular and may be affected by illness, emotional upset, change in climate, and other factors, the calendar method is not considered one of the most effective means of family planning. Also called rhythm method. (*Compare* BASAL BODY TEMPERATURE METHOD OF FAMILY PLANNING; OVULA-

TION METHOD OF FAMILY PLANNING; *See also* CONTRACEPTION.)

calf N. thick part at the back of the leg below the knee that contains the gastrocnemius muscle, which flexes when one stands on the toes.

calf bone *See* FIBULA, TIBIA.

caliber (kăl′ə-bər) N. diameter of a tube or vessel (e.g., a blood vessel).

calisthenics (kăl′ĭs-thĕn′ĭks) N. exercises usually done as a group, with provided cadence or rhythm and under the direction of a leader, as a means for developing or retaining flexibility, strength, and muscle tone (*compare* AEROBIC EXERCISE).

callus (kăl′əs) N.
1. hardened area of skin as on the bottom of the foot.
2. tissue formed around a bone fracture. ADJ. callous

calorie (kăl′ə-rē) N.
1. amount of heat needed to raise 1 gram of water 1 degree on the Celsius scale. Also called small calorie.
2. amount of heat equal to 1,000 small calories. Also called large calorie.
3. unit equal to 1 large calorie, denoting the heat expenditure of an organism and the energy or fuel value of a food. ADJ. caloric

calvaria (kăl-vâr′ē-ə) N. dome of the skull that varies in shape (e.g., oval, circular) from one individual to another. ADJ. calvarial

cAMP *See* CYCLIC AMP.

camphor (kăm′fər) N. chemical, derived from the plant *Cinnamomum camphora* or made artificially, having a penetrating smell and sometimes used for the treatment of skin conditions (although the effectiveness of such treatment is in question). Camphor is poisonous if swallowed and can be life-threatening.

canal (kə-năl′) N. relatively narrow tube, generally for conducting materials other than blood or lymph (e.g., the alimentary canal, for carrying food from the mouth to the stomach and intestines for digestion and for expelling wastes through the canal's end, the anus).

canalization (kăn′ə-lĭ-zā′shən) N. formation of channels or passages through tissue.

cancellous (kăn-sĕl′əs, kăn′sə-ləs) ADJ. containing a latticework type of structure; often used to describe the microscopic architecture of bones such as the vertebrae, femur, and calcaneus (heel).

cancer (Ca) N. abnormal, malignant growth of cells that invade nearby tissues and often spread (metastasize) to other sites in the body, interfering with the normal function of the affected sites. Although the basic cause of cancer remains unknown, most forms of cancer can be traced to a specific causal or precipitating factor (e.g., cigarette smoking, exposure to cancer-producing chemicals (carcinogens) or ionizing radiation, or overexposure to the sun); viruses are associated with some cancers and genetic (familial) susceptibility plays a role in certain forms of the disease. The incidence of different types of cancer varies greatly with age, sex, ethnic group, and geographic location. In the United States cancer is second to heart disease as a cause of death, with breast cancer and lung cancer leading the statistics. Older persons are much more prone to cancer (at age 25, the probability of developing cancer within 5 years is 1 in 700, at age 65, it is 1 in 14). The parts of the body most often affected by cancer are the breast, lungs, colon, uterus, oral cavity, and bone marrow. Major signs of cancer include a change in bladder or bowel habits; a sore that does not heal; a persistent cough or hoarseness; unusual bleeding or discharge; thickening or lump in the breast or other part of the body; indigestion or difficulty in swallowing; unexplained loss of weight; and change in a wart or mole. The treatment of cancer may involve surgery, the irradiation of affected parts, and/or chemotherapy. The prognosis depends on the type and site of the cancer, the promptness of initial treatment, and other factors; about one-third of patients with newly diagnosed cancers are ultimately permanently cured. (*See also* CARCINOMA; BONE CANCER; LEUKEMIA; LIVER CANCER; and other specific types of malignancies.)

cancer bodies *See* RUSSELL'S BODIES.

cancer of the blood *See* LEUKEMIA.

candida (kăn′dĭ-də) N. yeastlike fungus that may infect the mouth (as in thrush), skin (as in diaper rash), intestines, or vagina. Rarely, invasion of the bloodstream may occur. Treatment is with antifungal drugs. *See also* CANDIDIASIS.

candidiasis (kăn′dĭ-dī′ə-sĭs) N. infection caused by a Candida species of fungus (e.g., *Candida albicans*), affecting most often the skin, mouth, and vagina, and causing itching, peeling, whitish exudate, and some-

times easy bleeding. Common forms of candidiasis include thrush and some types of vaginitis and diaper rash. Treatment is by oral and topical antifungal drugs (e.g., nystatin) and sometimes use of gentian violet.

canine (kā′nīn) N. any of the four teeth, two in each jaw, flanking the incisors and projecting beyond the level of the other teeth.

canker (kăng′kər) N. ulcerlike sore, esp. of the mouth (*compare* CHANCRE).

cannabis (kăn′ə-bĭs) N. psychoactive substance derived from the leaves of the plant *Cannabis sativa* and related Cannabis species and found in marihuana and other hallucinogens; it is sometimes used in the care of some cancer patients as an antiemetic to counter nausea and vomiting associated with chemotherapy.

cannula (kăn′yə-lə) N. flexible tube inserted into a cavity for transferring fluids or other materials into or out of it (e.g., as in amniocentesis to withdraw amniotic fluid).

cannulation (kăn′yə-lā′shən) N. insertion of a cannula into a body cavity or duct (e.g., trachea); also called cannulization.

canthus (kăn′thəs) N., *pl.* canthi, angle formed by the upper eyelid with the lower eyelid, one being inner (nasal) and the other outer (temporal). ADJ. canthal

capacity N.
1. amount of material an organ or other part can hold when filled (e.g., lung capacity).
2. ability to perform an action (capability).

capillary N.
1. tiny blood vessels connecting arterioles and venules. Through

the one-cell-layer-thick walls (approx. 0.008 mm diameter) of capillaries, oxygen and nutrients are passed from arterioles to body tissues, and carbon dioxide and other wastes are passed from body tissues to venules.
2. any other small, hairlike tube for carrying lymph or other material.

capitate N. one of the eight bones of the wrist.

capitation N. payment mechanism in which a provider is paid, in advance, a set fee for medical services regardless of the amount or intensity of medical services rendered to a patient. *See* TABLE OF MANAGED CARE TERMS.

Capoten N. trade name for the antihypertensive captopril.

capsid N. cover (a protein) of a simple virus particle (virion).

capsule (kăp′səl) N.
1. envelope-like structure enclosing an organ or part (e.g., Bowman's capsule, which encloses a glomerulus in the kidney).
2. membrane that surrounds a microorganism (e.g., covering around a bacterium).
3. a medicine-containing shell of gelatin or other material that can dissolve in the stomach, releasing the capsule's contents. ADJ. capsular

captopril (kăp′tə-prĭl′) N. one of a class of drugs that block the formation of angiotensin in the kidney, leading to vasodilation. Sold under the trade name Capoten, this agent is used in the treatment of hypertension, congestive heart failure, and acute myocardial infarction. Adverse effects include kidney abnormalities and an elevated potassium level.

caput (kăp′o͝ot) N.
1. head.
2. enlarged or headlike part of an organ (e.g., caput humeri, head of the humerus, which fits into a cavity in the scapula).

car sickness N. nausea from acceleration, deceleration, and other motions experienced while riding in a car (*compare* AIRSICKNESS; MOTION SICKNESS; SEASICKNESS).

Carafate N. trade name for the antiulcer agent sucralfate.

carbohydrate (kär′bō-hī′drāt′) N. any of a group of organic compounds (containing the elements carbon, hydrogen, and oxygen, including starches and sugars, that are the chief energy sources of the body. Carbohydrates from foods result in production of glucose which is then metabolized to release energy, stored as adenosine triphosphate (ATP). Carbohydrates are synthesized by green plants (through the

CARBOHYDRATE METABOLISM

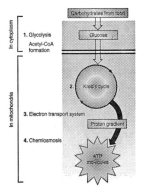

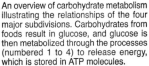

An overview of carbohydrate metabolism illustrating the relationships of the four major subdivisions. Carbohydrates from foods result in glucose, and glucose is then metabolized through the processes (numbered 1 to 4) to release energy, which is stored in ATP molecules.

process of photosynthesis), consumed by humans in the forms of cereals, flour products, fruits, and vegetables, and either absorbed immediately or stored in the form of glycogen. *See also* ACETYL CO-A; CHEMIOSMOSIS; ELECTRON TRANSPORT SYSTEM; KREBS CYCLE; GLYCOLYSIS.

carbon N. nonmetallic element present in virtually all living things and all organic matter. *See also* TABLE OF IMPORTANT ELEMENTS.

carbon dioxide N. colorless, odorless gas (CO_2) given off from the lungs as a waste product of respiration. Carbon dioxide levels in the blood regulate the breathing rate, and the acid-base balance of the blood and other body fluids is influenced by the levels of carbon dioxide and its compounds. *See also* APNEA; HYPERVENTILATION.

carbon monoxide N. colorless, odorless gas (CO) formed by the incomplete burning of organic materials (e.g., automotive fuel). Carbon monoxide is extremely toxic; by combining with hemoglobin, it can cause loss of oxygen transport to tissues, paralysis, and death. *See also* CARBON MONOXIDE POISONING.

carbon monoxide poisoning N. toxic condition caused by the inhalation and absorption of carbon monoxide gas, which is often generated during a fire or in the presence of a poorly functioning gas heating device. The carbon monoxide combines with hemoglobin in the blood, displacing oxygen, and causes loss of oxygen to body tissues. Symptoms include headache,

CARBON DIOXIDE TRANSPORT IN THE BLOOD

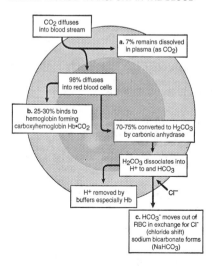

CO_2 diffuses into blood stream

a. 7% remains dissolved in plasma (as CO_2)

98% diffuses into red blood cells

b. 25-30% binds to hemoglobin forming carboxyhemoglobin Hb•CO_2

70-75% converted to H_2CO_3 by carbonic anhydrase

H_2CO_3 dissociates into H^+ to and HCO_3

H^+ removed by buffers especially Hb

Cl^-

c. HCO_3^- moves out of RBC in exchange for Cl^- (chloride shift) sodium bicarbonate forms ($NaHCO_3$)

shortness of breath, confusion, drowsiness, unconsciousness, and, if continued, death. Treatment involves removal of the person from the carbon monoxide environment, high concentrations of oxygen, and sometimes the use of a hyperbaric (oxygen) chamber.

carbonic anhydrase (an-hī-drāz) N. enzyme found in the stomach, pancreas, kidneys, and red blood cells that catalyzes the interconversion of carbon dioxide (CO_2) and water (H_2O) into carbonic acid (H_2CO_3), protons (H^+), and bicarbonate ions (HCO_3^-): $CO_2 + H_2O \leftrightarrow H_2CO_3 \leftrightarrow H^+ + HCO_3^-$. It enables red blood cells to transport carbon dioxide from the tissues to the lungs, the stomach and pancreas to secrete massive amounts of acid and bicarbonate, respectively, and the kidneys to maintain acid-base and fluid balance. *See also* ACID-BASE BALANCE.

carbuncle (kär′bŭn′kəl) N. cluster of boils or abscesses (resulting from infection with Staphylococcus bacteria) deep under the skin from which pus escapes to the skin surface. Treatment is by surgical drainage, antibiotics, and compresses.

carcin-, carcino- comb. forms indicating an association with cancer, specifically a carcinoma (e.g., carcinolysis, the breakdown of cancer cells, as by a drug).

carcinoembryonic antigen (CEA) (kär′sə-nō-ěm′-brē-ŏn′ĭk) N. antigen present only in very small amounts in normal tissues. Used as a screening test for cancer and as a tool to monitor the success of therapy (e.g.,

surgery, radiotherapy, chemotherapy).

carcinogen (kär-sĭn′ə-jən, kär′sə-nə-iĕn′) N. specific substance or chemical that gives rise to a cancer, a cancer-forming agent. ADJ. carcinogenic

carcinoma (kär′sə-nō′mə) N. malignant growth of epithelial cells that arises in the coverings and linings of the body parts (e.g., skin and mucous membranes) and in glands; these cells tend to invade adjacent tissues and to spread (metastasize) to other parts of the body via the lymphatic channels and/or bloodstream (*compare* LEUKEMIA; LYMPHOMA; SARCOMA).

carcinoma in situ N. small cluster or nest of malignant cells that has not yet invaded the deeper epithelial tissue layers or spread to other parts of the body; preinvasive cancer (e.g., carcinoma in situ of the uterine cervix). Treatment at this early stage is often successful. Also called preinvasive cancer.

card-, cardio- comb. forms indicating an association with the heart (e.g., cardioaortic, pert. to the heart and aorta).

cardia N.
1. that part of the stomach that connects with the esophagus.
2. obsolete term for heart.

cardiac ADJ. pert. to the heart (e.g., a cardiac disorder such as mitral valve prolapse); to the cardiac, or upper, part of the stomach; or, colloquially, to someone with a heart condition.

cardiac arrest N. sudden cessation of cardiac output and blood circulation, usually caused by ventricular fibrillation or other serious abnormality in heart ventricle function, and leading to oxygen lack, buildup of carbon dioxide, acidosis, and, if untreated, to kidney, lung, and brain damage and death. Treatment is by immediate cardiopulmonary resuscitation (CPR). Also called cardiopulmonary arrest. *Compare* RESPIRATORY ARREST.

cardiac arrhythmia N. abnormal rate of muscle contraction in the heart, caused by malfunction of impulse-conducting fibers in the heart or inability of the heart to respond to stress (e.g., fever, excessive exercise, altered metabolic balance). Types of arrhythmia include bradycardia, heart block, and tachycardia.

cardiac cycle N. cycle of events during which an electrical impulse is conducted through special fibers in the heart muscle, causing contraction of the atria followed by contraction of ventricles, which action pumps blood through the body. The cycle can be shown on an electrocardiogram as a series of waves, termed P, Q, R, S, and T waves; changes in wave patterns indicate abnormalities in the cardiac cycle.

cardiac conduction system N. specialized tissue that carries the nerve impulse for contraction from its origin, in the sinoatrial node, through the atria, to the atrioventricular node. From here it passes through the bundle of His into the ventricles via Purkinje fibers of the left and right bundle branches. Small, terminal Purkinje fibers deliver the stimulus at a cellular level. *See also* ELECTROCARDIOGRAM.

THE CONDUCTION SYSTEM OF THE HEART

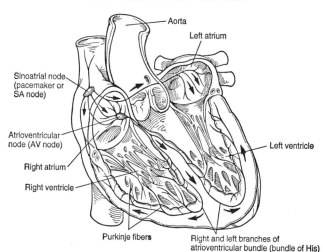

Aorta

Left atrium

Sinoatrial node (pacemaker or SA node)

Atrioventricular node (AV node)

Right atrium

Right ventricle

Left ventricle

Purkinje fibers

Right and left branches of atrioventricular bundle (bundle of His)

cardiac massage N. repeated, rhythmic compression of the heart through the chest wall or, during surgery, directly to the heart in an effort to maintain circulation during cardiac arrest as part of cardiopulmonary resuscitation.

cardiac monitor N. device for continual observation of the function of the heart. It may include electrocardiograph, oscilloscope, and other recordings of heart function; there may be an alarm to alert medical personnel to abnormal changes.

cardiac murmur *See* HEART MURMUR.

cardiac muscle N. special striated muscle of the heart, involuntary in function; one of three major types of muscle (the other two are smooth muscle and striated muscle). The heart's striated muscle is unusual because involuntary muscle is usually smooth.

cardiac output N. amount of blood expelled by the ventricles of the heart in a given period of time. A normal resting adult has a cardiac output of 2.5 to 4.2 liters per minute per square meter (L/min/m^2).

cardiac resuscitation *See* CARDIOPULMONARY RESUSCITATION.

cardiac tamponade N. condition in which accumulated pericardial effusion compresses the heart, leading to an inability to properly fill with blood; the heart is then unable to pump out sufficient volumes of blood for the body's normal functions and shock develops.

cardiectasis N. dilatation of the heart.

cardiogram (kär′dē-ə-grăm′) N. electronic recording of the rhythm and changes in the heart. *See also* ELECTROCARDIOGRAPHY.

cardiography (kär′dē-ə-ŏg′rə-fē) N. technique of electronically recording the activity of the heart to produce a cardiogram; also called electrocardiography.

cardiohepatomegaly N. enlargement of both the heart and the liver.

cardiologist N. physician who specializes in cardiology.

cardiology (kär′dē-ŏl′ə-jē) N. medical specialty that involves the study of the heart and the diagnosis and treatment of its diseases.

cardiomegaly (kär′dē-ō-měg′ə-lē) N. enlargement of the heart, usually due to some form of cardiac disease (e.g., hypertension, coronary artery disease, cardiomyopathy). Mild cardiomegaly may be normal in some very athletic individuals.

cardiomyopathy (kär′dē-ō-mī-ŏp′ə-thē) N. general term referring to primary disease of the muscle of the heart (myocardium). Causes range from congenital factors to viral infection to coronary artery disease.

cardiopulmonary arrest (kär′dē-ō-pŏŏl′mə-něr′ē) *See* CARDIAC ARREST.

cardiopulmonary resuscitation (CPR) N. emergency procedure, consisting of external cardiac massage and artificial respiration, used as the first treatment for a person who has collapsed, is unresponsive, has no pulse, and has stopped breathing. The purpose is to restore blood circulation and prevent death or brain damage due to lack of oxygen. CPR may be performed as a one- or two-person technique. Currently, the American Heart Association recommends that lay people be taught only the one-person method, which involves cardiac compressions at a rate of 80–100 per minute with two artificial breaths interspersed every 15 compressions. As a rule, CPR should not be performed by untrained individuals, though emergency dispatchers have successfully given instructions over the phone to people at the bedside of cardiac arrest victims. A portion of every CPR class is also dedicated to teaching the treatment of airway obstruction. *See also* HEIMLICH MANEUVER.

CARDIOPULMONARY
RESUSCITATION

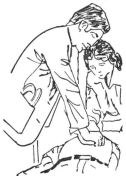

Note: This diagram is not intended for instructional purposes.

cardiospasm N. spasm of the cardiac sphincter (the valve between the distal end of the esophagus and the stomach), which prevents the normal passage of food into the stomach.

cardiovascular system N. body parts, including the heart and blood vessels, involved in the pumping of blood and transport of nutrients, oxygen, and waste products throughout the body. *Compare* CIRCULATORY SYSTEM.

cardioversion (kär′dē-ō-vûr′zhən) N. reestablishment of heart rhythm by means of electric shock. Typically used in abnormal but not acutely life-threatening rhythm disorders, such as rapid atrial fibrillation. In more acute situations, defibrillation is used.

carditis (kär-dī′tĭs) N. inflammation of the heart, usually resulting from infection (e.g., rheumatic fever, streptococcal sore throat), which causes pain, impaired circulation, and possibly damage to the heart muscle. *See also* ENDOCARDITIS; MYOCARDITIS; PERICARDITIS.

Cardizem N. trade name for the calcium blocker, diltiazem. *See* TABLE OF COMMONLY PRESCRIBED DRUGS—TRADE NAMES.

Cardura N. trade name for the oral antihypertensive, doxazosin. *See* TABLE OF COMMONLY PRESCRIBED DRUGS—TRADE NAMES.

caries (kâr′ēz) N. breakdown and death of tooth tissue, resulting in soft, discolored areas. Studies suggest that eating sugary foods tends to produce tooth decay, as does failure to brush the teeth and remove food particles whereas fluoridation (e.g., in water, toothpaste) tends to prevent it. Also called dental caries.

carina N. branch point of the windpipe (trachea) into the right and left mainstem bronchi.

carisoprodol N. *See* TABLE OF COMMONLY PRESCRIBED DRUGS—GENERIC NAMES.

carminative (kär-mĭn′ə-tĭv) N. chemical (e.g., simethicone) that prevents the formation of stomach gas (flatus) or eases its passing.

carotene (kăr'ə-tēn') N. red or orange pigment (a hydrocarbon), common to such foods as carrots, yams, and egg yolks, which is converted to vitamin A in the body; also used as a food coloring. An excess of carotene in the blood (carotinemia; also called xanthemia) may cause the skin to turn yellow.

carotid artery (kə-rŏt'ĭd) N. either of two main arteries of the neck, supplying the head and neck. ADJ. carotid. *See* MAJOR ARTERIES AND VEINS OF THE BODY, in Appendix.

carpal tunnel syndrome N. common disorder of the wrist and hand, caused by compression of the median nerve in the wrist area and manifested by pain, tingling, burning, and muscular weakness, sometimes spreading to the arm and shoulder. It is more common in women, esp. during pregnancy and menopause, but may also occur in both sexes as a result of trauma, rheumatoid arthritis, diabetes mellitus, or other disorder. Treatment involves pain relief (sometimes by the use of corticosteroids), the splinting and support of the wrist (esp. at night), and surgery if the condition persists.

carpus (kär'pəs) N. *See* WRIST. ADJ. carpal

carrier (kăr'ē-ər) N. person, generally in apparent good health, who harbors organisms that can infect and cause disease in others (*compare* VECTOR). Probably the most notorious carrier was Typhoid Mary.

cartilage (kär'tl-ĭj) N. tough supporting connective tissue serving to protect and connect body parts; and found chiefly in body tubes (e.g., trachea) and joints; in the embryo, the parts of the skeleton that develop into bone. Cartilage has no nerves or blood supply of its own. ADJ. cartilaginous

cartilaginification N. abnormal formation of cartilage from other tissues.

cascade (kă-skād') N. progression of a process through a series of steps; each step initiates the next one, until the final step is reached.

case history N. complete patient history up to the time of admission or treatment. Includes the medical, family, and social history, as well as information regarding the present complaint.

casein (kā'sēn') N. chief protein of milk, the basis of curds and cheese.

cast (kăst) N.
1. firm covering or bandage, often made with plaster of paris or similar substance, used to stabilize an injured body part during healing (e.g., a fractured leg).
2. mold used to copy a body part (e.g., a mold of teeth and jaws for fitting dentures).

castration (kă-strā'shən) N. surgical removal of the testes or ovaries, usually done to inhibit hormone secretion in cases of breast cancer in women, prostate cancer in men. Bilateral castration produces sterility.

castration anxiety N. unrealistic fear of injury to or loss of the sexual organs, sometimes the result of guilt over forbidden sexual desire or some threatening experience; in children the fear often involves being hurt by a parent (for boys, the father; for girls, the mother) because of one's sexual feelings toward the parent of the opposite sex. *See also* OEDIPUS COMPLEX.

CAT, CAT scan *See* COMPUTED TOMOGRAPHY.

cata- comb. form meaning downward, under, against (e.g., catabasis, decline of a disease).

catabiosis N. normal aging of cells.

catabolism (kə-tăb′ə-lĭz′əm) N. phase of metabolism in which complex chemicals are reduced to simpler forms (*compare* ANABOLISM). ADJ. catabolic

catalepsy (kăt′l-ĕp′sē) N. trance-like state in which the voluntary muscles become rigid and the body does not react to stimuli or change in position; occurs in psychotic patients and occasionally in persons under hypnosis. ADJ. cataleptic. *Compare* CATAPLEXY.

catalyst (kăt′l-ĭst) N. chemical (e.g., an enzyme) that speeds up the rate of a chemical reaction but is itself not permanently changed in the process. ADJ. catalytic

catamenia *See* MENSTRUATION.

cataphasia (kăt′ə-fā′zē-ə) N. speech disorder characterized by repetition of the same word several times in succession.

cataplexy (kăt′ə-plĕk′sē) N. sudden brief loss of muscle control brought on by strong emotion; may result in collapse, though the victim remains fully conscious. Spells last from a few seconds to several minutes. Seventy percent of patients with narcolepsy also have cataplexy. The drug imipramine may reduce the frequency of cataplexic attacks.

Catapres N. trade name for the antihypertensive clonidine. *See* TABLE OF COMMONLY PRESCRIBED DRUGS—TRADE NAMES.

cataract (kăt′ə-răkt′) N. eye disorder in which the lens becomes less transparent (more opaque) so that light rays cannot reach the retina and there is progressive painless loss of vision. Most cataracts are caused by degenerative changes after age 50, but some may be caused by trauma to the eye or exposure to certain chemicals; some are hereditary and some congenital (due perhaps to viral infection during pregnancy). Treatment is removal of the lens and use of special contact lenses or eyeglasses or the implantation of an intraocular lens (IOL); in children soft cataracts may be removed by fragmentation (via ultrasound) and drainage. *See also* EPIKERATOPHAKIA.

catarrh (kə-tär′) N. mucous membrane infection, esp. of the nose. ADJ. catarrhal

catastrophic illness (kăt′ə-strŏf′ ĭk) N. severe illness resulting in the need for prolonged hospitalization, extended recuperation, or both. After recovery, there may be persistent residual disability.

catatonia (kăt′ə-tō′nē-ə) N. syndrome in which motor behavior is disturbed, usually characterized by body rigidity and stupor but sometimes by impulsive and purposeless activity. It is usually associated with mental illness, esp. schizophrenia, but occasionally occurs in other disorders (e.g., encephalitis). ADJ. catatonic

catecholamine (kăt′ĭ-kō′lə-mēn′) N. any of a group of chemicals, including epinephrine, dopamine, and norepinephrine, produced in the medulla of the adrenal gland and also manufactured synthetically for use as drugs. They function in the body's response to stress and affect many physiological and metabolic activities (e.g., heartbeat, nerve responses, muscle activity). Both norepinephrine and dopamine act as neurotransmitters.

catgut (kăt′gŭt′) N. chemically treated suture (sewing) material made from the tissues of mammals and used in surgery; also shortened to gut.

catharsis (kə-thär′sĭs) N.
1. purging the body of chemical or other material (e.g., by the use of a cathartic [laxative] to stimulate bowel evacuation).
2. in psychology, method of relieving anxiety by recalling and communicating a buried memory. *See also* ABREACTION.

cathartic (kə-thär′tĭk) *See* LAXATIVE.

catheter (kăth′ĭ-tər) N. flexible, usually rubber or soft plastic, tube inserted into the body for removing or instilling fluids for diagnosis or treatment purposes. In its most common use a catheter is inserted through the urethra into the bladder to withdraw urine and empty (e.g., before surgery) or irrigate the bladder. v. catheterize

cathexis (kə-thĕk′sĭs) N. emotional attachment to an idea, object, or person. ADJ. cathectic

cation (kăt′ī′ən) N. positively charged atom.

cat-scratch disease N. disease from the scratch or bite of a cat, characterized by inflammation and pustule formation of the affected skin; lymph node swelling and sometimes fever and malaise can occur.

The etiologic agent is thought to be a virus. Usually no treatment is necessary; the symptoms spontaneously abate. Also called cat scratch fever.

cauda (kô′də) N., *pl*. caudae, taillike structure (e.g., cauda equina, bundle of nerves in the lower part of the spinal cord)

caudal (kôd′l) ADJ. pert. to the lower part; inferior in position.

caudal anesthesia N. type of regional anesthesia involving the injection of an anesthetic into the tail end (the small-of-the-back part) of the spinal canal to prevent pain in that region, as during the delivery of a baby or during anal or genitourinary surgery; now largely replaced by other forms of regional anesthesia, esp. epidural anesthesia; also called caudal block.

caul (kôl) N. intact amniotic sac surrounding the fetus at birth that must be broken to allow the baby to breathe.

causal ADJ. Responsible for bringing about a particular effect, condition, or result. For example, there is a documented causal link between cigarette smoking and an increased risk of coronary artery disease.

causalgia (kô-săl′jē-ə) N. burning feeling in a limb, usually associated with skin changes and resulting from nerve injury.

caustic N. agent that produces a burn or destroys tissue by chemical action (e.g., silver nitrate).

cauterize (kô′tə-rīz′) v. to destroy tissue for medical reasons (e.g., the removal of a wart) by burning with a hot iron, electron current, or chemical. N. cauterize.

caverna N. cavity or cavernlike structure.

THE TWO MAJOR BODY CAVITIES AND
THEIR SUBDIVISIONS AND COMPONENTS

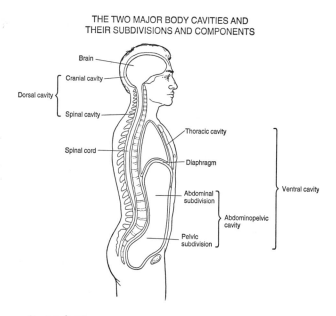

cavity (kăv′ĭ-tē) N.
1. hollow, cavelike structure (e.g., cranial cavity, the inside of the skull).
2. general term for dental caries.

CDC *See* CENTERS FOR DISEASE CONTROL.

CEA N. abbrev. for carcinoembryonic antigen.

cecum (sē′kəm) N. any part ending in a cul-de-sac; specifically, the closed, pocketlike beginning of the large intestine in the lower right part of the abdomen; the appendix is an offshoot of the cecum. ADJ. cecal

Cefizox N. trade name for the parenteral cephalosporin antibiotic ceftizoxime, which is used in moderate to severe intraabdominal infections. Adverse effects include minor liver abnormalities.

Cefobid N. trade name for the cephalosporin antibiotic cefoperazone.

cefoperazone (sĕf′ō-pĕr′ə-zōn′) N. parenteral cephalosporin antibiotic (trade name Cefobid) used for severe infections. Adverse effects include bleeding (due to vitamin K deficiency), diarrhea, and disulfiram-like reactions in patients ingesting alcohol concomitantly.

cefotaxime (sĕf′ō-tăk′sēm′) N. parenteral cephalosporin antibiotic (trade name Claforan) used for severe infections of the lungs, ears, skin, urinary tract, and throat. It is generally well tolerated.

cefoxitin (sə-fŏk′sĭ-tĭn) N. broad-spectrum cephalosporin antibiotic agent (trade name Mefoxin) used in the parenteral treatment of moderate to severe infections.

cefpodoxime N. cephalosporin antibiotic for oral use in mild to moderate respiratory infections (e.g., community-acquired pneumonia, otitis media, and pharyngitis); side effects are unusual and mostly consist of mild diarrhea.

cefprozil N. *See* TABLE OF COMMONLY PRESCRIBED DRUGS— GENERIC NAMES.

ceftazidime (sĕf-tăz′ĭ-dēm′) N. parenteral cephalosporin antibiotic (trade names Fortaz and Tazicef) used in the treatment of moderate to severe infections. The incidence of adverse effects is low.

Ceftin N. *See* TABLE OF COMMONLY PRESCRIBED DRUGS— TRADE NAMES.

ceftriaxone N. parenteral cephalosporin antibiotic (trade name Rocephin) indicated for severe infections of the lungs, ears, skin, urinary tract, and throat. Also used in the treatment of sexually transmitted diseases. Potential adverse effects include rash, eosinophilia, diarrhea, and liver abnormalities.

cefuroxime N. oral/parenteral cephalosporin antibiotic (trade name Zinacef; oral tablets sold under the name Ceftin) indicated for moderately severe infections of the lungs, urinary tract (including gonorrhea), ears, throat, and, in some cases, the meninges. *See* TABLE OF COMMONLY PRESCRIBED DRUGS —GENERIC NAMES.

Cefzil N. *See* TABLE OF COMMONLY PRESCRIBED DRUGS—TRADE NAMES.

-cele suffix indicating a swelling or tumor (e.g., cystocele, a protrusion of the bladder through the wall of the vagina).

Celebrex N. *See* TABLE OF COMMONLY PRESCRIBED DRUGS— TRADE NAMES.

celecoxib N. *See* TABLE OF COMMONLY PRESCRIBED DRUGS— GENERIC NAMES.

celiac disease N. disorder of children and adults caused by inability to tolerate gluten (wheat protein) and characterized by diarrhea (stools are pale, frothy, and foul-smelling),

DIAGRAM OF A CELL

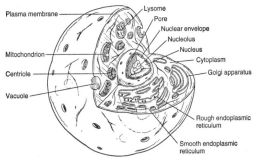

Plasma membrane
Lysome
Pore
Nuclear envelope
Nucleolus
Nucleus
Mitochondrion
Cytoplasm
Centriole
Golgi apparatus
Vacuole
Rough endoplasmic reticulum
Smooth endoplasmic reticulum

loss of weight, abdominal distension, and lethargy. It is often accompanied by lactose (milk sugar) intolerance. Treatment is a high-protein, gluten-free and, if necessary, milk-free diet. *See also* SPRUE.

celio- comb. form indicating an association with the abdomen (e.g., celioma, abdominal tumor).

celiocentesis N. hollow-needle puncture into the abdomen to remove materials for diagnostic examination.

celioscopy (sē'lē-ŏs'kə-pē) N. examination of the abdomen by means of an instrument (endoscope) inserted through an incision in the abdomen wall.

cell (sĕl) N. individual living unit, the basic structure for tissues and organs, made up of an outer membrane, the main mass (cytoplasm), and the nucleus, which controls the cell's metabolism and reproduction; a single living part (e.g., a red blood cell) or organism (e.g., a protozoan). ADJ. cellular

TYPES OF CELLS

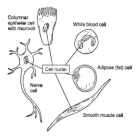

Columnar epithelial cell with microvilli

White blood cell

Cell nuclei

Adipose (fat) cell

Nerve cell

Smooth muscle cell

cell division *See* MEIOSIS; MITOSIS.

cellulitis (sĕl'yə-lī'tĭs) N. inflammation of tissue, esp. that below the skin, characterized by redness, pain, and swelling. Treatment is by antibiotics.

cellulose (sĕl'yə-lōs', -lōz') N. basic constituent (a polysaccharide) of plant fiber, providing bulk necessary for proper intestinal function. Fruit, bran, and green vegetables provide cellulose.

Celsius (sĕl'sē-əs) ADJ. pert. to a temperature scale in which the freezing point of water is 0° and the boiling point is 100°, as compared with 32° and 212°, respectively on the Fahrenheit scale. The name, commonly abbreviated as C, honors Anders Celsius, who devised it. Also called centigrade.

cementum (sĭ-mĕn'təm) N. layer of specialized tissue (modified bone) in a tooth, covering the root and neck.

center (sĕn'tər) N.
1. midpoint.
2. group of cells that have a special function (e.g., the speech center in the left brain hemisphere); also called centrum.

Centers for Disease Control (CDC) N. U.S. government agency, centered in Atlanta, Georgia, concerned with the investigation, diagnosis, and control of disease. New and unusual diseases (e.g., toxic shock syndrome, acquired immune deficiency syndrome — AIDS) are often intensively investigated by the CDC in cooperation with state and local health departments and private researchers and clinicians.

centesis (sĕn-tē'sĭs) N. puncture (by hollow needle) of a cavity or organ to draw out fluid (e.g., amniocentesis).

centigrade (sĕn'tĭ-grād') *See* CELSIUS.

central nervous system N. one of the two main divisions of the human nervous system (the

THE CENTRAL NERVOUS SYSTEM

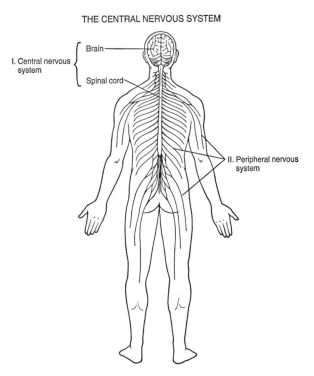

I. Central nervous system
Brain
Spinal cord
II. Peripheral nervous system

other being the peripheral nervous system), consisting of the brain and the spinal cord. The main coordinating and controlling center of the body, the central nervous system processes information to and from the peripheral nervous system. The system is made up of gray matter (mostly nerve cells and associated parts) and white matter (mostly nerve fibers and contains protective cerebrospinal fluid).

centralis ADJ. toward or at the center.

centrifugation N. separation of media or particles by spinning

them in suspension, the heavier materials being whirled to the outer part of the container; used, e.g., to separate blood cells from plasma in unclotted blood. ADJ. centrifugal

cephal-, cephalo- comb. forms indicating an association with the head (e.g., cephalocaudal, pert. to head and tail, or along that axis).

cephalalgia (sĕf′ə-lăl′jə) N. *See* HEADACHE.

cephalexin (sĕf′ə-lĕk′sĭn) N. oral cephalosporin antibiotic (trade names include Keflex and Keftab), commonly prescribed for mild to moderately severe in-

CEREBRAL HEMISPHERES

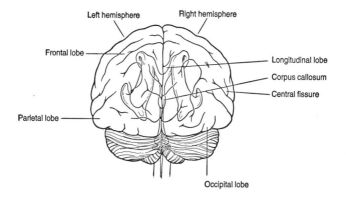

Left hemisphere

Right hemisphere

Frontal lobe

Longitudinal lobe

Corpus callosum

Central fissure

Parietal lobe

Occipital lobe

fections of the lungs, ears, skin, urinary tract, and throat. Adverse effects include diarrhea, nausea, and vomiting. *See* TABLE OF COMMONLY PRESCRIBED DRUGS—GENERIC NAMES.

cephalhematoma (sĕf′əl-hē′mə-tō′mə) N. collection of blood beneath the scalp of a newborn caused by pressure during birth.

cephalic index (sə-făl′ĭk) N. measurement used to determine whether the head is of normal shape. The index is a ratio of the width of the head (measured where the width is greatest) multiplied by 100 and divided by the length of the head (measured where it is greatest). A number of 74.9 or less indicates a head much longer than it is wide; 75–80, one that has a medium length; and more than 80, one that is disproportionately short.

cephalosporin (sĕf-ə-lə-spôr′ĭn) N. any of a group of broad-spectrum antibiotics obtained

from microorganisms (including fungi of the genus *Cephalosporium*) and used for treating infections caused by a wide variety of bacterial agents.

cerebellum (sĕr′ə-bĕl′əm) N. that part of the brain located behind the cerebrum and above the pons and concerned with the coordination and control of voluntary muscular activity. ADJ. cerebellar

cerebral (sĕr′ə-brəl) ADJ. pert. to the cerebrum of the brain (e.g., cerebral hemisphere, one of the halves of the cerebrum).

cerebral cortex N. thin layer of gray matter, with many folds on the surface of the cerebrum, that is the center for higher mental functions, perception, behavioral responses, and other functions. It is classified into many areas, each with specific functions (e.g., speech center).

cerebral dominance N. intrinsic property of one of the two hemispheres of the human brain such that it often exerts greater control over various bodily functions. Handedness, for example, may be determined by whether the left or the right hemisphere is dominant. In teaching and psychology, the left hemisphere ("left brain") is felt to be responsible for more detail-oriented tasks (e.g., mathematics, science) while the right hemisphere ("right brain") provides imagination and abstract thinking ability. There is much overlap, however, and the terms "left brained" and "right brained" are often used somewhat metaphorically.

cerebral hemorrhage N. flow of blood from a ruptured blood vessel in the brain; causes include high blood pressure, head injuries, and aneurysm. Symptoms, which depend on the site of the bleeding and the type of blood vessels involved, may include numbness and diminished mental function or, if severe, coma and death. *See also* CEREBROVASCULAR ACCIDENT.

cerebral palsy N. loss or deficiency of muscle control due to permanent, nonprogressive brain damage occurring before or at the time of birth. Symptoms include difficulty in walking, poor coordination of the limbs, lack of balance, speech or other sense organ difficulties, and sometimes mental retardation. Treatment depends on the difficulties present and may include leg braces, speech therapy, and antispasmodic or muscle-relaxing drugs.

cerebral thrombosis N. blood clot in a cerebral vessel.

cerebration (sĕr′ə-brā′shən) N. mental activity, thinking.

cerebri-, cerebro- comb. forms indicating an association with the cerebrum, specifically the cerebral hemispheres (e.g., cerebrovascular).

cerebrospinal (sĕr′ə-brō-spī′nəl) ADJ. pert. to the brain and spinal cord.

cerebrospinal fluid (CSF) N. normally clear liquid, produced in the ventricles of the brain, that fills and protects the cavities in the brain and spinal cord. In the adult there is normally about 140 milliliters of cerebrospinal fluid. Samples of the fluid, obtained by lumbar puncture, may be used to diagnose certain diseases. Also called spinal fluid.

cerebrovascular (sĕr′ə-brō-văs′kyə-lər) ADJ. pert. to the blood vessels of the brain.

cerebrovascular accident (CVA) N. abnormal condition in which hemorrhage or blockage of the blood vessels of the brain leads to oxygen lack and resulting symptom—sudden loss of ability to move a body part (as an arm or parts of the face) or to speak, paralysis, weakness, or, if severe, death. Usually only one side of the body is affected. Physical therapy and speech therapy can result in some degree of recovery. Also called stroke.

cerebrum (sĕrē′-brəm) N. main mass of the human brain; the two cerebral hemispheres that control conscious activity. ADJ. cerebral

cerumen (sə-roō′mən) N. earwax: soft, waxy, yellow-brown material secreted by the sebaceous glands of the external ear.

cervic-, cervico- comb. forms indicating an association with the neck (e.g., cervicofacial, pert. to the neck and face) or with the cervix of the uterus (e.g., cervicovesical, pert. to the uterine cervix and the bladder).

cervical (sûr′vĭ-kəl) ADJ.
1. pert. to the neck area (e.g., one of the cervical vertebrae).
2. pert. to the cervix of the uterus (e.g., cervical cancer usually means cancer of the cervix of the uterus) or to a constricted necklike part of another organ.

cervical cap N. contraceptive device consisting of a small rubber cap fitted over the cervix to block the entrance of sperm into the uterus. It may be left in place days or weeks at a time and is reported to be similar to the diaphragm in contraceptive efficacy.

cervical disc syndrome N. abnormal condition caused by compression of cervical (neck region) nerve roots, resulting from trauma or degenerative disease or other factors, that produces pain in the neck region, often radiating to the shoulder, arm, and hand, paresthesia, and some muscular weakness. Treatment may involve analgesics, immobilization of the area to allow rest, traction, and, if severe, surgery. Also called cervical root syndrome.

cervical smear N. small amount of the secretions and superficial cells of the cervix of the uterus, which are examined microscopically to detect the presence of any abnormal cells; the smear is taken with a special instrument inserted through the vagina. *See also* PAPANICOLAOU TEST.

cervical vertebrae N. any of the first seven segments of the ver-

tebral column, located in the neck region. *See also* ATLAS: AXIS.

cervicitis (sûr′vĭ-sī′tĭs) N. inflammation of the cervix of the uterus, often caused by fungal or bacterial infection, characterized by redness, vaginal discharge, pelvic pain, slight bleeding on intercourse, itching, and burning. Treatment is by antibiotics, topical ointments, or cautery.

cervix (sûr′vĭks) N. neck or necklike part of the organ, esp. the neck of the uterus, that part of the uterus that extends into the vagina; dilation of the cervix permits the passage of the fetus in childbirth. ADJ. cervical

Cesarean section (sĭ-zâr′ē-ən) N. surgical incision through the abdomen and uterus for removal of a fetus, commonly performed when conditions (e.g., maternal hemorrhage, premature separation of the placenta, fetal distress, fetus too large for passage through the mother's pelvis) for normal vaginal delivery are deemed hazardous for mother or baby. However, it is not uncommon for a Cesarean section to take place because it is easier for the mother, who for economic or employment reasons can choose the exact date that she will have her baby. The rate of Cesarean deliveries in the United States has increased to 24.1% of all births and is the highest in the world. Economics and the current medical-legal environment are largely responsible for this high rate. Hazards include those of major surgery for the mother and the possibility of too-early birth of the baby. Though vaginal birth after Cesarean (VBAC) is possible, this once popular procedure is losing favor due to recent reports of uterine rupture following delivery. Also called Caesarean, C-section. *See also* VAGINAL BIRTH AFTER CESAREAN.

cestode (sĕs'tōd') *See* TAPEWORM.

chafing N. irritation of the skin by friction, from clothing or from one sweaty body part (e.g., an inner thigh) rubbing against another.

Chagas disease (shä'-gəs) N. disease, caused by a parasite (usually *Trypanosoma cruzi*) transmitted by the bite of an insect and characterized by a lesion at the site of the bite, fever, enlarged lymph glands, rapid heartbeat, and, in chronic form, abnormalities of the heart muscle, esophagus, or colon. The acute form usually resolves itself without treatment.

chalasia (kə-lā'zē-ə) N. abnormal relaxation of a muscle or opening esp. of the sphincter muscle between the esophagus and stomach, resulting in reflux of stomach contents into the esophagus and regurgitation. Treatment involves a diet of frequent small meals and, in infants, feeding in the upright position.

chalazion (ka-lā'zē-on) N. nonmalignant small swelling on the eyelid that often requires surgical removal; also called meibomian cyst.

challenge (chăl'ənj) V. to inject an antigen into the body to determine the immunological result. N. immunological test of antigen reactivity.

chamber (chām'bər) N. enclosed area (e.g., aqueous chamber, humor-filled part of the eyeball); the heart chambers (auricles and ventricles).

chancre (shăng'kər) N. painless sore, esp. that associated with syphilis, which has the appearance of a hard ulceration (*compare* CANKER).

chancroid (shăng'kroid') N. contagious venereal ulcer; it usually appears as a papule on the skin of the genitalia that then ulcerates and, if untreated, produces buboes in the groin. Caused by the bacterium *Haemophilus ducreyi*, it is usually treated with sulfa drugs.

change of life *See* MENOPAUSE.

characteristic (kăr'ək-tə-rĭs'tĭk) N. distinguishing feature of an organism (e.g., a Mendelian, or inherited, characteristic).

charleyhorse (chär'lēhôrs') N. colloquial term for muscle cramp or soreness, esp. in the thigh or calf, usually after strenuous activity. Treatment is by heat application and a gradual stretching of the affected muscle.

checkup (chĕk'ŭp') N. colloquial term for a thorough physical examination, which may include an electrocardiogram, blood and urine tests, and other special procedures and laboratory tests, depending on the age, sex, and general health of the person.

cheek (chēk) N. side of the face below the eye including the lateral wall of the mouth.

cheil-, cheilo- comb. forms indicating an association with the lip (e.g., cheiloplasty, surgical correction of a lip defect).

cheilitis (kē-lī'tĭs) N. inflammation and cracking of the skin of the lips due to overexposure to the sun, vitamin deficiency, or allergic reaction to cosmetics. *See also* CHEILOSIS.

cheiloschisis (kī-lŏs′kĭ-sĭs) *See* HARELIP.

cheilosis (kī-lō′sĭs) N. disorder of the lips and mouth marked by fissures and scales and caused by a deficiency of riboflavin; also called perliche. *See also* CHEILITIS.

cheir-, cheiro- comb. forms indicating an association with the hand (e.g., cheiroplasty, surgical correction of a hand defect).

cheiromegaly N. condition in which the hands are abnormally large.

chelation N. chemical bonding used to remove some substances (e.g., metals) from tissues. Legitimately used against some types of toxicity (e.g., lead, iron), chelation has also been falsely promoted as an effective treatment for atherosclerosis.

chem-, chemo- comb. forms indicating an association with chemicals or chemistry (e.g., chemocautery, tissue destruction by chemicals).

chemiosmosis N. major form of energy production during cellular respiration where protons are pumped across mitochondral membranes. Once a gradient is established, enzymes use the energy of the protons to generate adenosine triphosphate (ATP).

chemoreceptor (kē′mō-rĭ-sĕp′tər) N. nerve ending outside of the central nervous system that reacts to certain chemical stimuli; may be part of a sensory organ (e.g., taste bud) or function independently (e.g., chemoreceptors in the aorta and other large blood vessels detect changes in flow and blood pressure).

chemosis (kē-mō′sĭs) N. edema of the mucous membrane of the eyeball and eyelid lining, resulting from injury, infection, or certain systemic diseases (e.g, anemia, kidney disease).

chemosurgery (kē′mō-sûr′jə-rē) N. destruction of malignant or otherwise diseased tissue by use of chemicals (e.g., in the treatment of skin cancer).

chemotaxis (kē′mō-tăk′sĭs) N. movement by a cell or organism toward (positive) or away from (negative) a chemical stimulus.

chemotherapy (kē′mō-thĕr′ə-pē) N. treatment of disease by chemical agents. The term includes the use of drugs (e.g., antibacterials, antifungals) to harm or kill disease-causing microorganisms but is most commonly used to refer to the use of drugs to treat cancer. Anticancer (antineoplastic) drugs generally inhibit the proliferation of cells and include alkylating agents (e.g., chlorambucil), antimetabolites (e.g., fluorouracil), periwinkle plant derivatives (e.g., vincristine), antineoplastic antibiotics (e.g., adramycin, mithramycin), and radioactive isotopes (e.g., iodine-131, phosphorus-32, gold-198). All these agents are associated with side effects, the most common of which are nausea and vomiting, suppression of bone marrow function, and loss of hair. ADJ. chemotherapeutic.

chest (chĕst) N. upper part of the torso, the thorax; also called pectus.

Cheyne-Stokes respiration (chān′) N. abnormal pattern of respiration with slow, shallow breathing alternating with periods of deep, rapid breathing; most often seen in central nervous system disorders; also called periodic breathing.

chiasm (kī′ăz′əm) N. X-shaped structure; the crossing of two lines or tracts, esp. chiasma opticum, crossed fibers of the optic nerve.

chicken pox N. acute contagious disease, caused by herpes varicella zoster virus, characterized by a rash of vesicles on the face and body. Chicken pox is a common childhood disease; it is usually mild in otherwise healthy children but may be serious in babies, children weakened by other diseases, and in adults. After an incubation period of two to three weeks, the disease usually begins with slight fever and malaise, after which itchy macules develop, often first on the back and chest; followed by fluid-containing vesicles that break easily and become encrusted. Treatment consists of fever-reducing drugs, lotions to relieve itching, and rest. One attack usually confers life-long immunity, but the virus lies dormant in nerve cells, sometimes to be reactivated, causing shingles. Also called varicella. *See also* HERPES ZOSTER.

chigger (chĭg′ər) N. parasitic mites that attack animals and humans by attaching to the skin surface. They inject a substance that breaks down the skin, resulting in itching and swelling. Chiggers do not feed on blood; the symptoms are due to the injected saliva; rather, they eat the broken-down skin.

chilblain (chĭl′blān′) N. redness and swelling, sometimes accompanied by burning and itching, of the skin due to exposure to cold; also called pernio (*compare* FROSTBITE).

child abuse N. physical, emotional, or sexual maltreatment of a child, often resulting in serious and often permanent injury or impairment and sometimes in death. It may be overt, as in severely beating a child, or covert, as in depriving the child of needed affection and emotional support. Child abuse occurs in all socio-economic levels (though it is probably reported more among the poor who visit hospital clinics or social agencies) and among children and parents of all ages, but certain factors are thought to increase the risk of child abuse; among these are parents who were themselves abused as children; parents involved in marital strife; emotionally unstable parents or those undergoing extreme stress (e.g., unemployment); and children who are very young (particularly in cases of beatings and physical abuse), are difficult by temperament, or have emotional or physical handicaps. *See also* CHILD NEGLECT.

child neglect N. failure of parents or others entrusted with the care of the child to provide adequate physical and emotional care, so that the child's health and development are endangered. *See also* CHILD ABUSE.

childbed fever *See* PUERPERAL FEVER.

childbirth N. act or process of giving birth to an offspring; labor (*See also* BRADLEY METHOD OF CHILDBIRTH, LAMAZE METHOD OF CHILDBIRTH, LEBOYER METHOD OF CHILDBIRTH, NATURAL CHILDBIRTH; READ METHOD OF CHILDBIRTH).

chill (chĭl) N. 1. feeling of cold due to cold environment. 2.

shivering and sensation of cold, often marking the start of an infection and development of a fever.

chimera (kī-mēr′ə) N. double-egg twin whose blood cells have mixed during development with those of the other twin; prior to the mix, each twin had a different blood type. Following the mix, each now has a combination type (mixed type). ADJ. chimerism. Recently, one hospital performed the first combined kidney and bone marrow transplantation to treat multiple myeloma. Chimerism of the bone marrow was deliberately induced, meaning that the patient's new blood cells were a mix of her previous type and the donor type. Since she received the bone marrow transplant in the first place because her own bone marrow was devoid of any cells, her new blood and tissue type is now functionally the same as the donor. The result was complete remission of the multiple myeloma, as well as a markedly reduced need for immunosuppressive drugs.

Chinese restaurant syndrome N. headache, feeling of tingling and burning, and sometimes of facial pressure, caused by eating food containing mono-sodium glutamate (MSG), which is often used in Chinese cooking.

chiralgia N. pain in the hand, esp. of nontraumatic origin.

chiropody (kĭ-rŏp′ə-dē) *See* PODIATRY.

chiropractic N. system of diagnosis and treatment based on the belief that many diseases are caused by pressure on nerves due to misalignments (subluxations) of the spinal column and that such diseases can be treated by correction (e.g., by massage) of the misalignment (*compare* NAPRAPATHY; OSTEOPATHY).

Chlamydia (klə-mĭd′ē-ə) N. general term for a group (genus) of intracellular parasites that cause a wide variety of diseases. *C. pneumoniae* causes respiratory infections (e.g., pneumonia, bronchitis, sinusitis) and is transmitted by respiratory secretions. Most cases are relatively mild and respond to either tetracycline or erythromycin antibiotics. Serious infections may result, especially in the elderly. *C. psittaci* is common in birds and animals and may cause disease (psittacosis) in persons exposed to pets, poultry, and meat processing. Psittacosis is similar to a viral illness with fever and malaise, but may resemble mononucleosis. Untreated (with tetracycline-type drugs), the fatality rate may rise as high as 20%. *C. trachomatis* is the most common cause of sexually transmitted vaginal and urethral disease (vaginitis, urethritis) in both sexes in industrialized countries. A test for specific antibodies is available. The organism responds to several antibiotics; treatment is important as it may be transferred to the infant during birth, resulting in blindness.

chloasma (klō-ăz′mə) N. permanent or transient tan or brownish pigmentation, esp. of the face, associated with pregnancy or the use of oral contraceptives; also called mask of pregnancy; melasma.

chlor-, chloro- comb. forms indicating greenness (e.g., chlorophyll) or an association with chlorine (e.g., chloroform).

chloral hydrate N. sedative and sleep-inducing drug now seldom used in medicine because of its irritating (to skin and mucous membranes, esp. the stomach) and potentially addictive properties. (Combined with alcohol, it is known colloquially as knockout drops or a Mickey Finn.)

chlorambucil (klôr-ăm′byə-sĭl) N. drug (trade name Leukeran) used to treat some forms of cancer.

chloramphenicol (klôr′ăm-fĕn′ĭ-kôl′) N. antibacterial and antirickettsial agent (trade name Chloromycetin), effective in treating many serious infections (esp. typhoid fever) but associated with some serious reactions (e.g., bone marrow depression) and now used with caution.

chlordiazepoxide (klôr′dī-āz′ə-pŏk′sīd) N. minor tranquilizer (trade name Librium) used to treat anxiety.

chloride N. an ion form (negatively charged) of chlorine; one of the major blood electrolytes.

chlorination N. addition of small amounts of a compound of chlorine (e.g., chlorine dioxide) into a water supply to kill organisms that might otherwise cause disease. *See also* CHLORINE.

chlorine (klôr′ēn′) N. gaseous element important in certain body processes (e.g., in hydrochloric acid, a stomach secretion essential for digestion) and used as a disinfectant (e.g., in swimming pools). It has a strong odor and is irritating to the respiratory tract and poisonous if ingested. *See also* TABLE OF IMPORTANT ELEMENTS.

chloroform (klôr′ə-fôrm′) N. chloride-containing liquid used as a solvent, sedative, and anesthetic. Although widely used as a general anesthetic (the first inhalation anesthetic) in earlier times and still used in some Third World countries (largely because no sophisticated equipment is available), chloroform is now recognized as a dangerous drug (e.g., it can cause liver damage and low blood pressure) and has been largely replaced by safer anesthetics.

chlorophyll (klôr′ə-fĭl) N. pigment of green plants that absorbs light and converts it into energy for the synthesis of carbohydrates.

chloroquine (klôr′ə-kwīn′) N. antibiotic used in the treatment of malaria, amebic dysentery, and systemic lupus erythematosis (SLE).

chlorosis (klə-rō′sĭs) N. old term for iron-deficiency anemia, esp. in women.

chlorothiazide N. diuretic and antihypertensive (trade name Diuril) used in the treatment of high blood pressure (hypertension) and edema. Adverse effects include electrolyte imbalances.

chlorpromazine (klôr-prŏm′ə-zēn′) N. major tranquilizer and antiemetic (trade name Thorazine) used in the treatment of certain psychotic disorders and severe nausea and vomiting.

choking N. condition due to blocking of the airway to the lungs, as with food or other swallowed object or with swelling of the larynx. The victim is unable to speak, tries to cough, becomes red and then purplish in the face, and becomes increasingly desperate to breathe, usually pointing to the throat, and, if unrelieved, collapses. Emergency treatment involves removal of the obstruction if possible and resuscitation if necessary. *See also* HEIMLICH MANEUVER.

chol-, chole-, cholo- comb. forms indicating an association with bile or the bile ducts (e.g., cholangiolitis, inflammation of the smallest bile ducts).

cholangiography (kō-lăn′jē-ŏg′rə-fē) N. X-ray examination of the bile ducts, after a special contrast medium has been injected.

cholangitis (kō′lăn-jī′tĭs) N. inflammation of the bile ducts marked by pain in the upper right quadrant of the abdomen, intermittent fever, and sometimes jaundice. Caused by bacterial infection or an obstruction (e.g., calculi or tumor), it is treated by antibiotics or surgery.

cholecystectomy (kō′lĭ-sĭ-stĕk′tə-mē) N. surgical removal of the gallbladder to treat inflammation (cholecystitis) and/or presence of stones in the gallbladder (cholelithiasis).

cholecystitis (kō′lĭ-sĭ-stī′tĭs) N. inflammation of the gallbladder. In acute form, usually caused by a gallstone that cannot pass through the cystic duct, and characterized by upper right quadrant pain, vomiting, and flatulence. In the chronic form, pain is often felt after a fatty meal. Surgery is the usual treatment.

cholecystokinin-pancreozymin (CCK) N. hormone secreted into the blood by the small intestine; stimulates contraction of the gallbladder and secretion of pancreatic enzymes (pancreatic juices). It was formerly thought that a separate hormone, pancreozymin, stimulated the production of pancreatic enzymes, while cholecystokinin led to gallbladder contraction. Now, data show that a single hormone, cholecystokinin-pancreozymin (CCK), secreted by the upper small intestine, is responsible for both pancreatic and gallbladder stimulation. Receptors for CCK have also been found in the brain, though the exact function is unknown.

cholelithiasis (kō′lə-lĭ-thī′ə-sĭs) N. presence of gallstones in the gallbladder, which may cause no symptoms or cause vague abdominal discomfort, flatulence, and intolerance to certain foods. If severe pain or obstruction and inflammation occur, cholecystectomy is recommended.

cholelithotomy (kō′lə-lĭ-thŏt′ə-mē) N. removal of gallstones through an incision in the gallbladder.

cholemesis (kō-lĕm′ĭ-sĭs) N. vomiting of bile.

cholera (kŏl′ər-ə) N. acute infection with the bacterium *Vibrio cholerae*, characterized by severe diarrhea and vomiting, often leading to dehydration, electrolyte imbalances, and, if untreated, death. Spread by water and food contaminated with the feces of infected persons, it is endemic in some parts of the world and frequently occurs at times of natural disasters (e.g., earthquake, floods). Treatment is by antibiotics and electrolyte replacement; a vaccine is available.

cholestasis (kō′lĭ-stā′sĭs) N. interruption in bile flow, caused by hepatitis or other liver disorder, alcohol or drug use, or obstruction (e.g., by calculi or tumor) in bile ducts, and marked by pale, fatty stools, itching, and jaundice.

cholesterol (kə-lĕs′tə-rôl′) N. complex chemical present in all animal fats and widespread in the body, esp. in bile, the brain, blood, adrenal glands, and nerve-fiber sheaths. It also forms deposits in blood vessels (atherosclerosis) and forms gallstones. In the body, cholesterol is involved in the synthesis of certain hormones (e.g., cortisone, estrogen) and vitamin D and in the absorption of fatty acids. Many studies indicate that excessive cholesterol levels in the blood can clog arteries and predispose to heart attacks and strokes (cardiovascular accidents). Whether the level of cholesterol can be controlled by avoiding or limiting saturated fatty acids in the diet is still in dispute. There are two kinds of cholesterol. Cholesterol attaches to lipoproteins in the blood. Low-density lipoproteins (LDL) carry cholesterol that builds up plaque, so LDL-cholesterol is considered bad cholesterol. High-density lipoproteins (HDL), however, carry cholesterol to the liver, where the body can get rid of it, and are considered good cholesterol.

choline (kō′lēn′) N. vitamin of the B complex, found in most tissues of animals and important (as part of acetylcholine) in nerve impulse transmission and in liver function. Some recent evidence indicates that it may also be important in retaining mental function in the elderly.

cholinergic (kō-lə-nûr′jĭk) ADJ. having effects similar to those resulting from the action of acetylcholine (e.g., in nerve transmission) (*compare* ADRENERGIC).

chondroblast (kŏn′drə-blăst′) N. cell that forms cartilage.

chondrocyte (kŏn′drə-sīt′) N. cartilage cell.

chondrodystrophy (kŏn′drə-dĭs′trə-fē) *See* ACHONDROPLASIA.

chondroma (kŏn-drō′mə) N. benign, fairly common tumor of cartilage cells.

chondromalacia (kŏn′drō-mə-lā′shə) N. softening of cartilage, esp. of the knee, causing pain, swelling, and degenerative changes.

chondrosarcoma (kŏn′drō-sär-kō′mə) N. malignant neoplasm of cartilage cells, most often occurring in long bones, the scapula, or the pelvic girdle.

chorda N. cordlike structure; tendon. ADJ. chordal

chorditis (kôr-dī′tĭs) N. inflammation of the spermatic cord or of the vocal cords.

chorea (kô-rē′ə) N. disease of the nervous system characterized by involuntary, rapid, and spastic jerks, esp. of the shoulders, hips, and face. *See also* HUNTINGTON'S CHOREA.

choriocarcinoma (kôr′ē-ō-kär′sə-nō′mə) N. rare and highly malignant tumor, usually of the uterus but may also develop at the site of an ectopic pregnancy. May occur during normal pregnancy or as a complication of hydatid mole. Some cases of long-term survival have been reported using the chemotherapeutic agent methotrexate.

chorion (kôr′ē-ŏn′) N. outer membrane of the embryo sac, which gives rise to the placenta (the inner membrane is the amnion). ADJ. chorionic

chorionic gonadotropin (kôr'ē-än-ĭk gō-nad-ō-trō-pin) *See* HUMAN CHORIONIC GONADOTROPIN.

chorioretinitis (kôr'ē-ō-rĕt'nī'tĭs) N. inflammation of the cell layer (choroid) behind the retina and of the retina itself, resulting in blurred vision.

choroid (kôr'oid') N. membrane in the eye, between the retina and the sclera, having many blood vessels. ADJ. choroidal

Christmas disease *See* HEMOPHILIA.

chrom-, chromo- comb. forms indicating color (e.g., chromatic, pert. to color and its production).

chromatid (krō'mə-tĭd) N. one of the two identical strands of a chromosome, occurring as a result of the replication of the chromosome during cell division.

chromatin (krō'mə-tĭn) N. easily stained, gene-carrying part of the cell nucleus. It consists of DNA (deoxyribonucleic acid, the basic hereditary material) and protein (usually histone).

chromatism (krō'mə-tĭz'əm) N.
1. abnormal coloring or pigmentation.
2. hallucinatory perception of colored lights.

chromatography (krō'mə-tŏg'rə-fē) N. any of several techniques for analyzing compounds and mixtures by virtue of the differences in absorbency of the various components of the compound or mixture.

chromesthesia (krō'mĕs-thē'zhə) N.
1. color sense.

2. confusion of actual sensation (e.g., of taste or smell) with imaginary sensations of color.

chromoblastomycosis N. skin disease, caused by infection with a fungus, characterized by itchy, warty nodules in a break in the skin that sometimes spread and ulcerate. Treatment is by excision of the nodules and by topical antibiotics.

chromosomal aberration N. any change in the normal structure or number of chromosomes, often causing physical and mental abnormalities (e.g., Down's syndrome, Kleinfelter's syndrome).

chromosome (krō'mə-sōm') N. threadlike structure in every cell nucleus that carries the inheritance factors (genes) composed of DNA (deoxyribonucleic acid, the gene material) and a protein (usually histone). A human cell normally contains 46 chromosomes, or 22 homologous pairs and 1 pair of sex chromosomes; one member of each pair of chromosomes is derived from each parent. (*See also* DIPLOID; HAPLOID; KARYOTYPE.) ADJ. chromosomal

chromosome mapping *See* MAPPING.

chronic (krŏn'ĭk) ADJ. long-lasting or frequently recurring (e.g., pain) (*compare* ACUTE).

chronic bronchitis N. form of chronic lung disease, often existing concomitantly with emphysema, characterized by excess production of sputum by the mucous membranes of the airways, leading to chronic cough and obstruction to airway flow. *See also* EMPHYSEMA; CHRONIC OBSTRUCTIVE PULMONARY DISEASE.

chronic fatigue syndrome (CFS) N. debilitating and complex disorder characterized by profound fatigue that is not improved by bed rest and that may be worsened by physical or mental activity. Persons with CFS most often function at a substantially lower level of activity than they were capable of before the onset of illness. In addition, patients report various nonspecific symptoms, including weakness, muscle pain, impaired memory and/or mental concentration, insomnia, and post-exertional fatigue lasting more than 24 hours. In some cases, CFS can persist for years. The cause or causes of CFS have not been identified, and no specific diagnostic tests are available. Moreover, since many illnesses have incapacitating fatigue as a symptom, care must be taken to exclude other known and often treatable conditions before a diagnosis of CFS is made. Since no cause for CFS has been identified and the pathophysiology remains unknown, treatment programs are directed at relief of symptoms, with the goal of the patient regaining some level of preexisting function and well-being. Some proposed treatments are unproven and may be harmful.

chronic lymphocytic leukemia (CLL) N. neoplasm of blood-forming tissue, more common in men and with advancing age, with an insidious start, progressing to fatigability, anorexia, weight loss, and swelling of the lymph glands, spleen, and liver. Normal activities may be continued for many years, and remissions may be induced by chemotherapy or irradiation.

chronic myelocytic leukemia (CML) N. malignant neoplasm of blood-forming tissues, occurring most often in older people, with an insidious start, progressing to malaise, bleeding gums, heat intolerance, skin lesions, abdominal discomfort, and spleen enlargement; also called myeloid leukemia.

chronic obstructive pulmonary disease (COPD) N. general term for chronic, nonreversible lung disease that is usually a combination of emphysema and chronic bronchitis. Patients have often been heavy smokers. Treatment is with bronchodilators, corticosteroids, and antibiotics, when necessary. Oxygen may be helpful in advanced cases.

chronobiology (krŏn′ō-bī-ŏl′ə-jē) N. the study of processes that repeat themselves at regular intervals under control of an internal timing mechanism within the patient. The best known of these is the circadian rhythm, with periods matching the solar 24-hour day. Some aspects of therapy involve treatment given in context of temporal changes in cell and tissue receptivity—some organs and cells respond to treatment better at particular times of the day. Therapy can also involve manipulations of the internal clock itself, such as by resetting its phase. Most commonly, this is done by appropriately timed exposure to light, altering producing of the hormone melatonin.

chronological age (krŏn′ə-lŏj′ĭ-kəl) N. age of a person expressed as the period of time (e.g., months, years) that has elapsed since birth (*compare* BONE AGE; DEVELOPMENTAL AGE; MENTAL AGE).

chrysotherapy (krĭs′ə-thĕr′ə-pē) N. treatment of disease (e.g., rheumatoid arthritis) with chemicals containing gold; possible side effects include blood, skin, kidney, and liver disorders.

chyle (kīl) N. cloudy fluid product of digestion in the small intestines, made up of fats; it is absorbed through lacteals into the lymphatic system and from there passes into the blood.

chyme (kīm) N. thick, semifluid mixture, consisting of partly digested food and digestive juices, that passes from the stomach to the duodenum of the small intestine.

cicatrix (sĭk′ə-trĭks′) N. scar: mark left after the healing of a wound; tissue lacks color and usually appears contracted.

-cide suffix meaning killing (e.g., amebicide, substance that is fatal to amebae).

cilia N., *sing.* cilium
  1. eyelashes.
  2. hairlike projections from a cell, esp. in the upper respiratory tract where cilia move particles of dust or other materials.

ciliary body (sĭl′ē-ĕr′ē) N. thick part of a vascular membrane joining the iris and choroid of the eye.

ciliary movement N. rhythmic action of hairlike structures (cilia) in certain body parts (e.g., the lining of the bronchial tubes); the sweeping action helps to move mucus or remove foreign particles (e.g., dust) from the tissue.

cimetidine (sĭ-mĕt′ĭ-dēn′) N. drug (trade name Tagamet) used to treat peptic ulcers and certain other conditions in which decreased acid secretion in the stomach is desired.

Adverse effects include diarrhea, dizziness, and skin reactions. *See* TABLE OF COMMONLY PRESCRIBED DRUGS—GENERIC NAMES.

cingulum N., *pl.* cingula, encircling structure or part (e.g., the beltlike band at the base of a tooth).

Cipro N. trade name for the antibiotic ciprofloxacin. *See* TABLE OF COMMONLY PRESCRIBED DRUGS—TRADE NAMES.

ciprofloxacin (sĭp′rō-flŏx′sə-sĭn) N. oral antibiotic (trade name Cipro) effective against several serious bacterial infections of the respiratory tract, skin, urinary tract, bones, and joints. Adverse effects include nausea, vomiting, and diarrhea. *See* TABLE OF COMMONLY PRESCRIBED DRUGS—GENERIC NAMES.

circadian rhythm (sər-kā′dē-ən) N. biological clock or rhythm of an organism, such as the natural sleep-wake cycle in a person's 24-hour schedule. Changing that rhythm can effect biological, mental, and behavioral functions (e.g., causing jet lag).

circle N. structure or part with a closed, ringlike shape (e.g., circle of Willis, consisting of communicating arteries in the brain).

circulation (sûr′kyə-lā′shən) N. general term for the movement of the blood, lymph, or other fluids in a continuous path through the body, as in blood moving through the network of arteries and veins. ADJ. circulatory

circulatory failure N. failure of the cardiovascular system to supply adequate levels of blood to body tissues, as a result of hemorrhage, heart malfunction,

CIRCULATORY SYSTEM

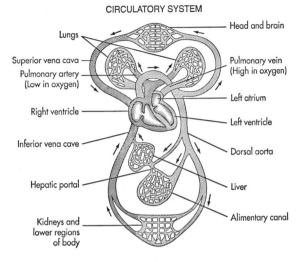

Lungs

Superior vena cava
Pulmonary artery
(Low in oxygen)

Right ventricle

Inferior vena cave

Hepatic portal

Kidneys and
lower regions
of body

Head and brain

Pulmonary vein
(High in oxygen)

Left atrium

Left ventricle

Dorsal aorta

Liver

Alimentary canal

or collapse of the peripheral vascular system.

circulatory system (sûr′kyə-lə-tôr′ē) N. network of channels through which a fluid passes around the body, esp., the network of arteries and veins transporting blood in the body. Also includes the thin-walled capillaries of the lymphatic system.

circum- comb. form meaning around (e.g., circumanal, pert. to the area around the anus).

circumcision (sûr′kəm-sĭzh′ən) N. surgical removal of the foreskin of the penis, widely performed on newborn boys (required in the Jewish and certain other religions) though its medical benefit is nonexistent and some risks (e.g., injury to the urethra, hemorrhage) are associated with the procedure. In adult males it is sometimes done to treat balanitis or phimosis.

circumduction (sûr′kəm-dŭk′shən) N. circular movement of a limb or eye.

cirrhosis (sĭ-rō′sĭs) N. chronic disease condition of the liver in which fibrous tissue and nodules replace normal tissue, interfering with blood flow and normal functions of the organ, including gastrointestinal functions, hormone metabolism, and alcohol and drug detoxification. The major cause of cirrhosis is chronic alcoholism. Symptoms include nausea, flatulence, light-colored stools, and abdominal discomfort. Treatment is by rest, a protein-rich diet, and abstinence from alcohol. If untreated, liver and kidney failure and gastrointestinal hemorrhage can occur, leading to death.

cisapride N. *See* TABLE OF COMMONLY PRESCRIBED DRUGS — GENERIC NAMES.

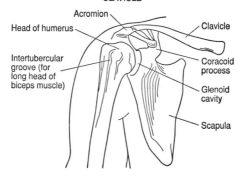

CLAVICLE

Acromion
Head of humerus
Clavicle
Intertubercular groove (for long head of biceps muscle)
Coracoid process
Glenoid cavity
Scapula

cisterna (sĭ-stûr′nə) N., *pl.* cisternae, reservoir, esp. for holding lymph or spinal fluid (e.g., cisterna chyli, chyle cistern).

citric acid (sĭt′rĭk) N. compound, derived from citrus fruits and fermented cane sugar, used to flavor foods and beverages and certain drugs, esp. laxatives.

Cl symbol for the element chlorine.

Claforan N. trade name for the cephalosporin antibiotic cefotaxime.

clairvoyance (klâr-voi′əns) N. ability to discern objects or persons not perceptible to the senses or to be aware of events that occur beyond the range of ordinary perception.

clamp (klămp) N. device used to grasp, compress, or support an organ, tissue, or other structure, esp. during surgery.

clarithromycin N. antibiotic (trade name Biaxin) related to both penicillin and to erythromycin; indicated in the treatment of mild to moderate respiratory infections; common side effects include diarrhea, nausea, and headache. *See* TABLE OF COMMONLY PRESCRIBED DRUGS—GENERIC NAMES.

Claritin N. *See* TABLE OF COMMONLY PRESCRIBED DRUGS—TRADE NAMES.

Claritin D 12HR N. *See* TABLE OF COMMONLY PRESCRIBED DRUGS—TRADE NAMES.

claudication (klô′dĭ-kâ′shən) N. limping or lameness. In intermittent claudication pain, esp. in the leg muscles, occurs with walking because the blood supply to these muscles is inadequate; the pain disappears with rest.

claustrophobia (klô′strə-fō′bē-ə) N. abnormal dread of being confined in closed rooms or small spaces; it is more common in women, can often be traced to an earlier traumatic experience, and is treated by psychotherapy and sometimes desensitization therapy.

claustrum N., *pl.* claustra, anatomical part that serves as a barrier, esp. a particular gray matter layer in the brain ADJ. claustral

clavicle (klăv′ĭ-kəl) N. collarbone: the long, curved horizontal bone just above the first rib that connects the scapula (shoulder blade) with the sternum (breastbone). ADJ. clavicular

clavulinic acid N. antibiotic, often used in combination with amoxicillin, to treat moderate to severe infections.

clawfoot N. deformity of the foot characterized by an abnormally high arch and hyperextension of the toes, giving the foot a clawlike appearance. Treatment depends on the severity of the condition; it may involve surgery. Also called pes cavus.

clear liquid diet N. diet that supplies fluid with minimal residue and includes clear and flavored drinks (e.g., ginger ale), fat-free broth, strained fruit juices, and gelatin desserts. It is not nutritionally adequate and can be used for only a limited time (e.g., one day postoperative).

clearance (klēr′əns) N. removal of something, as of wastes, from the blood by the kidney.

cleavage (klē′vĭj) N.
1. process of dividing, as of the fertilized egg into successive multiples of cells, from the single cell.
2. line formed by a groove between two parts.

cleft (klĕft) N. division, fissure, or cleavage, esp. one resulting in the nonunion of parts in the developing fetus (e.g., a cleft palate).

cleft foot N. abnormal condition in which the separation between the third and fourth toes extends into the foot.

cleft lip See HARELIP.

cleft palate N. congenital defect in which there is a fissure in the midline of the palate, either partial or extending through both hard and soft palates and into the nasal cavities, often associated with cleft in the upper lip. A common birth defect (occurring in about 1 in 2,500 births and more frequently in females), it is treated by special feeding techniques, reconstructive surgery, care of any associated speech, hearing, and oral problems, and emotional support.

click-murmur syndrome See MITRAL VALVE PROLAPSE.

climacteric (kli-măk′tər-ĭk, klī′măk-tĕr′ĭk) N. time in a woman's life associated with changes in her endocrine system and other body systems often accompanied by emotional changes; it ends with menopause, when reproductive capability ceases; colloquially called change of life.

Climara N. See TABLE OF COMMONLY PRESCRIBED DRUGS—TRADE NAMES.

climax (klī′măks′) N.
1. severest stage of a disease.
2. the height of sexual excitement; orgasm.

clinic (klĭn′ĭk) N. health-care facility part of an institution or hospital, designed to treat walk-in patients and/or train medical personnel.

clinical (klĭn′ĭ-kəl) ADJ. pert. to bedside patient care (e.g., clinical medicine) in contrast to basic-science studies (e.g., experimental medicine).

clinocephaly N. congenital defect in which the top of the head appears to be pushed in (is concave); also called clinocephalism.

clinodactyly (klī′nō-dăk′tə-lē) N. congenital defect in which one or more fingers or toes are abnormally positioned or bent.

Clinoril N. trade name for the anti-inflammatory sulindac.

clitoris (klĭt′ər-ĭs) N. small, erogenous part made up of erectile tissue at the front of the female external genital organs between the labia minora. ADJ. clitoral.

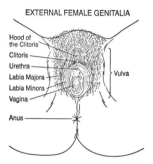

EXTERNAL FEMALE GENITALIA

Hood of the Clitoris
Clitoris
Urethra
Labia Majora
Labia Minora
Vagina
Anus
Vulva

CLL See CHRONIC LYMPHOCYTIC LEUKEMIA.

clofibrate (klō-fī′brāt) N. drug (trade name Atromid-S) used to lower high blood levels of cholesterol and triglycerides.

Clomid N. trade name for the fertility drug clomiphene citrate, the use of which has been associated with multiple births.

clonazepam N. See TABLE OF COMMONLY PRESCRIBED DRUGS —GENERIC NAMES.

clone (klōn) N. a group of genetically identical cells or organisms reproduced asexually from a single cell or individual. A few animals (e.g., sheep) have recently been cloned.

clonidine (klŏn′ĭ-dēn′) N. antihypertensive (trade name Catapres) that may be administered either orally or via transdermal patches; has also been used in heroin and alcohol withdrawal with variable success. Adverse effects include drowsiness, dry mouth, and, rarely, sexual dysfunction. See TABLE OF COMMONLY PRESCRIBED DRUGS—GENERIC NAMES.

clonus (klō′nəs) N. abnormal condition in which a skeletal muscle alternately contracts and relaxes; a rhythmical spasm often indicative of central nervous system disease. ADJ. clonic (as a clonic convulsion)

closed fracture See FRACTURE.

clot (klŏt) N. clump of material formed out of the contents of a fluid, as of blood. See also BLOOD CLOT; BLOOD COAGULATION.

clotrimoxazole/betamethasone N. See TABLE OF COMMONLY PRESCRIBED DRUGS—GENERIC NAMES.

clotting factor N. See COAGULATION FACTOR.

clotting time N. time required for blood to clot, usually determined by observing clot formation in a small sample of blood, used to diagnose some clotting disorders and to monitor anticoagulant drug therapy.

clubbing (klŭb′ĭng) N. condition of the fingers and toes in which their ends become wide and thickened; clubbing is often a symptom of disease, esp. heart or lung disease.

clubfoot (klŭb′fo͝ot′) N. congenital abnormality of the foot, esp. one in which the front part of the foot turns toward the inside of the heel. Less severe conditions can be treated by splints or casts applied during infancy; more severe conditions require surgery. See also TALIPES.

cluster headache (klŭs′tər) See HISTAMINE HEADACHE.

CML *See* CHRONIC MYELOCYTIC LEUKEMIA.

Co symbol for the element cobalt.

coagulation N. clotting process. *See* BLOOD COAGULATION.

coagulation factor (kō-ăg′yə-lā′shən) N. any of 13 factors in the blood, including fibrinogen and prothrombin, the actions of which are essential for blood coagulation. Also known as clotting factor.

coal miner's lung *See* BLACK LUNG DISEASE.

coalescence (kō′ə-lĕs′əns) N. fusion, as when the edges of a wound grow together.

coarctation (kō′ärk-tā′shən) N. constricting or narrowing, esp. with reference to a congenital defect of the aorta, which is usually repaired surgically.

coat (kōt) N. covering, esp. a membrane that forms a wall.

cobalt (kō′bôlt′) N. metallic element, the radioactive isotope of which (Co-60) is used in the treatment of cancer. Cobalt is contained in vitamin B_{12}. *See also* TABLE OF IMPORTANT ELEMENTS.

COBRA N. abbrev. for Consolidated Omnibus Budget Reconciliation Act; typically refers to the Federal Anti-dumping Law of 1985, and its subsequent amendments.

cocaine (kō-kān′, kō′kān′) N. white, crystalline powder, derived from the leaves of the coca plant (*Erythroxylon coca*) or prepared synthetically and used as a topical anesthetic, esp. for eye, ear, nose, and throat examinations. Cocaine is also a drug of abuse, used for its stimulating and anesthetic properties. Adverse reactions, esp. when used illicitly, include restlessness, euphoria, tremors, stroke, and myocardial infarction. It is addictive and associated with death due to heart attacks and cardiovascular accidents (strokes), even in young people.

coccidiomyocosis (kŏk-sĭd′ē-oi′dō-mī-kō′sĭs) N. infection caused by the fungus *Coccidioides immitis*, largely confined to the southwestern United States and Central and South America, where it is sometimes called desert rheumatism or valley fever. At first the symptoms resemble those of the common cold or influenza; after apparent recovery the disease may recur in a more serious form, with fever, weight loss, and arthritic pains. The initial infection often does not require treatment. Recurrent disease is treated by antifungal agents.

coccidiosis (kŏk-sĭd′ē-ō′sĭs) N. disease of tropical and subtropical areas, caused by the protozoan parasite *Isospora belli* or closely related species, characterized by watery diarrhea, fever, and malaise. It usually subsides within 2 weeks, rarely persisting to cause serious complications.

coccus (kŏk′əs) N., *pl.* cocci, round or generally round bacterium. ADJ. coccal

coccyx (kŏk′sĭks) N. four fused, partly developed vertebrae forming the tailbone in humans. ADJ. coccal

cochlea (kŏk′lē-ə, kō′klē-ə) N. snail-shaped part of the inner ear (*see also* LABYRINTH) whose sensory cells are stimulated by sound waves during hearing. ADJ. cochlear

cod liver oil N. oil from the liver of codfish and other fishes used to treat calcium and phosphorus deficiency and as a supplementary source of vitamins A and D.

codeine (kō′dēn) N. chemical (alkaloid), derived from opium or morphine, used as a pain reliever and cough suppressant. Adverse effects include nausea, constipation, and drowsiness; if taken in large amounts or for a long period, it is potentially addictive.

codependence N. addiction to an alcoholic, drug addict, or to any person. It is applied most often in the case of chemical dependence (drug or alcohol addiction) in which the chemical becomes the center of the family's life and every family member must adjust to it; this may involve pretending to be what the addict wants so there is as little confrontation as possible; often one addict or alcoholic parent is the focal point, while the other parent spends most of his or her time and energy trying to modify family life to the situation; codependence often results in serious psychological problems for all family members.

codon (kō′dŏn′) N. code for a specific amino acid, formed of three successive bases in a DNA (deoxyribonucleic acid) molecule.

coelom N. body cavity of an embryo that gives rise in humans to the pleural, pericardial, and peritoneal cavities.

coenzyme (kō-ĕn′zīm′) N. nonprotein substance (sometimes a vitamin) that functions to aid the action of an enzyme.

cofactor (kō′făk′tər) N. substance (e.g., a coenzyme) that must join with another to produce a given result.

coffee N. caffeine-containing beverage made from the seeds of the coffee plant.

cognition (kŏg-nĭsh′ən) N. mental faculty of knowing, including perceiving, thinking, recognizing, and remembering. ADJ. cognitive

cognitive behavioral therapy N. type of psychotherapy used to treat depression, anxiety, phobias, and other forms of mental disorder. It involves recognizing distorted thinking and learning to replace it with more realistic substitute ideas. Cognitive behavior therapy combines two kinds of psychotherapy—cognitive therapy and behavior therapy. Cognitive therapy teaches patients how certain thinking patterns cause their symptoms. Behavior therapy helps patients weaken the connections between troublesome situations and their habitual reactions to them. It also teaches patients how to relax physically and mentally, so they can feel better, think more clearly, and make better decisions. *See also* ANXIETY; ATYPICAL PSYCHOTICS; BIPOLAR DISORDER; PHOBIA.

cohesion (kō-hē′zhən) N. force of molecular attraction. ADJ. cohesive

coitus (kō′ĭ-təs) N. sexual union of a man and a woman in which the penis is inserted into the vagina, usually accompanied by excitement and often orgasm and ejaculation; also called intercourse; sexual intercourse. ADJ. coital

coitus interruptus N. contraceptive method during coitus in which the penis is removed from the vagina before ejaculation in an effort to prevent spermatozoa from entering the female's body. It is not considered a reliable method of contraception, however, because sperm are often released without sensation before ejaculation. Also called withdrawal method.

colchicine N. pain-relieving drug derived from the saffron plant, used to treat gout; common side effects include nausea, vomiting, and diarrhea.

cold (kōld) N. infection involving the nasal passages and upper part of the breathing system (not including the lungs) and including such symptoms as a runny nose, watery eyes, and a sore throat. Caused by one of many different viruses (mainly rhinoviruses), a cold may be treated with rest, decongestants and increased fluids, but usually not with antibiotics, which do not affect viruses (*compare* CORYZA, INFLUENZA, RHINITIS). Also called common cold, upper respiratory tract infection.

cold sore N. fever blister caused by herpes simplex virus, occurring on the skin or mucous membranes (e.g., at the corner of the mouth).

colic (kŏl′ĭk) N.
1. acute pain associated with spasm of smooth muscle, as occurs, for example, during passage of a kidney stone or gallstone.
2. in infants, recurrent (usually daily, often at the same time of day) episodes of persistent crying, usually accompanied by signs of abdominal distress; it may be caused by intestinal gas (from air swallowed with food),

though other explanations (e.g., neurological immaturity) have also been proposed. ADJ. **colicky**

colitis (kə-lī′tĭs) N. inflammation of the colon, either an episodic and functional condition (irritable bowel syndrome) or, more serious, chronic and progressive bowel disease (e.g., Crohn's disease, ulcerative colitis). Irritable bowel attacks, often precipitated by stress, are characterized by colicky pain and constipation or diarrhea; they are treated by stress avoidance and a bland diet. Chronic diseases lead to ulceration of intestinal tissue, bleeding, severe diarrhea, and other complications.

collagen (kŏl′ə-jən) N. protein of connective and other tissues (e.g., bone, cartilage). ADJ. **collagenous**

collagen disease N. any of several disorders (e.g., ankylosing spondylitis, arteritis nodosa, scleroderma, systemic lupus erythematosus) marked by disruption of connective tissue. Sometimes called collagen vascular disease.

collagen vascular disease *See* COLLAGEN DISEASE.

collagenase (kə-lăj′ə-nās′) N. enzyme that dissolves (lyses) the connective tissue protein collagen.

collagenolysis (kə′-lăj ən ō lī′-sus) N. breakdown (lysis) of the connective tissue protein collagen by a collagenase.

collapse (kə-lăps′) N.
1. general prostration.
2. state of extreme depression or exhaustion.
3. deflation, as of a lung.

collarbone (kŏl′ər-bōn′) *See* CLAVICLE.

colloid (kŏl′oid′) N. non-crystalline substance consisting of microscopic particles, often large single molecules, dispersed throughout a second substance such as a gel or liquid. Also refers to the gelatin-like substance of the thyroid gland that contains thyroid hormone.

colo- comb. form indicating an association with the colon (e.g., colorectal, pert. to the colon and rectum).

colon (kō′lən) N. segment of large intestine from the cecum to the rectum. ADJ. colonic

colon cancer N. malignant tumor of the colon. Symptoms may be minimal, consisting only of small amounts of blood in the stool. Treatment involves surgery and sometimes chemotherapy. Periodic rectal examinations and sigmoidoscopy are recommended for adults over 40 years of age so that the disease, if present, may be diagnosed and treated at an early stage.

colonic irrigation N. washing out of the lower part of the bowel by forcing large amounts of water or another cleaning medium into it.

colonoscopy (kō′lə-nŏs′kə-pē) N. procedure used to inspect the lining of the colon for polyps, tumors, and other abnormal lesions in which a fiberoptic endoscope is inserted into the colon by way of the rectum.

colony (kŏl′ə-nē) N. in microbiology, group of organisms grown from a single parent cell.

color blindness N. any of various abnormal conditions characterized by inability to distinguish colors. The most common form is daltonism, occurring mostly in males (approx. 8% of Caucasian males) as a sex-linked inherited trait characterized by an inability to distinguish red from green. Total color blindness, or achromatic vision, is rare and due to a defect of the retina.

Colorado tick fever N. generally mild viral infection, transmitted by the bite of a tick and common in the Rocky Mountain area of the United States; it is characterized by headache; pains in the legs, eyes, and back; and fever and chills, with the symptoms usually occurring in two episodes before final remission.

colostomy (kə-lŏs′tə-mē) N. surgical creation of an opening (stoma) in the abdominal wall to allow material to pass from the bowel through that opening rather than through the anus. A colostomy may be temporary, to allow an inflamed area of the intestine to heal, or permanent, as in cancer of the colon or rectum. (*Compare* ILEOSTOMY.)

colostrum (kə-lŏs′trəm) N. first fluid given off by the mother's breasts just before or after the birth of her baby; it contains white blood cells, protective antibodies, protein, and fat in a thin, yellow fluid.

colp-, colpo- comb. forms indicating an association with the vagina (e.g. colpitis, inflammation of the vagina).

colpocele (kŏl′pə-sēl′) N. hernia into the vagina.

colpocystitis (kŏl′pō-sĭ-stī′tĭs) N. inflammation of the vagina and bladder.

colposcopy (kŏl-pŏs′kə-pē) N. visual examination of the upper vagina-cervix through a special instrument (colposcope).

colpoxerosis (kŏl'pō-zĭ-rō'sĭs) N. condition in which the vagina is unusually dry.

column (kŏl'əm) N. pillarlike anatomical structure, esp. the spinal column and brain structures in the embryo.

coma (kō'mə) N. state of profound unconsciousness, from which the person cannot be aroused, resulting from drug action, toxicity (as in nephritis), brain injury, or disease. ADJ. comatose

combat fatigue N. any of various mental disorders, resulting from fatigue and the stress of combat, characterized by depression, anxiety, and often memory and sleep disorders; usually temporary but may occasionally lead to long-term emotional disorders; also called combat neurosis, shell shock.

comedo (kŏm'ĭ-dō') N., *pl.* comedones, accumulation, in a hair follicle or oil gland, of dead cells and oily substance; the basic lesion in acne vulgaris; commonly called blackhead.

comminuted fracture See FRACTURE.

Commission E Report N. report on herbal medicines by the German Federal Institute for Drugs and Medical Devices available in the United States through the American Botanical Council; widely regarded as authoritative because clear and convincing evidence for medical efficacy with reasonable certainty is the standard used for inclusion of herbs as part of the pharmacopoeia of the medical system in Germany.

commissure (kŏm'ə-shoōr') N. meeting place of two structures in the midline, such as the lips; also a band of nerve fibers passing across the midline within the central nervous system.

common bile duct N. duct, formed by junction of the hepatic and cystic ducts, that carries bile into the duodenum.

common cold See COLD.

communicable disease N. any disease transmitted from one person or animal to another, either directly through body discharges (e.g., nasal droplets, sputum, feces) or indirectly through substances or objects (e.g., contaminated drinking glasses, toys, bed linens) or vectors (e.g., flies, mosquitoes, ticks). Communicable diseases include those caused by viruses, bacteria, fungi, and parasites. Also called contagious disease. (*Compare* INFECTIOUS DISEASE.)

Compazine N. trade name for the antiemetic agent, prochlorperazine.

compensation (kŏm'pən-sā'shən) N.
1. adjustment after a change, to reattain balance or specific status for a part or function, as when the eye compensates for a change in light intensity by a corresponding change in pupil size.
2. making up for a physical injury or loss, as when a kidney enlarges after the other one is removed.
3. defense mechanism for adjusting to real or imagined inadequacies, as when a student who cannot master a foreign language works very hard for good science grades. ADJ. compensatory

complement (kŏm'plə-mənt) N. one of a series of enzymes, part of the immune-response mechanism in the blood serum, that works to break down invading microorganisms.

complement fixation N. immunologic response in which an antigen combines with an antibody and its complement, causing the complement to become inactive. This phenomenon is the basis of certain blood tests to determine the presence of antibodies against specific diseases.

complement fixation test N. blood test in which a sample of serum is exposed to a particular antigen and complement to determine whether antibodies to that particular antigen are present; used as a diagnostic aid (e.g., Wasserman test for syphilis).

complete blood count (CBC) N. determination of the number of red and white blood cells (erythrocytes and leukocytes) and sometimes platelets in 1 cubic milliliter sample of blood. One of the most common laboratory tests, it is an important aid to diagnosis (e.g., anemia, presence of infection). Hemoglobin levels may also be included in the test, as can determination of the numbers or percentages of the various types of white blood cells (differential blood count).

complete fracture *See* FRACTURE.

complex (kŏm'plĕks') N.
1. in psychology, related mental processes that interact to affect a person's behavior (e.g., inferiority complex).
2. group of chemicals or materials, related structurally or functionally, as in the immune system.
3. group of symptoms, a syndrome.

complex regional pain syndrome N. syndrome of unknown cause that often follows minor trauma, usually to an extremity. Numerous other conditions have also been associated with the syndrome including Lyme arthritis, barbiturate drugs, osteogenesis imperfecta, and various types of surgery (e.g., hip replacement surgery). Formerly known as reflex sympathetic dystrophy (RSD), signs and symptoms include sensory changes, autonomic nervous system dysfunction, skin atrophy, motor impairment, and psychological changes. The underlying pathological theme is an exaggerated inflammatory response to injury or surgery. Recent work suggests a genetic susceptibility. Prevention is important and includes early use of an injured extremity, physical therapy, and avoidance of smoking (decreases tissue blood supply). Sometimes, drug blockade of the sympathetic nervous system is effective in eliminating symptoms. *See also* ALLODYNIA; BISPHOSPHONATES; SYMPATHETIC NERVOUS SYSTEM.

complexion (kəm-plĕk'shən) N. texture, color, and appearance of the skin of the face.

compliance (kəm-plī'əns) N. degree to which a patient follows medical advice; noncompliant patients may fail to take medications as prescribed, refrain from smoking when advised, or not return for follow-up visits as requested.

complicated fracture *See* FRACTURE.

complication (kŏm'plĭ-kā'shən) N. any disease or other unwanted effect that occurs dur-

ing the course of or because of
another physical disorder (e.g.,
bedsores resulting from paralysis).

compound (kŏm′pound′) N. substance composed of two or
more elements chemically combined in definite proportions
and usually differing in properties from the elements considered separately; for example,
table salt, nonpoisonous at normal levels, consists of two
highly poisonous elements—
sodium and chloride; generally,
any combination of several
things (*compare* ELEMENT).

compound fracture *See* FRACTURE.

compress (kŏm′prĕs′) N. pad, usually of cloth or gauze (sometimes hot, cold, or medicated),
applied with pressure to an inflamed part or to a wound to
help control bleeding or to keep
parts from protruding through a
wound.

compression bandage (kəmprĕsh′ən) N. strip of cloth
wrapped around a part to stop
hemorrhage, immobilize the
part, or keep fluid from collecting in a limb.

compression fracture *See* FRACTURE.

compulsion (kəm-pŭl′shən) N.
persistent, irresistible urge to
do something that is usually
contrary to one's own standards
or wishes; a compelling impulse (*compare* OBSESSION).

computed tomography (CT)
(kəm-pyōō′tĭd) N. method for
examining the body's soft tissues (e.g., the brain) using X
rays, with the beam passing repeatedly (scanning) through a
body part, and a computer calculating tissue absorption at
each point scanned, from which

a visualization of the tissue is
developed. The technique enables the radiologist to study
normal structures as well as to
detect tumors, fluid buildup,
dead tissue, and other abnormalities. Formerly called computed (or computerized) axial
tomography (CAT). (*Compare*
NUCLEAR MAGNETIC RESONANCE,
POSITRON EMISSION TOMOGRAPHY.)

concave lens N. lens of glass or
hard plastic that has one or both
surfaces curved so that the
outer rim is thicker and the hollowed (caved) center is thinner;
used to improve the vision of
persons with nearsightedness
(myopia).

conception (kən-sĕp′shən) N.
1. fertilization of the female
egg cell (ovum) by a male
spermatozoon, the beginning of
pregnancy.
2. originating of a new idea.
3. concept.

conceptus (kən-sĕp′təs) N. product of conception, the fertilized
egg with its enclosing membranes in the uterus. *See also*
EMBRYO; FETUS.

concha (kŏng′kə) N., *pl.* conchae,
shell-shaped structure (e.g., the
concha auriculae, in the ear)
(*compare* COCHLEA).

concretion (kən-krē′shən) N.
1. stonelike formation within
an organ (e.g., the kidney).
2. abnormal joining of two
parts; solidification.

concussion (kən-kŭsh′ən) N. violent jarring or shaking, as from
a severe blow or shock, esp.
one to the head. A concussion
may cause a limited period of
unconsciousness.

condition (kən-dĭsh′ən) N.
1. a general term for the state
of a patient.

2. health disorder; abnormal state. v. to undergo physical training.

conditioned reflex (kən-dĭsh′ənd) N. reflex developed by training with a specific repeated stimulus, as in Pavlov's experiment, in which a dog salivates at the sound of a bell after a period in which each feeding is preceded by the ringing of a bell (*compare* UNCONDITIONED REFLEX).

conditioning (kən-dĭsh′ə-nĭng) N. psychological term for any of several types of learning that lead to specific responses to particular stimuli. *See also* OPERANT CONDITIONING.

condom (kŏn′dəm) N. thin sheath, usually of rubber or plastic, placed over the penis and used during coitus as a protection against sexually transmitted disease (venereal disease) and acquired immune deficiency syndrome (AIDS) and as a reasonably effective contraceptive.

conduction (kən-dŭk′shən) N. transport of energy through a system, as impulses through the nerves or as sound waves to the inner ear. For example, the cardiac conduction system carries the electrical impulse throughout the heart muscle, causing it to contract.

conduction anesthesia N. type of anesthesia produced by an anesthetic agent along the course of a nerve to inhibit the conduction of pain impulses to the area supplied by that nerve; also called nerve block anesthesia.

conductive hearing loss N. type of hearing loss caused by inadequate conduction of sound through the external and middle ear to the inner ear; an increase

in volume usually compensates for this defect (*compare* SENSORINEURAL HEARING LOSS).

condyle (kŏn′dīl′) N. rounded bump on a bone where it forms a joint with another bone or bones (as the rounded head of the femur into the cup-shaped acetabulum). ADJ. condylar

cone (kōn) N. light-sensitive cell in the retina of the eye; the cones are responsible for color vision and visual sharpness. ADJ. conic, conical

confinement (kən-fīn′mənt) N.
1. state of being restrained to a particular place to limit activity.
2. labor; childbirth.

conflict (kŏn′flĭkt′) N. state of mental struggle and frustration caused by the simultaneous presence of equally desirable, undesirable, or otherwise opposing or incompatible thoughts, drives, desires, or wishes.

confluent (kŏn′flōō-ənt) ADJ. merging, joining, running together (e.g., confluent tissues, pustules, or lesions).

confusion (kən-fyōō′zhən) N. state of mind in which one is unsure of the present time, place, or self-identity, causing bewilderment and inability to act decisively; it usually indicates organic mental disorder but may also occur in times of severe stress.

congenital (kən-jĕn′ĭ-tl) ADJ. present at birth.

congenital anomaly N. birth defect; abnormality, esp. a structural one, present at birth; may be inherited, acquired during pregnancy, or inflicted as the result of the birth process; two examples are Down's syndrome and cleft palate, resulting from incomplete development and union of the parts forming the palate.

congestion (kən-jĕs′chən) N. abnormal collection of blood or other fluid (e.g., mucus, bile), as in the lungs (pulmonary congestion). ADJ. congestive

congestive heart failure (kən-jĕs′tĭv) N. abnormal condition characterized by circulatory congestion and retention of salt and water by the kidneys; it is usually caused by a heart disorder and most often develops chronically with shortness of breath, due to fluid accumulation in the lungs, and edema of the extremities. Treatment includes rest, diuretics, vasodilators, digitalis, ACE inhibitors, and oxygen, if necessary.

conjoined twins (kən-joind′) *See* SIAMESE TWINS.

conjugated estrogens (kŏn′jə-gāt-ed) N. *See* TABLE OF COM-

CHARACTERISTICS OF CONNECTIVE TISSUES

Connective Tissue	Locations	Functions
Loose connective tissue	Beneath the skin, between muscles, beneath most epithelial layers	Binds organs together, holds tissue fluids
Dense connective tissue	Tendons and ligaments	Binds organs together
Reticular connective tissue	Walls of liver, spleen, and lymphatic organs	Support
Adipose tissue	Beneath the skin, around the kidneys, behind the eyeballs, on the surface of the heart	Protection, insulation, and storage of fat
Elastic connective tissue	Between adjacent vertebrae, in walls of arteries and airways	Provides elastic quality
Pigmented connective tissue	Eyes	Store pigment
Hyaline cartilage	Ends of bones, nose, and rings in walls of respiratory passages (trachea, bronchi)	Support, protection, provides framework
Elastic cartilage	Framework of external ear and part of the larynx	Support, protection provides framework
Fibrous cartilage	Between bony parts of backbone, pelvic girdle, and knee	Support, protection
Bone	Bones of skeleton	Support, protection, provides framework

TYPES OF CONNECTIVE TISSUE

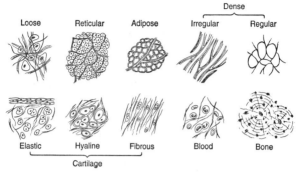

Loose   Reticular   Adipose   Dense — Irregular   Regular

Elastic   Hyaline   Fibrous   Blood   Bone

Cartilage

MONLY PRESCRIBED DRUGS—GENERIC NAMES.

conjugated estrogens/medroxy-progesterone N. *See* TABLE OF COMMONLY PRESCRIBED DRUGS—GENERIC NAMES.

conjunctiva (kŏn'jŭngk-tī'və) N. thin, transparent membrane that lines the eyelids and portions of the underlying eyeball.

conjunctivitis (kən-jŭngk'tə-vī'tĭs) N. inflammation of the mucous membrane lining of the eyelids and the front of the eye, caused by bacterial or viral infection, allergy, or irritation. The eyes look pink; the eyelids are stuck together in the morning, and there is discomfort, but usually not pain. Treatment depends on the cause. Also called pinkeye.

connective tissue (kə-nĕk'tĭv) N. material that supports and binds other tissues and parts of the body; it includes skin, bone, tendons, ligaments, and interlacing fibrils. Many diseases of connective tissue are difficult to cure (e.g., systemic lupus erythematosus, rheumatoid arthritis, and scleroderma).

Conn's syndrome N. disorder of the cortex of the adrenal gland (most often due to a benign tumor, rarely to another cause), in which excess secretion of aldosterone leads to disturbances in salt-water balance and symptoms of weakness, convulsions, muscular cramps and twitching, abnormal skin sensations (e.g., burning, itching), and sometimes paralysis.

consanguinity (kŏn'săn-gwĭn'ĭ-tē) N. relationship by common ancestry (bloodline); blood relationship.

conscious (kŏn'shəs) ADJ. alert, aware, or attentive, able to perceive and respond.

conscious sedation N. anesthetic procedure where intravenous medication is used to help relax the patient during a procedure, without inducing total unconsciousness. Usually utilized with procedures that are anxiety-producing for the patient, such as suturing a laceration in a child or endoscopy.

constipation (kŏn'stə-pā'shən) N. difficulty in having bowel movements because of loss of muscle tone in the intestine, very hard stools, or other causes (e.g., diverticulitis, intestinal obstruction). An increase in roughage (fruits, vegetables, bran) in the diet, along with plenty of water, often helps this condition.

constitution (kŏn'stĭ-too'shən) N. person's physical and mental makeup, including inherited qualities and general physique.

constriction (kən-strĭk'shən) N. narrowing, squeezing, or tightening.

consult v. to discuss with or seek advice from, esp. in deciding on diagnosis or treatment of a medical problem. N. consultation

contact dermatitis N. skin rash resulting from exposure to an irritant such as an alkali or acid (in, e.g., a cleaning product) or to a substance to which one has an allergic response (e.g., poison ivy).

contact lens N. small, curved, glass or plastic lens placed on the eye to correct vision or deliver medication. The lens is fitted to the individual's eye and made to float on a tear film. Contact lenses must be inserted carefully and periodically removed and cleaned. Soft contact lenses, made of a hydrophilic plastic, are more comfortable and can be worn for longer periods than the earlier glass contact lenses.

contagion (kən-tā'jən) N. passing of disease from a sick person to others. *See also* COMMUNICABLE DISEASE.

contagious disease (kən-tā'jəs) *See* COMMUNICABLE DISEASE.

contamination (kən-tăm'ə-nā'shən) N. inclusion, intentionally or accidentally, of unwanted substances or factors; pollution.

continence (kŏn'tə-nəns) N.
1. self-restraint or moderation, as in eating or in sexual activity.
2. ability to hold urine and feces and to voluntarily control their passage from the body.

contra- prefix meaning against (e.g., contraindication) or opposite (e.g., contrafissure, fracture opposite the site of the blow).

contraception (kŏn'trə-sĕp'shən) N. process or technique for the prevention of pregnancy. Methods include total abstinence from coitus; coitus interruptus (withdrawal); periodic abstinence or the rhythm method (refraining from coitus during a woman's fertile time, the time around ovulation, which is determined by the ovulation method, the calendar method, or the basal body temperature method); the use of mechanical devices to block sperm from moving up the female genital tract (including the condom, diaphragm, intrauterine device (IUD, cervical cap, sponge)), biochemical methods (birth control pill or oral contraceptive, hormonal injections); chemical means (spermicidal creams, jellies, foams, and suppositories); and sterilization (vasectomy in men, tubal ligation in women).

contraceptive (kŏn'trə-sĕp'tĭv) N. means of preventing fertilization mechanically (e.g., by condom, diaphragm, intrauterine device (IUD, sponge, cervical cap) by blocking the passage of sperm in the female reproductive tract; chemically by killing or immobilizing the sperm with spermicidal jellies, foams, creams, or suppositories; or biochemically by creating hormonal conditions in the female that make pregnancy impossible (e.g., oral contraceptive pill).

contraction (kən-trăk'shən) N.
1. shortening, or tension increase, as in muscle action; a persistent abnormal shortening.
2. in labor, rhythmic tightening of the upper uterine musculature that decreases the size of the uterus and pushes the fetus through the birth canal; uterine contractions typically begin mildly and then increase in severity and frequency, sometimes coming at a rate of one every 2 minutes and lasting about 1 minute.

contracture (kən-trăk'chər) N. abnormal, usually permanent contraction of a muscle due to atrophy of muscle fibers, extensive scar tissue over a joint, or other factors. *See also* DUPUYTREN'S CONTRACTURE.

contraindication (kŏn'trə-ĭn'dĭ-kā-shən) N. any factor prohibiting the use of a particular procedure or drug for a specific patient because of the likelihood of unwanted results. For example, the administration of penicillin is contraindicated if the person has had a severe allergic reaction to the drug.

contralateral ADJ. located on the opposite side. The left arm is contralateral to the right arm.

contrast medium N. substance, administered orally, intravenously, or via enema, that is radiopaque when exposed to X rays. The administration of such a compound allows for examination by a radiologist of the tissue or organ being filled.

contrecoup (kŏn'trə-kōō') N. injury to one side that results from a blow to the opposite side

(as a blow to the forehead causing damage to the back of the skull or rear part of the brain).

control (kən-trōl') N. in experimental design, standard used for comparison, as a placebo-receiving group of subjects in a drug-efficacy study.

contusion (kən-tōō'zhən) N. bruise; a superficial, nonlacerating injury from a blow. ADJ. contusive

convalescence (kŏn'və-lĕs'əns) N. period of recovery from injury, illness, or surgery, generally the time after the crisis has passed until health is regained.

conversion (kən-vûr'zhən) N. unconscious defense mechanism by which emotional conflicts are repressed and turned into physical symptoms having no organic basis (e.g., pain, numbness).

conversion hysteria N. emotional disorder in which emotional conflicts are converted into physical symptoms (e.g., blindness, paralysis, pain). Treatment is by psychotherapy. Also called conversion disorder; conversion reaction.

convolution (kŏn'və-lōō'shən) N. turn, fold, or coil of anything; also, convex fold or ridge in the surface of the brain.

convulsion (kən-vŭl'shən) N. sudden, involuntary, and violent contraction of a group of muscles, sometimes with loss of consciousness. Sometimes called a seizure, it may occur in a seizure disorder (e.g., epilepsy) or after head injury; sometimes caused by high fever in otherwise healthy infants and young children (febrile seizure). Convulsions are also associated with meningitis, brain tumors, and alcohol withdrawal syndrome.

Cooley's anemia (koo′lēz) *See* THALASSEMIA.

coordination (kō-ôr′dn-ā′shən) N. working together of parts in performing a function, esp. of the muscles in body movements.

COPD *See* CHRONIC OBSTRUCTIVE PULMONARY DISEASE.

coping N. adjustment of one's activities to overcome stress in the environment without change in goals.

copper (kŏp′ər) N. metallic element essential to normal body function. *See also* TABLE OF IMPORTANT ELEMENTS.

coprolalia (kŏp′rə-lā′lē-ə) N. repetitive use of obscenities in speech, as may occur involuntarily in Gilles de la Tourette syndrome.

copulation (kŏp′yə-lā′shən) *See* COITUS.

cor pulmonale (kôr) N. enlargement of the heart's right ventricle due to disease of the lungs (e.g., chronic obstructive pulmonary disease, emphysema) or pulmonary vascular system. Symptoms include chronic cough, shortness of breath on exertion, fatigue, and other signs of oxygen lack to the body tissues.

cord (kôrd) N. elongated, flexible part (e.g., the umbilical cord, vocal cords, and spinal cord). ADJ. cordal

Cordarone N. trade name for the antiarrhythmic amiodarone.

corditis N. inflammation of the spermatic cord, caused by infection, hydrocele, tumor, or injury to the groin and characterized by pain and sometimes swelling and tenderness in the testes.

corectopia N. unnatural placement of the pupil of the eye toward one side, rather than the center, of the iris.

Corgard N. trade name for the antihypertensive nadolol.

corium (kôr′ē-əm) N. *See* DERMIS.

corn (kôrn) N. horny mass of epithelial cells overlying a bone, usually on the toes and result-

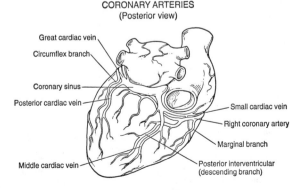

CORONARY ARTERIES
(Posterior view)

Great cardiac vein
Circumflex branch
Coronary sinus
Posterior cardiac vein
Small cardiac vein
Right coronary artery
Marginal branch
Middle cardiac vein
Posterior interventricular
(descending branch)

ing from chronic pressure (e.g., from ill-fitting shoes). Treatment includes paring or peeling of the hard tissue and relief of the pressure.

cornea (kôr′nē-ə) N. outer, transparent portion of the eye, consisting of five layers through which light passes to the retina. ADJ. corneal

corneal transplant (graft) N. replacement of a diseased or damaged cornea with one taken from a donor eye, usually from a person who recently died.

corneum N. outermost, horny layer (stratum corneum) of the skin; upper layer of the epidermis.

cornu N., *pl.* cornua, hornlike part (e.g., the ethmoid cornu of the nose). ADJ. cornual

corona (kə-rō′nə) N., *pl.* coronae, crown or crownlike structure or part, as the enamel covering of a tooth (dental crown). ADJ. coronal (as the coronal suture of the skull).

coronary (kôr′ə-něr′ē) ADJ. surrounding, as a crown, esp. the coronary arteries surrounding the heart. N. *See* MYOCARDIAL INFARCTION.

coronary artery N. one of a pair of arteries that branch from the aorta and supply the heart. Any malfunction or disease of these arteries (coronary atherosclerosis) can seriously affect the heart (e.g., depriving it of necessary oxygen and nutrients).

coronary artery bypass N. type of open-heart surgery in which a section of a blood vessel (e.g., the saphenous vein) is grafted from the aorta onto a coronary artery in an effort to improve the blood supply to the heart by bypassing a diseased or blocked

section of the coronary artery. If effective, better cardiac function and reduced angina should be expected. Depending on the location and severity of the coronary artery disease, the patient's life expectancy may be increased, though the operation does not ensure the prevention of future myocardial infarction. Since grafts have been shown to develop atherosclerosis after several years, the patient must also control any cardiac risk factors that may be present (e.g., smoking, hypertension, diabetes, and elevated cholesterol). Angioplasty techniques have eliminated the need for some of these operations.

CORONARY ARTERY BYPASS

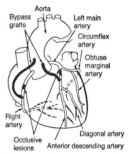

The grafts run from the aorta to the occluded vessel.

coronary artery disease *See* ATHEROSCLEROSIS.

coronary care unit (CCU) N. hospital area specially equipped and staffed to treat patients with serious, life-threatening cardiac problems.

coronary insufficiency N. abnormally limited blood flow through the arteries supplying the heart muscle, which can cause chest pain (angina).

coronary occlusion N. obstruction of a coronary artery, caused by a blood clot or progressive atherosclerosis.

coronary thrombosis N. presence of a blood clot in any of the arteries supplying the heart muscle, thereby obstructing the flow of blood to the heart. *See also* THROMBUS.

coroner (kôr′ə-nər) N. government official who investigates the cause of death in a person, especially if the reason is unclear or potential criminal activity is suspected. Depending on local laws, the coroner may or may not be a physician. The medical examiner is a physician, usually a pathologist, with specific training in death investigation. The coroner and medical examiner may be one individual, or the medical examiner may work for the coroner's office.

corpus (kôr′pəs) N., *pl.* corpora, specialized part that can be distinguished from the surrounding tissues (e.g., corpus callosum, white-matter bridge between the two hemispheres of the brain). ADJ. corporeal

corpus luteum N., *pl.* corpora lutea, so-called yellow body in the ovary; it is endocrine tissue that fills the space left by a released egg and is shed in menstruation if the egg (ovum) is not fertilized but remains to produce progesterone if fertilization occurs.

corpuscle (kôr′pə-səl) N. any small body, esp. a red blood cell (erythrocyte) or a white blood cell (leukocyte). ADJ. corpuscular

correlation N. degree or extent to which two measures (variables) occur together. Statisticians report a correlation (symbol *r*) as ranging from +1.0 (absolute direct agreement) to −1.0 (absolute inverse relationship), with .0 being an uncorrelated, fully random relationship.

cortex (kôr′tĕks′) N. outer part of an organ, esp. that of the brain (cerebral cortex), kidney (renal cortex), or adrenal gland (adrenal cortex) (*compare* MEDULLA). ADJ. cortical

cortic-, cortico- comb. forms indicating an association with an outer covering (cortex) (e.g., corticospinal, pert. to the brain's cortex and the spinal cord).

corticosteroid (kôr′tĭ-kō-stēr′oid′) N. any of a group of hormones, including cortisol and corticosterone and other glucocorticoids as well as mineralocorticoids, produced in the adrenal cortex and important for the metabolism of carbohydrates and proteins, for water and salt balance, and for the function of the cardiovascular system, the kidneys, and other organs. These hormones are also produced synthetically, for use as drugs in the treatment of a very large variety of diseases, including deficiency of natural adrenal production and many inflammatory conditions (e.g., rheumatoid arthritis). Large doses and/or prolonged use of the drugs is associated with many side effects, including increased susceptibility to infection, fluid retention, emotional changes, and peptic ulcer.

corticosterone (kôr′tĭ-kŏs′tə-rōn′) N. hormone of the adrenal cortex that promotes sodium (salt) retention.

corticotropin (kôr′tĭ-kō-trō′pən) *See* ADRENOCORTICOTROPIC HORMONE.

cortisol (kôr′tĭ-sôl′) N. adrenal-cortex hormone used in the treatment of rheumatoid arthritis and other inflammatory conditions; also called hydrocortisone.

cortisone (kôr′tĭ-sōn′) N. hormone of the adrenal cortex that functions in carbohydrate metabolism and which, as a drug, is used to treat inflammatory conditions.

coryza (kə-rī′zə) *See* RHINITIS.

cosmetic surgery (kŏz-mĕt′ĭk) N. any surgical procedure to improve the appearance of a part, esp. to remove scar tissue, a birthmark, or excessive tissue, as on the face (face-lifting) or the nose (rhinoplasty). *See also* PLASTIC SURGERY.

cost-, costi-, costo- comb. forms indicating an association with a rib (e.g., costochondral, pert. to a rib and its cartilage).

costa (kŏs′tə) N., *pl.* costae, one of the 12 pairs of ribs forming the general shape of the chest (thorax). ADJ. costal

costochondritis (kŏs′tō-kŏn-drī′tĭs) N. inflammation at the junction of a rib and its cartilage. Usually viral in nature, this is commonly associated with chest pain (worsened on inspiration) and point tenderness, and may mimic the pain associated with diseases of the heart or lung. Patients with costochrondritis may hyperventilate, leading to a sensation of shortness of breath (dyspnea).

cough (kôf) N. sudden, forceful, and audible expulsion of air from the lungs that clears the air passages of irritants and helps to prevent aspiration of foreign particles into the lungs. It is a common symptom of a cold or other upper respiratory infection, of bronchitis, pneu-

monia, tuberculosis, or other lung disease, and of some forms of heart disease. Treatment depends on the cause; it may include use of antitussives.

Coumadin N. trade name for the anticoagulant warfarin. *See* TABLE OF COMMONLY PRESCRIBED DRUGS—TRADE NAMES.

coumarin N. anticoagulant drug used to prevent and treat a thrombus or embolus.

count (kount) N. numerical indication of the number of items (e.g., blood cells, bacteria) in a particular unit or sample. *See also* BLOOD COUNT.

covalent bond *See* BONDING.

cowpox (kou′pŏks′) N. mild disease characterized by a pustular rash and caused by vaccinia virus transmitted to humans from infected cattle. Cowpox infection confers immunity to smallpox, which is caused by a similar virus. Also called vaccinia.

coxa (kŏk′sə) N., *pl.* coxae, hip, hip joint.

coxsackievirus N. any of a group of viruses that produce a variety of symptoms and diseases including the common cold, meningitis, pericarditis, and myocarditis. Infection occurs primarily in the summer months.

Cozaar N. *See* TABLE OF COMMONLY PRESCRIBED DRUGS—TRADE NAMES.

CPR *See* CARDIOPULMONARY RESUSCITATION.

crab louse N. body louse (*Phthirus pubis*) that infects the hair of the genital region and is often transmitted venereally.

crack N. street term for an illicit preparation of cocaine that is far more potent, addictive, and dangerous than the typical nasally inhaled powder form. Crack has precipitated strokes and heart attacks in young, previously healthy individuals, sometimes resulting in death.

cradle cap N. common dermatitis of infants, characterized by thick, yellow, greasy scales on the scalp. Treatment is by oils and ointments to soften the scalp and by frequent shampoos.

cramp (krămp) N. painful, often spasmodic, uncontrollable tightening of a muscle (e.g., in the calf), usually relieved by pulling the end of the affected part (e.g., the foot) in the opposite direction, stretching the involved muscle; pain resembling a muscular cramp.

crani-, cranio- comb. forms indicating an association with the cranium or skull (e.g., craniocerebral, pert. to the skull and cerebrum).

cranial (krā′nē-əl) ADJ. referring to the head, brain, or portion of the skull bones that encloses the brain.

cranial nerves N. 12 pairs of nerves, each pair having sensory or motor functions, or both, that extend from the brain without passing through the spinal cord. (The eleventh pair arises from both the brain and the upper spinal cord.)

craniotomy (krā′nē-ŏt′ə-mē) N. surgical opening into the skull, performed to control bleeding, remove tumors, or relieve pressure inside the cranium.

cranium (krā′nē-əm) N. skull; specifically the bony enclosure of the brain; it is composed of eight bones (frontal, occipital, sphenoid, ethmoid, two temporal, and two parietal).

creatine (krē′ə-tēn′) N. compound produced in the body and found in muscle and blood, the phosphate form (phosphocreatine) of which is an energy source for muscle flexion.

creatinine (krē-ăt′n-ēn′) N. breakdown product of phosphocreatine, an energy source for muscle contraction; small amounts are normally found in the blood and urine. In kidney failure, creatinine abnormally accumulates in the body. *See* CREATINE.

crepitation (krĕp′ĭ-tā′shən) N.
1. grating sound, as made by the rubbing of the ends of a fractured bone.
2. crackling chest sound heard with the stethoscope. ADJ. crepitant

crepitus (krĕp′ĭ-təs) N.
1. noisy release of bowel gas (flatus) from the intestine.
2. grating or crackling sound (crepitation).

cretinism (krēt′n-ĭz′əm) N. severe, congenital hypothyroidism characterized by dwarfism, mental retardation, coarse dry skin and features, and muscular incoordination. It results from thyroid deficiency or inadequate iodine intake by the mother while the fetus is developing. Relatively rare in the United States, the disorder occurs mainly in areas where the diet lacks sufficient iodine and goiter is prevalent.

Creutzfeldt-Jakob disease (kroits′ fĕlt) N. rare, fatal abnormality of the brain; the most likely cause is a prion, an abnormal form of a normal protein known as a cellular prion protein. It typically occurs in middle age, producing symptoms of progressive dementia, difficulty in speech,

CRANIAL NERVES

Number	Name	Type	Function
I	olfactory	sensory	sense of smell
II	optic	sensory	sense of sight
III	oculomotor	motor	eye movements; pupil contractions
IV	trochlear	motor	eye movements
V	trigeminal	motor and sensory	facial sensation; jaw motions
VI	abducens	motor	eye movements
VII	facial	motor and sensory	facial expression; sense of taste
VIII	vestibulocochlear (auditory)	sensory	balance; sense of hearing
IX	glossopharyngeal	motor and sensory	swallowing; sense of taste
X	vagus	motor and sensory	swallowing; speech; sense of taste
XI	(spinal) accessory	motor	swallowing; speech; head/shoulder movements
XII	hypoglossal	motor	tongue movements; proprioceptors

CRANIAL NERVES

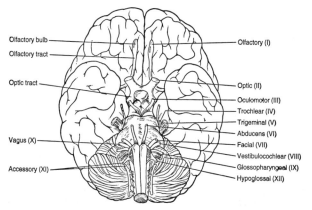

muscle wasting, and involuntary movements, and leading to death, usually within 1 year. *See also* KURU; PRION.

crib death *See* SUDDEN INFANT DEATH SYNDROME.

crisis (krī′sĭs) N., *pl.* crises
1. turning point in a disease, after which the patient either improves or gets worse.
2. turning point in events affecting a person emotionally.

crisis intervention N. in psychiatry, treatment to help resolve an immediate problem or reduce an emotional trauma, the aim being to restore the person to the precrisis level of functioning.

critical (krĭt′ĭ-kəl) ADJ.
1. being in or approaching a state of crisis in a disease.
2. being at risk or in uncertain condition.

Crohn's disease (krōnz) N. chronic inflammatory condition affecting the colon and/or terminal part of the small intestine and producing frequent episodes of diarrhea (the feces are typically nonbloody and semisoft), abdominal pain, nausea, fever, weakness, and weight loss. Treatment is by anti-inflammatory agents; antibiotics, if necessary, to control infection; and adequate nutrition. Also called regional enteritis. (*Compare* ULCERATIVE COLITIS.)

cromolyn N. inhaled powder (trade name Intal) used in the long-term treatment of asthma; use during an acute attack may markedly aggravate the patient's condition.

crossed eye *See* STRABISMUS.

crossmatching N. procedure used by blood banks to determine the compatibility of a donor's blood with that of a potential transfusion recipient after initial typing has been done.

croup (kro͞op) N. disease of infants and young children, characterized by harsh coughing, hoarseness, fever, and difficulty in breathing, usually due to viral infection. Mild cases can be relieved by the use of vaporizers, humidifiers, or steam from hot running water (to relieve spasm of muscles in the larynx), but children with high fever or severe respiratory distress should be hospitalized. ADJ. croupy

crus (kro͞os, krŭs) N., *pl.* crura, leg from the knee to the foot. ADJ. crural

crutch (krŭch) N. wooden or metal staff, usually reaching from the ground almost to the armpit, used as an aid in walking (e.g., with a broken leg).

cry-, cryo- comb. forms indicating an association with cold (e.g., cryogen, chemical that freezes and destroys diseased tissue).

cryesthesia (krī′ĭs-thē′zhə) N. hypersensitivity to cold.

cryoanesthesia (krī′ō-ăn′ĭs-thē′zhə) N. insensibility resulting from deep cold.

cryocautery (krī′ō-kô′tə-rē) N.
1. instrument for destroying tissue by freezing it.
2. application of a substance (e.g., carbon dioxide) that freezes and destroys tissue.

cryoglobulin (krī′ō-glŏb′yə-lĭn) N. abnormal protein that separates from a solution (precipitates), such as blood, when cooled and dissolves when reheated to body temperature. Cryoglobulins are found in the blood in conjunction with certain tumors, as well as some types of pneumonia.

cryopreservation (krī′ō-prĕz′ər-vā′shən) N. preserving of any body tissue or fluid at low temperature so that it may be used again in the future. Commonly used to preserve sperm for artificial insemination procedures.

cryosurgery (krī′ō-sûr′jə-rē) N. use of extreme cold (e.g., liquid nitrogen) to destroy unwanted tissue (e.g., warts, cataracts, skin cancer). The cooling agent is applied by means of a metal probe; temperatures as low as −160°C can be achieved.

crypt (krĭpt) N. pocketlike structure, as in a part with deep indentations.

cryptococcosis (krĭp′tə-kŏ-kō′sĭs) N. disease, caused by the fungus *Cryptococcus neoformans,* in which jellylike nodules develop in internal tissues, often first in the lungs, causing coughing; and then spreading to the nervous system, causing headache and visual and speech difficulties. In North America, middle-aged men in the southeastern states are the prime victims. Treatment is by antifungal agents.

cryptorchidism (krĭp-tôr′kĭ-dĭz′əm) N. failure of one or both testes to move into the scrotum as the male fetus develops; also called cryptorchidy, cryptorchism; undescended testis. ADJ. cryptorchid

C-section *See* CESAREAN SECTION.

CSF *See* CEREBROSPINAL FLUID.

CT *See* COMPUTED TOMOGRAPHY.

Cu symbol for the element copper.

cubitus (kyōō′bĭ-təs) N.
1. elbow.

2. arm from the elbow to the fingertips. ADJ. cubital

cuboid bone N. tarsal (ankle) bone on the lateral side of the foot.

cul-de-sac N. one-entry, pouchlike structure; blind pouch (e.g., the appendix).

culdoscopy (kŭl-dŏs′kə-pē) N. technique for visually examining the pelvic organs of a woman by insertion of a culdoscope (special instrument) through the vagina; *compare* LAPAROSCOPY.

culture (kŭl′chər) N. deliberate growing of microorganisms in a solid or liquid medium (e.g. agar, gelatin), as of bacteria in a Petri dish.

cuneus N. wedge-shaped part of the back lobe of the brain.

cunnilingus (kŭn′ə-lĭng′gəs) N. stimulation of the female genitalia with the mouth and tongue.

cupping (kŭp′ĭng) *See* TABLE OF ALTERNATIVE MEDICINE TERMS.

cupula N. part shaped like a small inverted cup (e.g., cupula pleurae, roof of the pleural cavity).

curanderismo *See* TABLE OF ALTERNATIVE MEDICINE TERMS.

curare (kōō-rä′rē) N. substance, derived from the tropical Strychnos plant, that is a powerful muscle relaxant used as an adjunct to anesthesia; in large doses it may cause paralysis and death.

curet N. scoop-shaped instrument used to remove material from a surface or cavity (e.g., the uterus) by scraping; also called curette.

curettage (kyōōr′ĭ-täzh′) N. scraping of a cavity, esp. the inside of the uterus or other surface, either to remove a tumor or other unwanted material or to obtain a sample of tissue for analysis. *See also* DILATATION AND CURETTAGE.

curvature (kûr'və-choŏr') N. outline of a part or structure, esp. the spinal column, that is not in a straight line.

Cushing's disease (koŏsh'ĭngz) N. disorder in which excessive secretion of adrenocorticotropic hormone (ACTH) by the pituitary (due, e.g., to a tumor) causes increased secretion of hormones by the adrenal cortex, leading to fat deposition on the face, back, and chest; edema; high blood sugar levels; muscle weakness; and increased susceptibility to infection. Treatment involves removal of ACTH-secreting tissue in the pituitary or, if this is not possible, removal of the adrenal glands. Also called hyperadrenalism. (*Compare* CUSHING'S SYNDROME.)

Cushing's syndrome N. disorder caused by excessive cortisol; symptoms include a moon face, mental or emotional disturbances, high blood pressure, weight gain, and, in women, abnormal growth of facial and body hair. The syndrome may be due to overproduction of cortisol by the adrenal glands or by prolonged administration of certain drugs. Also called hyperadrenocorticism. (*Compare* CUSHING'S DISEASE.)

cusp (kŭsp) N.
1. tapered point, esp. those on the tops of the teeth.
2. any of the small flaps or leaflike divisions of the valves of the heart. ADJ. cuspid

cutaneous (kyoō-tā'nē-əs) ADJ. pert. to the skin.

cuticle (kyoō'tĭ-kəl) N.
1. layer of skin at the base of the nail.
2. epidermis.

cutis (kyoō'tĭs) *See* SKIN.

CVA *See* CEREBROVASCULAR ACCIDENT.

cyan-, cyano- comb. forms indicating blueness (e.g., cyanoderma, bluish discoloration of the skin).

cyanide poisoning (sī'ə-nīd') N. poisoning from the ingestion or inhalation of cyanide (found in bitter almond oil and wild cherry syrup; common in smoke from fires and as an industrial chemical); causes rapid heart rate, drowsiness, convulsions, and frequently death within 15 minutes. Treatment involves oxygen and a specific group of antidotes.

cyanocobalamin (sī'ə-nō'kō-băl'ə-mĭn) N. vitamin of the B-complex group essential for normal metabolism, nerve function, and blood formation; rich sources are liver, kidney, eggs, and other meats and dairy products; used to prevent and treat pernicious anemia and certain other anemias. Also called vitamin B_{12}; antipernicious anemia factor.

cyanosis (sī'ə-nō'sĭs) N. bluish discoloration of the skin and mucous membranes, occurring when the oxygen in the blood is sharply diminished, as in asphyxia. ADJ. cyanotic

cycle (sī'kəl) N. series of steps or events that occur regularly (e.g., the menstrual cycle). ADJ. cyclic

cyclic adenosine monophosphate (sik-lik ə-děn-ə sēn mono-fäs-fāt) *See* CYCLIC AMP.

cyclic AMP (cAMP; cyclic adenosine monophosphate) N. small, ring-shaped molecule derived from adenosine triphosphate (ATP). Acts as a chemical signal, termed a second messenger, for intracellular signal transduction, such as transferring the effects of hormones like glucagon and adrenaline, which cannot get through the cell membrane. It is one of the most common second messengers in the body, mediating a large number of biochemical reactions, as well as the actions of numerous medications. *See also* SECOND MESSENGER; SIGNAL TRANSDUCTION.

cyclobenzaprine (sī′klō-bĕn′zə-prēn′) N. *See* TABLE OF COMMONLY PRESCRIBED DRUGS—GENERIC NAMES.

cyclopia (sī-klō′pē-ə) N. developmental abnormality in which there is only one eye.

cyclopropane N. flammable anesthetic gas that provides good anesthesia and skeletal muscle relaxation with minimal side effects, but has been largely replaced by safer, nonflammable anesthetic agents.

cyproheptadine (sī′prō-hĕp′tə-dēn′) N. antihistamine (trade name Periactin) used to treat some allergic reactions. Adverse effects include drowsiness, dry mouth, rapid heart rate, and hypersensitivity reactions.

cyst (sĭst) N.
  1. closed, fluid-filled sac embedded in tissue (as in the breast) that is abnormal or results from disease.
  2. anatomically normal sac (e.g., the gallbladder or the dacrocyst, the tear sac in the eye).

cyst-, cysti-, cysto- comb. forms indicating an association with a cyst or with the bladder (e.g., cystolith, stone in the bladder).

cysteine (sĭs′tē-ēn′) N. essential (not produced by the body, required in the diet) amino acid.

cystic breast disease *See* FIBROCYSTIC DISEASE OF THE BREAST.

cystic duct (sĭs′tĭk) N. tube that carries bile from the gallbladder toward the intestine; it joins with the hepatic duct from the liver to form the common bile duct, which empties into the duodenum.

cystic fibrosis N. inherited disease, usually recognized in infancy or early childhood, in which the glands, esp. those of the pancreas, lungs, and intestines, become clogged with thick mucus. The sweat is typically salty, containing high levels of sodium and chloride. Respiratory infections are common and can lead to death. Life expectancy has improved markedly, and many victims now reach adulthood. Also called fibrocystic disease of the pancreas; mucoviscidosis.

cystic mastitis *See* FIBROCYSTIC BREAST DISEASE.

cystitis (sĭ-stī′tĭs) N. inflammation of the urinary bladder and ureters, characterized by pain, urgency and frequency of urination, and blood in the urine. More common in women, it may be caused by bacterial infection, stones, tumor, or trauma. Treatment depends on the cause and may include increased fluid intake and antibiotics.

cystocele (sĭs′tə-sēl′) N. condition, sometimes occurring after childbirth, in which the urinary bladder bulges through the wall of the vagina.

cystogram (sĭs′tə-grăm′) N. X ray of the bladder, usually obtained following injection of contrast media through a catheter placed into the bladder via the urethra.

cystoplegia (sĭs-tə-plē′jē-ə) N. bladder paralysis.

cystoscopy (sĭ-stŏs′kə-pē) N. examination of the urinary bladder by means of an instrument (cytoscope) inserted into it through the urethra.

cyt-, cyto- comb. forms indicating an association with a cell (e.g., cytocide, substance that destroys cells).

cytochromes (sī′tə-krōmz′) N. iron-containing proteins found in human cells; involved in cellular metabolism.

cytogenesis (sī′tō-jĕn′ĭ-sĭs) N. developmental process in cell formation.

cytogenetics N. study of cell formation, structure, and function (cytology) as it relates to heredity (genetics). Modern techniques have proven that genetic information is carried on chromosomes, which contain genes (codes for individual characteristics). On a molecular basis, genes are made up of deoxyribonucleic acid (DNA). Cytogenetic techniques employed

on amniotic fluid are frequently used to diagnose fetal abnormalities within the first few weeks of gestation.

cytology (sī-tŏl′ə-jē) N. science of cells, their development and functions. ADJ. cytologic

cytolysis (sī-tŏl′ĭ-sĭs) N. breakdown of cells, esp. by the destruction of the cell's outer membrane.

cytomegalovirus (CMV) (sī′tə-mĕg′ə-lō-vī′rəs) N. any of a group of herpes viruses that normally produce disease only in humans with impaired or immature immune systems, including newborns, those being treated with immunosuppressive drugs (e.g., transplant patients), and those with acquired immune deficiency syndrome (AIDS).

cytoplasm (sī′tə-plăz′əm) N. all of the substance of a cell outside the nucleus. ADJ. cytoplasmic

cytotoxic (sī-tə-tŏk′sĭk) ADJ. pert. to the destruction of cells.

cytotoxic drug N. drug commonly used in chemotherapeutic treatment of cancer to inhibit the proliferation of cells.

D

D and C N. *See* DILATATION AND CURETTAGE.

D vitamin N. several chemicals (e.g., calciferol) contained naturally in fish-liver oil and egg yolk, and essential to health, esp. the absorption of calcium and phosphorus. *See also* VITAMIN; TABLE OF VITAMINS.

dacry-, dacryo- comb. forms indicating an association with tears (e.g., dacryorrhea, excessive flow of tears).

dacryocystitis (dăk′rē-ō-sĭ-stī′tĭs) N. inflammation of the lacrimal sac (tear sac), due to obstruction of the tube draining the tears into the nose and characterized by tearing and discharge from the eye. Treatment is by antibiotics.

dacryopyosis (dăk′rē-ō-pī-ō′sĭs) N. condition in which pus is present in the tear duct or gland.

dactyl (dăk′təl) N. finger or toe.

dactyl-, dactylo- comb. forms indicating an association with the fingers or toes (e.g., dactyledema, excessive fluid in a finger, causing it to puff up).

dactylomegaly (dăk′tə-lō-měg′ə-lē) N. abnormally large fingers and/or toes.

Dalmane N. trade name for the sedative-hypnotic flurazepam hydrochloride.

Daltonism N. sex-linked, inherited form of color blindness characterized by inability to distinguish red from green. *See also* COLOR BLINDNESS.

dander (dăn′dər) N. small scales from animal skins or hair or bird feathers, which may cause an allergic reaction in some persons.

dandruff (dăn′drəf) N. condition in which scales of white flaky or grayish waxy material (dead skin) are shed by the scalp. Treatment involves regular use of a detergent shampoo.

dapsone (dăp′sōn′) N. drug used to treat leprosy and certain skin disorders.

dark adaptation (därk) reflex changes in the eye to allow vision in decreased light (e.g., in dim light after being in normal light); it involves a dilation of the pupil so that more light enters (*compare* LIGHT ADAPTATION).

Darvocet N. trade name for a fixed-combination drug containing the pain-reliever and fever-reducer acetaminophen and the pain reliever propoxyphene hydrochloride (Darvon).

Darvocet N N. *See* TABLE OF COMMONLY PRESCRIBED DRUGS—TRADE NAMES.

Darvon (där′vŏn) N. trade name for the widely used prescription analgesic propoxyphene hydrochloride.

Darvon compound N. trade name for a fixed-combination prescription analgesic containing propoxyphene hydrochloride, aspirin, and caffeine; it is used to treat mild to moderate pain.

Datril N. trade name for the pain-reliever and fever-reducer acetaminophen.

day blindness *See* HEMERALOPIA.

Daypro N. trade name for the anti-inflammatory drug, oxaprozin. *See* TABLE OF COMMONLY PRESCRIBED DRUGS—TRADE NAMES.

deaf (dĕf) ADJ. unable to hear.

deafness (dĕf′nĭs) N. partial or complete loss of hearing in one or both ears, caused by the absence or incomplete development of the ear, the auditory nerve, or parts of the brain, by damage to the hearing apparatus (e.g., from infection or injury); or by degeneration (from aging) of the hearing apparatus. In assessing deafness, the degree of hearing loss, the types of sounds that can be discriminated, and the cause of the impairment generally classified as conductive hearing loss or sensorineural hearing loss are determined; treatment depends on these findings and may involve the use of a hearing aid.

death (dĕth) N. state of the body in which brain function ceases and heart function can be maintained only artificially; the state at which loss of brain and heart function is not reversible. In brain death, which has recently become of legal importance, normal reflexes (e.g., respiration) are absent and consciousness cannot be recovered; organs may then be removed for transplantation before the heartbeat has stopped.

death instinct N. in psychoanalytic (Freudian) theory, unconscious urge to die.

death wish N. desire, conscious or unconscious, for oneself or another to die.

debility (dĭ-bĭl′ĭ-tē) N. weakness, lack of strength.

debridement (dā′brēd-män′, dĭ-brēd′mənt) N. removal of non-healthy tissue and foreign material from a wound or burn to prevent infection and permit healing.

Decadron N. trade name for the corticosteroid dexamethasone.

decalcification N. loss of calcium from bone or teeth.

decay (dĭ-kā′) N.
1. gradual breakdown of dead tissue or other dead organic material, due to the action of microorganisms.
2. process of decline or aging.

decerebrate N. person subjected to cutting of the spinal cord at the level of the brainstem, usually as a result of severe trauma; also refers to body position assumed by patients with severe brain damage (decerebrate rigidity or posturing) with the extremities stiff and extended, and the head retracted; opposite is decorticate rigidity with arms flexed, fists clenched, and legs extended.

decibel N. unit of measurement expressing the intensity or loudness of sound relative to that of a standard; intensity of sound in bels is the logarithm of the ratio

DECIBEL

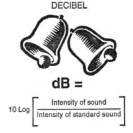

$$dB = 10 \, Log \left[\frac{\text{Intensity of sound}}{\text{Intensity of standard sound}} \right]$$

of the intensity of that sound and a standard sound. A decibel (dB) is one-tenth of a bel.

decidua (dĭ-sĭj′o͞o-ə) N. epithelial tissue of the endometrium, the lining of the uterus, that is shed in menstruation and after the birth of a baby. ADJ. decidual, deciduous

deciduoma (dĭ-sĭj′o͞o-ō′mə) N. tumor of the uterus consisting of decidual tissue; may be benign or malignant.

deciduous tooth (dĭ-sĭj′o͞o-əs) N. any of the 20 teeth that appear during infancy and early childhood and are later shed, generally between the ages of 6 and 13, to be replaced by the permanent teeth; also called milk tooth; primary tooth.

decoagulant N. *See* ANTICOAGULANT.

decompensation (dē′kŏm-pən-sā′shən) N. process of deterioration from a healthier to a less healthy state; often used in reference to chronic congestive heart failure when the patient is no longer able to maintain normal cardiac function, despite medications and restriction of activity. Persons with severely decompensated heart failure may require heart transplantation to survive.

decomposition (dē-kŏm′pə-zĭsh′ən) N. normal decay process of dead tissue. In plants, this is often referred to as rotting. The formal term for human and animal tissue is putrefaction.

decompression sickness (dē′kəm-prĕsh′ən) *See* BENDS.

decongestant (dē′kən-jĕs′tənt) N. drug (e.g., phenylephrine) that reduces congestion; decongestants may be applied as nasal sprays or drops or taken by mouth.

decorticate ADJ. position assumed by patients with severe brain damage (decorticate rigidity or posturing) with arms flexed, fists clenched, and legs extended; opposite is decerebrate rigidity with the extremities stiff and extended, and the head retracted.

decortication (dē-kôr′tĭ-kā′shən) N. removal of all or part of the outer layer (cortex) of an organ or structure.

decrudescence (dē′kro͞o-des′əns) N. lessening of the severity of symptoms.

decubitus (dĭ-kyo͞o′bĭ-təs) N. reclining position, as in a bed.

decubitus ulcer N. inflammation or sore on the skin over a bony prominence (e.g., shoulder blade, elbow, hip, buttocks, heel), resulting from prolonged pressure on the area, usually from being confined to bed. Most frequently seen in elderly and immobilized persons, decubitus ulcers may be prevented by frequent change of position, early ambulation, cleanliness, and use of skin lubricants and a water or air mattress; once present, the ulcers must be washed and dried carefully, and a sterile dressing with moisturizing oil applied; if severe, debridement and drainage may be necessary. Also called bedsore; pressure sore.

decussation (dĕk′ə-sā′shən) N. natural crossing over of fibers, esp. nerve fibers, or other parts from opposite sides of the body, to form an X shape.

defecation (def-ĕ-kā′shŭn) N. passage of feces out of the body; bowel movement.

defecation reflex *See* RECTAL REFLEX.

defect (dē′fĕkt′) (dĭ-fĕkt′) N. abnormality, either the absence of a part, ability, or function or its imperfect presence. A congenital defect is an imperfection, not necessarily inherited, present at birth.

defense (dĭ-fĕns′) N. ability to resist or impede an attack of disease infection, or other phenomenon.

defense mechanism N. psychological, unconscious reaction or process for avoiding or controlling anxiety and emotional conflict. *See also* COMPENSATION.

defervescence (dē′fər-vĕs′əns) N. time that marks the decline of fever to normal temperature. ADJ. defervescent

defibrillation (dē-fĭb′rə-lā′shən) N. stopping, usually by electric shock, of heart muscle contractions that are out of normal rhythm (are fibrillating). In this common emergency procedure, a defibrillator delivers an electric shock (of preset voltage) to the heart through the chest wall in an attempt to restore normal heart rhythm. *See* VENTRICULAR TACHYCARDIA, VENTRICULAR FIBRILLATION. *Compare* CARDIOVERSION.

defibrillator (dē-fĭb′rə-lā′tər) N. electronic device used to apply electrical shocks to the heart via paddles or pads placed on the patient's chest (defibrillation); used in the treatment of ventricular tachycardia and ventricular fibrillation. During cardioversion, the same device is employed, but utilized in a different manner. *See* CARDIOVERSION.

deficiency disease (dĭ-fĭsh′ən-sē) N. any disease resulting from lack of a vitamin, mineral, or other essential nutrient. Scurvy, rickets, and night blindness are examples of deficiency diseases. *See also* TABLE OF IMPORTANT ELEMENTS; TABLE OF VITAMINS.

deficit (dĕf′ĭ-sĭt) N. reduction, from the normal level, in the amount of a substance or in a level of function (e.g., oxygen deficit, a condition caused by strenuous exercise, that exists in cells during temporary oxygen shortage).

deformity (dĭ-fôr′mĭ-tē) N. condition in which the body in general or any part of it (e.g., the hand) is misshapen, distorted, or malformed. A deformity may result from injury, disease, or birth defect (e.g., Arnold-Chiari deformity, in which part of the brain protrudes through the skull).

degeneration (dĭ-jĕn′ə-rā′shən) N. physical and/or mental decline that involves tissue and cellular changes and the loss of specialized function; the extreme result is death of the parts involved and loss of their function. ADJ. degenerative

degenerative disorder (dĭ-jĕn′ər-ə-tĭv) N. any of several conditions that lead to progressive loss of function (e.g., chorea, Parkinsonism).

deglutition (dē′gloo-tĭsh′ən) N. process of swallowing.

degustation (dē′gŭ-stā′shən) N. *see* GUSTATION.

dehiscence (dē-hĭs′əns) N. splitting open of an organ, part, or surgical wound.

dehydration (dē′hī-drā′shən) N. extreme loss of water from the body tissues, often accompanied by imbalance of sodium, potassium, chloride, and other electrolytes in the body. Dehydration may occur in prolonged diarrhea, vomiting, or perspiration and is of more concern in infants and young children. Symptoms include thirst, dry skin, cracked lips, and dry mouth. Treatment involves restoring the fluid and electrolyte balance either by having the person drink liquids or by the intravenous administration of water and salts.

déjà vu (dā′zhä vü′) N. sense that what one is seeing or experiencing has been encountered before, when actually it has not. Déjà vu occurs in normal persons but it is more frequent in certain disorders (e.g., some forms of epilepsy). (*Compare* JAMAIS VU.)

delirium (dĭ-lēr′ē-əm) N. state, usually brief, of incoherent excitement, confused speech, restlessness, and hallucinations. It may occur in high fever, ingestion of certain toxic substances and drugs, nutritional deficiencies, endocrine imbalance, or severe stress (e.g., postoperative) or mental illness. Treatment includes bed rest, quiet, the use of drugs to quiet the patient, and treatment of the underlying cause. (*Compare* DEMENTIA.) ADJ. delirious

delirium tremens (DTs) (trē′mənz) N. acute and severe (15% mortality) physical and mental disturbance caused by withdrawal from alcohol use after prolonged drinking. Symptoms include loss of appetite and restlessness, followed by excitement, disorientation, sweating, shaking, anxiety, extreme perspiration, and terrifying hallucinations. The acute episode is a true medical emer-gency. Treatment includes hospitalization, sedative drugs (often in high doses), adequate fluid and nutritional supplementation, and vitamins. *See also* KORSAKOFF'S PSYCHOSIS.

delivery (dĭ-lĭv′ə-rē) N. in obstetrics, birth of a child.

delta rhythm (dĕl′tə) N. brainwave frequency of high voltage that is characteristic of dreamless, deep sleep from which an individual is not easily aroused; also called delta wave. It is the slowest of the four brainwave patterns (*compare* ALPHA RHYTHM; BETA RHYTHM; THETA RHYTHM).

Deltasone N. *See* TABLE OF COMMONLY PRESCRIBED DRUGS— TRADE NAMES.

deltoid muscle N. large, thick, triangular muscle that covers the shoulder and is involved in arm movements.

DELTOID MUSCLE

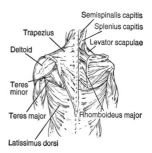

delusion (dĭ-loo′zhən) N. false belief; a continuing irrational idea that cannot be changed by logical argument. Delusions common in mental illness include delusion of grandeur, of persecution by others, and of affliction with disease. ADJ. delusional

demand feeding (dǐ-mǎnd′) N. giving food to a baby or animal whenever it shows a need, in contrast to schedule feeding, in which feedings are given according to a fixed, preset schedule (e.g., every 4 hours).

dementia (dǐ-měn′shə) N. progressive state of mental decline, esp. of memory function and judgment, often accompanied by disorientation, stupor, and disintegration of the personality. It may be caused by certain metabolic diseases, drug intoxication, or injury, in which cases it is often reversible once the underlying cause is treated. If, however, it is caused by a disease such as Alzheimer's disease, by brain injury, or by degeneration brought about by aging (senile dementia), the changes that occur are irreversible. (*Compare* DELIRIUM.)

dementia praecox N. obsolete term for schizophrenia.

Demerol (děm′ə-rôl′) N. trade name for the prescription narcotic analgesic meperidine.

demineralization N. loss of mineral salts, esp. from bone, as can occur in hyperparathyroidism and osteomalacia.

demulcent (dǐ-mŭl′sənt) N. oil, salve, or other agent that soothes and relieves skin discomfort.

Demulen N. trade name for an oral contraceptive.

demyelination (dē-mī′ə-lə-nā′shən) N. process of destruction or removal of the myelin covering of some nerve fibers, resulting in their impaired function; it occurs in multiple sclerosis and some other disorders.

dendrite (děn′drīt′) N. one of the branching processes or treelike parts of a nerve cell that conveys impulses to the nerve cell body (*compare* AXON). ADJ. dendritic

dengue (děng′gē) N. virus-caused disease, rare in the United States, that is transmitted by the Aedes mosquito mostly in tropical and subtropical areas; it is marked by fever, muscle and joint pain, headache, and rash. Symptoms recur after a brief interval and the patient may require some time to recover.

dens N. upward bony protrusion (odontoid process) of the second cervical vertebra (axis) towards the first (atlas); this articulation forms the joint about which the head rotates, as when saying no.

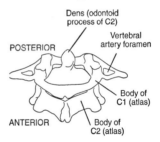

C2

Dens (odontoid process of C2)

Vertebral artery foramen

POSTERIOR

Body of C1 (atlas)

ANTERIOR　　Body of C2 (atlas)

density N. degree of compactness or relative weight of a substance compared with a reference standard; in radiology, the ability of a material to absorb X rays. Materials that are radiodense or radiopaque absorb much X ray, allowing very little to pass through to the film. They appear as white shadows on standard X-ray films. Radiolucent materials have low X-ray density, permitting many X rays to pass and strike the film. They appear as darker shadows on standard films.

dent-, denta-, denti-, dento- comb. forms indicating an association with the teeth (e.g., dentalgia, toothache).

dental (dĕn′tl) ADJ. pert. to a tooth or teeth.

dental caries *See* CARIES.

dentin (dĕn′tĭn) N. bonelike major tissue found in a tooth, covering the pulp and being itself covered by the enamel above the gums; also called dentine.

dentition (dĕn-tĭsh′ən) N.
1. development and eruption of teeth (*see* TEETHING).
2. number, type, and arrangement of teeth in the mouth.

denture (dĕn′chər) N. manufactured, removable replacement for one or more natural teeth; also called plate.

denudation (dē′nōo-dā′shən) N. removal of a layer or cover through surgery, disease, or trauma; often used in reference to the skin. Severe skin infections may cause loss or sloughing of skin; the affected area is said to be denuded. A person without protective gear who falls off a motorcycle may denude portions of the body. Sometimes, a superficial layer of skin is removed by sandpaper or chemical means to treat acne or remove a tatoo (dermabrasion).

deossification (dē-ŏs′ə-fĭ-kā′ shən) N. loss or removal of the mineral content of bone tissue.

deoxyribonucleic acid (DNA) (dē-äk-si-rī-bō-nōo-kla-ik) N. large molecule shaped like a double helix and found primarily in the chromosomes of the cell nucleus; it contains the genetic information of the cell. The genetic information is coded in the sequence of sub-units (nucleotides) making up the DNA molecule. Nucleotides contain one of four bases (adenine, guanine, cytosine, or thymine), a sugar (deoxyribose), and a phosphate (phosphorus-containing) group; they are held together by hydrogen bonds. *See also* GENE; HYDROGEN BONDS.

THE DOUBLE HELIX STRUCTURE OF THE DNA MOLECULE

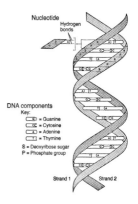

Nucleotide
Hydrogen bonds

DNA components
Key:
Guanine
Cytosine
Adenine
Thymine
S = Deoxyribose sugar
P = Phosphate group

Strand 1   Strand 2

Depakote N. *See* TABLE OF COMMONLY PRESCRIBED DRUGS—TRADE NAMES.

dependence (dĭ-pĕn′dəns) N. state in the habitual use of a drug or other product at which adverse symptoms result upon withdrawal from use. Dependence may be physical (caused by habitual use of, e.g., alcohol or heroin) in which case withdrawal symptoms may include sweating, nausea and vomiting, or tremors; or psychological (involving repeated use of tobacco or some soft drugs, such as amphetamines), in which case withdrawal may cause restlessness, sleeplessness, or depression. ADJ. dependent

depersonalization (dē-pûr′sə-nə-lĭ-zā′shən) N. sense of dreamlike unreality and a loss of the sense of one's own identity, often resulting from stress or anxiety.

depilatory (dĭ-pĭl′ə-tôr′ē) N. chemical or other agent that removes hair. ADJ. depilatory

depolarization (dē-pō′lər-ĭ-zā′shən) N. loss, reduction, or change in the chemical or electrical polarity of a part such as occurs in the transmission of an impulse along a nerve or muscle fiber. *See* ACTION POTENTIAL, RESTING POTENTIAL.

depressant (dĭ-prĕs′ənt) N. drug that decreases or slows the function or activity of a body part or system (e.g., a cardiac depressant slows the heartbeat).

depressed fracture (dĭ-prĕst′) *See* FRACTURE.

depression (dĭ-prĕsh′ən) N.
1. in anatomy, hollow or depressed area, downward placement.
2. in physiology, decrease in function or activity.
3. in psychology, dejected state of mind with feelings of sadness, discouragement, and hopelessness, often accompanied by reduced activity and ability to function, unresponsiveness, apathy, and sleep disturbances. The condition may be mild and temporary, a sign of emotional disorder, or severe and long-lasting, a sign of serious psychosis. Treatment depends on the severity of the condition and may include psychotherapy, antidepressants, and occasionally electroconvulsive therapy. Evidence indicates that a tendency toward some forms of depression may be inherited.

derangement (dĭ-rānj′mənt) N. disturbance of the mind or body; in orthopedics, refers to disruption of the normal relationships between joint structures (e.g., internal derangement of the knee).

dereism N. fantasy state in which thinking is removed from reality and logic, sometimes manifested in severe form in schizophrenia. ADJ. dereistic

derm-, derma-, dermo-, dermato- comb. forms indicating an association with the skin (e.g., dermovascular, pert. to blood vessels of the skin).

derma (dûr′mə) N. *See* SKIN. ADJ. dermal

dermabrasion (dûr′mə-brā′zhən) N. removal of scars, tattoos, and other marks by sanding or wire-brushing off some of the outer skin layer while the skin surface is anesthetized.

dermatitis (dûr′mə-fī′tĭs) N. acute or chronic inflammation of the skin, which becomes red and itchy and may develop blisters or other eruptions. There are many causes, including allergy, disease (e.g., eczema), and infection. Treatment depends on the cause.

dermatoglyphics N. study of the patterns of lines (as whorls, loops, and arches in the fingertips, forming the fingerprints) on the hands and feet, which are unique to each person. Of interest to criminologists, these patterns are also significant in the study of genetic disorders.

dermatologist (dûr′mə-tŏl′ə-jist) N. physician who specializes in dermatology.

dermatology (dûr′mə-tŏl′ə-jē) N. medical specialty concerned with the skin and its development, function, diseases, and treatment. ADJ. dermatologic, dermatological

dermatome (dûr′mə-tōm′) N.
1. surgical instrument for cutting thin slices of tissue for skin graft.
2. area of the skin that receives innervation from a particular portion of the spinal cord.

dermatomycosis (dûr′mə-tō-mī-kō′sĭs) N. fungus infection of the skin, esp. on moist parts protected by clothing, as the groin or feet (e.g., athlete's foot); also called dermatophytosis.

dermatosis (dûr′mə-tō′sĭs) N. disorder of the skin, esp. one in which there is no inflammation (e.g., occupational dermatosis, skin disease caused by exposure to irritants on the job).

dermis (dûr′mĭs) N. layer of skin below the epidermis; it consists of several layers and contains blood vessels, lymph vessels, hair follicles, glands, and nerves; also called (colloq.) corium.

dermoid cyst (dûr′moid′) N. tumor, usually benign, with an epithelium-lined wall and a cavity containing fatty material or bits of bone, hair, and cartilage.

DES (dē′ē-ĕs′) *See* DIETHYLSTILBESTEROL.

descending aorta (dĭ-sĕn′dĭng) N. main part of the aorta that runs from the aortic arch into the trunk of the body, consists of the thoracic and abdominal aortas, and from which arteries supplying many parts of the body (e.g., esophagus, ribs, stomach) branch.

descending colon N. that part of the colon extending from the end of the transverse colon on the left side of the abdomen in the region of the spleen downward to the sigmoid colon in the pelvis.

descensus N. fall or drop, as of an organ from its original or normal position (e.g., descensus uteri, dropping of the uterus until it protrudes from the vagina).

desensitization (dē-sĕn′sĭ-tĭ-zā′shən) N.
1. removal of the sensation of pain, as by cutting a nerve.
2. in immunology, relief from an allergic reaction to a specific foreign material (allergen or immunogen), as in desensitizing injections for hay fever sufferers.
3. in psychology, a treatment method for modifying fear-induced behavior, involving a gradual facing of the cause (e.g., being among animals) until it fails to induce fear or anxiety (*compare* RECIPROCAL INHIBITION).

desert rheumatism *See* COCCIDIOMYCOSIS.

desiccation (dĕs′ĭ-kā′shən) N. process of drying, often to an abnormal extent.

desmosome N. thickened patches of cell membranes that bind adjacent cells together.

desquamation (dĕs′kwə-mā′shən) N. normal loss of bits of outer skin in the form of scales.

Desyrel N. trade name for the antidepressant trazodone. *See* TABLE OF COMMONLY PRESCRIBED DRUGS — TRADE NAMES.

detached retina N. separation of the retina from the choroid in the back of the eye, usually resulting from internal changes in the eye, sometimes from severe injury. Symptoms include the sensation of flashing lights as the eye is moved, the appearance of floating spots in front of the eye, and loss of vision in the affected part of the retina. Treatment is by surgery. Also called retinal detachment.

detoxification N.
1. process of removing a poison (toxin) or neutralizing its effect, normally a function of the liver.
2. process of removing the physiological effects of a drug from an addict.

devascularization (dē-văs′kyə-lər-ĭ-zā′shən) N. loss of blood supply, either via surgery, trauma, or disease. Also refers to draining of some blood from an area of the body, as in preparation for surgery, to reduce bleeding.

development (dĭ-vĕl′əp-mənt) N. gradual change from a simple to a more complex level; physical, mental, and emotional changes an individual organism undergoes from its earliest form through its adult form. ADJ. developmental.

developmental age N. measure of a child's developmental progress in, e.g., body size, motor skills, or psychological functioning, expressed as an age. *See also* BONE AGE; CHRONOLOGICAL AGE; MENTAL AGE.

deviant (dē′vē-ənt) ADJ. varying from a normal state, esp. in behavior.

deviated septum N. abnormal shift in position of any wall-like part that separates two chambers, most often referring to the nasal cavity. Deviated nasal septum is a common condition, causing symptoms of obstructed nasal passages, sinusitis, recur-

rent infection, nosebleeds, and difficulty in breathing. Treatment is by surgery.

deviation (dē′vē-ā′shən) N.
1. movement away from a normal course of activity, as an abnormal deflection of the line of sight.
2. in ophthalmology, abnormal position of an eye or the eyes.

dexamethasone (dĕk′sə-mĕth′ə-sōn′) N. corticosteroid drug (trade name Decadron) used to treat allergic reactions and inflammatory conditions. Adverse effects include electrolyte and hormonal imbalances.

Dexedrine (dĕk′sĭ-drĭn) N. trade name for a central nervous system stimulant (dextroamphetamine sulfate) used in the treatment of narcolepsy and some attention deficit disorders; it was formerly used to reduce appetite in the treatment of obesity. Adverse effects include restlessness, increased blood pressure, and other signs of central nervous system excitation, as well as nausea and loss of appetite. It must be used with caution by persons with hypertension, cardiovascular disease, and many other disorders. It is potentially addictive.

dextr-, dextro- comb. forms indicating a position to the right or a right-hand direction, motion, tendency, or relationship (e.g., dextrocerebral, pert. to right-brain-hemisphere dominance) (*compare* LEVO-).

dextrality (dĕk-străl′ĭ-tē) *See* RIGHTHANDEDNESS.

dextrocardia (dĕk′strō-kär′dē-ə) N. condition in which the heart is positioned toward the right side of the chest. This may be a congenital defect, sometimes accompanied by reversal of the arrangement of other body parts (transposition), or it may be caused by disease.

dextrose (dĕk′strōs′) N. simple sugar, also called glucose, used in intravenous feeding; table sugar (sucrose) is broken down to dextrose in the body.

dhobie itch N. skin infection, caused by the fungus *Tinea cruris* and marked by ringed lesions in folds of the skin of the thigh region; it is aggravated by obesity, tight clothing, and warmth. Treatment is by antifungal agents and cold compresses.

di- prefix meaning two (e.g., diphasic, having two phases).

Diabeta N. trade name for the oral antidiabetic glyburide.

diabetes (dī′ə-bē′tĭs) N. either of two disorders—diabetes insipidus and diabetes mellitus. Used alone, the term usually refers to diabetes mellitus.

diabetes insipidus N. uncommon metabolic disorder characterized by extreme thirst and the passing of very large amounts of urine; it is caused by failure of the pituitary gland to produce or secrete sufficient amounts of antidiuretic hormone (ADH, vasopressin) or, less often, by failure of the kidneys to respond to ADH. The pituitary (or kidney) malfunction may be due to trauma, surgery, or lesion, but in many cases the cause is unknown. Treatment is by removal of the underlying cause, if possible, and by administration of vasopressin (ADH) and careful monitoring to prevent dehydration and electrolyte imbalance, esp. in the young. Diabetes insipidus differs from diabetes mellitus in that in the former excessive sugar is not present in the blood or urine. *See also* NEPHROGENIC DIABETES INSIPIDUS.

diabetes mellitus N. complex and chronic disorder of metabolism due either to partial or total lack of insulin secretion by the pancreas (specifically by the beta cells of the islets of Langerhans in the pancreas) or to the inability of insulin to function normally in the body. Symptoms include excessive thirst and urination, weight loss, and the presence of excessive sugar in the urine and the blood. The disease is common, and evidence suggests that the incidence is increasing. There are two major forms: ketoacidosis prone and nonketoacidosis prone. Ketoacidosis prone, or Type I, diabetes was formerly known as juvenile-onset diabetes; Nonketoacidosis prone, or Type II, diabetes, as adult-onset diabetes. Both forms have a hereditary predisposition and are without known cure at the present time. Type I tends to appear at a younger age. Type II disease may be precipitated by obesity, severe stress, pregnancy, menopause, or other factors. Treatment depends on the severity of the disease; mild forms may be managed with diet alone, but other cases require the use of drugs to lower blood sugar levels (oral antidiabetics) or injections of insulin. Severe and/or untreated cases frequently lead to serious complications, including premature atherosclerosis, often affecting the legs and leading to ulcers of the feet, early coronary artery disease; kidney disorders; eye disorders, sometimes leading to blindness; and nerve problems (neuropathy). (*See also* DIABETIC COMA, INSULIN SHOCK.) ADJ. diabetic (as in diabetic diet).

diabetic coma (dī′ə-bĕt′ĭk) N. decreased level of consciousness that can occur in diabetes mellitus as a result of failure to take prescribed insulin or in the presence of some stress (e.g., infection, surgery) that increases the need for insulin. Warning signs include great thirst, headache, nausea, and vomiting. If untreated, the condition can lead to death. Treatment includes the administration of insulin and steps to correct dehydration and electrolyte imbalances. Also called diabetic ketoacidosis. (*Compare* INSULIN SHOCK.)

diagnosis (dī′əg-nō′sĭs) N. identification of a disease or other condition by evaluating the patient's appearance, symptoms, and history; by physical examination; and, if needed, by analyzing the results of laboratory tests (e.g., urinalysis, blood count) and other procedures (e.g., X rays) (*See also* DIFFERENTIAL DIAGNOSIS). ADJ. diagnostic

diagnosis-related groups (DRG) N. federal system of classification of diseases into groups. This is used by Medicare Part A under the prospective payment system to determine the payment to hospitals for inpatient services. *See* TABLE OF MANAGED CARE TERMS.

dialectical behavioral therapy (DBT) N. form of cognitive behavioral therapy developed as a tool for persons with self-harm behaviors such as cutting and suicide attempts, especially in persons with borderline personality disorder. DBT maintains that some people, due to invalidating environments during upbringing and due to biological factors as yet unknown, react abnormally to emotional stimulation. Their level of arousal goes up much more quickly, peaks at a higher level, and takes more time to return to baseline. This explains why borderlines are known for crisis-strewn lives and extreme emotional lability (emotions that shift rapidly). Because of their past invalidation, patients do not have any methods for coping with these sudden, intense surges of emotion. DBT is a method for teaching skills that will help in this task. *See also* BORDERLINE PERSONALITY DISORDER (*compare* COGNITIVE BEHAVIORAL THERAPY).

dialysis (dī-ăl′ĭ-sĭs) N.
1. method, involving a semipermeable membrane, used to separate smaller particles from larger ones in a liquid mixture.
2. medical procedure for filtering waste products from the blood of some kidney-disease patients or for removing poisons or drugs.

Diamox N. trade name for the drug acetazolamide.

diapedesis (dī′ə-pĭ-dē′sĭs) N. passage of blood cells through the intact walls of the vessels that contain them.

diaper rash (dī′ə-pər) N. reddening of the skin and eruption of spots and raised lesions in the diaper area of infants, caused by irritation from ammonia produced by the breakdown of urine or by irritation from feces or warmth. Treatment includes frequent diaper changes; care-

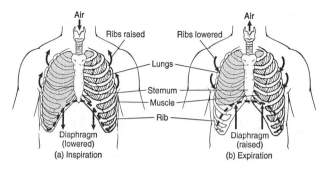

Changes in the volume of the thoracic cavity as the breathing muscles contract and relax

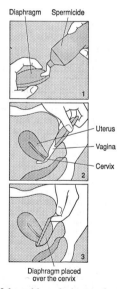

Diaphragm placed over the cervix

ful washing, drying, and ventilation of the affected area, and the use of antimicrobial agents.

diaphoresis (dī′ə-fə-rē′sĭs) N. perspiration, esp. profuse perspiration associated with fever, stress, physical exertion, or exposure to heat. ADJ. diaphoretic

diaphragm (dī′ə-frăm′) N.
1. muscular partition that divides the chest from the abdomen and functions in respiration, moving downward during inspiration (breathing in) to increase the volume of the thoracic (chest) cavity and moving upward during expiration (breathing out) to decrease the volume. During inspiration the diaphram moves downward, as the ribs move forward and outward, enlarging the chest cavity. Air then rushes in. During expiration the diaphragm rises, the chest cavity becomes smaller and air is forced out of the lungs.
2. rubber or plastic dome-shaped cup that fits over the cervix of the uterus and that is used, with spermicidal jelly, as a contraceptive; it acts as a barrier to the passage of spermatozoa upward in the female reproductive tract.

diaphragmatic hernia (dī′ə-frăg-măt′ĭk) See HIATUS HERNIA.

diaphysis (dī-ăf′ĭ-sĭs) N., pl. diaphyses, shaft of a long bone (compare EPIPHYSIS).

diarrhea (dī′ə-rē′ə) N. frequent passage of loose, watery stools (the stools may contain mucus, blood, or excessive fat), sometimes accompanied by nausea, vomiting, abdominal cramps, and feelings of malaise and weakness. Diarrhea may be a symptom of a viral or bacterial infection (mild or severe), food poisoning, disorder of the colon (e.g., colitis), gastrointestinal tumor, metabolic disorder, or other disease. Untreated, it can lead to dehydration, electrolyte imbalance, and weakness. Treatment depends on the cause, but the symptom itself may be treated with an antidiarrheal drug (e.g., Lomotil).

diastole (dī-ăs′tə-lē) N. period between two contractions of the heart, when the chambers widen and fill with blood. On heart muscle contraction (systole), the blood is pumped through the heart and into the arteries. In blood pressure readings, diastole is the second (or lower) number given. ADJ. diastolic

diathermy (dī′ə-thûr′mē) N. use of high-frequency, ultrasound or microwaves to raise the temperature of a part of the body (e.g., the arm); sometimes used to treat deep-seated pain.

diazepam (dī-ăz′ə-păm′) N. minor tranquilizer (trade name Valium) used to treat anxiety and tension and as a skeletal muscle relaxant in cases of muscle spasm, and as an anticonvulsant in some cases of epilepsy; it is commonly prescribed for many conditions. The drug may cause drowsiness and fatigue, and withdrawal symptoms may occur after discontinuance of prolonged or high-dosage use. *See* TABLE OF COMMONLY PRESCRIBED DRUGS—GENERIC NAMES.

Dick test (dĭk) N. skin test for determining susceptibility to scarlet fever. The toxin responsible for scarlet fever is injected through the skin; if an inflammation appears, the person is not immune to the disease.

diclofenac sodium N. anti-inflammatory drug used in the treatment of arthritis and ankylosing spondylitis; side effects include stomach irritation and intestinal bleeding.

dicloxacillin N. antibacterial drug used to treat staphylococcal infections, esp. those resistant to penicillin.

diet (dī′ĭt) N.
1. food and drink a person normally takes (*see also* BALANCED DIET).
2. special schedule of food and drink to meet particular needs (as in the treatment of diabetes mellitus) (*See also* BLAND DIET; CLEAR LIQUID DIET; AND OTHER SPECIAL DIETS). V. to lower one's calorie intake, or to eat only certain foods, for a specific purpose, usually to lose weight.

diethylstilbestrol (DES) (dī-ĕth′əl-stĭl-bĕs′trôl) N. synthetic nonsteroidal estrogen used to treat problems of menopause and menstruation and to limit milk production in the breasts, as well as in the treatment of prostate cancer. It was formerly used in cases of threatened abortion but was found to be associated with a higher-than-normal incidence of vaginal cancer (and other cancers of the reproductive tract) in the daughters of women so treated during pregnancy. Also called stilbestrol.

differential blood count (dĭf′ə-rĕn′shəl) N. enumeration (numbers or percentages) of the specific types of white blood cells (leukocytes) found in a given volume (usually 1 cubic milliliter) of blood; used as an aid to diagnosis.

differential diagnosis N. systematic method for diagnosing a disorder that lacks unique signs or symptoms; for example, headache may have many causes and the patient's other symptoms as well as the results of laboratory tests and other procedures must be considered in arriving at a correct diagnosis.

differentiation (dĭf′ə-rĕn′shē-ā′shən) N. process of changing from an original unspecialized form to a different, more specialized, form or function, e.g., cell differentiation in the developing embryo.

diffusion (dĭ-fyōō′zhən) N. movement of particles from an area of high concentration to an area of low concentration to produce an even distribution in the available space.

Diflucan N. *See* TABLE OF COMMONLY PRESCRIBED DRUGS—TRADE NAMES.

diflunisal N. nonsteroidal anti-inflammatory (trade name Dolobid) used in the treatment of osteoarthritis, rheumatoid arthritis, and other inflammatory conditions, and for the relief of mild pain. Adverse

THE DIGESTIVE SYSTEM

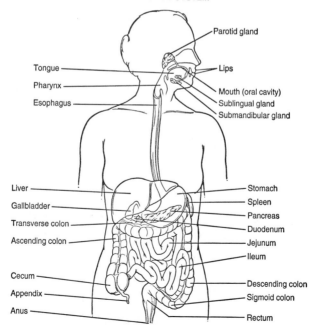

MAJOR DIGESTIVE ORGANS AND THEIR FUNCTIONS

Organ	Important Functions
Mouth	Mixes food with salivary secretions; taste, chewing
Salivary glands	Produce buffers and enzymes that begin digestion
Pharynx	Passageway shared with respiratory system, leads to esophagus
Esophagus	Delivers food to stomach
Stomach	Secretes acids and digestive enzymes that break down proteins
Small intestine	Secretes enzymes and other factors for nutrient digestion; absorbs nutrients
Liver	Secretes biles (required for lipid digestion), synthesizes blood proteins, stores lipid carbohydrate reserves
Gallbladder	Stores biles for release into small intestine
Pancreas	Secretes digestive enzymes and buffers into small intestine
Large intestine	Removes water from nondigested material; stores wastes
Anus	Opening to exterior for discharge of feces

effects include gastrointestinal bleeding and nausea.

digestion (dī-jĕs′chən) N. process of breaking down food, by mechanical (e.g., chewing, churning) and chemical (e.g., the action of enzymes) means, into substances that can be absorbed and used by the body. Chemical digestion begins in the mouth with the action of saliva but takes place largely in the stomach and small intestine.

digestive system (dī-jĕs′tĭv) N. those parts of the body that function in a coordinated manner for the digestion and absorption of food. The digestive system includes the digestive tube and accessory organs (e.g., gallbladder, liver) that secrete enzymes used in digestion. Also: digestive tract.

digestive tube N. tube, of mucous membrane and muscle tissue, about 8.3 meters (27 feet) long in the adult, extending from the mouth through the pharynx, esophagus, stomach, small intestine, and large intestine to the anus; also called alimentary canal.

digitalis (dĭj′ĭ-tăl′ĭs) N. any of several drugs (e.g., digoxin, digitoxin) derived from foxglove plants (*Digitalis genera*) and sold under various trade names, used to strengthen heart muscle contraction and regulate cardiac arrhythmias.

digitate ADJ. having fingers or fingerlike projections.

digitoxin (dĭj′ĭ-tŏk′sĭn) N. drug; a digitalis preparation, sold under various trade names (e.g., Crystodigin), used to treat congestive heart failure and cardiac arrhythmias.

digoxin (dǐj-ŏk′sǐn) N. drug; a digitalis preparation sold under various trade names (e.g., Lanoxin) used to treat congestive heart failure and cardiac arrhythmias. *See* TABLE OF COMMONLY PRESCRIBED DRUGS —GENERIC DRUGS.

Dilacor XR N. trade name for a long-acting preparation of the oral calcium blocker, diltiazem.

Dilantin N. trade name for the nonsedative, anticonvulsant drug diphenylhydantoin used in the treatment of epilepsy. *See* TABLE OF COMMONLY PRE-SCRIBED DRUGS—TRADE NAMES.

dilatation (dǐl′ə-tā′shən) N. enlargement of an organ or an opening, occurring as a normal physiologic response (e.g., widening of the pupil of the eye as a response to decreased light, widening of the uterine cervix during labor to allow passage of the fetus) or produced deliberately, as in the use of drugs to widen the pupil of the eye or the use of a dilator to open the cervix.

dilatation and curettage (D&C) N. enlargement of the cervix of the uterus and scraping of the endometrium (lining) of the uterus. It is a common procedure, usually performed using local anesthetic, to remove uterine tissue for examination and diagnosis, to stop prolonged or heavy bleeding, to remove the products of conception (a method of abortion), to remove retained fragments of the placenta after childbirth or abortion, and to remove small tumors.

Dilaudid N. trade name for the narcotic pain reliever hydromorphone hydrochloride.

diltiazem (dǐl-tī′ə-zěm′) N. drug of the calcium-blocker class useful in the treatment of hypertension, angina, and heart failure. Diltiazem is sold under the trade name Cardizem. Adverse effects include cardiac arrhythmias, hypotension, and liver damage. *See* TABLE OF COMMONLY PRESCRIBED DRUGS—GENERIC NAMES.

dilution (dī-loō′shən) N. decrease in the amount of a substance in a solution for each unit of volume, usually the result of adding water to increase the volume.

Dimetane N. trade name for the antihistamine brompheniramine maleate used to treat hypersensitivity reactions, including rhinitis, itching, and skin reactions. Adverse effects include drowsiness, dry mouth, and rapid heartbeat.

Dimetapp N. trade name for a fixed-combination drug containing two decongestants (phenylephrine hydrochloride and phenylpropanolamine hydrochloride) and an antihistamine (brompheniramine maleate—Dimetane); it is used to relieve nasal congestion and to treat certain hypersensitivity reactions such as rhinitis.

dimethyl sulfoxide (DMSO) (dī-měth′əl-sŭl-fŏk′sīd′) N. anti-inflammatory agent used topically to treat some injuries, or in combination with other drugs to facilitate their absorption through the skin.

Diovan N. *See* TABLE OF COMMONLY PRESCRIBED DRUGS—TRADE NAMES.

dioxin (dī-ŏk′sǐn) N. ingredient in an herbicide used to control plant growth and causally linked to many cancers. Dioxin was a primary ingredient in Agent Orange, which was used by the U.S. military during the Vietnam War. It is no longer available in the United States.

diphenhydramine N. antihistamine drug (trade name Benadryl) used to treat hay fever and other allergic reactions involving the nasal passages and also, sometimes, to treat motion sickness and to produce sedation.

diphenylhydantoin N. medication (trade name Dilantin) that can be given either orally or parenterally to suppress and prevent, to some extent, the occurrence of convulsions. Also known as phenytoin.

diphtheria (dĭf-thēr′ē-ə) N. acute, contagious infection caused by bacterium *Corynebacterium diphtheriae,* which produces a toxin affecting the whole body and characterized by severe inflammation of the throat and larynx with production of a membrane lining the throat, along with fever, chills, malaise, brassy cough, and, in some cases (esp. if untreated or unusually severe), by impaired function of the heart muscle and peripheral nerves. More common in children and once epidemic in many parts of the world, it is now rare in the United States because of routine immunization (DPT vaccine) against the disease. Treatment is by diphtheria antitoxin, antibiotics, rest, increased fluid intake, and tracheostomy, if necessary. *See also* SCHICK TEST.

diploid ADJ. pert. to an individual or cell that has two complete sets of homologous chromosomes, one set from each parent; the diploid chromosome number is found in somatic (body) cells, not in gametes (sex cells), and is characteristic for each species, being 46 in normal human body cells (*compare* HAPLOID).

diplomate N. specialist whose competence has been certified by the appropriate professional group (e.g., the American Board of Internal Medicine).

diplopia (dĭ-plō′pē-ə) N. double vision, in which a single object is seen as two objects. If one eye is covered, diplopia often disappears.

dipole N. molecule in which each end has an equal, but opposite, electrical charge; may also refer to oppositely charged poles of a magnet.

dipsomania N. intense, persistent desire to drink alcoholic beverages to excess; alcoholism.

dis- prefix meaning reversal, removal, exclusion, separation (e.g., disarticulation, separation of two bones in a joint).

disability N. weakness, defect, disorder, or other impairment that results in reduction or loss of mental or physical function; incapacity. As defined by the U.S. Department of Health, Education, and Welfare, disability is inability, caused by medically determined physical or mental impairment expected to last for at least 12 months, to engage in substantial gainful employment. Determination of disability is a legal one encompassing both medical and other issues. Impairment, on the other hand, is a purely medical determination.

disc N. flattened, rounded part, esp. referring to the cushioning tissues between the vertebrae; also called disk. Also intervertebral disc.

discharge N.
1. substance that is excreted from an organ or part.
2. electrical action of a nerve cell.

discoid lupus erythematosus (DLE) N. chronic, recurrent disease, thought to be an auto-immune disease and occurring primarily in women between 20 and 40 years of age, characterized by a butterfly-shaped eruption of scale-covered red lesions over the cheeks and bridge of the nose (sometimes in other areas). Treatment includes avoidance of the sun or use of a sunscreen and use of steroid and antimalarial drugs. (*Compare* SYSTEMIC LUPUS ERYTHEMATOSUS.)

disease N.
1. impairment of health or condition of abnormal functioning.
2. disorder with recognizable symptoms (e.g., fever, inflammation) that result from infection, improper diet, or other cause.

disequilibrium N. loss or weakness of balance, as may occur, e.g., in cases of inner ear disease.

disinfect V. to kill germs that may cause infection. N. disinfectant.

disinhibition N. elimination or countering of restraint or abstinence; in psychiatry, loss of the conscious suppression of unacceptable thoughts or desires resulting in socially or culturally unacceptable behavior.

disk *See* DISC.

dislocation N. displacement of a part, esp. a bone, from its normal position, as in a shoulder or the vertebral column.

disorder (dĭs-ôr′dər) N. disturbance of normal function of the mind or body; disease.

disorganized schizophrenia *See* HEBEPHRENIA.

disorientation (dĭs-ôr′ē-ĕn-ta′shən) N. mental confusion, characterized by a loss of awareness of space, time, or personal identity; it may be caused by drugs, severe stress, or organic disease.

dispensary (dĭ-spĕn′sə-rē) N.
1. place, such as a physician's office or pharmacy, where medicines and other curative materials are given to patients.
2. free clinic for outpatients.

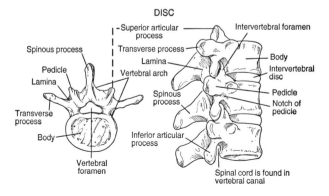

DISC

Spinous process
Pedicle
Lamina
Transverse process
Body
Vertebral foramen

Superior articular process
Transverse process
Lamina
Vertebral arch
Spinous process
Inferior articular process

Intervertebral foramen
Body
Intervertebral disc
Pedicle
Notch of pedicle
Spinal cord is found in vertebral canal

displaced fracture *See* FRAC-TURE.

displacement (dĭs-plās′mənt) N.
1. shifting of something out of its normal position.
2. unconscious transfer of feeling or action from the original object to another, more acceptable one (a defense mechanism), for example, pounding a pillow instead of chastizing a child.

dissection (dĭ-sĕk′shən) N. separation of body tissues, usually along natural divisions, by cutting or probing, for visual or microscopic examination.

disseminated lupus erythematosus (dĭ-sĕm′ə-nā′tĭd) *See* SYSTEMIC LUPUS ERYTHEMATOSUS.

disseminated multiple sclerosis *See* MULTIPLE SCLEROSIS.

dissociation (dĭ-sō′sē-ā′shən) N.
1. reversible separation of chemical molecules into simpler forms.
2. in psychiatry, separation of certain ideas, thoughts, or emotions from the consciousness, often as a defense mechanism.

dissociative disorder N. neurosis in which repressed emotional conflict causes a separation in the personality with confusion in identity. Marked by symptoms of amnesia, dream state, or multiple personality, it is treated with psychotherapy, hypnosis, and antianxiety drugs.

dissolution N. breakup in the normal anatomical state of part or parts of an organism.

distal ADJ.
1. away from the center, toward the far end of something.
2. farthest from the point of origin (*compare* PROXIMAL).

distension (dĭ-stĕn′shən) N. state of being stretched out or enlarged, as abdominal distension from gas (flatus). ADJ. distended.

distilled water N. water cleansed of impurities and microorganisms by converting it into steam and then condensing it again (usually several times) as a liquid. It has many uses, as for mixing chemicals and irrigating body parts.

disulfiram (dī-sŭl′fə-răm′) N. alcohol deterrent, commonly known under the trade name Antabuse, used in the treatment of alcoholism. It causes nausea, abdominal cramping, and sweating if alcohol is ingested. Adverse reactions, which can be extremely severe, include neuritis and polyneuritis; drowsiness and skin eruptions occur in some patients. The drug interacts with many other drugs and must be used with caution in those taking drugs for many disorders.

diuresis (dī′ə-rē′sĭs) N. increased excretion of urine, usually due to drinking large amounts of liquid or to the action of a diuretic (e.g., Diuril, Lasix) or occurring as a symptom of disease (e.g., diabetes mellitus).

diuretic (dī′ə-rĕt′ĭk) N. drug that promotes the production and excretion of urine; it is commonly used in the treatment of edema, hypertension, and congestive heart failure. There are several types of diuretics, including thiazides (e.g., chlorothiazide—Diuril and hydrochlorothiazide—Esidrix), loop diuretics (furosemide—Lasix), and others (spironolactone—Aldactone). Several adverse reactions are common to diuretics, chiefly electrolyte (esp. sodium and potassium) imbalances.

Diuril N. trade name for the diuretic chlorothiazide.

diverticulitis (dī'vûr-tĭk'yə-lī'tĭs) N. inflammation of an abnormal sac (diverticulum) at a weakened point in the digestive tract, esp. the colon. Symptoms include cramplike abdominal pain, fever, and diarrhea or constipation. Treatment is by rest and antibiotics; severe cases may require surgery. (*Compare* DIVERTICULOSIS.)

diverticulosis (dī'vûr-tĭk'yə-lō'sĭs) N. presence of abnormal pouchlike sacs (diverticula) through the muscular layers of the colon. The condition, increasingly common in persons over the age of 50, produces few or no symptoms, except occasional rectal bleeding. (*Compare* DIVERTICULITIS.)

DIVERTICULA OF THE COLON

Inflamed diverticulum

Diverticula

diverticulum (dī'vûr-tĭk'yə-ləm) N., *pl.* diverticula, pouchlike herniation through the muscular wall of a tubular organ, esp. the colon.

dizygotic twins N. fraternal twins: twins who developed from two separate fertilized eggs. Dizygotic twins may be of the same or opposite sex; they do not contain the same genetic makeup and differ from each other in the same way as other siblings with the same parents do. (*Compare* MONOZYGOTIC TWINS; SIAMESE TWINS.)

dizziness (dĭz'ē-nĭs) N. sensation of unsteadiness, faintness, or whirling in space, often with inability to maintain balance; it has many causes, including middle-ear disorder, drug (including alcohol) intoxication, and hypertension. A dizzy person is in danger of falling and therefore should be placed on a bed or the floor. *Compare* VERTIGO.

DLE *See* DISCOID LUPUS ERYTHEMATOSUS.

DMSO *See* DIMETHYL SULFOXIDE.

DNA *See* DEOXYRIBONUCLEIC ACID.

DNA polymerase *See* POLYMERASE.

DOA N. abbreviation for dead on arrival, a term used by physicians, ambulance personnel, and others to signify that a patient was dead on arrival at the hospital or other healthcare facility.

Dolobid N. trade name for the nonsteroidal anti-inflammatory diflunisal.

dolor (dō'lər) N. pain. ADJ. dolorific

dominance (dŏm'ə-nəns) N. ability of a specific genetic characteristic to appear at the expense of another (*compare* RECESSIVE GENE).

Donnatal N. fixed-combination drug, containing a sedative (phenobarbital) and several other agents, used to decrease gastrointestinal spasm.

donor (dō'nər) N. person who gives living tissue (e.g., eye, blood, semen) to be used in another person (*compare* HOST).

dopamine (dō′pə-mēn′) N. chemical found in the brain and elsewhere in the body that functions as a neurotransmitter. As a drug also known under the trade name Intropin it is used to treat shock and hypotension.

Doriden N. trade name for the sedative glutethimide.

dorsal (dôr′səl) ADJ. pert. to the back or posterior (*compare* VENTRAL).

dorsi-, dorso- comb. forms indicating an association with the back (dorsum), e.g., dorsolateral, pert. to the back and sides.

dorsiflexion (dôr′sə-flĕk′shən) N. bending backward of a part.

dorsum (dôr′səm) N., *pl.* dorsa, 1. back. 2. back surface of any part, e.g., the dorsum of the hand. ADJ. dorsal, dorsalis

dosage (dō′sĭj) N. schedule of how much and how frequently a drug or other therapeutic agent (e.g., vitamins) is to be administered.

dose (dōs) N. amount of a medication or other substance, or of radiation, to be given at one time. *See also* LETHAL DOSE.

dosimetry N. 1. measurement of the dose of radiation emitted by a radioactive source. 2. calculation of the appropriate dose of radiation to treat a particular condition in a particular patient.

double pneumonia N. pneumonia of both lungs at the same time.

double vision N. *See* DIPLOPIA.

double-blind study N. experiment in which neither the investigator nor the subject knows whether the subject received the experimental variable (e.g., a drug) or a placebo, thus eliminating any influence such knowledge might have on the reactions of the subject and the expectations or interpretations of the investigator.

douche (do͞osh) N. introduction of a jet of water or special fluid into or around a given part, esp. the vagina, to cleanse or free the part from odor-causing contents, or to treat infection.

Down's syndrome N. congenital defect, usually caused by the presence of an extra No. 21 chromosome (trisomy) and characterized by mental retardation (the I.Q. averages 50–60); oblique placement of the eyes; a small head flattened at the back; a large, furrowed tongue; short stature; bowel defects; and heart abnormalities. The syndrome, the most common of the chromosomal abnormalities, is associated with advanced maternal age, esp. over age 35 (1 in 80 offspring of women over 40 will be affected); it can be detected through amniocentesis. Care of a Down's syndrome child involves both the prevention of physical problems (e.g., respiratory infections, to which these children are especially prone) and long-range programs to promote mental and motor skills. A less common form of the disease, caused by a translocation of a chromosome, is an inherited (genetic) defect, not associated with maternal age.

doxazosin N. oral antihypertensive agent (trade name Cardura), administered once daily; the most common side effect is orthostatic hypotension. *See*

TABLE OF COMMONLY PRESCRIBED DRUGS—GENERIC NAMES.

doxepin N. tricyclic antidepressant (trade names Sinequan and Adapin) used to treat depression. Adverse effects include sedation, dry mouth, and gastrointestinal, cardiovascular, and neurologic disturbances.

doxycycline N. tetracycline antibiotic (trade name Vibramycin) effective against many infections.

DPH N. abbrev. for the anticonvulsant medication diphenylhydantoin.

DPT vaccine N. abbreviation for diphtheria and tetanus toxoids and pertussis (whooping cough) vaccine. The combination vaccine is usually given in a series of injections during infancy and early childhood.

drain (drān) N. tube inserted into a body cavity, sometimes during surgery, to remove unwanted material.

drainage (drā′nĭj) N. drawing off of fluid from a body cavity, usually fluid that has accumulated abnormally.

Dramamine (drăm′ə-mēn′) N. trade name for a drug (dimenhydrinate) used to prevent and treat nausea, esp. that due to motion sickness.

drive (drīv) N. natural force that compels a person to an action as the hunger drive directs one to eat. The basic drives are sex, hunger, and thirst. A secondary drive is a learned or acquired drive, not directly related to satisfying a physical need (e.g., a striving for recognition).

Drixoral N. trade name for a fixed-combination drug containing an antihistamine and a vasoconstrictor; it is used to treat upper respiratory congestion.

drop foot (drŏp) N. condition in which the foot is flexed toward the sole (plantar surface) or droops and cannot be voluntarily flexed toward a normal position.

dropsy (drŏp′sē) *See* EDEMA.

drosophilia N. type of fly, including the common fruit fly.

drug (drŭg) N.
1. substance taken by mouth, injection, or applied locally to prevent or treat a disorder (e.g., to ease pain).
2. chemical substance introduced into the body to cause pleasure or a sense of changed awareness, as in the nonmedical use of lysergic acid diethylamide (LSD).

drug abuse N. use of a drug for nontherapeutic purposes (e.g., to alter one's sense of awareness, as with lysergic acid diethylamide—LSD). Commonly abused substances include barbiturates, alcohol, sedatives, and amphetamines. Drug abuse can lead to physical and mental damage, and with some substances, to drug dependence and addiction. Drug abuse and drug addiction are serious problems in our society today. Particularly worrisome is the growing incidence in elementary and secondary school-aged children.

drug addiction N. condition marked by an overwhelming desire to take a drug to which one has become habituated because of long-term use and by the development of withdrawal symptoms (mental and/ or physical) if the drug is not taken. Heroin and barbiturates are common addictive drugs.

drug dependence N. condition in which one craves or depends on a particular drug that one is accustomed to taking.

dry socket (drī) N. inflammation at the site of an extracted tooth, characterized by pain, pus, and frequently infection.

DTs *See* DELIRIUM TREMENS.

Duchenne's muscular dystrophy *See* MUSCULAR DYSTROPHY.

duct (dŭkt) N. tubelike channel for carrying fluids or other materials from one organ or part to another (e.g., the bile duct, which carries bile to the duodenum).

duct gland *See* EXOCRINE GLAND.

ductless glands (dŭkt′lĭs) *See* ENDOCRINE GLANDS.

ductule (dŭk′tool′) N. small duct, e.g., one of the small tubes found in the tear glands.

ductus arteriosus N. blood vessels in the fetus connecting the pulmonary artery directly to the ascending aorta, thus bypassing the pulmonary circulation. It normally closes at birth; failure to close—patent ductus arteriosus—often requires surgical correction.

ductus deferens N. duct about 45 centimeters (18 inches) long, leading from testis looping around the bladder, and ending in the ejaculatory duct. *See also* VAS DEFERENS.

dumb ADJ. mute; lacking the ability to speak. Colloq. stupid, of low intelligence.

dumbness N. lack of the ability to speak. Colloq. stupidity.

dumdum fever *See* KALA-AZAR.

dumping syndrome (dŭm′pĭng) N. group of symptoms, including nausea, dizziness, sweating, and faintness, occurring after a meal, particularly a meal rich in carbohydrates, in patients who have had stomach surgery; it is due to a too-rapid emptying of the stomach contents and the development of low sugar levels in the blood.

duodenal ulcer N. ulcer in the duodenum; it is the most common type of peptic ulcer.

duodeno- comb. form indicating an association with the duodenum (e.g., duodenocholangitis, inflammation of both the duodenum and the common bile duct).

duodenum (doo′ə-dē′nəm) N. first part of the small intestine; it receives material from the stomach (through the pyloric valve) and passes it to the jejunum, the medial part of the small intestine. The duodenum plays a vital role in digestion, receiving acid chyme from the stomach, bile from the bile duct, pancreatic juices from the pancreas, and intestinal juices—all of which function in the chemical breakdown of food molecules. ADJ. duodenal

Dupuytren's contracture N. painless condition in which the fourth and fifth fingers bend into the palm of the hand and resist extension because of progressive thickening of tissue beneath the skin in the palm. Of unknown cause, it primarily affects middle-aged men. Treatment involves surgical excision of excess tissue.

dura mater (door′ə) N. thickest and outermost of the three membranes (meninges) that enclose the brain and spinal cord (the others being the pia mater and the arachnoid membrane).

durable power of attorney N. written advanced directive whereby a mentally competent patient designates a surrogate, typically a relative or close friend, to make medical decisions if the patient loses his or her decision-making capacity; the surrogate should base decisions on the patient's previously expressed preferences, if known, or what is considered to be in the patient's best interest, if his or her previous wishes are not known; the durable power of attorney applies to all medical situations in which the patients are incapable of making their own decisions, not just terminal illness. The living will, on the other hand, applies only in case of a terminal illness.

dwarfism (dwôr′fĭz′əm) N. underdevelopment of the body, characterized primarily by abnormally short stature, often with underdeveloped limbs and other defects. Causes include genetic defects, pituitary or thyroid malfunctioning, kidney disease, and certain other disorders. *See also* ACHONDROPLASIA; HOMUNCULUS; PITUITARY DWARF; PRIMORDIAL DWARF.

dyadic ADJ. pert. to a relationship involving two persons, e.g., that of doctor and patient in therapy, esp. psychotherapy.

Dyazide N. trade name for a fixed-combination drug containing two diuretics (hydrochlorothiazide and triamterene); it is used to treat hypertension and edema. *See* TABLE OF COMMONLY PRESCRIBED DRUGS—TRADE NAMES.

Dynacirc N. trade name for the calcium channel blocker, isradipine.

dynamo- comb. form indicating force or strength (e.g., dynamogenesis, energy development).

dys- comb. form meaning bad, abnormal, difficult, adverse (e.g., dysethesia, distorted sense, esp. of touch).

dysaphia (dĭs-ā′fē-ə) N. defect in the sense of touch.

dysarthria (dĭs-är′thrē-ə) N. difficulty in pronouncing words clearly or correctly, usually because of poor control over the speech muscles.

dysautonomia (dĭs-ô′tə-nō′mē-ə) N. rare hereditary disease resulting in autonomic nervous system dysfunction, most commonly in Ashkenazi Jews. Symptoms include mental retardation, lack of coordination, vomiting, frequent infections, and seizures.

dyschezia (dĭs-kē′zē-ə) N. difficulty in passing stools, usually from long-continued, voluntary suppression of the urge to defecate.

dyscrasia (dĭs-krā′zhə) N. any diseased or imbalanced state of the body or its systems (e.g., blood dyscrasia, any abnormal condition of the blood). ADJ. dyscratic

dysentery (dĭs′ən-tĕr′ē) N. intestinal inflammation caused by bacteria, protozoa, parasites, or chemical irritants, and marked by abdominal pain; frequent, bloody stools, and rectal spasms. Treatment includes replacement of lost fluids and sometimes antibiotics. ADJ. dysenteric

dysequilibrium N. any abnormality in the sense of balance.

dysfunction (dĭs-fŭngk′shən) N. state in which the proper response or activity of a part (e.g., a muscle) or organ is weak, absent, or otherwise abnormal. ADJ. dysfunctional

dysfunctional uterine bleeding N. uterine bleeding due to hormonal imbalance, not a diseased condition (e.g., uterine tumor).

dysgenesis (dĭs-jĕn′ĭ-sĭs) N. abnormal development of an organ or part, esp. in the embryo stage. ADJ. dysgenic

dysgraphia (dĭs-grăf′ē-ə) N. impairment of the ability to write correctly, due to a brain or motor disorder.

dyskinesia (dĭs′kə-nē′zhə) N. difficulty in carrying out voluntary movements. *See also* TARDIVE DYSKINESIA. ADJ. dyskinetic

dyslexia (dĭs-lĕk′sē-ə) N. impairment of ability to read in which letters and words are reversed. Dyslexia, which affects more boys than girls, is usually linked to a central nervous system disorder, although some experts believe that it represents a complex of problems, possibly including visual defects, impaired hearing, stress, and inadequate instruction. ADJ. dyslexic

dyslogia (dĭs-lō′jē-ə) N. impairment of the power to think logically and rationally.

dysmenorrhea (dĭs-mĕn′ə-rē′ə) N. painful menstruation. Primary dysmenorrhea, intrinsic to the process of menstruation and not the result of any other disease or condition, is very common. Typically, cramplike pain in the lower abdomen, sometimes accompanied by nausea, vomiting, intestinal cramps, and other discomfort begins just before or with the onset of menstrual flow. Oral contraceptives and antiprostaglandins lessen the discomfort but for some women in whom the pain is severe potent analgesics may be needed. Secondary dysmenorrhea, caused by a specific disorder (e.g., uterine tumor, pelvic infection, endometriosis), is usually marked by pain that lasts longer and is often accompanied by bladder or bowel discomfort; treatment depends on the underlying cause.

dysosmia (dĭs-ŏz′mē-ə) N. condition in which the sense of smell is impaired.

dyspareunia (dĭs′pə-rōō′nē-ə) N. abnormal condition in women in which sexual intercourse is painful; it may be caused by abnormality of the genitalia, psychophysiological reactions, inadequate sexual arousal, or other factors.

dyspepsia (dĭs-pĕp′shə) N. stomach upset; a disorder of the digestive function, marked by vague discomfort, heartburn, or nausea. ADJ. dyspeptic

dysphagia (dĭs-fā′jə) N. condition in which swallowing is difficult or painful, due to obstruction of the esophagus or muscular abnormalities of the esophagus or pharynx.

dysphasia (dĭs-fā′zhə) N. speech impairment, usually due to brain injury, stroke, or tumor.

dysphonia (dĭs-fō′nē-ə) N. difficulty in speaking due to impairment of the voice. ADJ. dysphonic

dysplasia (dĭs-plā′zhə) N. general term for any abnormal change or development, as in the shape or size of cells. ADJ. dysplastic

dyspnea (dĭsp-nē′ə) N. shortness of breath or labored, difficult breathing; causes include strenuous activity, lung disorders, heart disease, and extreme stress or tension (*compare* HYPERPNEA).

dyspraxia (dĭs-prăk′sē-ə) N. decrease in proper function (as of an organ) or of ability to coordinate muscular actions.

dystocia (dĭs-tō′sē-ə) N. difficult labor, due to unusually large fetus, abnormal position of the fetus, contracted or obstructed birth canal, or other factor.

dystonia (dĭs-tō′nē-ə) N. abnormal muscle tone, esp. sudden muscle spasms due to a rare inherited disease (dystonia musculorum deformans) or sometimes to drug reaction.

dystrophy (dĭs′trə-fē) N. degeneration or defective development of a tissue, esp. muscles, which loses strength and decreases in size (*see also* MUSCULAR DYSTROPHY). ADJ. dystrophic

dysuria (dĭs-yo͞or′ē-ə) N. painful or difficult urination; it may be caused by inflammation of the bladder (cystitis) or urethra (urethritis) or other disorders.

E

E vitamin N. any of a group of fat-soluble vitamins (tocopherols) important in reproductive function and blood cell production; rich sources are vegetable oils, nuts, soybeans, and eggs. *See also* VITAMIN; TABLE OF VITAMINS.

ear (ēr) N. hearing and balance organ, including three general structures; the outer (external) ear; the middle ear, including the eardrum cavity and the three tiny bones that transmit the hearing vibrations; and the inner (internal) ear, including the main organ of hearing (the organ of Corti) and the balance mechanism.

earache (ēr′āk′) N. pain in the ear; it may be caused by ear disease or by infection or disease of the nose, mouth region, throat, and other nearby areas; also called otalgia.

eardrum (ēr′drŭm′) *See* TYMPANIC MEMBRANE.

earwax (ēr′wăks′) *See* CERUMEN.

eating disorder N. serious disturbances in eating behavior, such as extreme and unhealthy reduction of food intake or severe overeating, as well as feelings of distress or extreme concern about body shape or weight. Eating disorders are not due to a failure of will or behavior; rather, they are real, treatable medical illnesses in which certain maladaptive patterns of eating take on a life of their own. The main types of eating disorders are anorexia nervosa and bulimia. A third type, binge eating disorder, has been suggested but has not yet

THE EAR

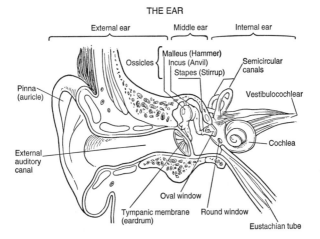

External ear | Middle ear | Internal ear

Ossicles { Malleus (Hammer)
Incus (Anvil)
Stapes (Stirrup)

Semicircular canals

Pinna (auricle)

Vestibulocochlear

External auditory canal

Cochlea

Oval window

Tympanic membrane (eardrum)

Round window

Eustachian tube

been approved as a formal psychiatric diagnosis. *See also* ANOREXIA NERVOSA; BINGE EATING DISORDER; BULIMIA.

EBV *See* EPSTEIN-BARR VIRUS.

eccentric (ĭk-sĕn′trĭk) ADJ. peripheral; located away from the center.

ecchymosis (ĕk′ĭ-mō′sĭs) N. bruise; discolored (purplish) spot resulting from an accumulation of blood under the skin's surface caused by injury or fragility of the blood vessel walls. *See also* PETECHIA.

eccrine (ĕk′rĭn) ADJ. pert. to sweating or sweat glands.

eccrine gland N. type of sweat gland distributed over much of the body; its secretion is clear, has only a slight odor, and functions in cooling the body (*compare* APOCRINE GLAND).

ECF *See* EXTRACELLULAR FLUID.

ECG *See* ELECTROCARDIOGRAM.

echino- comb. form indicating an association with spines or spinyness (e.g., echinosis, state in which the red blood cells have an irregular appearance).

echinococcosis (ĭ-kī′nə-kə-kō′sĭs) N. infection with a tapeworm (*Echinococcus*), usually transmitted through contact with infected dogs (esp. their stool). It is characterized by cyst formation in tissue, esp. the liver; symptoms depend on the tissue affected. Treatment involves surgical excision of the cysts. Also called hydatid disease.

echo virus (ĕk′ō) N. any of a group of small viruses, some of which are responsible for human illnesses.

echocardiography (ĕk′ō-kär′dē-ŏg′rə-fē) N. diagnostic procedure using ultrasound waves to study the heart, its structure and motions. It is used to assess disorders of cardiac muscle function or valve function, or other abnormalities. N. echocardiogram.

echoencephalography (ĕk′ō-ĕn-sĕf′ə-lŏg′-rə-fē) N. diagnostic procedure using ultrasound waves to study the brain; it may reveal expanding lesions or expansion of brain ventricles.

echolalia (ĕk′ō-lā′lē-ə) N. in psychiatry, automatic and meaningless repetition of another's words, sometimes occurring in schizophrenia and other neurological and mental disorders.

eclampsia (ĭ-klămp′sē-ə) N. rare (approx. 0.2% of all pregnancies in the United States) and serious pregnancy disorder. Eclampsia is characterized by convulsions, coma, high blood pressure, protein in the urine, and edema; signs of impending convulsions include headache, blurred vision, epigastric pain, and anxiety. Once the convulsions are controlled and emergency treatment of the pregnant woman is completed, delivery of the fetus is usually necessary (fetal mortality is 25%). (*See also* TOXEMIA OF PREGNANCY.) ADJ. eclamptic

ecstasy N. emotional state marked by exalted delight, exhilaration, extreme joy. ADJ. ecstatic

ECT *See* ELECTROCONVULSIVE THERAPY.

ectasia (ĕk-tā′zē-ə) N. dilatation or distension of a part or organ (e.g., alveolar ectasia, abnormal expansion of the air sacs in the lungs); also ectasis (*compare* ATELECTASIS).

ecto- comb. form meaning outer, outside, (e.g., ectogenous, coming from the outside, as disease-causing germs) (*compare* ENDO-).

ectoderm (ĕk'tə-dûrm') N. in the embryo, outside layer of cells from which the nervous system, skin, special sense organs (e.g., eyes, ears), and certain other body parts arise. (The two other cell layers are the inner endoderm and the middle mesoderm.) ADJ. ectodermal, ectodermic

ectomorph (ĕk'tə-môrf') N. person whose physique is thin, fragile, and generally nonmuscular (*compare* ENDOMORPH; MESOMORPH). ADJ. ectomorphic

-ectomy suffix indicating surgical removal of a part or organ (e.g. appendectomy, removal of the appendix).

ectopia (ĕk-tō'pē-ə) N. abnormal positioning of a part or organ, esp. at the time of birth. ADJ. ectopic

ectopic pregnancy (ĕk-tŏp'ĭk) N. abnormal pregnancy, occurring in about 2% of all pregnancies, in which the fertilized egg (conceptus, embryo) implants outside of the uterus, most often (90%) in the fallopian tube (tubal pregnancy) but occasionally in the ovary (ovarian pregnancy) or abdominal cavity (abdominal pregnancy). As the embryo develops the tube ruptures or other complications arise, usually causing hemorrhage and requiring immediate surgery. Also called extrauterine pregnancy.

ectro- comb. form indicating congenital absence (e.g., ectromelia, congenital absence or marked shortening of the long bones of one or more limbs).

ectrodactyly N. congenital absence of some fingers or toes.

ectrogeny (ĕk-trŏj'ə-nē) N. congenital absence of any body part or organ.

ectropion N. turning outward (eversion) of an edge or margin, esp. of the eyelid, as a result of injury, facial nerve paralysis, or atrophy of eye tissue.

eczema (ĕk'sə-mə) N. inflammation of the skin that usually produces itching and the development of small blisterlike formations that release fluid and then form a crust. It may be caused by contact with a specific irritant or occur without apparent cause. Treatment usually involves topical corticosteroids. ADJ. eczematous

Edecrin N. trade name for the diuretic ethacrynic acid.

edema (ĭ-dē'mə) N. abnormal collection of fluid in spaces between cells, esp. just under the skin or in a given cavity (e.g., peritoneal cavity) or organ (e.g., the lungs—pulmonary edema). Causes include injury, heart disease, kidney failure, cirrhosis, and allergy. Treatment depends on the cause but often involves bedrest, diuretics, and restriction of salt. Formerly known as dropsy; also called hydrops. ADJ. edematous

edentulous ADJ. without teeth, as when all the natural teeth have been removed.

EDTA N. ethylenediaminetetraacetic acid; chelating agent used in treatment of heavy metal poisoning. Also used by some alternative care practitioners to treat coronary artery disease; this practice is considered highly controversial by many conventional health care providers.

EEG *See* ELECTROENCEPHALOGRAM.

EES *See* ERYTHROMYCIN.

effacement N. shortening of the cervix and thinning of its walls as it is stretched and dilated during labor.

effector (ĭ-fĕk′tər) N. organ that becomes active in response to stimulation; nerve fiber that terminates on a muscle or gland and stimulates contraction.

efferent (ĕf′ər-ənt) ADJ. carrying outward, away from the center, as a nerve carrying impulses from the brain to a muscle, gland, or other effector organ, or as a vessel (e.g., a blood or lymphatic vessel) carrying fluid (e.g., blood, lymph) away from an organ or part (*compare* AFFERENT).

effervescent ADJ. giving off bubbles; charged naturally or artificially with carbon dioxide or other gas.

Effexor N. *See* TABLE OF COMMONLY PRESCRIBED DRUGS—TRADE NAMES.

effleurage N. rhythmic, firm or gentle stroking, as in massage. Effleurage of the abdomen is commonly used in the Lamaze method of childbirth.

effusion (ĭ-fyōō′zhən) N. escape of fluid (e.g., blood, lymph, serum) into a body cavity, often associated with circulatory or kidney disorders.

egg (ĕg) N. ovum; sex cell (gamete) of the female, which, when fertilized by the male spermatozoon, becomes a zygote.

ego (ē′gō) N. term used by Freud and now generally accepted to mean the self, esp. the conscious self (*compare* ID; SUPEREGO).

ego- comb. form indicating a relationship to the self (e.g., egocentric, selfish, focusing especially or exclusively on oneself).

egomania (ē′gō-mā′nē-ə) N. abnormally excessive self-regard.

Ehlers-Danlos syndrome (ā′lərs-dăn′lŏs) N. inherited disorder in which the elastic connective tissue, especially that of the joints and of the aorta, becomes abnormally loose; results in excessive motion of the joints, and at times, aneurysm of the aortic arch.

Einthoven N. Dutch physiologist who devised the first electrocardiograph; he was the first to link this recording of the heart's electrical activity with its mechanical contraction. The original electrocardiogram (EKG, ECG) had three leads, or points of reference, which could be drawn as a triangle (Einthoven's Triangle).

ejaculate (ĭ-jăk′yə-lāt′) N. sperm-containing fluid (semen) emitted during ejaculation. The fluid volume of each ejaculation is usually between 2 and 5 milliliters, and it contains 50,000,000 to 150,000,000 spermatozoa.

ejaculation (ĭ-jăk′yə-lā′shən) N. sudden discharge of something, esp. of semen during coitus, masturbation, or nocturnal emission. The sensation of ejaculation is called orgasm. *See also* PREMATURE EJACULATION.

ejaculatory duct (ĭ-jăk′yə-lə-tôr′ē) N. duct about 2 centimeters (1 inch) long, behind the bladder that transports sperm from the ductus deferens to the urethra.

EKG *See* ELECTROCARDIOGRAM.

elastic (ĭ-lăs'tĭk) ADJ. having the ability to resume the original shape once the force that changed that shape is removed.

elastin (ĭ-lăs'tĭn) N. connective tissue protein that forms elastic fibers in tissue, particularly the middle layer of arteries (media).

elastosis (ĭ-lă-stō'sĭs) N. condition in which elastic tissue breaks down.

Elavil (ĕl'ə-vĭl) N. trade name for the commonly used antidepressant amitriptyline hydrochloride. *See* TABLE OF COMMONLY PRESCRIBED DRUGS—TRADE NAMES.

elbow (ĕl'bō') N.
1. joint at which the upper arm (humerus) and forearm (specifically the ulna and radius of the forearm) meet; it is a common site of inflammation and injury. *See also* TENNIS ELBOW.
2. any L-shaped part or angle, as in an apparatus tube.

elbow bones *See* RADIUS, ULNA.

elective (ĭ-lĕk'tĭv) ADJ. decided on by the patient and/or the physician, esp. with relation to procedures (e.g., surgery) that are not essential.

electric ADJ. pertaining to, involving, or caused by electricity. Evidence shows that electric current may guide the development of embryos and the regeneration of tissue, including bone; the sources for this electric current are in dispute.

electric burn N. burn caused by heat generated by an electric current. *See also* BURN.

electric shock N. traumatic state caused by the passage of an electric current through the body. It usually results from accidental contact with exposed circuits in household appliances but may also result from contact with high-voltage wires or from being struck by lightning. The damage to the body depends on the type, intensity, and duration of the current; it commonly includes burns, heart rhythm abnormalities, and unconsciousness.

electric(al) healing N. use of electricity to increase the rate of natural repair of damaged tissues (e.g., fractures). Research suggests the electricity may keep the parathyroid hormone (which can destroy bone tissue) from acting on cells at the repair site.

electrical potential (ĭ-lĕk'trĭ-kəl) N. difference in electrical charge between two differently charged bodies. Normally, the inside of heart cells is negatively charged (−90 millivolts) in comparison to the outside. When nerve impulses pass through the heart, the cells become more positive inside due to an influx of sodium and calcium ions, which are positively charged (called depolarization). This change in electrical potential leads to contraction of the cardiac muscle cells. Following contraction, the intracellular chemical milieu returns to baseline and the electrical potential returns to −90 millivolts.

electro- (ĭ-lĕk'trō) comb. form indicating an association with electricity (e.g., electrocoagulation, the clotting of blood by applying an electric instrument—electrocautery).

electroanesthesia (ĭ-lĕk'trō-ăn'ĭs-thē'zhə) N. loss of sensation resulting from application of an electric current to the body or to a part.

electrocardiogram (ECG, EKG) (ĭ-lĕk'trō-kär'dē-ə-grăm') N.

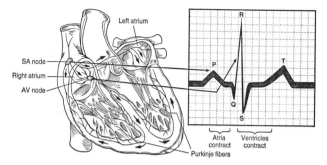

The electrical activity of the heart as seen in the waves of an electrocardiogram.

graphic recording, produced by an electrocardiograph, of the electrical activity of the heart. It permits the detection of abnormalities in the transmission of the cardiac impulse through the heart muscle via the cardiac conduction system and serves as an important aid in the diagnosis of heart ailments. *See also:* CARDIAC CONDUCTION SYSTEM.

electrocardiograph (ĭ-lĕk′trō-kär′dē-ə-grăf′) N. device used to record the electrical activity of the heart. The patient is asked to lie down and rest quietly on a table, and electrodes, called leads, are positioned, usually using an adhesive gel, on certain sites on the chest and extremities. The leads detect the electrical impulses of the heart and transmit them to the recording device. ADJ. electrocardiographic

electrocardiography (ĭ-lĕk′trō-kär′dē-ŏg′rə-fē) *See* CARDIOGRAPHY.

electrocautery (ĭ-lĕk′trō-kô′tə-rē) N. application of a needle or snare heated by an electric current to destroy tissue (e.g., to remove warts).

electrochemical N. changes in the electrical charge within or between cells or membranes due to movement of chemicals, usually electrolytes such as sodium, potassium, or calcium.

electroconvulsive therapy (ECT) (ĭ-lĕk′trō-kən-vŭl′sĭv) N. treatment for certain mental disorders, esp. severe depression, in which a brief convulsion is induced by passing an electric current through the brain. The patient is placed in a comfortable supine position, and a state of general anesthesia induced. Electrodes are placed on both sides of the forehead, and an electric current is delivered for a very brief time (less than one-half second). The patient then experiences involuntary muscle contractions (convulsions) for a short period and awakens with no memory of the shock. Electroconvulsive therapy is now less commonly used than it once was, having been largely replaced by psychoactive drugs. Also called electroshock therapy; shock therapy.

electrode (ĭ-lĕk′trōd′) N. conductor used to make electrical contact with some nonmetallic part of a surface or circuit; often used in conjunction with monitoring of the heart rhythm by electrodes held to the skin by adhesive.

electroencephalogram (EEG) (ĭ-lĕk′trō-ĕn-sĕf′ə-lə-grăm′) N. graphic recording, produced by an electroencephalograph, of the electric activity of the brain. Electroencephalograms are helpful in detecting and locating brain tumors and in diagnosing epilepsy.

electroencephalograph (ĭ-lĕk′trō-ĕn-sĕf′ə-lə-grăf′) N. device for receiving and recording the electrical activity of the brain. In most cases electrodes are attached to various areas of the head and the patient is asked to remain quiet while the brain-wave activity is recorded; during neurosurgery electrodes may be placed directly on the surface of or within the brain. ADJ. electroencephalographic

electrolysis (ĭ-lĕk-trŏl′ĭ-sĭs) N.
1. electrical action that causes a chemical (e.g., a salt) to break down into simpler forms.
2. passing of an electric current into a hair root to remove superfluous or unwanted hair. ADJ. electrolytic

electrolyte (ĭ-lĕk′trə-līt′) N. chemical (element or compound) in the body that when dissolved produces ions, conducts an electric current, and is itself changed in the process. The proper amount and equilibrium of certain electrolytes (e.g., calcium, sodium, potassium) in the body is essential for normal health and functioning.

electrolyte balance N. equilibrium between electrolytes in the body that is essential for normal functioning, with a deficiency or excess of a particular electrolyte usually producing char-

acteristic symptoms. The normal electrolyte balance may be disturbed by many disorders, including prolonged diarrhea or vomiting, kidney malfunction, or malnutrition, or by disturbed activity of the adrenal cortex, pancreas, pituitary, or other gland.

electromyogram (EMG) (ĭ-lĕk′trō-mī′ō-grăm′) N. recording of the electrical activity occurring when voluntary (skeletal) muscles work; it is helpful in diagnosing muscle and nerve abnormalities.

electron (ĭ-lĕk′trŏn′) N. extremely small particle with a negative electrical charge that revolves about the center (nucleus) of an atom.

electron microscope N. instrument that is similar to a light microscope but uses a beam of electrons, not light, to scan surfaces and create an image; magnification 1,000 times that of an optical microscope is possible.

electron transport system N. series of compounds located within the inner membrane of the mitochondrion; high-energy electrons generated in the Krebs cycle pass from compound to compound, sequentially imparting their energy to each. Energy from the high-energy electrons is used to move protons (H^+) from the mitochondrial matrix through the membrane via a proton pump (specialized protein) to the opposite side. Protons that have accumulated outside of the inner membrane then return to the matrix via a specialized enzyme (ATP synthetase). This sequential movement of protons generates a force that, using oxygen, allows ATP synthetase to catalyze chemiosmo-

ELECTRON TRANSPORT SYSTEM

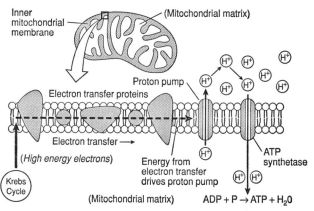

High energy electrons generated during the Krebs cycle pass from the mitochondrial matrix to electron transfer system proteins within the inner mitochondrial membrane. Energy released as electrons are transferred between the proteins drives the proton pump, forcing protons (H^+) outside of the membrane. When enough protons accumulate, the concentration gradient forces some back into matrix, through ATP synthetase. Energy released during this process is used to convert ADP to ATP and water (H_2O). Oxygen is required to complete the process of chemiosmosis.

sis—the reaction that generates adenosine triphosphate (ATP) from adenosine diphosphate (ADP) and also produces water (H_2O). Also called electron transport chain. *See also* ADENOSINE DIPHOSPHATE (ADP), ADENOSINE TRIPHOSPHATE (ATP), CHEMIOSMOSIS, KREBS CYCLE.

electronegative ADJ. having a negative electric charge.

electronic fetal monitor (ĭ-lĕk-trŏn'ĭk) *See* FETAL MONITOR.

electrophoresis (ĭ-lĕk'trō-fə-rē'sĭs) N. movement of charged particles in a liquid medium in response to changes in an electric field. The technique allows the separation of component parts of a substance and is widely used to analyze certain substances (e.g., determining the proteins present in a sample of serum).

electroretinogram (ĭ-lĕk'trō-rĕt'n-ə-grăm') N. graphic recording of the electrical activity of the retina; made by flashing a light into the eye and recording the effects on the retina with special devices attached to the eye and the back of the head; it is used to help diagnose retinal disease.

electroshock therapy (ĭ-lĕk'trō-shŏk') *See* ELECTROCONVULSIVE THERAPY.

electrosleep N. sleep that is brought about by applying a controlled electric current to the head. The procedure has been used in treating mental and emotional disorders (e.g., anxiety, depression, insomnia).

electrosurgery (ĭ-lĕk-trō-sûr′jə-rē) N. surgery performed using electrical devices (e.g., electrically wired needles).

element (ĕl′ə-mənt) N. simplest chemical form, in which only one kind of atom is contained (e.g., oxygen) (*compare* COMPOUND).

elementary particles N. particle of which other, larger particles are composed. For example, atoms are made up of smaller particles known as electrons, protons, and neutrons. The proton and neutron, in turn, are composed of more elementary particles known as quarks. *See also* LEPTONS; PARTICLE PHYSICS; QUARKS.

elephantiasis (ĕl′ə-fən-tī′ə-sĭs) N. condition characterized by enormous enlargement of certain body parts, esp. the legs and scrotum, often with a thickening and coarsening of the skin. It is the end stage of the disease filariasis and is due to blockage of the lymphatic vessels by infiltration of filarial worms.

elimination (ĭ-lĭm′ə-nā′shən) N. process of getting rid of material, as of waste products through the urine.

elixir (ĭ-lĭk′sər) N. sweetened, flavored liquid, usually containing a small amount of alcohol, used in compounding medicines to be taken by mouth.

Elixophyllin N. trade name for the drug aminophylline.

elongation N. act of lengthening something, particularly a muscle, ligament, or tendon. Also, the condition of being lengthened.

elution N. separation of one material from another by washing; used in chemistry in reference to washing ions from ion-exchange resins.

emaciation (ĭ-mā′shē-ā′shən) N. excessive thinness, due to disease (e.g., tuberculosis, cancer) or poor nutrition.

emasculation (ĭ-măs′kyə-lā′shən) N.
1. surgical removal of the penis and/or testes. *See also* CASTRATION.
2. loss of a feeling of masculinity or of having male characteristics.

embalming (ĕm-bäm′) N. preserving a dead body or body parts, usually for burial, by injecting a preservative solution such as formaldehyde. Usually done within 48 hours of death.

embolectomy (ĕm′bə-lĕk′tə-mē) N. surgical removal of an embolus, usually from an artery.

embolism (ĕm′bə-lĭz′əm) N. blockage of a blood vessel, esp. an artery, by an embolus. Treatment depends on the nature of the embolus, the degree of obstruction, and the blood vessels affected.

embolus (ĕm′bə-ləs) N., *pl.* emboli, clot of blood (thrombus), foreign object, bit of tissue, or air or gas bubble that moves through the bloodstream until it becomes lodged in a vessel, causing an embolism.

embryo (ĕm′brē-ō′) N. early developing organism, from the zygote to the fetal stage; in humans, from week 3 to week 8 after conception, at which time the main organ systems have formed, at least in their early stages. ADJ. embryonic

embryo- comb. form indicating an association with an embryo (e.g., embryotrophy, nourishment of the embryo).

embryogenesis (ĕm′brē-ō-jĕn′ĭ-sĭs) N. growth and development of an embryo.

embryology (ĕm-brē-ŏl′ə-jē) N. study of the growth and development of an embryo into the final organism.

emergency (ĭ-mûr′jən-sē) N. occasion of urgency; situation that arises suddenly and requires immediate action to save the life or health of a person (e.g., as when someone has swallowed poison).

emergency medical technician (EMT) N. person specially trained in prehospital care of the sick or injured patient; although the level of baseline education is specified by the Department of Transportation and typically is limited to basic life support (e.g., cardiopulmonary resuscitation, splinting, bandaging, extrication, spinal immobilization), certain states and localities allow EMTs to perform more advanced life support skills (e.g., administration of epinephrine to victims of anaphylactic shock, defibrillation); nationally, there is a strong trend to train all basic EMTs in defibrillation.

Emergency Medical Treatment and Active Labor Act *See* ANTI-DUMPING LAW OF 1985.

emergency medicine N. medical specialty concerned with the diagnosis and prompt treatment of injuries, trauma, or sudden illnesses.

emesis (ĕm′ĭ-sĭs) *See* VOMITING.

emetic (ĭ-mĕt′ĭk) N. substance that induces vomiting (e.g., ipecac), used in the treatment of some cases of drug overdose and in certain types of poisonings.

Emetrol N. trade name for a fixed-combination drug containing fructose, glucose (sugars), and phosphoric acid, used to treat nausea and vomiting.

EMG N. *See* ELECTROMYOGRAM.

Eminase N. trade name for the thrombolytic agent, APSAC.

eminence (ĕm′ə-nəns) N. raised, bumplike projection on a part, esp. on a bone (e.g., the deltoid eminence, a rise on the shaft of

MEMBRANES OF THE EMBRYO

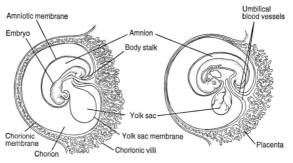

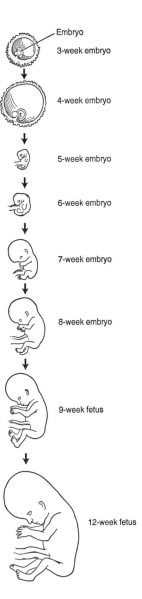

Embryo
3-week embryo
4-week embryo
5-week embryo
6-week embryo
7-week embryo
8-week embryo
9-week fetus
12-week fetus

the upper arm bone, where the deltoid muscle attaches).

emissary veins N. small blood vessels in the skull that drain blood from sinuses in the dura mater to veins outside the skull.

emission (ĭ-mĭsh′ən) N. release of something, esp. the uncontrolled discharge of semen during sleep (nocturnal emission). Also a component of the male sexual response, leading to ejaculation.

emmenagogue (ĭ-mĕn′ə-gôg′) N. drug used to bring on menstruation.

emmetropia (ĕm′ĭ-trō′pē-ə) N. state of normal vision, in which there is proper focus of light onto the retina. ADJ. emmetropic

emollient (ĭ-mŏl′yənt) N. agent that soothes or softens the skin (e.g., lanolin).

emotion (ĭ-mō′shən) N. intense feeling; a state of arousal, pleasant or unpleasant, often accompanied by physical changes such as release of epinephrine from the adrenal glands. Emotions include fear, anger, and love. ADJ. emotional

empathy (ĕm′pə-thē) N. ability to recognize and relate to, and to some extent share in, the emotions of another. ADJ. empathetic

emphysema (ĕm′fĭ-sē′mə) N. abnormal condition of the lungs in which there is overinflation of the air sacs (alveoli) of the lungs, leading to a breakdown of their walls, a decrease in respiratory function, and, in severe cases, increasing breathlessness. Emphysema appears to be associated with chronic bronchitis, smoking, and advancing age; one form that occurs early in life is related to a hereditary lack of an enzyme. Early symptoms of emphysema include dyspnea, cough, rapid heart rate; advanced cases are marked by signs of oxygen insufficiency (restlessness, weakness, confusion) and frequently by complications of pulmonary edema and congestive heart failure. Breathing exercises, drugs such as bronchodilators, and the prevention of respiratory infections may be helpful; severe cases may require oxygen.

empiric ADJ. pert. to treatment of disease based on observation and experience, not on knowledge of the specific causes or mechanisms of the disease.

Empirin N. trade name for a drug containing aspirin (a pain-reliever and a fever-reducer).

empyema (ĕm'pī-ē'mə) N. pus in the lung cavity or other body cavity, usually due to bacterial infection; treatment is by antibiotics and surgical drainage of the pus.

EMT N. abbrev. for emergency medical technician.

EMTALA *See* ANTI-DUMPING LAW OF 1985.

emulsify v. form into an emulsion, a mixture of two liquids that are not totally soluble within each other.

emulsion (ĭ-mŭl'shən) N. combination of two liquids (e.g., oil and water) dispersed one in the other.

E-mycin N. trade name for the antibiotic erythromycin.

en bloc ADJ. as a whole, in one piece.

enalapril (ĭ-năl'ə-prĭl) N. one of a class of drugs that block the formation of angiotensin in the kidney, leading to vasodilation. Sold under the trade name

Vasotec, enalapril is used in the treatment of hypertension, congestive heart failure, and myocardial infarction. Adverse effects include kidney problems and elevated potassium levels. *See* TABLE OF COMMONLY PRESCRIBED DRUGS—GENERIC NAMES.

enamel (ĭ-năm'əl) N. hard white covering above the gum line of a tooth.

enanthema N. eruption on a mucous membrane (e.g., the inside of the mouth).

enarthrosis (ĕn'är-thrō'sĭs) *See* BALL-AND-SOCKET JOINT.

encainide N. antiarrhythmic drug (trade name Enkaid) used in the treatment of life-threatening arrhythmias. Adverse effects include the exacerbation of arrhythmias and diarrhea. It is generally recommended that administration of this agent be started in a hospital.

encanthis N. a small growth at the inner angle of the eyelids.

encapsulation N. process of enclosing something in a covering; the condition of being enclosed in a capsule, as the tendons or nerves are enclosed in membranous sheaths.

encephal-, encephalo- comb. form indicating an association with the brain (e.g., encephalospinal, pert. to the brain and spinal cord).

encephalitis (ĕn-sĕf'ə-lī'tĭs) N. inflammation of the brain, usually due to viral infection but sometimes occurring as a complication of another infection (e.g., influenza, measles) or resulting from poisoning. Symptoms include headache, drowsiness, neck pain, nausea, and fever, followed sometimes by neurologic disturbances such as seizures, paralysis, and personality changes. The outcome depends on the cause, extent of the brain inflammation, and general condition of the patient. *See also* ENCEPHALOMYELITIS.

encephalocele (ĕn-sĕf′ə-lō-sēl′) N. protrusion of the brain through a congenital fissure in the skull.

encephalogram (ĕn-sĕf′ə-lə-grăm′) N. X ray of the brain made by withdrawing cerebrospinal fluid and replacing it with a gas (e.g., oxygen). It is a risky procedure, used when computed tomography is not definitive, and used in diagnosis of hydrocephalus and other abnormalities.

encephalomyelitis (ĕn-sĕf′ə-lō-mī′ə-lī′tĭs) N. acute inflammation of the brain and spinal cord, marked by fever, headache, neck and back pain, and vomiting; in severe cases and in weak or aged persons seizures, coma, and death may result. *See also* ENCEPHALITIS.

encephalon (ĕn-sĕf′ə-lŏn′) N. *See* BRAIN.

encephalopathy (ĕn-sĕf′ə-lŏp′ə-thē) N. any brain disease or disorder.

enchondroma (ĕn′kŏn-drō′mə) N. benign, slow-growing tumor of cartilage cells at the ends of tubular bones, esp. those of the hands and feet.

encopresis (ĕn′kŏ-prē′sĭs) N. condition, not caused by physical illness or defect, in which the passing of feces occurs without control.

encysted ADJ. surrounded by a capsule or membrane.

end-, endo- comb. form meaning inward, within (e.g., endocranial, within the skull) (*compare* ECTO-).

endarteritis (ĕn′där-tə-rī′tĭs) N. inflammation of the inner lining of an artery or arteries, often associated with advanced syphilis and causing progressive thickening and blocking of the vessel.

endemic (ĕn-dĕm′ĭk) ADJ. indigenous (native) to a given population or area; occurring frequently in a given group or community, esp. pert. to a disease.

endemic typhus *See* MURINE TYPHUS.

endocarditis (ĕn′dō-kär-dī′tĭs) N. inflammation of the membrane (endocardium) lining the inside of the heart and the heart valves, caused by bacterial infection. Symptoms include fever and changes in heart rhythms; damage to heart valves may occur. Treatment consists of bed rest, antibiotics, and surgery, if necessary, to treat damaged valves.

endocardium (ĕn′dō-kär′dē-əm) N. membrane that lines the chambers of the heart and the heart valves.

endocervicitis N. inflammation of the epithelium and glands of the cervix of the uterus.

Endocet N. *See* TABLE OF COMMONLY PRESCRIBED DRUGS— TRADE NAMES.

endocranium (ĕn′dō-krā′nē-əm) N. membrane lining the inside of the skull.

endocrine gland (ĕn′də-krĭn) N. any ductless gland (e.g., pituitary gland) that releases its secretion—a hormone—directly into the bloodstream, through which it moves to specific target organs to produce an effect.

endocrine system N. network of endocrine glands that produce and secrete hormones directly into the bloodstream for transport to specific target organs, where they exert their effect. Along with the nervous system, the endocrine system coordinates and regulates many of the activities of the body, including growth, metabolism, sexual development, and reproduction. *See* MAJOR ORGAN SYSTEMS; MAJOR ENDOCRINE GLANDS in Appendix.

endocrinologist N. physician who specializes in the diagnosis and treatment of diseases affecting the endocrine system.

endocrinology (ĕn′də-krə-nŏl′ə-jē) N. study of the structure, function, and diseases of the endocrine system. ADJ. endocrinologic

endoderm (ĕn′də-dûrm′) N. in the embryo, the inner layer of cells, from which the epithelium of the trachea, bronchi, lungs, gastrointestinal tract, and many other organs arise and from which the lining of body cavities and the covering of internal organs arises. (The other cell layers are the outer ectoderm and the middle mesoderm.)

endogenous (ĕn-dŏj′ə-nəs) ADJ. developed within an organism; arising within; for example, endogenous obesity is caused by an endocrine or metabolic disorder, not by overeating (*compare* EXOGENOUS).

endogenous depression N. serious and persistent form of depression believed due to a complex interrelationship of biochemical, genetic, and psychological factors and frequently not traceable

to a specific extrinsic event (e.g., death of a spouse).

endometrial ADJ. pert. to the endometrium, the mucous membrane lining of the uterus (e.g., endometrial carcinoma, cancer of uterine lining).

endometriosis (ĕn′dō-mē′trē-ō′sĭs) N. condition marked by the presence, growth, and function of endometrial tissue outside of its normal location (lining of the uterus) in such sites as the uterine walls, the fallopian tubes, the ovaries, and other sites within the pelvis or, rarely, out of the pelvic region. Endometriosis is fairly common (est. 15% of women), esp. in childless women and women who have children late in life. Symptoms depend on the size and location of the displaced tissue but commonly include painful menstruation, painful coitus, and sometimes painful urination and defecation and premenstrual staining. Endometriosis is a common cause of infertility. Treatment includes analgesics to relieve pain, hormones to decrease the size and number of lesions and, in severe cases, surgery.

ENDOCRINE GLANDS

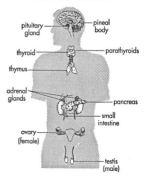

pituitary gland
pineal body
thyroid
parathyroids
thymus
adrenal glands
pancreas
small intestine
ovary (female)
testis (male)

ENDOCRINES AND THEIR HORMONES

Name of Gland	Location	Hormone	Normal Functions	Excess Secretion	Diminished Secretion
Anterior pituitary	Base of brain, forward portion	Growth hormone (STH)	Affect skeletal growth, protein synthesis, blood glucose concentration	Gigantism acromegaly	Dwarfism
		Trophic hormones TSH ACHT FSH LH	Stimulate target glands thyroid adrenal cortex ovarian follicles; testes gonads	Oversecretion of target glands	Undersecretion of target glands
Posterior pituitary	Base of brain, hind portion	Vasopressin	Control of blood pressure; reabsorption of water by kidney tubules	Increased blood pressure; glycogen converted to sugar	Decreased blood pressure; excess sugar changed to fat; kidney tubules not reabsorbing water
		Oxytocin	Contractions of uterus		
Thyroid	Two lobes on either side of larynx	Throxin (65% iodine)	Controls rate of oxidation in cells	Increased oxidation; nervous exophthalmic goiter	Lowered oxidation; in a child—cretinism; in an adult—myxedemic goiter due to lack of iodine in drinking water

ENDOCRINES AND THEIR HORMONES (CONTINUED)

Name of Gland	Location	Hormone	Normal Functions	Excess Secretion	Diminished Secretion
Parathyroid	Four glands above thyroid	Parathormone	Regulates amount of calcium in blood	Trembling due to lack of muscular control	Contraction of muscles (tetany); death
Stomach	Mucous lining	Gastrin	Stimulates secretion of gastric juices	Promotes ulceration of stomach wall	Inhibits gastric digestion
Small intestine	Mucous lining	Secretin	Activates the liver and pancreas to secrete and release their secretions	Excessive pancreatic and liver secretions	Diminished pancreatic and liver secretion
Adrenal medulla	Two glands above kidney	Adrenalin	Controls release of sugar from liver; contraction of arteries; clotting	Increases blood pressure; promotes clotting; releases glycogen; strengthens heart beat	
Adrenal cortex		Glucocorticoids	Affect normal functioning of gonads; help maintain normal blood sugar levels	Cushing's disease	Addison's disease; muscular weakness, darkening of skin, low blood pressure; death
		Mineralo-corticoids	Stimulate kidney tubules to reabsorb sodium	Hyperaldo-steronism	

ENDOCRINES AND THEIR HORMONES (CONTINUED)

Name of Gland	Location	Hormone	Normal Functions	Excess Secretion	Diminished Secretion
Isles of Langerhans	Embedded in pancreas	Insulin	Regulates storage of glycogen in liver; accelerates oxidation of sugar in cells	Hypoglycemia	Diabetes; unused sugar remains in blood and is excreted with urine
Gonads	Abdominal region	Testosterone (males) Estrogen, progesterone (females)	Regulates normal growth and development of sex glands; regulates reproduction; controls sex characteristics	Premature development of gonads; effects on secondary sex characteristics	Interference with normal reproductive functions; diminished growth of sex characteristics
Thymus	Chest region	Thymosin	Stimulates immunological activity of lymphoid tissue		Breakdown of immune system
Pineal	Base of brain	Melatonin	Regulates gonadotropins by anterior pituitary		

endometritis (ĕn′dō-mĭ-trī′tĭs) N. acute or chronic inflammation of the endometrium, usually caused by bacterial infection and most commonly occurring after childbirth, abortion, or the fitting of an intrauterine device (IUD). Symptoms include fever, abdominal pain, enlargement of the uterus, and vaginal discharge (often foul-smelling). Treatment includes antibiotics and rest; untreated, endometritis may lead to blockage of the fallopian tubes and resultant ectopic pregnancy or infertility.

endometrium (ĕn′dō-mē′trē-əm) N. mucous membrane lining of the uterus, which, under hormonal control, changes in thickness and complexity during the menstrual cycle, and if pregnancy does not occur is mostly shed during menstruation. ADJ. endometrial

endomorph (ĕn′də-môrf′) N. person whose body tends to be more heavily developed in the torso than in the limbs, with fat accumulations giving the body a generally round and soft appearance (compare ECTOMORPH; MESOMORPH). ADJ. endomorphic

endomyocarditis (ĕn′dō-mī′ō-kär-dī′tĭs) N. acute or chronic inflammation of the heart muscle (myocardium) and the inner lining (endocardium) of the heart, due to disease or infection. See also ENDOCARDITIS.

endoneurium (ĕn′dō-no͝or′ē-əm) N. fragile tissue covering the separate fibers in a nerve.

endorphin (ĕn-dôr′fĭn) N. any of several naturally occurring chemicals (proteins) in the brain, believed to be involved in reducing or eliminating pain and in enhancing pleasure. Studies show that acupuncture may induce activation of endorphins. (Compare ENKEPHALIN.)

endoscopy (ĕn-dŏs′kə-pē) N. inspection of the inside of a body cavity by means of a special instrument (endoscope), usually inserted through a natural body opening (e.g., the mouth, anus, urethra) but sometimes through an incision. ADJ. endoscopic

endosteum (ĕn-dŏs′tē-əm) N. membranous lining of a cavity inside a bone.

endothelium (ĕn′dō-thē′lē-əm) N. layer of flat cells that lines the heart, blood and lymph vessels, and some body cavities. ADJ. endothelial

endotoxin (ĕn′dō-tŏk′sən) N. toxin confined within a bacterium or other microorganism and released only when the microorganism is broken down or dies. Endotoxins may cause fever, chills, shock, and other symptoms in the infected person. (Compare EXOTOXIN.) ADJ. endotoxic

ENDOTRACHEAL TUBE

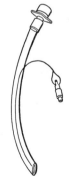

endotracheal tube (ĕn′də-trā′kē-əl) N. catheter inserted through the mouth or nose into the trachea to maintain an open airway (e.g., in severe inflammation and swelling of the pharynx), to deliver oxygen, to permit suctioning of mucus, or to prevent aspiration of stomach contents.

end-plate N. end of the fiber of a motor nerve in a muscle that receives a stimulus (neurotransmitter) from a motor nerve fiber.

Enduron N. trade name for a diuretic and antihypertensive.

enema (ĕn′ə-mə) N. insertion of liquid into the rectum to remove feces, to help diagnose certain gastrointestinal disorders (barium enema), or to administer drugs or nourishment.

enervation N.
1. weakness, loss of strength or energy.
2. surgical removal of a nerve.

enflurane N. nonflammable gas used as a general anesthetic.

engagement (ĕn-gāj′mənt) N. in obstetrics, fixation of the presenting part of the fetus, usually the head, in the maternal pelvis; it usually occurs in late pregnancy, after which fetal movements are curtailed.

engorge (ĕn-gôrj′) v. to fill to the limit of expansion.

enkephalin (ĕn-kĕf′ə-lĭn) N. any of a group of brain chemicals (proteins) that influence mental activity and behavior (sometimes grouped with the endorphins as natural opiates). Evidence shows that these chemicals influence the body's immune system and help fight disease. (*Compare* ENDORPHIN.)

enoderm *See* ENDODERM.

enophthalmos (ĕn′ŏf-thăl′məs) N. condition in which the eyeball is displaced back in the eye

socket, because of injury or developmental defect.

Enovid N. trade name for an oral contraceptive containing the estrogen mestranol and the progestin norethynodrel.

enter-, entero- comb. forms indicating an association with the intestine (e.g., enterogastric, pert. to the intestine and stomach).

enteric (ĕn-tĕr′ĭk) ADJ. pert. to the intestines.

enteric-coated N. referring to pills or tablets; covered with an outer layer of film that does not dissolve until the medication reaches the small intestine. As a result, the lining of the stomach is not exposed to the underlying medication. Enteric coating is commonly used to reduce stomach inflammation from known irritants, such as aspirin.

enteritis (ĕn′tə-rī′tĭs) N. inflammation of the intestine, esp. the small intestine, due to viral or bacterial infection or other disorder, usually marked by diarrhea (*compare* GASTROENTERITIS).

enterobiasis (ĕn′tə-rō-bī′sĭs) N. infection of the large intestine with the pinworm *Enterobius vermicularis,* occurring esp. in children. The females deposit eggs around the anus, which cause itching; if the patient scratches the area and then puts the fingers in or near the mouth, reinfection occurs. Treatment is by anthelmintics (agents that destroy worms).

enterocolitis (ĕn′tə-rō-kō-lī′tĭs) N. general term for infection of both the small intestine and the colon; symptoms may include nausea, vomiting, diarrhea, and fever. Both viruses and bacte-

THE ACTIVITY OF ENZYMES

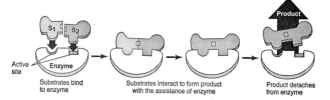

Substrates bind to enzyme • Active site Enzyme • Substrates interact to form product with the assistance of enzyme • Product detaches from enzyme • Product

ria cause enterocolitis. Infection with either may result in severe illness and dehydration.

enterolithiasis (ĕn′tə-rō-lĭ-thī′ə-sĭs) N. presence of stonelike formations in the intestines.

enteropathic ADJ. capable of causing disease in any part of the intestine.

enteroptosis (ĕn′tə-rŏp-tō′sĭs) N. unusually downward position of the intestine in the abdominal cavity.

enterospasm N. excessive, abnormal contraction of muscles in the intestine, usually causing pain.

enterostomy (ĕn′tə-rŏs′tə-mē) N. surgical creation of a permanent opening into the intestine through the abdominal wall performed in the treatment of cancer, Crohn's disease, and sometimes malnutrition (*compare* COLOSTOMY).

enterotoxin (ĕn′tə-rō-tŏk′sĭn) N. poison produced by or originating in the intestinal contents; often refers to a toxin made by bacteria under various disease conditions such as food poisoning or toxic shock syndrome.

Entozyme N. trade name for a fixed-combination drug containing bile salts and digestive enzymes (pepsin and pancreatin).

entropion (ĕn-trō′pē-ŏn′) N. abnormal inward turning of an edge, esp. the eyelid toward the eyeball, resulting from spasm or from scar tissue on the conjunctiva.

entropy N. degree of randomness, chaos, or disorder in any system; chemically, energy in a system that is not available to perform mechanical work, but may be used internally.

enucleation N. surgical removal of a whole tumor or whole organ (e.g., the eyeball).

enuresis (ĕn′yə-rē′sĭs) N. passing of urine without control, esp. during sleep (bedwetting). The condition can be caused by a urinary tract disorder but is usually a childhood phenomenon that is outgrown. Restriction of fluids, esp. near bedtime, and the use of a device that rings a bell to awaken the child when urination begins are sometimes helpful. (*Compare* NOCTURIA; *see also* INCONTINENCE.) ADJ. enuretic

enzyme (ĕn′zīm) N. protein produced in cells that acts as a catalyst speeding up the rate of biological reactions without itself being used up. Many enzymes are involved in digestion (e.g., lipase helps to break down fat) and respiration. The names of many enzymes end in

-ase. *See also* SUBSTRATE. ADJ. enzymatic

eosin (ē′ə-sən) N. red dye commonly used to stain cells, bacteria, and other materials for examination under the microscope.

eosinopenia (ē′ə-sĭn′ə-pē′nē-ə) N. decrease in the number of eosinophils in the blood.

eosinophil (ē′ə-sĭn′ə-fĭl′) N. white blood cell readily stained with eosin. Eosinophils, normally about 1–3% of the total white blood cell count, are believed to function in allergic responses and in resisting some infections.

eosinophilia (ē′ə-sĭn′ə-fĭl′ē-ə) N. increase in the number of eosinophils in the blood; it commonly occurs in allergic reactions and in some inflammatory conditions.

ep-, epi- prefix meaning on or above (e.g., epipial, on the brain's inner covering, the pia mater).

ependyma N. very thin membrane that lines the ventricles of the brain and the central spinal canal; helps to form cerebrospinal fluid.

ephedrine (ĭ-fĕd′rĭn, ĕf′ĭ-drēn′) N. bronchodilator; drug that widens the air passages of the lungs and is used to treat asthma, bronchitis, and other conditions. Adverse effects include headache, nervousness, and insomnia.

epicanthus (ĕp′ĭ-kăn′thəs) N. vertical fold of skin on the inner aspect of the eye, normal in Oriental persons and sometimes occurring also in Down's syndrome; also called epicanthic fold. ADJ. epicanthal, epicanthic

epicardia (ĕp′ĭ-kär′dē-ə) N. that part of the esophagus between the diaphragm and the stomach.

epicardium (ĕp′ĭ-kär′dē-əm) N. innermost of the two layers of the pericardium, the membranous covering of the heart.

epicondyle (ĕp′ĭ-kŏn′dīl) N. projection on a bone, above another part, the condyle.

epicondylitis (ĕp′ĭ-kŏn′dl-ī′tĭs) N. painful inflammation of the muscles and soft tissue around the elbow, usually caused by excessive strain, as in tennis or golf, or by carrying a heavy load. Treatment includes rest and injection of pain-relieving drugs into the joint area. *See also* TENNIS ELBOW.

epicranium (ĕp′ĭ-krā′nē-əm) N. all layers of the scalp; the coverings of the skull.

epidemic (ĕp′ĭ-dĕm′ĭk) N. outbreak of infectious disease (e.g., influenza) in which many people in a given geographic area are readily affected with the disorder. ADJ. affecting a large number of people at the same time (*compare* ENDEMIC; PANDEMIC).

epidemiology (ĕp′ĭ-dē′mē-ŏl′ə-jē) N. study of the causes, occurrences, and control of disease.

epidermis (ĕp′ĭ-dûr′mĭs) N. superficial, outer layers of the skin that contain numerous nerve endings but no blood vessels. Made up of squamous epithelium tissue, the epidermis is divided into two layers. The outer stratum corneum contains dead cells that are sloughed off as new cells from the inner stratum germinativum push upward; other layers are also sometimes found esp. in thick skin (e.g., the palms and soles). ADJ. epidermal, epidermoid.

THE LAYERS OF THE EPIDERMIS

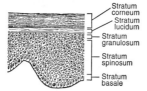

Stratum corneum
Stratum lucidum
Stratum granulosum
Stratum spinosum
Stratum basale

epididymis (ĕp′ĭ-dĭd′ə-mĭs) N. long, coiled tube along the back side of the testis that connects the seminiferous tubules of the testis to the vas deferens. Sperm mature as they pass through the epididymis and are then stored before ejaculation. ADJ. epididymal

epididymitis (ĕp′ĭ-dĭd′ə-mī′tĭs) N. acute or chronic inflammation of the epididymis, producing tenderness, pain in the groin, chills and fever; it may result from sexually transmitted disease, inflammation of the prostate, or urinary tract infection. Treatment includes rest, support of the area, and antibiotics, if appropriate.

epidural (ĕp′ĭ-doŏr′əl) ADJ. outside the dura mater, the outermost membranous covering of the brain and spinal cord; also called extradural.

epidural anesthesia N. injection of local anesthesia into the epidural space of the spinal column to achieve regional anesthesia of the abdominal, genital, or pelvic area; widely used in vaginal childbirth, Cesarean delivery, and gynecologic surgery.

epigastric (ĕp′ĭ-găs′trĭk) ADJ. above the stomach; in the epigastrium, the region of the abdomen just below the chest.

epiglottis (ĕp′ĭ-glŏt′ĭs) N. flap of mucous-membrane-covered cartilage at the back of the mouth cavity that covers the opening to the windpipe during swallowing, thereby preventing choking.

epiglottitis (ĕp′ĭ-glŏ-tī′tĭs) N. inflammation of the epiglottis, characterized by severe sore throat (pharyngitis), difficulty in swallowing (dysphagia), and fever. If untreated, complete airway obstruction with respiratory failure and death may result. It is most common in children 3–5 years old, but may also occur in adults. The cause is a bacterial infection (Hemophilus influenza). Treatment involves hospitalization, intravenous antibiotics, and possibly, placement of an endotracheal tube for breathing.

epikeratophakia (ĕp′ĭ-kĕr′ə-tō-fā′kē-ə) N. shaping of a piece of donated cornea to the eye of a patient who has had a cataract removed. Called a living contact lens, the added tissue bends the light to focus on the retina. The technique has been used on babies born with cataracts and also for correction of keratoconus and myopia.

epilation (ĕp′ə-lā′shən) N. removal of hair by the roots.

epilepsy (ĕp′ə-lĕp′sē) N. neurological disorder characterized by recurrent episodes (ranging from several times a day to once in several years) of convulsive seizures, impaired consciousness, abnormal behavior, and other disturbances produced by uncontrolled electrical discharges from nerve cells in the brain. Trauma to the head, brain tumor, chemical imbalances, and other factors may be associated with epilepsy, but in

LAYERS OF THE EPIDERMIS

Stratum (Layer)	Characteristics
Stratum basale (stratum germinativum)	Deepest layer; single layer of cuboidal or columnar cells; site of continuous cellular reproduction; contains the only cells of the epidermis that receive nutrition; cells are constantly undergoing division and being pushed up to the body surface.
Stratum spinosum	Many keratinocytes with spiny appearance; some keratin.
Stratum granulosum	Three to five rows of flat cells; site of keratohyalin and keratin formation.
Stratum lucidum	Only in the thick skin of the palms and soles; consists of clear, flat, dead cells; cells contain eleidin.
Stratum corneum	Outermost layer of epidermis; 25 to 30 rows of flat, dead cells filled with keratin; continuously shed and replaced.

most cases the cause is unknown. Treatment depends on the severity and frequency of episodes and usually involves anticonvulsant drugs. Common types of epilepsy are grand mal and petit mal. ADJ. epileptic.

epimysium (ĕp'ə-mĭz'ē-əm) N. fibrous tissue surrounding a muscle.

epinephrine (ĕp'ə-nĕf'rĭn) N.
1. hormone of the adrenal medulla that acts as a powerful stimulant in times of fear or arousal and has many physiological effects; these include increasing breathing, heart, and metabolic rates to provide quick energy, constricting blood vessels, and strengthening muscle contraction; also called adrenaline.
2. synthetic drug used in the treatment of bronchial asthma to reduce bronchospasm and dilate air passageways in the treatment of anaphylactic shock, hypotension, and cardiac arrest.

epineurium N. connective tissue sheath surrounding a nerve fiber.

epiphysis (ĭ-pĭf'ĭ-sĭs) N., *pl.* epiphyses.
1. end portion of a long bone, separated by cartilage from the shaft (the diaphysis) until the bone stops growing, at which time the shaft and head unite.
2. *See* PINEAL GLAND. ADJ. epiphyseal

episcleritis N. inflammation of the sclera (the white of the eye) and overlying tissues.

episiotomy (ĭ-pĭz'ē-ŏt'ə-mē) N. incision made to enlarge the opening of the vagina during a difficult birth or forceps delivery. The purpose is to make the delivery easier or to hasten it, and to avoid stretching and tearing adjacent muscle and tissue.

epispadias (ĕp'ĭ-spā'dē-əs) N. congenital abnormality in males in which the opening for passing urine (the urethra) is on the upper surface of the penis.

epistaxis (ĕp'ĭ-stăk'sĭs) N. bleeding from the nose; causes include a blow or other injury, violent sneezing, high blood pressure, and fragile mucous membranes. The bleeding may be controlled by applying pressure to the sides of the nose, by inserting cotton or gauze, or by holding an ice compress over the nose. Also called nosebleed.

epithelium (ĕp'ə-thē'lē-əm) N. cell layers covering the outside body surfaces as well as forming the lining of hollow organs (e.g., the bladder) and the passages of the respiratory, digestive, and urinary tracts. ADJ. epithelial

eponym N. name for a structure, condition, or process that includes or is formed from the name of a person (e.g., Meniere's disease, Parkinsonism).

epsom salt (ĕp'səm) N. bitter-tasting chemical (magnesium sulfate) commonly dissolved in water and swallowed to treat heartburn and constipation. It may also be prescribed to prevent seizures (esp. in preeclampsia) and is used as a soaking solution for treatment of inflammations.

Epstein-Barr virus (EBV) (ĕp'stīn) N. virus that causes infectious mononucleosis and in parts of Africa is associated with Burkitt's lymphoma.

Epstein's pearls N. small, white, pearl-like cysts occurring on the hard palate of a newborn that disappear within a few weeks.

equilibrium (ē'kwə-lĭb'rē-əm) N. state of balance, in which opposing forces (e.g., body chemicals such as calcium and phosphorus) exactly counteract each other.

A COMPARISON OF EPINEPHRINE AND NOREPINEPHRINE

Body Organ or Function Affected	Epinephrine	Norepinephrine
Heart	Rate increases Force of contraction increases	Rate increases Little or no effect on force of contraction
Blood vessels	Vessels in skeletal muscle vasodilate, thereby decreasing resistance to blood flow	Vessels in skeletal muscles vasoconstrict, thereby increasing resistance to blood flow
Systemic blood	Some increase due to increased cardiac output	Great increase due to vasoconstriction
Airways	Dilation	Less effect
Reticular formation of brain	Activated	Little effect
Liver	Promotes change of glycogen to glucose—increasing blood sugar	Little effect on blood sugar
Metabolic rate	Increases	Little or no effect

equine encephalitis N. infection characterized by inflammation of the brain and spinal cord, fever, headache, nausea, vomiting, and neurological symptoms (e.g., tremor, visual disturbances). It is caused by a virus transmitted by a mosquito from an infected horse.

Erb's palsy N. paralysis of the arm due to injury to the brachial plexus, most often during childbirth, also called Erb-Duchenne paralysis.

erectile dysfunction (ED) N. condition where the penis does not harden and expand when a man is sexually excited, or when he cannot keep an erection. ED can be a total inability to achieve erection, an inconsistent ability to do so, or a tendency to sustain only brief erections. The word "impotence" may also be used to describe other problems that interfere with sexual intercourse and reproduction, such as lack of sexual desire and problems with ejaculation or orgasm. Using the term "erectile dysfunction" makes it clear that those other problems are not involved. In older men, ED usually has a physical cause, such as disease, injury, or side effects of drugs. The incidence of ED increases with age, but it is not an inevitable part of aging. Any disorder that causes injury to the nerves or impairs blood flow in the penis has the potential to cause ED. Surgery (especially radical prostate and bladder surgery for cancer) can injure nerves and arteries near the penis, causing ED. Psychological factors such as stress, anxiety, guilt, depression, low self-esteem, and fear of sexual failure cause 10 to 20% of ED cases. Drugs for treating ED can be taken orally, injected directly into the penis, or inserted into the urethra at the tip of the penis. While oral medicines (e.g., Viagra, Cialis, or Levitra) improve the response to sexual stimulation, they do not trigger an automatic erection as injections do.

TYPES OF EPITHELIAL TISSUE

Simple squamous

Simple cuboidal

Simple columnar

Pseudostratified columnar

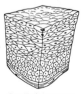

Stratified squamous

Transitional

Many men achieve stronger erections by injecting drugs into the penis, causing it to become engorged with blood. Drugs such as papaverine hydrochloride, phentolamine, and alprostadil (Caverject) widen blood vessels. These drugs may create unwanted side effects, however, including persistent erection (known as priapism) and scarring. Nitroglycerin, a muscle relaxant, can sometimes enhance erection when rubbed on the penis. A system for inserting a pellet of alprostadil into the urethra is marketed as Muse. The system uses a prefilled applicator to deliver the pellet about an inch deep into the urethra. An erection will begin within 8 to 10 minutes and may last 30 to 60 minutes.

erectile tissue (ĭ-rĕk′təl) N. type of spongy tissue (e.g., that found in the penis or clitoris) having large spaces within it that can fill with blood to stiffen the structure in which it is contained.

erection (ĭ-rĕk′shən) N. state of rigidity, esp. of the penis, which becomes enlarged and elevated when its tissues fill with blood usually as a result of sexual arousal but also occurring normally during sleep and as a result of physical stimulation. Erection of the penis enables the penis to enter the vagina during coitus.

erethism (ĕr′ə-thĭz′əm) N. state of abnormal irritation, sensitivity, or excitement.

ergo- comb. form indicating an association with work or exertion (e.g., ergocardiogram, record of heart action during exertion).

ergocalciferol (ûr′gō-kăl-sĭf′ə-rôl′) See CALCIFEROL.

ergonomics (ûr′gə-nŏm′ĭks) N. study and analysis of work as it relates to human physical and physiological processes.

ergonovine N. ergot preparation used to contract the uterus to prevent or treat hemorrhage following childbirth or abortion.

ergot (ûr′gət) N. fungus (*Claviceps purpurea*) that infects wheat, rye, and other cereal grains. It produces several alkaloids (ergonovine, ergotamine) used in medicine. Ingestion of food contaminated with ergot causes ergotism.

ergotamine (ûr-gŏt′ə-mēn′) N. ergot alkaloid that causes constriction of blood vessels and contraction of uterine muscles and is used to treat migraine and postpartum lack of muscle tone in the uterus.

ergotism N. ergot poisoning, resulting from prolonged or excessive use of ergot-containing drugs or from accidental ingestion of ergot-contaminated food. Symptoms include excessive thirst, diarrhea, nausea, vomiting, cramping, abnormal cardiac rhythms, and, if severe, seizures and gangrene of the extremities.

Ergotrate maleate N. trade name for ergonovine.

erogenous (ĭ-rŏj′ə-nəs) ADJ. pert. to stimulation of the sexual instinct, esp. to the areas of the body (erogenous zones) where such stimulation leads to sexual arousal.

erosion (ĭ-rō′zhən) N. wearing away of a surface, esp. a mucous membrane or epidermal surface, due to inflammation, injury, friction, or other factor.

eroticism (ĭ-rŏt'ĭ-sĭz'əm) N.
1. sexual instinct or desire.
2. unusually strong or persistent sexual drive.

eructation (ĭ-rŭk-tā'shən) N. act of bringing up air from the stomach with a characteristic noise; belching.

eruption (ĭ-rŭp'shən) N.
1. act of breaking out and becoming visible, esp. a rash or other skin lesion.
2. emergence of a tooth as it breaks through the gum.

erysipelas (ĕr'ĭ-sĭp'ə-ləs) N. acute skin disease, caused by infection with bacteria of the genus streptococcus (esp. *Streptococcus pyogenes*) and characterized by redness, swelling, fever, pain, and skin lesions. Treatment is by antibiotics.

erysipeloid (ĕr'ĭ-sĭp'ə-loid') N. infection of the hands, characterized by reddish nodules and sometimes erythema. It is usually acquired by handling meat or fish infected with *Erysipelothrix rhusiopathiae*. Treatment is by antibiotics.

Ery-Tab N. *See* TABLE OF COMMONLY PRESCRIBED DRUGS—TRADE NAMES.

erythema (ĕr'ə-thē'mə)N. abnormal redness of the skin resulting from dilatation of the capillaries, as occurs in sunburn. ADJ. erythematous

erythema multiforme (mŭl'tə-fôr'mē) N. a red, slightly raised rash occurring on the body as a hypersensitivity reaction to a disease, drug, or other allergen. Treatment depends on the cause.

erythema nodosum N. tender, reddened nodules on the shins, legs, and occasionally other body areas, often accompanied by fever, muscle and joint pain, and malaise; it occurs in certain diseases, as a drug reaction, and in certain allergic reactions.

erythro- comb. form meaning red (e.g., erythroclasis, splitting of red blood cells).

erythroblast (ĭ-rĭth'rə-blăst') N. nucleated cell passing through maturation stages to become a mature erythrocyte. Erythroblasts are normally found in bone marrow, but they may appear in the blood circulation in certain diseases.

erythroblastosis fetalis (ĭ-rĭth'rō-blă-stō'sĭs) N. severe anemia in newborn babies, resulting from an incompatibility between fetal and maternal blood, specifically involving the Rh factor. It typically occurs in the Rh-positive infant (the Rh factor being inherited from the father) of an Rh-negative mother, the mother transmitting to the fetal bloodstream antibodies against the Rh antigen that cause destruction of the fetal blood. The disorder rarely occurs in a first-born (unless the mother has already been sensitized to Rh antigen by a transfusion with Rh-positive blood), but the risk increases with each succeeding pregnancy. The condition can be diagnosed before birth through amniocentesis and treated by intrauterine transfusion. In some cases the development of Rh antibodies by the mother may be prevented by administration of anti-RH gamma globulin (RhoGAM) following birth or abortion of an Rh-positive fetus.

Erythrocin N. trade name for the antibacterial erythromycin.

erythrocyte (ĭ-rĭth′rə-sīt′) N. mature red blood cell (RBC), which contains the pigment hemoglobin, the main function of which is to transport oxygen to the tissues of the body. A red blood cell is a biconcave disc with no nucleus. It is the main cellular element in the blood; in 1 cubic milliliter of blood there are usually 4,500,000–5,000,000 erythrocytes in males, 4,000,000–4,500,000 in females.

erythrocyte sedimentation rate (ESR) N. rate at which red blood cells settle out in a tube (usually a 10-centimeter or 200-milliliter tube) of unclotted blood under standardized conditions. An ESR higher than normal usually indicates the presence of inflammation, and the test can be used as a diagnostic aid and for monitoring the course of an inflammatory process (e.g., in chronic infections, rheumatic disorders). Colloquially called sed rate.

erythrocythemia N. massive and abnormal increase in the numbers of circulating red blood cells (erythrocytes); often due to a tumor of the bone marrow, such as polycythemia vera. *Compare* ERYTHROCYTOSIS.

erythrocytosis (ĭ-rĭth′rō-sī-tō′sĭs) N. any abnormal increase in the numbers of red blood cells, but to a lower extent and due to many different conditions (e.g., emphysema, cigarette smoking, living at altitude). *Compare* ERYTHROCYTHEMIA.

erythroderma (ĭ-rĭth′rō-dûr′mə) N. any skin disorder associated with abnormal redness (*compare* ERYTHEMA).

erythromycin (ĭ-rĭth′rə-mī′sĭn) N. antibiotic, known under several trade names (e.g., E-Mycin, Erythrocin) used to treat infections caused by a wide variety of bacteria and other microorganisms. Adverse side effects are uncommon but may include nausea and diarrhea or, rarely, hypersensitivity reactions and liver inflammation. *See* TABLE OF COMMONLY PRESCRIBED DRUGS—GENERIC NAMES.

erythropoiesis (ĭ-rĭth′rō-poi-ē′sĭs) N. process of erythrocyte production; it normally occurs in the bone marrow.

erythropoietin (ĭ-rĭth′rō-poi-ē′tĭn) N. protein produced by the kidneys and liver that stimulates the bone marrow to produce red blood cells (erythrocytes). Since only 15% of the body's erythropoietin is manufactured by the liver, a patient with kidney failure inevitably becomes anemic. The gene for this hormone has been cloned and recombinant (genetically engineered) erythropoietin produced in animal cells is available for clinical use. It has also been used illegally in athletes seeking a competitive advantage.

eschar (ĕs′kär′) N. scab or crust that forms on the skin after a burn.

Esidrix N. trade name for the diuretic hydrochlorothiazide. *See* TABLE OF COMMONLY PRESCRIBED DRUGS—TRADE NAMES.

-esis suffix indicating an action or condition (e.g., enuresis).

Eskalith N. trade name for the antipsychotic lithium carbonate.

esmolol (ĕs′mə-lôl′) N. intravenous beta-blocking drug (trade name Brevibloc) with short duration of action, used primarily for rate control in cardiac arrhythmias.

esophag-, esophago- comb. forms indicating an association with the esophagus (e.g., esophagectomy, surgical removal of the esophagus).

esophagitis (ĭ-sŏf'ə-jī'tĭs) N. inflammation of the esophagus, most often caused by backflow of acid stomach contents (gastro-esophageal reflux) often associated with hiatus hernia but sometimes caused by infection or irritation.

esophagoscope (ĭ-sŏf'ə-gə-skōp') N. special optical instrument used to examine the esophagus, to dilate the canal, or to remove a foreign object or material for biopsy.

esophagus (ĭ-sŏf'ə-gəs) N. gullet; the muscular canal, about 24 centimeters (10 inches) long, that connects the pharynx and stomach; food passes through it by waves of peristalsis. ADJ. esophageal

esotropia (ĕs'ə-trō'pē-ə) N. condition in which one or both eyes appear to turn inward, cross-eye (*see also* STRABISMUS).

ESP *See* EXTRASENSORY PERCEPTION.

ESR *See* ERYTHROCYTE SEDIMENTATION RATE.

essential amino acid (ĭ-sĕn'shəl) *See* AMINO ACID.

essential hypertension N. high blood pressure (hypertension) for which no specific cause can be found.

EST *See* ELECTROCONVULSIVE THERAPY.

Estar N. trade name for a coal tar preparation used to treat eczema, psoriasis, and other skin conditions.

Estrace N. *See* TABLE OF COMMONLY PRESCRIBED DRUGS—TRADE NAMES.

Estraderm N. *See* TABLE OF COMMONLY PRESCRIBED DRUGS—TRADE NAMES.

estradiol (ĕs'trə-dī'ôl') N. most powerful naturally occurring female hormone. *See also* ESTROGEN; TABLE OF COMMONLY PRESCRIBED DRUGS—GENERIC NAMES.

Estratab N. trade name for an estrogen preparation.

estriol (ĕs'trī-ôl') N. naturally occurring, rather weak estrogen.

estrogen (ĕs'trə-jən) N. general term for the female hormones (including estradiol, estrone, estriol) produced in the ovaries (and in small amounts in the testes and adrenals). In women estrogen functions in the menstrual cycle and in the development of secondary sex characteristics (e.g., breast development in adolescence). As a synthetic preparation, sold under many trade names, estrogen drugs are used to treat menstrual irregularities, to relieve symptoms of menopause, to treat cancer of the prostate, and in oral contraceptives. Long-term use of estrogen has been associated with some blood-clotting disorders and some forms of cancer and is controversial.

estrone (ĕs'trōn') N. form of estrogen.

Estronol N. trade name for an estrone preparation.

estrus (ĕs'trəs) N. periodic occurrence of sexual activity in female mammals, marked by acceptance of the male (commonly known as being in heat).

The term is not used in reference to human sexuality.

ethacrynic acid N. diuretic (trade name Edecrin) used to treat edema. Adverse effects include muscle weakness, electrolyte imbalance, and hearing disorders.

ethanol (ĕth'ə-nôl') N. ethyl alcohol: the alcohol found in alcoholic beverages and the alcohol used in solution as an antiseptic. *See also* ALCOHOL.

ether (ē'thər) N. liquid used as a solvent and general anesthetic. It is generally safe and provides excellent pain relief and muscle relaxation without greatly depressing the respiratory and circulatory systems. However, it is explosive and highly flammable, has an irritating odor, and frequently causes postoperative nausea and vomiting. For these reasons it has been largely replaced by safer anesthetic drugs.

ethical drug (ĕth'ĭ-kəl) N. prescription drug; drug available only by prescription (e.g., Demerol).

ethmoid (ĕth'moid') N. one of the eight bones of the cranium; a small bone filled with air spaces that is between the eye sockets. ADJ. ethmoidal

ethmoid sinus N. cavity in the ethmoid bone behind the bridge of the nose.

ethosuximide N. anticonvulsant (trade name Zarontin), used to treat petit mal epilepsy. Adverse effects include blood abnormalities and gastrointestinal disturbances.

Ethrane N. trade name for the inhalation general anesthetic enflurane.

ethyl alcohol *See* ETHANOL; ALCOHOL.

ethyl chloride N. highly flammable topical anesthetic used in the treatment of skin irritations and in minor skin surgery. Adverse effects include pain and muscle spasm.

ethylene N. gas sometimes used as a general anesthetic. Nausea and vomiting commonly occur after its use.

etiology (ē'tē-ôl'ə-jē) N. study of the causes of disease. ADJ. etiologic

etodolac N. nonsteroidal anti-inflammatory agent used in the treatment of arthritis and for pain; side effects include stomach irritation and intestinal bleeding.

Etrafon N. trade name for a fixed-combination drug containing a tranquilizer (perphenazine) and an antidepressant (amitriptyline).

eu- prefix meaning good, well (e.g., eucapnia, optimal level of carbon dioxide in the arteries).

eucapnia N. presence of normal amounts of carbon dioxide in the blood.

eugenics (yōō-jĕn'ĭks) N. study concerned with controlling the characteristics of future generations through selective breeding techniques.

eukaryote (yōō-kăr'ē-ōt) N. organism containing cells that have true nuclei (*compare* PROKARYOTE). ADJ. eukaryotic

eunuch (yōō'nək) N. male whose testes have been removed; a eunuch shows signs of lack of male hormone (testosterone), such as feminine voice and lack of facial hair.

euphoria (yoo-fôr′ē-ə) N.
1. feeling or state of well-being and optimism.
2. exaggerated and unreal sense of well-being, commonly seen in some mental disorders.

eustachian tube (yoo-stā′shən) N. mucous-membrane-lined tube that connects the nasopharynx and the middle ear; it allows pressure in the inner ear to be equalized with that of the atmosphere. Increased pressure in the tube, occurring, e.g., in a plane that is ascending, can usually be relieved by swallowing. Also called auditory tube.

euthanasia (yoo′thə-nā′zhə) N. the act of deliberately causing another's death to relieve suffering. This may be done either actively by the use of artificial means (e.g., drugs) or passively by withholding treatment necessary for the prolongation of life. Also called mercy killing.

eventration (ē′věn-trā′shən) N.
1. protrusion of the intestine through the abdominal wall.
2. surgical removal of the organs in the abdomen.

eversion (ĭ-vûr′zhən, -shən) N. act of turning something inside out or turning it (e.g., a foot) outward.

evisceration (ĭ-vĭs′ə-rā′shən) N. surgical removal of an organ or the contents of the eyeball. *See also* EVENTRATION; EXENTERATION).

evoked potential (ĭ-vōkt′) N. electrical response produced in the central nervous system by an external stimulus (e.g., a flash of light). The response can be monitored on recording equipment (*see also* ELECTROENCEPHALOGRAM) and used to verify the integrity of nerve connections.

Ewing's sarcoma N. malignant tumor developing in bone marrow, usually in long bones or the pelvis; it occurs most often in adolescent boys and produces pain, swelling, and an increase in white blood cells. Treatment is by radiotherapy and surgical removal (sometimes amputation). Also called Ewing's tumor.

ex- prefix meaning away from, from, out of, outside (e.g., exsufflation, process of withdrawing the air from a cavity or organ, esp. the lungs).

exacerbation (ĭg-zăs′ər-bā′shən) N. increase in the seriousness of a disease or disorder, usually marked by a worsening of the symptoms.

examination (ĭg-zăm′ə-nā′shən) N. act of viewing and studying the body, using various procedures, techniques and equipment to ascertain the general health of the person and the presence or absence of any disease or disorder. The examination may include palpation (e.g., of the abdomen), percussion (tapping fingers or special instrument on a body surface to detect the presence of fluid or determine the borders of an internal organ); auscultation (e.g., use of a stethoscope on the chest); the taking of tissue samples or body fluids (e.g., blood) for laboratory analysis; the analysis of X rays or other diagnostic procedures involving the internal organs; and the evaluation of subjective complaints (symptoms) of the patient.

exanthem (ĭg-zăn′thəm) N.
1. any disease that includes fever and skin eruptions, such as measles.

2. skin rash, such as that seen in rubella, measles, or chicken pox.

exchange transfusion (ĭks-chānj′) N. removal of a person's blood in small amounts and its replacement with equal amounts of donor blood, esp. exchange transfusion of the fetus (intrauterine exchange transfusion) or the newborn to treat erythroblastosis fetalis (neonatorum) by removing the Rh and ABO antibodies and lysed erythrocytes (red blood cells) and substituting blood with normal oxygen-carrying capacity.

excision (ĭk-sĭzh′ən) N. surgical removal of a part or organ. V. excise.

excoriation N. injury to the surface of the skin caused by scratching, scraping, chemicals, or other means.

excrement (ĕk′skrə-mənt) *See* FECES.

excrescence (ĭk-skrĕs′əns) N. abnormal projection or outgrowth (e.g., a wart).

excretion (ĭk-skrē′shən) N.
1. discharge of waste from an organ or from the body.
2. waste matter such as feces or urine (*compare* SECRETION). ADJ. excretory, V. excrete.

exenteration N.
1. surgical removal of the organs within a body cavity, as those of the pelvis (*see also* EVISCERATION).
2. removal of the entire contents of the eye socket.

exercise (ĕk′sĕr-sīs) N. activity to condition the body, maintain fitness, or correct a deformity. *See also* AEROBIC EXERCISE; ISOMETRIC EXERCISE; ISOTONIC EXERCISE.

exfoliation (ĕks-fō′lē-ā′shən) N. scaling off of dead skin; this occurs naturally but may be increased in some skin diseases and severe sunburn.

exhalation (ĕks′hə-lā′shən) N. process of breathing out, expelling air from the lungs. V. exhale

exhaustion (ĭg-zôs′chən) N. extreme fatigue; complete lack of energy. *See also* HEAT EXHAUSTION.

exhibitionism (ĕk′sə-bĭsh′ə-nĭz′əm) N. psychosexual disorder marked by exposure of the genitals to another person, usually of the opposite sex, for self-gratification in a socially unacceptable situation.

exo- (ĕk′sō) prefix meaning outer, outside, outward (e.g., exoenzyme, enzyme whose action is outside the originating cell).

exocrine gland (ĕk′sə-krĭn) -krēn, -krĭn′) N. gland that discharges its secretion usually through a duct, to an adjacent epithelial surface, as the sweat glands discharge onto the skin surface. Included among the exocrine glands are the sudoriferous (sweat) glands, sebaceous glands, certain glands involved in digestion (e.g., ducts secreting pancreatic juice in the pancreas), lacrimal (tear) glands, salivary glands, wax-producing glands of the ear, and mammary glands. Also sometimes called duct gland. (*Compare* ENDOCRINE GLAND.)

exogenous (ĕk-sŏj′ə-nəs) ADJ. originating or developing from outside the body; for example, exogenous obesity is caused by overeating, not by bodily malfunction (*compare* ENDOGENOUS).

exomphalos (ĕk-sŏm′fə-lŏs′, -ləs) N. umbilical hernia, in which some organs in the abdomen push into the umbilical cord.

exophthalmic goiter (ĕk′səf-thăl′mĭk) N. exophthalmos occurring in association with goiter. Symptoms may include, protruding eyeballs, tachycardia, higher rate of metabolism, and anemia. The condition is more likely to occur in freshwater regions because of the lack of iodine in fresh water. Also called Grave's disease; thyrotoxicosis.

exophthalmos (ĕk′səf-thăl′məs) N. abnormal protrusion of one or both eyeballs, due to goiter, injury, or disease of the eyeball or socket. Treatment depends on the cause.

exophytic ADJ. growing outward (e.g., a tumor that grows on the surface of an organ).

exostosis (ĕk′sŏ-stō′sĭs) N. benign outgrowth from a bone, usually covered with cartilage.

exotoxin (ĕk′sō-tŏk′sĭn) N. poison produced by a living microorganism and secreted into the surrounding medium (*compare* ENDOTOXIN).

exotropia (ĕk′sə-trō′pē-′ə) N. outward turning of one eye relative to the other. *See also* STRABISMUS.

expander N. substance that increases the size, volume, or quantity of another substance (e.g., plasma expander, used to add to blood plasma volume in emergencies).

expectorant (ĭk-spĕk′tər-ənt) N. agent that promotes expectoration.

expectoration N. process of raising material (e.g., mucus or phlegm) from the respiratory tract by coughing and then spitting it out of the mouth. V. expectorate

expiration (ĕk′spə-rā′shən) N.
1. act of breathing out air from the lungs.
2. death. V. expire

exploration (ĕk′splə-rā′shən) N. thorough examination of an area of the body, esp. in exploratory surgery.

expression (ĭk-sprĕsh′ən) N. act of forcing something out by pressing or squeezing (e.g., expressing milk from a breast). In genetics, refers to exhibition of one or more traits carried by a gene.

exsanguination N. severe blood loss.

extended care facility N. institution that provides nursing, medical, and custodial care for a prolonged period, as in a chronic illness or rehabilitation from acute illness.

extension (ĭk-stĕn′shən) N. stretching; action of moving two joined parts away from one another (*compare* FLEXION).

extensor (ĭk-stĕn′sər) N. muscle that, when flexed, causes extension of a joint, or straightening of an arm or leg.

exteriorize (ĭk-stēr′ē-ə-rīz′) V. to place an internal organ or part of it (e.g., part of the colon in a colostomy) on the outside of the body.

external ear (ĭk-stûr′nəl) N. outer structure of the ear, consisting of the fleshy auricle and the canal (external acoustic meatus) leading to the tympanic membrane (eardrum).

externalize V. in psychology, to turn inner problems outward and express them in social relationships.

extinction N. in psychology, loss of a learned response because of nonreward or nonreinforcement.

extirpation (ĕk'stər-pā'shən) N. surgical removal of an entire part, organ, or growth.

extra- comb. form meaning additional, beyond, outside (e.g., extracorporeal, outside the body).

extracellular (ĕk'strə-sĕl'yə-lər) ADJ. located on or outside a cell.

extracellular fluid (ECF) N. protein-and electrolyte-containing fluid (e.g., potassium, chloride) in blood plasma and interstitial fluid that helps control water and electrolyte movement in the body. Normally, the body has about 14 liters (15 quarts) of ECF. (*Compare* INTRACELLULAR FLUID.)

extraction (ĭk-străk'shən) N. act of pulling out, as a tooth.

extrasensory perception (ESP) (ĕk'strə-sĕn'sə-rē) N. awareness or knowledge obtained by means other than the five senses. *See also* CLAIRVOYANCE; TELEPATHY.

extrasystole (ĕk'strə-sĭs'tə-lē) N. premature contraction of the heart; depending on the site of origin and the clinical picture, may be a normal variant or may indicate organic and potentially severe heart disease. Colloq. skipped beats.

extrauterine pregnancy *See* ECTOPIC PREGNANCY.

extravasation N. leakage of fluid (e.g., blood) to the tissues outside the vessel normally containing it; this may occur in injuries, burns, and allergic reactions.

extremity (ĭk-strĕm'ĭ-tē) N. any of the limbs; an arm or a leg.

extrication N. process whereby a victim is freed from entrapment, such as a wrecked motor vehicle, a collapsed hole in the ground, a building destroyed by an earthquake.

extroversion (ĕk'strə-vûr'zhən) N. directing of feelings and interests toward external things and the outside world rather than toward oneself; the person so inclined is an extrovert. Also called extraversion (*compare* INTROVERSION).

extrusion (ĭk-strōo'zhən) N. act of pushing something out by force.

THE TWO MAJOR FLUID COMPARTMENTS OF THE BODY

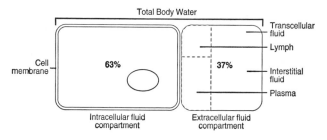

exudation (ĕks'yoŏ-dā'shən) N. slow escape (oozing) of fluids and cellular matter from blood vessels or cells through small pores or breaks in the cell membranes, sometimes the result of inflammation. v. exude.

eye (ī) N. either of two organs of sight located in a bony socket at the front of the skull. The outer coat of the eye is made of the anterior transparent cornea and the posterior opaque sclera (white of the eye). Light enters through the cornea, passes through a fluid-filled anterior chamber, then passes through the opening (pupil) in the iris (colored portion of the eye) and finally through the lens and vitreous humor to strike nerve cells (rods and cones) in the retina of the eye. The impulse is then transmitted from the retina through the optic nerve to the brain.

eye strain (ī'strān') N. tiredness of the eyes brought about by prolonged close work or occurring in a person with an uncorrected eye problem; symptoms are aching and burning of the eyes, often accompanied by headache; also called asthenopia.

eyebrow (ī'brou') N. arch above the eye in the frontal bone, separating the eye socket from the forehead.

eyelash (ī'lăsh') N. one of many hairs growing along the margin of the eyelid. Collectively called cilia, their movement helps to keep the eye free of debris.

eyelid (ī'lĭd') N. movable fold of skin over the eye.

STRUCTURES OF THE EYE

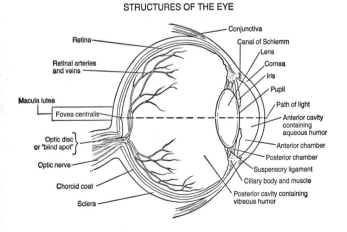

EYE MOVEMENT

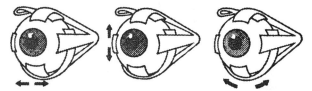

Six muscles attached to the outside of the eye control eyeball movement.

EYE STRUCTURES AND THEIR FUNCTIONS

Structure	Function
Cornea	Refracts light; important in focusing light onto the retina
Sclera	Maintains shape of eye and protects eye; also serves as site of muscle attachment
Iris	Controls amount of light passing through the pupil
Cilliary body	Changes shape of lens (accommodation) and secretes aqueous humor
Choroid	Absorbs light; contains blood vessels for eye structures
Retina	Absorbs light and stores vitamin A; receives light and forms image for transmission to brain
Lens	Refracts light; important in accommodation
Anterior cavity	Maintains shape of eye and refracts light through its aqueous humor
Posterior cavity	Maintains shape of eye and refracts light through its vitreous humor
Aqueous humor	Fills anterior cavity, helping to maintain shape of eye; refracts light; maintains intraocular pressure
Vitreous humor	Fills posterior cavity and maintains intraocular pressure; lends shape to eye and keeps retina firmly pressed against choroid; refracts light

F

F
1. symbol for the element fluorine
2. abbreviation for the Fahrenheit temperature scale.

face (fās) N. front of the head, from the hairline to the chin, and including the forehead, eyes, nose, cheeks, and jaw. ADJ. facial

face lift (fās′lĭft′) *See* RHYTIDOPLASTY.

facet (făs′ĭt) N. distinct feature or element; anatomically, refers to a small smooth area on a bone or other surface, such as the facet joints of the vertebral column.

facial nerve N. one of a pair of mixed sensory and motor nerves, the seventh cranial nerves, that innervate much of the face, with sensory fibers extending from taste buds in the tongue and motor fibers extending to the scalp, muscles of facial expression, and some of the lacrimal (tear) and salivary glands.

facilitation (fə-sĭl′ĭ-tā′shən) N. in neurology, phenomenon that occurs when two or more impulses, individually not powerful enough to produce a response in a neuron, combine to bring about a response (action potential) (*compare* INHIBITION).

factor (făk′tər) N. something that produces or influences a result (e.g., factor S, sleep-promoting substance isolated from human urine).

factor I—factor XIII N. blood clotting proteins, most of which are present in blood plasma, involved in the process of blood coagulation *See also* FIBRINOGEN; PROTHROMBIN; THROMBOPLASTIN; CLOTTING FACTORS.

facultative (făk′əl-tā′tĭv) ADJ. able to adjust to different environments or conditions (e.g., facultative anaerobe, organism that normally lives without air but can survive in air).

faculty (făk′əl-tē) N. ability to do something specific (e.g., the faculty of hearing).

Fahrenheit (făr′ən-hīt′) ADJ. pert. to a temperature scale, commonly abbreviated as F, on which water freezes at 32° and boils at 212°, as compared to 0° and 100°, respectively, on the Celsius scale.

failure (fāl′yər) N. loss of ability to function normally. *See also* HEART FAILURE; RENAL FAILURE.

faint (fānt) V. to become unconscious, usually as a result of insufficient blood flow to the brain, as a reaction to emotional or physical shock, or to pain, hunger, or fear. *See also* SYNCOPE.

falciform ADJ. sickle-shaped.

falciform ligament N. ligament attaching part of the liver to the diaphragm and abdominal wall.

fallopian tube (fə-lō′pē-ən) N. either of two tubes or ducts, each of which extends from the uterus to the region of an ovary. The tube serves as passage for

A FRONTAL VIEW OF THE FEMALE REPRODUCTIVE TRACT

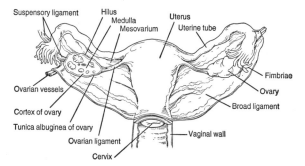

the movement of an ovum from the ovary (after ovulation) to the uterus and for the movement of sperm from the uterus upward toward the ovary. Fertilization normally occurs in the fallopian tube. Also called oviduct.

Fallot's syndrome (fǎ-lōz′) **(tetralogy)** *See* TETRALOGY OF FALLOT.

false labor *See* BRAXTON-HICKS CONTRACTIONS.

false-negative N. test or procedure result indicating a normal or negative result when, in fact, an abnormal condition is actually present. A test is said to be sensitive when it has a low false-negative rate. An insensitive test has a high false-negative rate and should not be relied upon to exclude abnormality or disease. For example, an electrocardiogram for heart disease is relatively insensitive—many patients with coronary artery disease, including acute heart attacks, have a negative result. Other tests, such as nuclear medicine treadmill scans, are far more sensitive due to a much lower percentage of false-negative results.

false-positive N. test or procedure result indicating a positive or abnormal result when, in fact, no abnormal condition is actually present. A specific test has a low false-positive rate. A nonspecific test has a high false-positive rate and should not be relied upon to suspect or diagnose an abnormality or disease. Some types of urine pregnancy tests are very nonspecific—any type of contaminant (such as dirt, blood, or vaginal secretions) may give a false-positive result when, in reality, the patient is not pregnant. A serum pregnancy test is both sensitive and specific.

familial (fə-mĭl′yəl) ADJ. pert. to some factor (e.g., a disease or characteristic), usually but not always inherited, that is present in some families but not in others, occurring in family members more frequently than would be expected by chance (*compare* ACQUIRED; CONGENITAL; HEREDITARY).

familial hypercholesterolemia (hī′pər-kə-lĕs′tər-ə-lē′mē-ə) N.

inherited disorder characterized by a high level of serum cholesterol and early development of atherosclerosis that places affected individuals at a high risk for certain types of heart disease.

family history N. part of a patient's medical history in which questions are asked about the incidence and prevalence of specific diseases and disorders in his/her family in an attempt to ascertain whether the patient has a hereditary or familial tendency toward a particular disease.

family planning N. deliberate limiting or spacing of the number of children born to a couple (*see also* CONTRACEPTION).

family therapy N. in psychiatry, treatment that focuses on the individual as a family member; in the same session two or more family members or the whole family may meet together with the therapist to discover how the various family members interact.

famotidine (fə-mō′tĭ-dēn′) N. oral/parenteral H_2 histamine blocker (trade name Pepcid) used in the treatment of peptic ulcers, gastritis, and gastroesophageal reflux. *See* TABLE OF COMMONLY PRESCRIBED DRUGS —GENERIC NAMES.

fantasy (făn′tə-sē, -zē) N. 1. free play of the imagination. 2. conversion of disliked reality into invented, imagined experiences in order to fulfill hidden desires or express unconscious conflicts.

farmer's lung (fär′mərz) N. respiratory disorder caused by an allergic response to inhaled fungi from moldy hay and characterized by coughing, difficult breathing, nausea, chills, fever, and rapid heartbeat.

farsightedness (fär′sī′tĭd-nĭs) *See* HYPEROPIA.

FAS *See* FETAL ALCOHOL SYNDROME.

fascia (făsh′ē-ə) N., *pl.* fasciae, fibrous connective tissue that supports soft organs and sheaths structures such as muscles.

fascicle (făs′ĭ-kəl) N., *pl.* fasciculi, small bundle of nerve, muscle, or tendon fibers; also called fasciculus. ADJ. fasicular

fasciitis (făsh′ē-ī′tĭs) N. inflammation of fascia anywhere in the body; most commonly refers to painful, but non-life-threatening inflamation of the plantar fascia on the sole of the foot. Necrotizing fasciitis of the tissue surrounding the hip or back muscles, however, may be fatal.

fascioliasis N. infection with the liver fluke *Fasciola hepatica,* obtained by eating aquatic plants (e.g., watercress) with encysted forms of the flukes and common in many parts of the world, including the southern United States. Symptoms include fever, abdominal pain, loss of appetite, jaundice, vomiting, and diarrhea; liver damage sometimes occurs. Treatment is by bithionol (TBP).

fasciolopsiasis N. intestinal infection common in the Far East and caused by eating aquatic plants (e.g., water chestnuts) contaminated with *Fasciolopsis buski* flukes. Symptoms include abdominal pain, diarrhea, and, in severe cases, edema. Treatment is by anthelmintics.

fast V. to go without all or certain food (*compare* ANOREXIA; DIET).

fat N.
1. water-soluble substance derived from fatty acids and found in animal tissues, where it serves as a source of energy.
2. type of body tissue (adipose) containing stored fat that serves as a source of energy as insulation, and as a protective cushion for vital organs.

fat embolism N. serious circulatory disease in which a fat embolus blocks an artery; the embolus enters the circulation after fracture of a long bone or traumatic injury to adipose (fatty) tissue or a fatty liver.

fat metabolism (mǐ-tăb′ə-lǐz′əm) N. biochemical processes in the body by which fats ingested in the diet are broken down (first into fatty acids and glycerol and then into simpler compounds) into substances that can be used by the cells of the body. Fats are a major energy source, providing approximately 9 kilocalories per gram, compared with about 4 kilocalories per gram for carbohydrates.

fatality rate (fā-tăl′ǐ-tē) N. number of deaths during a given period for a stipulated population (e.g., the percentage of people in the United States who die of a particular disease in 1 year).

fatigability N. a tendency to become easily tired or to lose strength.

fatigue (fə-tēg′) N.
1. exhaustion, weariness, loss of strength resulting from hard or prolonged mental or physical work.
2. temporary inability of tissues (e.g., muscle) to respond to stimuli that normally produce a response.

fatigue fracture (fə-tēg′) (frăk′chər) N. break that results from excessive physical activity, not from a specific injury; sometimes occurs in the metatarsal bones of runners; also called stress fracture.

fatty acid (făt′ē) (ăs′ĭd) N. organic (carbon-containing) acid; fatty acids are the building blocks of many lipids. Some fatty acids are manufactured by the body; others, the essential fatty acids, must be supplied by the diet.

fatty liver (făt′ē) (lĭv′ər) N. accumulation of certain fats (triglycerides) in the liver, due to alcoholic cirrhosis or exposure to certain drugs or toxic substances, or occurring as complication of certain conditions (e.g., kwashiorkor, pregnancy); symptoms include enlarged liver, loss of appetite, and abdominal discomfort. Treatment depends on the cause.

fauces (fô′sēz′) N. opening at the back of the mouth into the pharynx.

favism (fā′vĭz′əm) N. anemia resulting from eating fava beans or breathing in the plant's pollen. It occurs in the Mediterranean area (e.g., Italy); victims have an inherited blood abnormality and enzyme deficiency. Symptoms include dizziness, headache, fever, vomiting, and diarrhea. Blood transfusions may be required.

favus (fā′vəs) N. contagious fungal infection of the scalp, producing honeycomblike crusts, a musty odor, and itching. The condition occurs chiefly in the Middle East and Africa.

FDA *See* FOOD AND DRUG ADMINISTRATION.

Fe symbol for the element iron.

febrile (fĕb′rəl, fē′brəl) ADJ. pert. to or characterized by an elevated body temperature (fever).

febrile seizure (sē′zhər) *See* CONVULSION.

fecal impaction (fē′kəl) N. accumulation of hardened feces in the rectum or lower part of the colon which the person is unable to move. Treatment is by enemas and manual breaking of the stool with a gloved finger. Prevention includes a diet containing bulk foods, adequate water intake, exercise, and sometimes use of stool softeners.

fecalith (fē′kə-lĭth′) N. hard mass of feces in the colon, evacuated manually or by means of an oil enema.

feces (fē′sēz) N. material discharged from the bowel in defecation. Formed in the colon, feces consist of water, undigested food residue, bacteria, and mucus. Also called stool. ADJ. fecal

fecundity (fĭ-kŭn′dĭ-tē) N. ability to produce offspring, esp. in large numbers in a short period. ADJ. fecund

feeblemindedness *See* MENTAL RETARDATION.

feedback (fēd′băk′) N. coupling of the output of a gland or process to the input; return of some portion of the energy or effect of a process to the originating source in order to regulate its further output. For example, a feedback mechanism controls the release of thyroxine from the thyroid gland, the level of thyroxine in the circulating blood is detected by the pituitary gland, which then responds to maintain the level at normal range, releasing a factor (thyroid-stimulating hormone) to stimulate the thyroid to release more thyroxine if needed.

feeding (fē′dĭng) N. taking in of food or offering of food (*See also* BREAST FEEDING, DEMAND FEEDING; FORCED FEEDING).

fee-for-service (FFS) ADJ. payment mechanism in which a provider is paid for each service rendered to a patient. *See* TABLE OF MANAGED CARE TERMS.

Fehling's solution N. solution of copper sulfate, potassium tartrate, and sodium hydroxide used to test for sugar (esp. glucose) in the urine, which, when present, turns the solution reddish.

Feldene N. trade name for the anti-inflammatory piroxicam.

fellatio (fə-lā′shē-ō′) N. sucking the penis or otherwise stimulating it with the mouth.

felodipine N. *See* TABLE OF COMMONLY PRESCRIBED DRUGS—GENERIC NAMES.

female (fē′māl′) ADJ. pert. to the sex that bears young (*compare* MALE). N. woman or girl.

feminization (fĕm′ə-nĭ-zā′shən) N. development of womanlike changes (e.g., breast enlargement, loss of facial hair) in a male because of endocrine (hormonal) disorder or the administration of certain drugs.

femoral artery (fĕm′ər-əl) (är′tə-rē) N. main artery of the thigh, arising from the external iliac artery in the inguinal region and running down two thirds of the thigh, after which it divides into several branches. *See* MAJOR ARTERIES AND VEINS OF THE BODY, in Appendix.

femoral nerve (fĕm′ər-əl) (nûrv) N. main nerve of the anterior (front) part of the thigh, receiving sensory impulses from the front and inner thigh and supplying the muscles of the anterior thigh; also called anterior crural nerve.

femoral pulse (fĕm′ər-əl) (pŭls) N. pulse of the femoral artery, felt in the groin.

femur (fē′mər) N. thighbone, the longest and strongest bone in the body, extending from the hip to the knee. Largely cylindrical, the femur has a large rounded head that fits into the acetabulum of the hipbone; a neck and shaft with projections and ridges for the attachment of muscles; and an expanded distal end that articulates with the tibia of the lower leg. Also called thigh bone. ADJ. femoral

fenestra (fə-nĕs′trə) N. windowlike opening, sometimes closed by a membrane. The fenestra ovalis (*fenestra vestibuli*), or oval window, and the fenestra rotonda (*fenestra cochleae*), or round window, are two openings in the ear.

fenestration (fĕn′ĭ-strā′shən) N. 1. surgical procedure in which a windowlike opening is created in the inner ear to restore

LOWER EXTREMITY BONES

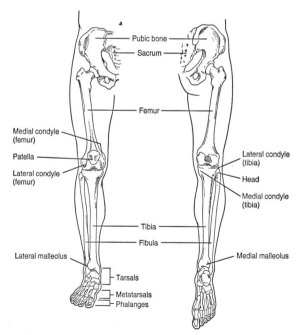

hearing lost because of osteo-sclerosis.

2. any surgical procedure in which an opening is created to gain access to a cavity within an organ or bone.

fenoprofen N. anti-inflammatory used in the treatment of arthritis and other painful inflammatory disorders. Adverse side effects include gastrointestinal upsets, dizziness, and drowsiness.

Feosol N. trade name for an iron-containing drug used to treat some types of anemia.

Fergon N. trade name for an iron-containing compound used to treat some types of anemia.

fermentation (fûr′mən-tā′shən) N. breakdown of complex substances, esp. sugar and other carbohydrates, by enzymes or microorganisms.

-ferous comb. form meaning bearing, yielding (e.g., lipoferous, carrying fat).

ferr-, ferri-, ferro- comb. form indicating an association with iron (e.g., ferrokinetics, the rate of change in iron levels in the body).

ferritin (fĕr′ĭ-tĭn) N. iron compound found in the intestines, liver and spleen, it contains more than 20% iron and is one of the chief forms in which iron is stored in the body.

fertile (fûr′tl) ADJ. capable of reproducing, of bearing young. N. fertility

fertile period N. that time in the menstrual cycle in which fertilization is most likely to occur. Attempts to determine a woman's fertile period are based on knowledge of when ovulation (the release of an ovum, or egg from the ovary) occurs (usually 14 days before onset of a period), of how long the ovum will survive (usually 24 hours), and of how long sperm will survive in the female genital tract (usually 48–72 hours). Thus the fertile period begins 2 or 3 days before ovulation and lasts 2 or 3 days afterward, but to allow for possibly longer survival times of sperm and egg it is usually considered to last 7 or 8 days around ovulation. Knowledge of the fertile period is used by some to help prevent conception and by others to try to increase the chance of conception. *See also* BASAL BODY TEMPERATURE METHOD OF FAMILY PLANNING; CALENDAR METHOD OF FAMILY PLANNING; OVULATION METHOD OF FAMILY PLANNING; CONTRACEPTION.

fertilization (fûr′tl-ĭ-zā′shən) N. union (fusion) of the male and female sex cells (gametes, the spermatozoon and ovum) to form a single cell (zygote) that then divides to eventually form the fetus. *See also* TEST TUBE BABY. Fertilization takes place in the fallopian tube of the female.

fester (fĕs′tər) V. colloq. to become inflamed and form pus.

festination (fĕs′tə-nā′shən) N. involuntary quickening and shortening of steps in walking, as occurs in some diseases (e.g., PARKINSONISM).

fetal (fēt′l) ADJ. pert. to a fetus.

fetal age N. age of the conceptus counted from the time of fertilization. Since in most cases pregnancy is counted from the first day of the last menstrual period but fertilization occurs about 2 weeks thereafter, the fetal age is often about 2 weeks less than the calculated length of the pregnancy. Also called fer-

FERTILIZATION

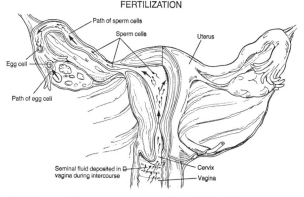

Path of sperm cells

Sperm cells

Uterus

Egg cell

Path of egg cell

Seminal fluid deposited in
vagina during intercourse

Cervix

Vagina

tilization age. (*Compare* GESTA-
TIONAL AGE.)

fetal alcohol syndrome (fēt′l)
(ăl′kə-hôl′) (sĭn′drōm′) N. a
condition in which mental ability, body formation, and facial
development may be defective
in a fetus as the result of the
mother's consumption of alcohol (ethanol) while pregnant.
The fetus may also be stillborn
as a result. *See also* TERATOGEN.

fetal circulation N. system of
blood vessels and special structures through which blood
moves in the fetus. The fetus is
attached to the mother's placenta through the umbilical
cord. Maternal oxygenated
blood from the placenta travels
through the umbilical vein to
the liver of the fetus and from
there through the inferior vena
cava to the right atrium of the
heart. It then passes through the
foramen ovale into the left
atrium and from there to the left
ventricle and circulation
through the head and upper
body parts. The returning blood
flows through the superior vena
cava into the right atrium, from
which at low pressure it flows
into the right ventricle and then

through the pulmonary artery to
the descending aorta and circulation through the lower body
parts. The wastes of the fetus
are carried by the blood through
the umbilical arteries back to
the placenta, where they diffuse
into the mother's bloodstream
for eventual excretion. This
system, which differs in many
ways from the circulatory path
in an adult, allows oxygen and
nutrients to be supplied to the
fetus and wastes to be carried
away. At birth several changes
occur, including closure (at
least partial) of the foramen
ovale so that blood no longer
flows from the right atrium to
the left atrium. Circulation
through the baby's lungs begins
with the first breath.

fetal distress N. compromised or
abnormal condition of the
fetus, usually characterized by
abnormal heart rhythm and discovered during pregnancy or
labor, sometimes through the
use of a fetal monitor. If possible, the cause of the problem is
determined and corrected; otherwise, immediate Cesarean
delivery may be indicated.

fetal heart rate N. number of heartbeats in the fetus during a given time, normally between 100 and 160 beats per minute but varying with cycles of rest and activity and maternal condition. The fetal heart rate is detected through the use of a fetoscope or fetal monitor.

fetal membranes N. collectively, the amnion, chorion, and umbilical cord (which includes the yolk stalk, allantois, and blood vessels), all of which function for the protection, nourishment, respiration, and excretion of the developing fetus. The placenta, of both fetal and maternal tissue, also serves these functions.

fetal monitor N. device used during pregnancy, labor, and childbirth to observe the fetal heart rate and maternal uterine contractions. The device may be applied externally on the abdomen of the mother or, less commonly, inserted into the uterus through the vagina.

fetal movement N. motion of the fetus itself within the uterus. The motion is usually first detected by a woman pregnant for the first time at about the 16th week of pregnancy, somewhat earlier in those who have had previous pregnancies.

fetid (fet-əd) ADJ. having a foul odor.

fetishism (fĕt′ĭ-shĭz′əm) N. transfer of sexual or love interest to an object (fetish), either an inanimate object (e.g., underwear) or a part of the body not usually associated with sex (e.g., the foot). Partial fetishism or auxiliary fetishism refers to use of an object to heighten interest in heterosexual intercourse (e.g., the wearing of particular articles of clothing).

fetishist N. one who engages in fetishism.

feto- comb. form indicating an association with a fetus (e.g. fetoplacental, pert. to the fetus and the placenta).

fetology (fē-tŏl′ə-jē) N. that branch of medicine concerned with the fetus in the uterus, including the diagnosis and treatment of abnormalities.

fetometry (fē-tŏm′ĭ-trē) N. measurement of a fetus, esp. the diameter of the head.

fetoprotein (fē′tə-prō′tēn) N. antigen that occurs naturally in the fetus and sometimes in adults with certain cancers. A greater-than-normal amount of alpha fetoprotein (AFP) in the fetus often indicates an abnormality of the neural tube (e.g., hydrocephalus or spina bifida).

fetor (fē′tər, -tôr′) N. bad smell. ADJ. fetid

fetoscope (fē′tə-skōp′) N. stethoscope placed on the mother's abdomen to detect the fetal heartbeat.

fetoscopy N. procedure that allows direct observation of the fetus in the uterus and the withdrawal of fetal blood for analysis by way of a fetoscope introduced through a small incision in the pregnant woman's abdomen.

fetus (fē′təs) N. live offspring while it is inside the mother (in utero); in humans, from the beginning of the third month of pregnancy until birth. ADJ. fetal

fever (fē′vər) N. rise in the temperature of the body. Normal body temperature is 98.6° Fahrenheit (37.0° Celsius) taken orally, somewhat higher rectally. A rise in temperature can sometimes be caused by severe

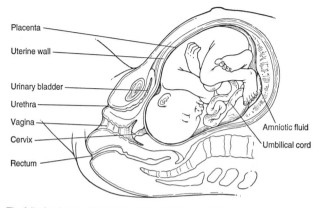

Placenta
Uterine wall
Urinary bladder
Urethra
Vagina
Cervix
Rectum
Amniotic fluid
Umbilical cord

The fully developed child in place immediately before birth.

stress, strenuous exercise, or dehydration, but fever is most often a sign of infection (bacterial, viral, or other) or other disease. Fever is often accompanied by headache, chills, and feeling of malaise; high fevers can cause delirium and convulsions (esp. in young children). The onset, course, and duration of a fever vary with the cause; certain diseases are associated with characteristic rising and falling curves that may aid in diagnosis. Also called pyrexia. (*See* HYPERPYREXIA.) ADJ. febrile

fever blister N. cold sore caused by herpes virus (*see also* HERPES SIMPLEX).

fexofenadine N. *See* TABLE OF COMMONLY PRESCRIBED DRUGS —GENERIC NAMES.

fiber (fī′bər) N.
1. long, threadlike structure (e.g., nerve fiber, collagen fiber).
2. food content that adds roughage to the diet and is considered by some to help prevent such diseases as diverticulosis,

appendicitis, and colon cancer. Foods rich in fiber include whole-grain cereals, nuts, fruits, and leafy and root vegetables.

fiberoptics N. technique in which thin, flexible, glass or plastic fibers in special instruments called fiberscopes are used to view inner parts of the body; the fibers transmit light and relay a magnified image of the body part.

fiberscope (fī′bər-skōp′) N. flexible instrument containing light-carrying glass or plastic fibers used to view internal body structures. Fiberscopes are especially designed for examination of particular body parts. For example, the bronchoscope is designed for viewing the tracheal and bronchial region; the gastroscope, for viewing the interior of the stomach; the duodenoscope, for viewing the duodenum.

fibril (fī′brəl, fīb′rəl) N. very small fiber or thread of a fiber (e.g., myofibrils of muscle fiber).

fibrillation (fĭb'rə-lā'shən) N. recurrent, involuntary, and abnormal muscular contraction in which a single or a small number of fibers act separately rather than as a coordinated unit, esp. in the heart, as in atrial or ventricular fibrillation. The primary cause is ischemia of the heart muscle. The treatment consists of prompt defibrillation, or drugs (e.g., lidocaine, diltiazem).

fibrin (fī'brĭn) N. insoluble protein in the blood that combines with similar molecules, red and white blood cells, and platelets to form a blood clot. Fibrin is formed by the action of thrombin on its precursor fibrinogen. *See also* BLOOD COAGULATION.

fibrinogen (fī-brĭn'ə-jən) N. protein present in the blood plasma and essential to the process of blood coagulation; the factor (Factor I) converted into fibrin by thrombin in the presence of calcium ions during the process of blood coagulation.

fibrinolysis (fī'brənō-lī'-sĭs) N. process in which protein fibrin is dissolved, resulting in the breakup and removal of small blood clots; this is a normal, ongoing process in the body. The principles of fibrinolysis have been utilized therapeutically via administration of drugs that dissolve blood clots associated with disease (e.g., as occurs in a coronary artery during an acute myocardial infarction). *See also* THROMBOLYSIS; THROMBOLYTIC THERAPY.

fibroadenoma (fī'brō-ăd'n-ō' mə) N. benign nontender, movable, and firm tumor of the breast, most common in young women and caused by high estrogen levels.

fibroblast (fī'brə-blăst') N. cell that gives rise to connective tissue; produces collagen, elastin, and reticular protein that are the precursors of bone, collagen, and other connective tissue cells.

fibrocartilage (fī'brō-kär'tl-ĭj) N. type of connective tissue found in intervertebral discs consisting of thick bundles of collagen fibers.

fibrocystic disease of the breast N. common condition among women characterized by the presence of one or more cysts in the breast. The cysts are benign but should be watched carefully for any changes in size or consistency; women with fibrocystic breast disease have a higher-than-average likelihood of developing breast cancer later in life. In many cases no treatment is necessary; in other cases aspiration of the cyst with/without a biopsy is performed. Some investigators believe that consumption of caffeine (e.g., in coffee, soft drinks) in large amounts is associated with fibrocystic breast disease. Also called cystic breast disease, cystic mastitis.

fibrocystic disease of the pancreas *See* CYSTIC FIBROSIS.

fibroid tumor (fī'broid') N. benign tumor (fibroma) containing fibrous tissue, esp. that of the uterus. Fibroid tumors of the uterus are common and in many cases do not require treatment; if, however, they cause discomfort or hemorrhage, surgical removal is necessary.

fibroma (fī-brō'mə) N. nonmalignant tumor of connective tissue.

fibromyalgia (fī′brō′mī′al-jēə) N. nonarticular rheumatic condition, sometimes called fibromyalgia syndrome (FMS), characterized by widespread musculoskeletal aching, stiffness, and tenderness on palpation of characteristic sites (tender points). The typical patient is a mid-forties female, with a mean symptom duration of 6 years, though it may also occur in children and adolescents. Associated complaints are common and include generalized fatigue, morning stiffness, and sleep disturbances. Patients have evidence of cognitive impairment on formal testing, probably due to their diffuse pain, sleepiness, fatigue, and negative mood. Anxiety, headaches, and irritable bowel syndrome are frequent. Affected women have a significantly increased incidence of gynecological disease (e.g., bleeding disorders, chronic pelvic pain, pelvic inflammatory disease) than healthy women of the same age group without fibromyalgia. The cause is unknown. Recent work has shown metabolic abnormalities in muscles of affected patients. Nearly 50% of fibromyalgia patients also have symptoms compatible with multiple chemical sensitivity syndrome. A multidisciplinary approach to treatment is often required. Response to treatment (physical therapy, nonsteroidal anti-inflammatory drugs [NSAIDs], antidepressant drugs) varies. Symptoms may last up to 15 years, despite waxing and waning of discomfort. *See also* GROWTH HORMONE; MULTIPLE CHEMICAL SENSITIVITY SYNDROME; CHRONIC FATIGUE SYNDROME; PELVIC INFLAMMATORY DISEASE.

fibromyositis (fī′brō-mī′ə-sī′tĭs) N. any of a large number of disorders marked by local inflammation of muscle and connective tissue, stiffness, and joint or muscle pain. Fibromyositis may result from infection, trauma, or other cause. Treatment includes rest, pain-relieving drugs, and sometimes massage.

fibronectin (fī′brə-něk′tĭn) N. blood or tissue protein that may indicate premature labor.

fibroplasia (fī′brə-plā′zhə) N. development of fibrous connective tissue, such as in scar formation. Sometimes occurs in noninjured areas, such as the blood vessels, leading to narrowing and decreased flow. The reasons are unclear.

fibrosis (fī-brō′sĭs) N. increase in the formation of fibrous connective tissue, either normally as in scar formation, or abnormally to replace normal tissues, esp. in the lungs, uterus, or heart *See also* CYSTIC FIBROSIS.

fibrous (fī′brəs) ADJ. consisting of fibers.

fibrous joint N. immovable joint, such as those in the skull (*compare* SYNOVIAL JOINT).

fibula (fĭb′yə-lə) N. long, thin outer bone of the lower leg. It articulates with the tibia (the other lower leg bone) just below the knee and extends to the outer side of the ankle; also called calf bone.

field N.
1. area, as that seen through a microscope (microscopic field).
2. area seen by the fixed eye (visual field).
3. open area during surgery (operative field).
4. area of expertise (e.g., field of psychiatry).

fight-or-flight response N. action of certain hormones (e.g., epinephrine, norepinephrine) within the body that prepares the person to respond to stress—either face the threat (fight) or avoid the threat (flight). Also called the acute stress response, these actions were first described by physiologist Walter Cannon in the 1920s as a theory that animals (including humans) react to threats with a general discharge of the sympathetic nervous system. *See also* EPINEPHRINE; NOREPINEPHRINE; SYMPATHETIC NERVOUS SYSTEM.

filariasis (fĭl′ə-rī′ə-sĭs) N. disease, largely of the tropics, caused by filariae (long, threadlike worms) that enter the body through mosquito bites and infest primarily lymph glands and vessels. Symptoms include blockage of the lymph vessels and resultant swelling and pain in the limb distal to the blockage, which, over many years, may lead to elephantiasis. Treatment is by anthelmintics.

filiform (fĭl′ə-fôrm′) ADJ. thread-shaped.

fimbria (fĭm′brē-ə) N., *pl.* fimbriae, fringe or fringelike structure, such as the fingerlike projections around the ovarian end of the Fallopian tube.

finger (fĭng′gər) N. any of the five digits of the hand.

Fiorinal N. trade name for a fixed combination drug containing the pain-relieving, fever-reducing, and anti-inflammatory agent aspirin; the sedative-hypnotic butalbital; and the stimulant caffeine.

first aid N. immediate care given an injured or ill person before treatment by medically trained personnel. The most critical concerns are dealt with first: maintenance of adequate heart function, an open airway, and control of bleeding; after that, care depends on the nature of the injury or illness.

fission (fĭsh′ən) N. splitting, as in the asexual formation of new bacterial or protozoan cells or in the splitting of an atomic nucleus, with the release of energy.

fissure (fĭsh′ər) N.
1. any of the deep grooves of the outer covering of the brain.
2. cleft or groove in a part, whether normal or abnormal (e.g., anal fissure, a long ulcer-like groove at the anus).

fistula (fĭs′chə-lə) N., *pl.* fistulae, abnormal opening or channel connecting two internal organs or leading from an internal organ to the outside (e.g., urinary fistula, an abnormal channel of the urinary tract). Fistulas are due to ulceration, failure of a wound to heal, injury, tumors, or congenital defects. Surgical repair is not always possible. (*Compare* ANASTOMOSIS.) ADJ. fistular; fistulous

fit N. colloquial term for a sudden attack (e.g., a fit of coughing) or a seizure (e.g., in epilepsy).

fixation (fĭk-sā′shən) N.
1. process of securing a part, as by sewing with catgut or wire (suturing).
2. halt in personality growth at a particular stage of psychological development.
3. hardening and preservation of tissues for examination under a microscope.

fixed-combination drug N. preparation containing multiple ingredients in specific amounts;

it allows concomitant administration of two or more drugs.

flaccid (flăs'ĭd) ADJ. limp, soft, weak, or flabby (e.g., a muscle).

flaccid bladder N. type of malfunctioning bladder caused by interruption of the normal reflex arc associated with voiding; symptoms include absence of bladder sensation, overfilling of the bladder, and inability to urinate voluntarily (*compare* SPASTIC BLADDER).

flaccid paralysis N. abnormality characterized by weakness or loss of muscle tone due to disease or injury to the nerves affecting the involved muscles (*compare* SPASTIC PARALYSIS).

flagellation (flăj'ə-lā'shən) N. action of whipping someone else (*see also* SADISM) or of being whipped (*see also* MASOCHISM) for stimulation or sexual arousal.

flagellum (flə-jĕl'əm) N., *pl.* flagella, threadlike tail or other extension from an organism, as in a spermatozoon, to provide locomotion.

Flagyl N. trade name for the antiprotozoal metronidazole used to treat trichomoniasis (a vaginal infection), giardiasis, and certain other infections.

flank (flăngk) N. part of the body between the ribs and the upper border of the ilium.

flap (flăp) N. section of tissue used to cover a burn or other injury (e.g., pedicle flap, a tubular gathering of skin, one end of which is left attached in the original site while the other end is freed for attachment in another part of the body). When the flap has healed at the new site, the other end is also detached and the remaining skin is sewn in place.

flare N.
1. reddening of the skin around a lesion produced by an allergic reaction.
2. reddening of the skin spreading outward from a focus of irritation or infection.

flaring *See* NASAL FLARING.

flatfoot (flăt'foot') N. condition in which the instep is not arched and the bottom of the foot (plantar surface) is flat, sometimes causing pain and fatigue. Treatment, when needed, is by special shoes or other devices. Also called pes planus.

flatulence (flăch'ə-ləns) N. abnormal amount of abdominal gas, causing distension of the stomach or intestine and sometimes discomfort.

flatus (flā'təs) N. gas in the stomach and/or intestines. ADJ. flatulent

flavin (flā'vĭn) *See* B$_2$ (RIBOFLAVIN), TABLE OF VITAMINS.

flecainide (flĭ-kā'nīd') N. oral antiarrhythmic (trade name Tambocor) indicated in the treatment of highly symptomatic and/or life-threatening arrhythmias that have not responded to other agents. Adverse effects include visual disturbances, dizziness, shortness of breath, and exacerbation of arrhythmias and of congestive heart failure. Because of the high incidence of potentially dangerous adverse reactions, experts recommend that other agents be tried first.

Flexeril N. trade name for the muscle relaxant cyclobenzaprine, used for muscle spasm and acute injury. Adverse effects include drowsiness, dry mouth, and dizziness. *See* TABLE OF COMMONLY PRESCRIBED DRUGS—TRADE NAMES.

flexion (flĕk′shən) N. bending of a joint (e.g., the elbow) that causes two adjoining bones (e.g., those in the upper and lower arm) to come closer together (*compare* EXTENSION).

flexor (flĕk′sər) N. muscle that bends a joint (e.g., flexor hallucis brevis, the muscle that bends the great toe upward).

flexure (flĕk′shər) N. angle or fold, such as the hepatic flexure of the colon.

floater (flō′tər) N. spot that appears in the visual field when one stares at a blank wall. Floaters are due to bits of protein and other debris that move in front of the retina. Usually they are harmless, but a sudden increase in the number of floaters may indicate an abnormal condition (e.g., detached retina).

flocculation N. reaction in which material that is normally invisible in a solution forms a suspension or precipitate as a result of changes in the physical or chemical conditions. This reaction is the basis of flocculation tests used to diagnose certain diseases (e.g., syphilis).

Flonase N. *See* TABLE OF COMMONLY PRESCRIBED DRUGS—TRADE NAMES.

flosequinan N. vasodilator (trade name Manoplax) indicated in the treatment of congestive heart failure; potential side effects include headache, dizziness, palpitation, taste disturbance, tachycardia, and vomiting.

Flovent N. *See* TABLE OF COMMONLY PRESCRIBED DRUGS—TRADE NAMES.

floxuridine N. antineoplastic drug used to treat certain cancers. Adverse effects include alopecia, dermatitis, gastrointestinal disturbances, and depression of bone marrow function.

flu (floo) *See* INFLUENZA.

fluconazole N. *See* TABLE OF COMMONLY PRESCRIBED DRUGS—GENERIC NAMES.

fluke (flook) N. parasitic worm belonging to the class Trematoda; passes through numerous stages and may infect the blood, intestines, liver, or lung.

flumazenil N. injectable benzodiazepine antagonist (trade name Romazicon) that reverses sedation associated with either clinical use or abuse of these drugs; potential side effects include seizures, especially in patients who have overdosed on both benzodiazepines

flunisolide (floo-nĭs′ə-līd′) N. inhaled corticosteroid anti-inflammatory agent (trade name Aerobid) used in the treatment of asthma; side effects may include suppression of adrenal gland secretion during patient transfer from oral steroids.

fluorescein (floo-rĕs′ē-ĭn) N. dye used in ophthalmology to detect certain defects of the cornea (injuries and foreign bodies) and other abnormalities and to determine whether the fit of a contact lens is correct; appears a bright green color when visualized under an ultraviolet lamp.

fluorescence (floo-rĕs′ēns) N. emission of light by a material when it is exposed to certain types of radiation (e.g., X ray or ultraviolet). This property is used in fluoroscopy. ADJ. fluorescent

fluoridation (floŏr′ĭ-dā′shən) N. addition of fluorine to drinking water to prevent or reduce tooth decay. The fluorine compounds enhance the ability of the tooth to withstand acid breakdown, and their use (although controversial) has led to a decline in the prevalence of dental caries in the United States and other countries. Too much fluoride in the water, however, can lead to fluorosis.

fluorine (floŏr′ēn′) N. element that helps form bones and teeth. *See also* TABLE OF IMPORTANT ELEMENTS.

fluorocarbon N. any of several chemical compounds of fluorine and carbon, which, because of their ability to carry large amounts of oxygen, may become useful in artificial blood for humans who cannot have, or refuse for religious reasons, transfusions of human blood.

fluoroscopy (floŏ-rŏs′kə-pē) N. technique in which a special device (fluoroscope) allows the immediate projection of X-ray images of the body onto a special fluorescent screen. It eliminates the need for taking and developing X rays.

fluorosis (floŏ-rō′sĭs) N. condition resulting from excessive intake of fluorine, usually from too high concentrations in drinking water; it causes discoloration and pitting of tooth enamel in children and bone and joint changes in adults.

fluorouracil (floŏr′ō-yoŏr′ə-sĭl) N. antineoplastic drug used to treat certain cancers. Adverse effects include alopecia, bone marrow depression, and gastrointestinal disturbances.

fluoxetine hydrochloride (floŏ-ŏk′sĭ-tēn′) (hī′drə-klôr′īd′) N. antidepressant drug (trade name Prozac) used in the treatment of depression, obsessive-compulsive disorders, and in attention-deficit disorder. Although widely touted as being safer than its predecessors, some patients receiving this drug have developed insomnia, anorexia, and worsened depression. Whether these side effects are from the underlying depression itself or due to the drug is a matter of controversy. Many physicians feel that fluoxetine is safe when used under appropriate circumstances. *See* TABLE OF COMMONLY PRESCRIBED DRUGS—GENERIC NAMES.

fluphenazine N. tranquilizer used to treat psychotic disorders. Adverse effects include hypotension, liver toxicity, and blood abnormalities.

flurazepam (floŏ-răz′ə-păm′) N. minor tranquilizer used to treat insomnia. Adverse effects include drug hangover (next-day sleepiness), dizziness, and possibly the development of dependence.

flurbiprofen N. oral nonsteroidal anti-inflammatory agent (trade name Ansaid) used in the treatment of arthritis; side effects include stomach irritation and intestinal bleeding.

flush (flŭsh) N.
1. sudden reddening of the face.
2. sudden sensation of heat, common in certain mental disorders and during menopause.

fluticasone propionate N. *See* TABLE OF COMMONLY PRESCRIBED DRUGS—GENERIC NAMES.

flutter (flŭt′ər) N. rapid movement back and forth of a part, esp. of the heart chambers (atria and ventricles).

fluvastatin N. *See* TABLE OF COMMONLY PRESCRIBED DRUGS—GENERIC NAMES.

flux (flŭks) N. excessive flow of liquid from an organ or cavity (e.g., diarrhea); also, continuous change (e.g., things are in a state of flux).

focal distance (fō′kəl) N. in ophthalmology, distance between the lens and the point behind the lens at which light from a distant point is focused. In a normal-sighted person the point of focus is on the retina, but distortions in the shape of the eyeball may cause myopia (nearsightedness) or hyperopia (farsightedness).

focal seizure N. transitory disturbance in motor or sensory function, such as lip smacking, a tingling feeling, or convulsions in a certain body part, caused by abnormal electrical activity of nerve cells in a particular localized area of the brain; a limited form of epilepsy.

focus (fō′kəs) N., *pl.* foci
1. point at which light, sound, or other rays meet, as determined by positions of lenses and other devices; the point of convergence of light after passing through a convex lens is the place at which there is the clearest image.
2. main site of an infection or other diseased state. ADJ. focal

fold (fōld) N. doubling back or infolding (e.g., neural fold, which leads to development of the neural tube in the embryo).

folic acid (fō′lĭk, fŏl′ĭk) N. one of the B-complex vitamins, essential for cell growth and reproduction; it functions as a coenzyme with vitamins C and B_{12} in the metabolism of proteins and the formation of iron-carrying hemoglobin in red blood cells. Rich sources include green leafy vegetables, liver, kidney, and whole grain cereals. Also called folacin; pteroylglutamic acid.

folie (fô-lē) N. any of several abnormal reactions; mental disorder.

folk medicine *See* TABLE OF ALTERNATIVE MEDICINE TERMS.

follicle (fŏl′ĭ-kəl) N.
1. pouchlike cavity, as that in the skin enclosing a hair.
2. saclike gland e.g., sebaceous follicle, which secretes sebum.
3. Graafian follicle of the ovary, from which an ovum erupts. ADJ. follicular

follicle-stimulating hormone (FSH) N. substance given off by the anterior portion of the pituitary gland (one of the three gonadotropins—follicle-stimulating hormone [FHS], luteinizing hormone [LH], human chorionic gonadotropin [HCG]) that stimulates the growth and maturation of the graafian follicle in the ovary and spermatogenesis (formation of sperm) in the testes. FSH is sometimes administered to stimulate ovulation and sperm production. *See also* GRAAFIAN FOLLICLE; HUMAN CHORIONIC GONADOTROPIN; LUTEINIZING HORMONE.

folliculitis (fə-lĭk′yə-lī′tĭs) N. inflammation of a hair follicle.

fomentation (fō′mən-tā′shən) N. application of warm, wet coverings to relieve pain or inflammation.

fomes (fō′mēz) N., *pl.* fomites, any object (as a utensil, towel, money) that can support and transmit disease-causing organisms.

fontanel (fŏn'tə-nĕl') N. one of two membrane-covered soft spots in the skull of a newborn infant, which close as the cranial bones develop, usually by 18–24 months of age. Fontanels may be bulging and tender in infants with meningitis and depressed in those with dehydration. Also called fontanelle.

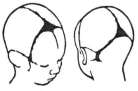

Diagram of fontanels

food allergy N. hypersensitivity reaction to an antigen, most often a protein, ingested in food. Symptoms may include rhinitis, diarrhea, nausea, vomiting, itchy skin eruptions, bronchial asthma, and colitis. Foods commonly associated with allergic reactions in sensitized people include eggs, wheat, milk, fish and seafoods, citrus fruits and tomatoes, and chocolate.

Food and Drug Administration (FDA) N. federal agency concerned with the enforcement of laws regulating the manufacture and distribution of food, drugs, and cosmetics.

food poisoning N. acute illness caused by eating food containing toxic substances (e.g., insecticide) or organisms (bacteria and fungi, esp. certain mushrooms) and the toxins produced by them. The bacteria most commonly responsible for food poisoning are *Clostridium botulinum, Salmonella,* and *Staphylococcus*; the mushrooms are *Amanita* species. Symptoms vary with the type of poison and may range from mild abdominal discomfort, nausea, and diarrhea to severe symptoms including paralysis, coma, and death. *See also* BOTULISM; GASTROENTERITIS; MUSHROOM POISONING; PTOMAINE; SALMONELLOSIS.

foot (fŏŏt) N. that part of the leg below the ankle; also called pes.

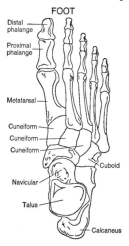

FOOT

Distal phalange
Proximal phalange
Metatarsal
Cuneiform
Cuneiform
Cuneiform
Cuboid
Navicular
Talus
Calcaneus

foot-and-mouth disease N. common viral disease of farm animals in Europe, Asia, and Africa that is sometimes transmitted to humans who come in contact with the animals and their products; symptoms include headache, fever, malaise, and small blisters on the oral membranes and tongue

footdrop N. abnormal condition in which the foot is not in its normal flexed position, but rather drags; it is usually due to damage to the nerves of the foot.

foramen (fə-rā'mən) N. hole or opening, esp. in a bone or membrane (e.g., foramen ovale, opening between the two atria of the fetal heart that closes after birth).

force-carrying particles N. in particle physics, all forces are due to interactions of elementary particles: gravitational, electromagnetic, strong, and weak. For each type of force there is an associated carrier particle that is vital in energy transfer. The carrier particle of the electromagnetic force is the photon; for gravity, the graviton (theoretical; never observed in a laboratory); for strong forces, gluons; for weak forces, bosons. *See also* ELEMENTARY PARTICLES; LEPTONS; PARTICLE PHYSICS; QUARKS.

forced feeding N. forcible administration of food (e.g., through a nasal tube) to someone who will not (e.g., as a political protest) or cannot otherwise eat.

forceps N. (fôr'səps) any of a large variety of surgical instruments used to grasp, handle, pull, or otherwise manipulate a body part or a fetus.

forceps delivery N. obstetrical procedure in which forceps are inserted through the vagina to grasp the head of the fetus and draw it through the birth canal, performed to shorten labor or quickly deliver a baby in distress. The forceps usually leaves marks on the baby's skull and sometimes causes injury; forceps deliveries have declined in recent years as the rate of Cesarean deliveries has increased.

forearm (fôr'ärm') N. that part of the upper extremity between the elbow and the wrist.

forebrain (fôr'brān') N. that part of the brain controlling sensation, perception, emotion, learning, thinking, and other intellectual functions and including the olfactory bulb and tracts,

FOREARM

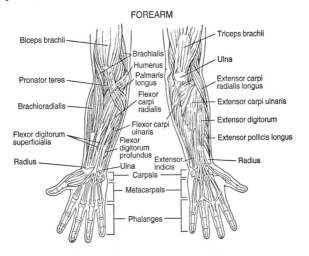

cerebral hemispheres, and nasal ganglia, optic tracts, and hypothalamus; also called prosencephalon.

forensic medicine (fə-rĕn′sĭk) N. branch of medicine concerned with the legal aspects of medical care, such as the cause of unexplained death; forensic pathology provides evidence used in the resolution of crimes involving human death.

foreplay (fôr′plā′) N. stimulation of sexual arousal between partners before actual intercourse.

foreskin (fôr′skĭn′) N. loose skin around the base of the head of the penis (glans) or clitoris; the prepuce; its removal constitutes circumcision.

formaldehyde (fôr-măl′də-hīd′) N. poisonous gas that, when dissolved in water, has many uses as a disinfecting and preserving agent.

formalin (fôr′mə-lĭn) N. solution of 37% formaldehyde, used to preserve tissue.

formication (fôr′mĭ-kā′shən) N. sensation that worms or insects are crawling on the skin; it is sometimes a symptom of drug intoxication.

formula (fôr′myə-lə) N.
1. simplified statement, using, as a rule, symbols and numerals that show the relationship among certain factors; for example, Fahrenheit temperature (F) can be converted to Celsius (C) by this formula: $C = \frac{5}{9}(F - 32)$, and water can be expressed as H_2O, signifying its makeup of two hydrogen (H) atoms and one oxygen (O) atom.
2. preparation, containing proteins, carbohydrates, fats, minerals, and vitamins, usually in proportions similar to those of breast milk, used to feed infants. Most infant formulas are based on cow's milk, but some based on soybean or other substances are available for infants who cannot tolerate milk products.

fornix (fôr′nĭks) N. part shaped like an arch, as the fornix cerebri in the hippocampus of the brain or the vaginal fornix.

Fosamax N. *See* TABLE OF COMMONLY PRESCRIBED DRUGS—TRADE NAMES.

fosinopril N. *See* TABLE OF COMMONLY PRESCRIBED DRUGS—GENERIC NAMES.

fossa (fŏs′ə) N., *pl.* fossae, channel or shallow depression (e.g., axillary fossa, the armpit).

fovea (fō′vē-ə) N. surface pit or small depression, esp. the pit in the center of the macula lutea of the retina; when light rays from an object converge on the fovea, the sharpest visual image is obtained.

fracture (frăk′chər) N. break, esp. of a bone. There are many kinds of fractures, including:
closed fracture N. bone break in which the skin is not broken.
comminuted fracture N. fracture in which there are several breaks in a bone, resulting in two or more fragments.
complete fracture N. break involving the entire width of the involved bone
complicated fracture N. bone break that results in injury to another organ, as, for example, when a broken rib pierces a lung.
compound fracture N. fracture in which the broken end(s) of the bone break through

the skin; also called open fracture.

VARIOUS TYPES OF FRACTURES

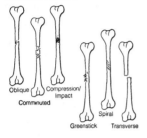

Oblique

Compression/Impact

Comminuted

Greenstick

Spiral

Transverse

compression fracture N. bone break that collapses the bone, esp. in short bones (e.g., vertebrae).

depressed fracture N. break in the skull with the bone pushed inward.

displaced fracture N. fracture in which the two ends of the broken bone are separated from each other.

greenstick fracture N. incomplete fracture in which the bone is bent and only the outer arc of the bend is broken; it occurs primarily in children and often heals quickly.

impacted fracture N. break in which one fragmented end is wedged into the other fragmented end.

incomplete fracture N. break that does not involve the entire width of the involved bone.

simple fracture N. uncomplicated closed fracture in which the skin is not broken.

frank breech N. position of the fetus within the mother's uterus in which the buttocks present at the maternal pelvic outlet, not the head as is normal for delivery.

fraternal twins (frə-tûr′nəl) *See* DIZYGOTIC TWINS.

freckle (frĕk′əl) N. small, flat, brown or tan discoloration on the skin, usually resulting from exposure to the sun; the tendency to freckle is hereditary and occurs primarily in redheaded persons and others with fair skin. Since these people tend to develop more serious skin changes, they should avoid overexposure to the sun.

free association N. in psychoanalysis, technique intended to reveal what is carried in the unconscious, whereby a person says spontaneously whatever comes to mind, esp. in giving the first word or thought that occurs when a word cue is given.

free radical N. group of atoms acting as a single unit, but unable to exist independently for more than a short period of time; contains an oxygen atom with a free electron. Free radicals may cause damage to a wide variety of tissues. They are implicated in aging, brain damage, Alzheimer's disease, and a variety of other conditions. These data form the basis for administration of antioxidant drugs and vitamins, which bind free radicals, eliminating them from the body.

fremitus (frĕm′ĭ-təs) N. flutter that can be felt by the hand of the examiner or by listening, as the chest vibrations that occur with speech or on coughing.

frenulum (frĕn′yə-ləm) N. band or fold of membrane that connects two organs and usually limits the movement of one, esp. the band of tissue (frenulum linguae) that extends from the floor of the mouth to the undersurface of the tongue, limiting the movement of the tongue. (If the frenulum is too short, tongue movement is impaired; this condition, known as tongue-tied, can usually be corrected surgically.) Also called frenum.

frequency (frē′kwən-sē) N.
1. need to have an action occur often (e.g., urinary frequency).
2. number of times a phenomenon occurs in a certain time period (e.g., the number of heartbeats per minute).
3. in statistics, number of events or instances of something for each unit (*compare* INCIDENCE).

Freudian (froi′dē-ən) ADJ. pert. to Sigmund Freud or his theories esp. those relating to sexual symbolism.

Friedman test N. reliable means for determining whether or not a woman is pregnant; it involves injecting some of her urine into an unmated female rabbit, and then, 2 days later, examining the ovaries of the rabbit. The finding of yellow bodies (corpora lutea) indicates that the woman is pregnant. Also called rabbit test. *See also* CORPUS LUTEUM.

Friedreich's ataxia (frēd′rīks) N. abnormal condition marked by muscular weakness, loss of muscular control, and an abnormal gait, usually beginning between the ages of 5 and 20, progressing to affect the upper extremities, and leading to severe disability and often death.

frigidity (frĭ-jĭd′ĭ-tē) N. sexual passivity or unresponsiveness, esp. in a woman; coldness; inability to reach the climax of sexual intercourse (orgasm). ADJ. frigid

frontal (frŭn′tl) ADJ. pert. to the forehead.

frontal lobe N. that part of the cerebral cortex in either hemisphere of the brain; found directly behind the forehead, it helps to control voluntary movement and is associated with the higher mental activities (e.g., planning, judgment) as well as with personality.

frontal sinus N. one of a pair of hollow spaces (sinuses) in the frontal bone above the eye socket.

frostbite (frôst′bīt′) N. tissue damage, esp. of the fingers, toes, ears, or nose, caused by freezing and generally due to prolonged exposure to very cold weather. The affected parts turn white and become numb. Gentle warming in tepid water, without rubbing, is the appropriate first aid measure. Severe freezing results in the death of the tissues, necessitating amputation of the affected part.

frottage (frô-täzh′) N. sexual gratification obtained by rubbing against a person of the opposite sex, as in a crowded train.

fructose (frŭk′tōs′, frook′-) N. simple sugar found in honey and some fruits; also called fruit sugar; levulose.

fructosuria (frŭk′tō-soor′ē-ə) N. presence of fructose (levulose) in the urine, a harmless condition.

FSH *See* FOLLICLE-STIMULATING HORMONE.

fugue (fyoog) N. state in which a person appears to be conscious of his/her actions but later has no recollection of them. If the condition lasts for a long time, the person may leave his/her usual surroundings and start a new life elsewhere. The condition is believed to be due to inability to handle a conflict or severe stress. Sometimes called fugue state.

fulminant (fo͝ol′mə-nənt) ADJ. occurring with suddenness and severity (e.g., disease, pain, fever). V. fulminate

Fulvicin N. trade name for the antifungal griseofulvin.

functional disorder N. condition in which a body part (e.g., an organ) functions (acts or works) abnormally, although it is physically normal; in other words, a disorder marked by symptoms and signs for which no anatomical or physiological cause can be identified (*compare* ORGANIC DISORDER).

fundus (fŭn′dəs) N., *pl.* fundi, base of a hollow organ; that part of a structure farthest from its opening, as the inside of the eye farthest from the pupil, or the wide end of the uterus opposite the cervix.

fungal infection N. inflammatory condition caused by a fungus. Common fungal infections are candidiasis, tinea (ring-worm), and coccidioidomycosis.

fungus (fŭng′gəs) N., *pl.* fungi, one of a group of simple plant-like organisms, including mushrooms and yeasts, some of which cause disease (fungal infection). ADJ. fungal

funiculitis (fyo͞o-nĭk′yə-lī′tĭs) N. inflammation of the spermatic cord or spinal cord.

funny bone N. colloquial term for the back of the elbow, where the ulnar nerve is near the surface. A sharp blow to the site causes a most unpleasant shock or tingle.

furosemide N. commonly used diuretic (trade name Lasix), used to treat hypertension and edema. Adverse effects include fluid and electrolyte imbalances. *See* TABLE OF COMMONLY PRESCRIBED DRUGS—GENERIC NAMES.

furry tongue *See* HAIRY TONGUE.

furuncle (fyo͝or′ŭn′kəl) N. boil: small, painful lump in the skin that has a core of dead tissue and surrounding inflammation. Caused by bacterial (staphylococcal) infection through a sweat gland or hair follicle, it produces pain, redness, and swelling. Treatment is by antibiotics, applications of moist heat, and surgical incision and drainage if necessary.

furunculosis (fyo͞o-rŭn′kyə-lō′sĭs) N. acute skin disease marked by presence of many furuncles.

fusiform ADJ. spindle-shaped, tapering at both ends.

fusion (fyo͞o′zhən) N.
1. normal or abnormal joining.
2. combining of images from both eyes to form one image (optical fusion).
3. surgical joining of two or more vertebrae (spinal fusion).
V. fuse

G

GABA *See* GAMMA-AMINOBUTY-
RIC ACID.

gabapentin N. *See* TABLE OF COM-
MONLY PRESCRIBED DRUGS—
GENERIC NAMES.

gag (găg) V. to feel like vomiting;
to retch. N. object used to hold
the mouth open during surgery
or to prevent swallowing of the
tongue during a seizure (e.g., in
epilepsy).

gag reflex N. normal retching reaction, which may be produced
by touching the soft palate at
the back of the mouth; also
called pharyngeal reflex.

gait (gāt) N. way in which a person walks.

galactagogue N. agent that promotes the flow of milk.

galactocele (gə-lăk′tə-sēl′) N.
1. breast cyst containing milk
and caused by closure of a milk
duct.
2. accumulation of milky fluid
in the sac surrounding the testis.

galactorrhea (gə-lăk′tə-rē′ə) N.
1. excessive flow of milk.
2. secretion of milk not associated with breast-feeding, sometimes a sign of a pituitary gland
disorder.

galactose (gə-lăk′tōs′) N. simple
sugar derived from milk sugar
(lactose) and found in other substances; it is readily absorbed in
the digestive tract and converted
into glycogen in the liver.

galactosemia (gə-lăk′tə-sē′mē-ə)
N. inherited (autosomal recessive) disease in which a deficiency in or absence of the

enzyme (galactose-1-phosphate
uridyl transferase) necessary for
the metabolism of galactose to
glucose results in galactose
accumulation, leading to mental retardation, spleen and liver
enlargement, cataract formation, and other abnormalities.
Symptoms of vomiting, diarrhea, and poor weight gain typically develop shortly after
birth. The disease can be diagnosed through blood and urine
tests; treatment is a galactose-
free diet.

gall (gôl) *See* BILE.

gallbladder N. pear-shaped organ,
about 8 centimeters (3 inches)
long and located on the lower
surface of the liver, that is a
reservoir for bile. Bile produced
in the liver passes (through the
hepatic duct) to the gallbladder,
where it is stored; the presence
of food, esp. fats, in the duodenum and hormonal influences
cause the gallbladder to contract, releasing the bile to the
common bile duct for transport
to the duodenum. The gallbladder is a common site of stone
formation (cholelithiasis) and
inflammation (cholecystitis).

gallop (găl′əp) N. abnormal heart
rhythm during which extra heart
sounds are heard during each
cardiac cycle; the combination
of normal and abnormal sounds
much like a horse galloping.
Sometimes called a gallop
rhythm.

gallop rhythm N. heart rhythm
characterized by the presence
of an extra sound on stetho-

GALLBLADDER

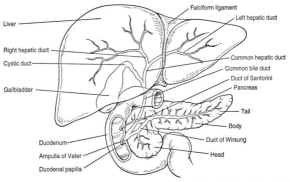

Falciform ligament
Left hepatic duct
Liver
Right hepatic duct
Cystic duct
Common hepatic duct
Common bile duct
Duct of Santorini
Gallbladder
Pancreas
Tail
Body
Duct of Wirsung
Duodenum
Ampulla of Vater
Head
Duodenal papilla

scopic examination; it may indicate a heart abnormality.

gallstone (gôl′stōn′) N. stonelike mass (calculus) in the gallbladder or in its duct. *See also* CHO-LELITHIASIS.

galvanic skin response (găl-văn′ĭk) N. change in the electrical resistance of the skin, measurements of which are used in some studies involving reactions to stress and other physiological variables.

Gamblers Anonymous N. fellowship based on the Twelve Step Program, designed to help persons unable to control their desire to gamble.

gamete (găm′ēt′, gə-mēt′) N. mature sex cell with the haploid number of chromosomes; either the spermatozoon in the male, or the egg (or ovum) in the female. Union of male and female gametes in fertilization results in the formation of a zygote with the diploid chromosome number.

gameto- comb. form indicating an association with sex (reproductive) cells (e.g., gametocyte,

cell capable of developing into a gamete).

gametocide N. agent able to kill sex cells.

gametogenesis (gə-mē′tə-jĕn′ĭ-sĭs) N. development and maturation of sex cells; it occurs through the process of meiosis. In males it is called spermatogenesis; in females, oogenesis.

gamma globulin (găm′ə) (glŏb′yə-lĭn) N. protein antibody formed in response to a foreign substance, such as a bacterial infection; synthetic gamma globulin preparations are also given to reduce the likelihood of contracting certain infections after exposure, such as hepatitis. Sometimes called immunoglobulin.

gamma ray N. electromagnetic wave of very short wavelength emitted by radioactive substances. Controlled radiation with gamma rays and rays of other wavelengths is used in medical diagnosis and in the treatment of some skin cancers and other cancers deep within the body.

gamma-aminobutyric acid (GABA) N. amino acid found

in the central nervous system, esp. the brain, that functions as an inhibitory neurotransmitter by slowing nerve transmission. GABA may have a role in prevention of seizures; the benzodiazepine drugs (e.g., Valium) exert their effect by increasing the brain's production of GABA. Experimentally, artificial forms of GABA have been used to prevent and to treat delirium tremens (DTs). Recent use of illicit preparations as a "date rape" drug, however, have limited the clinical use of GABA. *See* ROHIPNOL.

gammopathy (gă-mŏp′ə-thē) N. condition in which proteins having antibody activity (immunoglobulins) increase greatly in the blood.

gangli-, ganglio- comb. forms indicating an association with a ganglion (e.g., gangliocyte, ganglion cell).

ganglion (găng′glē-ən) N., *pl.* ganglia.
1. collection of nerve cells forming a knotlike shape and usually lying outside the brain and spinal cord; in the autonomic nervous system, chains of ganglia lie on either side of the spinal cord.
2. cyst that forms on a tendon, esp. in the wrist.

gangliosidosis (găng′glē-ō-sī-do′sĭs) *See* TAY-SACHS DISEASE.

gangrene (găng′grēn; găng-grēn′) N. tissue death resulting from lack of nutrition and oxygen when the blood supply to the affected part is decreased or lost because of disease (e.g., diabetes), injury, blood clot, tourniquet, frostbite, severe burn, or bacterial infection. The arms and legs are most commonly affected. Treatment includes antibiotics, a hyper-

baric chamber, and at times surgery. (*Compare* NECROSIS.) ADJ. gangrenous

Gantanol N. trade name for sulfamethoxazole, a sulfonamide antibacterial used to treat certain infections, esp. those of the urinary tract.

Gantrisin N. trade name for sulfisoxazole, a sulfonamide antibacterial used to treat urinary infections.

gap junction N. minute pores between cells; provide pathways for intercellular communication by means of transfer of ions and other molecules from one cell to another.

Garamycin N. trade name for the antibacterial gentamicin.

gargoylism (gär′goil′ĭz′əm) *See* HURLER'S SYNDROME.

gas N. basic form of matter; a gas lacks definite shape, and its volume depends on temperature and pressure.

gas embolism *See* AIR EMBOLISM.

gas gangrene N. form of gangrene in which the causative organism forms gas bubbles in the infected tissue.

gastr-, gastro- comb. forms indicating an association with the stomach (e.g., gastroesophageal, pert. to the stomach and esophagus).

gastrectomy (gă-strĕk′tə-mē) N. surgical removal of all or part of the stomach; it is usually done to stop hemorrhage from an ulcer or to remove a chronic ulcer or cancer.

gastric (găs′trĭk) ADJ. pert. to the stomach.

gastric digestion N. process of breaking down food (esp. protein) in the stomach through the action of chemicals in the gastric juice.

gastric juice N. secretions given off by the gastric glands of the stomach and consisting chiefly of hydrochloric acid, the lubricant mucin, and the enzymes pepsin and lipase.

gastric lavage (găs′trĭk) (lăv′ĭj, lä-väzh′) N. washing out the stomach with sterile water or a salt-water solution to remove the contents, either harmful materials (poisons) or blood (as from a bleeding ulcer); sometimes called pumping out the stomach.

gastric ulcer N. erosion or open sore of the lining of the stomach that may penetrate the muscle layers and wall of the stomach. Symptoms include burning pain, belching, and nausea; they tend to occur when the stomach is empty, after certain foods have been eaten, or when the patient is under stress. Treatment includes avoidances of irritating foods, and drugs to decrease the acidity of the stomach. If the ulcer perforates the stomach wall and hemorrhage occurs, surgery is usually needed. *See also* PEPTIC ULCER.

gastrin (găs′trĭn) N. hormone secreted by the pylorus (the upper part of the stomach) that stimulates the release of gastric juice from stomach glands and helps stimulate the secretion of bile and pancreatic juice.

gastritis (gă-strī′tĭs) N. inflammation of the lining of the stomach, characterized by loss of appetite, nausea, vomiting, and discomfort after eating. Acute gastritis may be caused by the ingestion of an irritating substance (e.g., aspirin, too much alcohol) or by bacterial or viral infection; chronic gastritis is often a symptom of gastric ulcer, stomach cancer, pernicious anemia, or other disorder. *Helicobacter pylori*, a spiral-shaped bacterium found in the stomach, is generally acknowledged as the main cause for most peptic ulcers and many cases of chronic gastritis. *See*

MAJOR COMPONENTS OF GASTRIC JUICE

Component	Source	Function
Pepsinogen	Chief cells of the gastric gland	Converts to pepsin
Pepsin	Formed from pepsinogen in the presence of hydrochloric acid	Protein-digesting enzyme capable of breaking down nearly all types of protein
Hydrochloric acid	Parietal cells of the gastric gland	Provides acidic environment; needed for converting pepsinogen into pepsin
Mucus	Goblet cells and mucous glands	Provides viscous, alkaline protective layer on the stomach wall
Intrinsic factor	Parietal cells of the gastric glands	Encourages the absorption of vitamin B_{12}

also HELICOBACTER PYLORI; PEPTIC ULCER; PERNICIOUS ANEMIA.

gastrocnemius (găs′trŏk-nē′mē-əs) N. superficial muscle in the back of the leg that forms the greater part of the calf. *See* MAJOR MUSCLES OF THE BODY, in Appendix.

gastroenteritis (găs′trō-ĕn′-tə-rī′tŭs) N. inflammation of the stomach and intestines. Symptoms include abdominal discomfort, loss of appetite, nausea, vomiting, and sometimes diarrhea. Causes include bacterial or viral infection, ingestion of toxic or irritating substances, allergic reactions to specific foods (e.g., milk intolerance), and other disorders. Treatment depends on the cause. *See also* INTESTINAL FLU.

gastroenterologist N. physician who specializes in the diagnosis and treatment of diseases affecting the gastrointestinal tract.

gastroenterology (găs′trō-ĕn′tə-rŏl′ə-jē) N. medical specialty concerned with the study of the gastrointestinal tract and the diseases that affect it.

gastroenterostomy (găs′trō-ĕn′tə-rŏs′tə-mē) N. surgical creation of an artificial opening between the stomach and the small intestines performed when the normal opening has been eliminated through removal of all or part of the stomach or of part of the small intestine.

gastroesophageal reflux N. backflow of the contents of the stomach into the esophagus, usually caused by malfunction of the sphincter muscle between the two organs; symptoms include burning pain in the esophagus, commonly known as heartburn. *See also* HIATUS HERNIA.

gastrogavage (găs′trō-gə-väzh′) N. artificial feeding of a nutrient solution through a tube inserted into a surgically created opening into the stomach; it is done in cases of prolonged unconsciousness or cancer of the esophagus; also called gastrostomy feeding.

gastrointestinal (GI) (găs′trō-ĭn-tĕs′tə-nəl) ADJ. pert. to the stomach and intestines.

gastrointestinal tract N. stomach and intestines; sometimes used more broadly to include the entire digestive tube from the mouth to the anus.

gastroscopy N. visual examination of the stomach (esp. the upper part) by means of a flexible fiberoptic instrument (gastroscope) inserted through the esophagus; photographs may be taken and specimens removed for analysis.

gastrostomy (gă-strŏs′tə-mē) N. surgical creation of an artificial opening into the stomach through the abdominal wall, done to allow artificial feeding (gastrogavage) in cases of prolonged unconsciousness or esophageal cancer.

gastrula (găs′trə-lə) N. early stage in embryo development occurring after the blastula stage; the gastrula is a hollow, cup-shaped structure consisting of an outer ectoderm layer and an inner layer that later differentiates into two layers (endoderm and mesoderm).

gatekeeper N. primary care or other health care provider who coordinates the utilization and delivery of medical services. *See* TABLE OF MANAGED HEALTH CARE TERMS.

Gaucher's disease (gō-shāz′) N. rare, familial disorder of fat metabolism that leads to spleen and liver enlargement and abnormal bone growth. Mortality is high in early childhood; those who survive through adolescence, however, may live for many years.

gavage (gə-väzh′) N. artificial feeding of liquid or semiliquid food through a tube, most commonly one extending from the nose to the stomach (nasogastric tube) See also GASTROGAVAGE.

gelatin (jĕl′ə-tn) N. a jellylike protein derived from connective tissues such as bones and ligaments and used as food, in medicinal preparations (e.g., suppositories, capsules), and as a medium for growing microorganisms; also called gel.

gemfibrozil N. oral agent (trade name Lopid) useful in the treatment of elevated serum triglyceride levels, with a variable effect on hypercholesterolemia. Although dietary measures should be tried first, this agent has been successful. See TABLE OF COMMONLY PRESCRIBED DRUGS—GENERIC NAMES.

gender (jĕn′dər) N. sex (male or female) of an animal.

gender identity N. awareness of knowing to which sex (male or female) one belongs; this awareness normally begins in infancy, continues through childhood, and is reinforced during adolescence.

gender role N. sexual identity that a person assumes and presents to others.

gene (jēn) N. basic unit of inheritance, basic unit of genetic material made up usually of DNA; that part of a chromosome that is considered to be a single unit of heredity and that codes for the production of a specific polypeptide chain of a protein. In humans and many other animals genes occur as paired alleles. These gene pairs control hereditary traits and are located in the same position on a pair of chromosomes. See also CHROMATIN; MUTATION.

gene splicing N. technique for recombining the chemical structures of a gene. See also RECOMBINANT DNA.

general anesthesia N. agent, usually given by inhalation or intravenous injection, that produces unconsciousness and complete loss of sensation throughout the body; it is used for major surgery (e.g., removal of a lung or of the stomach) (compare REGIONAL ANESTHESIA; LOCAL ANESTHESIA).

generalized seizure See GRAND MAL.

generic (jə-nĕr′ĭk) ADJ. pert. to the descriptive or nonproprietary (nontrade) name of a drug or other product; for example, diazepam is the generic name for Valium.

genesis (jĕn′ĭ-sĭs) N. origin, evolution or generation of something. ADJ. genetic

-genesis suffix meaning the production of something (e.g., psychogenesis, development of the mind) (compare -GENIC).

genetic (jə-nĕt′ĭk) ADJ.
  1. pert. to a gene or heredity.
  2. pert. to origin, birth, development.

genetic counseling N. process of determining the risk of a particular genetic disorder occurring within a family and providing information and advice based on that determination; used to help couples in family planning and in the care of children affected or thought to be affected with a particular genetic disorder. An accurate diagnosis is essential and may require special biochemical and cell studies; a careful and complete family medical history is also needed. The subjects of prenatal diagnosis (*See also* AMNIOCENTESIS), artificial insemination, sterilization, and termination of a pregnancy may be included in the counseling, depending on the particular disease and circumstances involved.

genetic disease N. any disorder or abnormality that results from inherited factors (genes) (e.g., Tay-Sachs disease, sickle-cell anemia) (also called inherited disorder).

genetic engineering N. process of altering and controlling the genetic makeup of an organism through manipulation and recombination of the genetic material deoxyribonucleic acid (DNA). *See also* RECOMBINANT DNA.

genetic marker N. specific gene that produces a recognizable trait and can be used in family or population studies, e.g., to determine susceptibility to a certain disease.

genetic screening N. process of analyzing a specific group of people to detect the presence of or susceptibility to a particular disease or diseases. Examples include the screening of all infants for phenylketonuria and the screening of certain racial or ethnic groups who have a high incidence of a particular disease, such as sickle-cell anemia among blacks and Tay-Sachs disease among Ashkenazic Jews. *See also* GENETIC COUNSELING.

genetics (jə-nĕt′ĭks) N. science that studies inherited characteristics; study of genes, their composition and function. ADJ. genetic

-genic suffix meaning producing, causing, forming (e.g., cytogenic, producing cells) (*compare* -GENESIS).

geniculum (jə-nĭk′yə-ləm) N., *pl.* genicula, kneelike bend in a small structure, such as a vein.

genital herpes (jĕn′ĭ-tl) *See* HERPES.

genital phase N. in psychoanalytic theory, the fifth stage in a person's development, occurring in adolescence and marked by interest and frequently participation in sexual activity (*compare* ORAL PHASE, ANAL PHASE, PHALLIC PHASE, LATENCY PHASE).

genitalia (jĕn′ĭ-tā′lē-ə) N. male or female reproductive organs, esp. the external ones; also called genitals. ADJ. genital

genitourinary (GU) (jĕn′ĭ-tō-yŏŏr′ə-nĕr′ē) ADJ. pert. to the genital and urinary systems of the body.

genome (jē′nōm′) N. complete set of hereditary factors (genes) contained in the chromosomes of each cell of an individual.

genotype (jĕn′ə-tīp′) N. complete genetic makeup or constitution of an individual organism or a related group (*compare* PHENOTYPE). ADJ. genotypic

gentamicin (jĕn′tə-mī′sĭn) N. antibiotic (trade name Garamycin) used to treat some severe infections. Adverse effects include kidney and hearing disturbances and hypersensitivity reactions.

gentian violet N. agent with antibacterial, antifungal, and anthelmintic properties used to treat pinworms and infections of the skin and vagina.

genu vulgum (jē′noo, jĕn′yoo) See KNOCKKNEE.

geographic medicine N. medical specialty concerned with the geographic distribution of diseases and their causes as related to climate, elevation, topography, and culture; also called geomedicine.

geriatrics (jĕr′ē-ăt′rĭks) N. medical specialty that deals with the problems of aging and the diagnosis and treatment of diseases affecting the aged. ADJ. geriatric

germ (jûrm) N.
1. microorganism, esp. one that causes disease.
2. unit from which a structure or part originates (e.g., germ layer, layer from which new tissue develops). ADJ. germinal

germ cell N. cell (spermatozoon or ovum) in any stage of its development (*compare* SOMATIC CELL).

German measles See RUBELLA.

gerontology (jĕr′ən-tŏl′ə-jē) N. scientific study of aging or of old age.

Gestaltism (gə-shtäl′tĭz′əm) N. school of psychology that maintains that the mind perceives integrated wholes, not discrete parts; for example, that a triangle is perceived as a triangle, not as three lines. In Gestaltism, behavior is seen as an integrated response to a situation, not as a series of sensations and reflexes. Also called

Gestalt psychology. (*Compare* APPERCEPTION.)

gestation (jĕ-stā′shən) N. period of time in humans and other viviparous animals from fertilization of the ovum to birth; the length of pregnancy. Human gestation averages 266 days, or about 280 days from the first day of the last menstrual period. *See also* PREGNANCY.

gestational age (jĕ-stā′shə-nəl) N. age of a fetus or newborn, usually expressed in weeks since the onset of the mother's last menstrual period (*compare* FETAL AGE).

GH *See* GROWTH HORMONE.

GHRF *See* GROWTH-HORMONE-RELEASING FACTOR.

GI *See* GASTROINTESTINAL.

GI series N. sequence of diagnostic tests involving the alimentary canal, esp. the stomach and intestines. It is usually done by inserting (e.g., by enema) a contrast medium (e.g., barium sulfate) into the parts to be studied, X-raying or otherwise obtaining images of those parts, and having films or other images reviewed by a radiologist to detect the presence of any abnormality (e.g., tumor, ulcer).

giardiasis (jē′är-dī′ə-sĭs) N. infection of the intestines with *Giardia lamblia*, a protozoan found in contaminated food and water throughout the world; symptoms include diarrhea, nausea, abdominal discomfort, and flatulence. Treatment is with the drug metronidazole (Flagyl).

gibbus (gĭb′əs) N. lump or protrusion on the body surface, esp. of the spine, resulting from fracture or collapse of a vertebra. ADJ. gibbous

gigantism (jī-găn′tĭz′əm) N. condition characterized by excessive size, caused most frequently by oversecretion of growth hormone from the pituitary gland. Treatment is by irradiation or removal of the pituitary gland. *See also* ACROMEGALY.

Gilles de la Tourette syndrome N. sometimes intermittent condition characterized by facial grimaces, tics, involuntary grunts, shouts, movements of the upper body, and compulsive use of obscene and offensive language (coprolalia). Treatment with agents that block the effects of the neurotransmitters dopamine and serotonin have been found effective. Also known as Tourette's syndrome.

gingiva (jĭn′jə-və) N., *pl.* gingivae, mucous membrane and fibrous tissue that encircles the neck of each tooth; also called gum. ADJ. gingival.

gingivitis (jĭn′jə-vī′tĭs) N. condition in which the gums are red, swollen, and bleeding. It most commonly results from poor oral hygiene and the development of bacterial plaque on the teeth, but is also common in pregnancy and may be a sign of another disorder (e.g., diabetes mellitus, vitamin deficiency).

girdle (gûr′dl) N. a ringlike arrangement or part (e.g., pelvic girdle).

glabella (glə-běl′ə) N. smooth bump between the eyebrows, most noticeable in men.

gland (glănd) N. any of numerous organs in the body (e.g., thyroid gland), each of which is made up of specialized cells that secrete or excrete materials not related to their own metabolism but needed by the body. There are two main types of glands: endocrine, or ductless, glands that secrete hormones directly into the bloodstream; and exocrine, or duct, glands that release materials into ducts or onto adjacent epithelial surfaces; included among the exocrine glands are sudoriferous (sweat) glands, sebaceous glands, and lacrimal (tear) glands.

glanders N. bacterial (*Pseudomonas mallei*) infection, endemic in Africa, Asia, and South America, where it is transmitted to humans from infected horses and other domesticated animals. Symptoms include purulent (pus-filled) inflammation of the mucous membranes and ulcerating skin lesions that, if untreated by antibiotics, may spread to internal tissues and lead to death.

glandular fever (glăn′jə-lər) *See* INFECTIOUS MONONUCLEOSIS.

glans (glănz) N. glandlike part, esp. that at the end of the clitoris or penis.

glaucoma (glou-kō′mə) N. disease in which elevated pressure in the eye, due to obstruction of the outflow of aqueous humor, damages the optic nerve and causes visual defects. Acute (angle-closure) glaucoma is a hereditary disorder with the iris blocking the flow of aqueous humor; symptoms, which may occur suddenly, include dilated pupil, red eye, blurred vision, and severe eye pain, sometimes accompanied by nausea and vomiting; if untreated by special eye drops or surgery, angle-closure glaucoma may result in permanent blindness within a few days. The much more common open-angle, or chronic, glaucoma, also hereditary, is one of the leading causes of blindness in the United States. Caused by blockage of the canal of Schlemm, it produces symptoms very slowly with gradual loss of peripheral vision over a period of years, sometimes with headache, dull pain, and blurred vision. Treatment involves the use of special eye drops. Glaucoma can also occur as a congenital defect or as a result of another eye disorder.

gleet (glēt) N. mucus or pus discharged from the penis or vagina, esp. after gonorrhea.

glenoid cavity N. socket of the shoulder joint into which the head of the humerus fits.

glia (glē′ə) See NEUROGLIA.

gliding joint (glī′dĭng) N. type of synovial joint in which the articulations of the bones allow only gliding motion; examples of gliding joints are the ankle and the wrist.

glimepiride N. See TABLE OF COMMONLY PRESCRIBED DRUGS—GENERIC NAMES.

glioma (glē-ō′mə) N. tumor of neuroglia cells.

glipizide (glĭp′ĭ-zīd′) N. oral antidiabetic (trade name Glucotrol) that works by stimulating the release of insulin from the pancreas. Adverse effects include hypoglycemia, gastrointestinal disturbances, and skin rashes. See TABLE OF COMMONLY PRESCRIBED DRUGS—GENERIC NAMES.

globin (glō′bĭn) N. protein in hemoglobin, the oxygen-carrying compound of red blood cells.

globulin (glŏb′yə-lĭn) N. any of a group of simple proteins found in the blood. See also IMMUNOGLOBULINS.

globus hystericus (glō′bəs) N. transitory feeling of a lump in the throat that cannot be swallowed or coughed up, often accompanying anxiety or emotional experience; it is thought to be due to a functional disturbance of nerves and muscles affecting the lower throat region.

glomerular capsule See BOWMAN'S CAPSULE.

glomerular filtration rate (GFR) N. speed at which plasma is filtered through capillaries of the kidney (at the glomerulus), removing waste products, conserving water as necessary, and forming urine. In a typical day, normal kidneys reabsorb more than 99% of the material filtered.

glomerulonephritis (glō-mĕr′yə-lō-nə-frī′tĭs) N. disease of the glomerulus of the kidney characterized by decreased production of urine, the presence of protein and blood in the urine, and edema; the cause is unknown, but it sometimes follows an acute upper respiratory infection, perhaps as an allergic reaction to the infective organism (e.g., streptococcal).

glomerulus (glō-mĕr′yə-ləs) N., pl. glomeruli, cluster, esp. the network of blood capillaries, contained in Bowman's capsule of a kidney nephron that is the main site where waste products from the blood are filtered into the kidney tubules. ADJ. glomerular

glomus (glō′məs) N. group of small arterial blood vessels, richly supplied with nerves, and connecting to veins.

glossa (glô′sə) See TONGUE.

glossalgia N. pain in the tongue; also called glossodynia.

glossitis (glô-sī′tĭs) N. inflammation of the tongue. Acute glossitis, characterized by swelling and pain, usually results from infection or injury. Chronic glossitis, with atrophy of tongue tissue, sometimes occurs in pernicious anemia. One superficial form of glossitis (Moeller's glossitis, or glossodynia exfoliativa), marked by irregular red patches on the tongue and sensitivity to hot and spicy foods, occurs in some middle-aged women.

glossolalia (glô′sə-lā′lē-ə) N.
1. repetitive nonsense speech, not related to the subject or situation involved.
2. speaking in an unknown language, speaking in tongues during a religious experience.

glossopharyngeal (glŏs′ō-fə-rĭn′jē-əl) ADJ. pert. to the tongue and pharynx.

glossopharyngeal nerve N. one of a pair of mixed sensory and motor nerves, the ninth cranial nerves, essential to taste, sensation in the palate, secretion of the parotid glands, and swallowing.

glossoptosis N. abnormal downward or backward placement of the tongue.

glossopyrosis N. burning sensation in the tongue.

glottis (glŏt′ĭs) N. voice-producing part of the larynx, consisting of the vocal cords and the opening (covered by the epiglottis) they form. ADJ. glottic

glucagon (gloo′kə-gŏn′) N. hormone produced in the pancreas that stimulates the conversion of glycogen in the liver to glucose; preparations of glucagon are sometimes used to treat certain hypoglycemic (low blood sugar) conditions.

glucocorticoid (gloo′kō-kôr′tĭ-koid′) N. any of several hormones, including cortisol, corticosterone, and cortisone, released by the cortex of the adrenal gland, that exert an anti-inflammatory effect and affect protein, fat, and carbohydrate metabolism to help the body respond to stress and avoid fatigue.

gluconeogenesis (gloo′kə-nē′ə-jĕn′ĭ-sĭs) N. de novo production of glucose (sugar) by the liver.

Glucophage N. *See* TABLE OF COMMONLY PRESCRIBED DRUGS—TRADE NAMES.

glucose (gloo′kōs′) N. simple sugar that is the major energy source in the body. Ingested in certain foods, esp. fruits, and produced by the breakdown of other carbohydrates, glucose is absorbed into the blood from the intestines; excess amounts are stored in the form of glycogen, chiefly in the liver. Determination of glucose levels in the blood is important in the diagnosis of many disorders, including diabetes mellitus. Pharmaceutical preparations of glucose (e.g., dextrose) are widely used in medicine.

glucose tolerance test N. test of the body's ability to metabolize carbohydrates, used in the diagnosis of diabetes mellitus, hypoglycemia, and other disorders. After an overnight fast, the level of glucose in the blood is measured; then the patient is given a 100-gram dose of glucose to drink, and glucose levels in the blood and urine are tested periodically during several hours. Other than in the diagnosis of pregnancy-induced diabetes, the glucose tolerance test is rarely used.

glucosuria (gloo'kə-soor'ĕ-ə) N. abnormal presence of glucose in the urine, resulting from ingestion of large amounts of carbohydrates, kidney disease, diabetes mellitus, or other metabolic disorder (*compare* GLYCOSURIA).

Glucotrol N. trade name for the oral antidiabetic glipizide. See TABLE OF COMMONLY PRESCRIBED DRUGS—TRADE NAMES.

glutamic acid (gloo-tăm'ĭk) N. nonessential amino acid, preparations of which are used in digestive aids.

gluteal (gloo'tē-əl, gloo-tē') ADJ. pert. to the buttocks (nates).

gluten (gloot'n) N. insoluble protein found in wheat, rye, and other grains; inability to handle gluten is the cause of celiac disease.

gluten-free diet N. diet used in the treatment of celiac disease and related disorders that eliminates products such as wheat, rye, oats, beans, cabbage, turnips, and cucumbers, which are rich in gluten.

glutethimide (gloo-tĕth'ə-mīd') N. sedative (trade name Doriden) used to treat some sleep disorders. Adverse effects include skin rashes and the possibility of dependence.

gluteus (gloo'tē-əs) N. any of three paired muscles in the buttocks involved in movements of the thigh. See MAJOR MUSCLES OF THE BODY, in Appendix.

glyburide N. oral antidiabetic (trade names DiaBeta and Micronase) that works by stimulating the release of insulin from the pancreas. Adverse effects

include hypoglycemia, gastrointestinal disturbances, and skin rashes. *See* TABLE OF COMMONLY PRESCRIBED DRUGS—GENERIC NAMES.

-glycemia (glī-sē'mē-ə) suffix meaning sugar in the blood (*see also* HYPOGLYCEMIA; HYPERGLYCEMIA).

glycerine (glĭs'ər-ĭn) N. sweet, colorless preparation of glycerol used as a moisturizing agent for chapped skin; in suppositories; and as a sweetening agent in drugs; also called glycerin.

glycerol (glĭs'ə-rôl, -rōl') N. alcohol found in fats. *See also* GLYCERINE.

glycine (glī'sēn', -sĭn) N. nonessential amino acid, widely found in proteins, preparations of which are used in antacids and in the treatment of some muscle disorders.

glycogen (glī'kə-jən) N. polysaccharide that is the principal form in which carbohydrates are stored in the body. Stored primarily in the liver and in muscle, glycogen is readily broken down to glucose when needed by the body.

glycogenesis (glī'kə-jĕn'ĭ-sĭs) N. formation of glycogen from glucose.

glycogenolysis (glī'kə-jə-nŏl'ĭ-sĭs) N. conversion of glycogen into glucose in the liver and skeletal muscles.

glycolysis (glī-kŏl'ə-sĭs) N. breakdown of glucose and other sugars through a series of enzyme-catalyzed reactions to either pyruvic acid (aerobic glycolysis in the presence of oxygen) or lactic acid (anaerobic glycolysis without oxygen), releasing energy for the body in the form of adenosine triphosphate (ATP).

glycosuria (glī′kə-soŏr′ē-ə) N. presence of abnormally high levels of sugar, esp. glucose, in the urine, due to ingestion of large amounts of carbohydrates, kidney disease, diabetes mellitus, or other metabolic disorder.

goiter (goi′tər) N. enlargement of the thyroid gland at the front of the neck; it may be caused by deficiency of iodine in the diet, by tumor, or by overactivity (exophthalmic goiter) or underactivity of the thyroid gland. Treatment depends on the cause and often involves surgical removal of all or part of the thyroid gland.

gold (gōld) N. metallic element; gold salts are sometimes used in the treatment of rheumatoid arthritis, and radioactive gold isotopes are used to treat some forms of cancer (*see also* TABLE OF IMPORTANT ELEMENTS).

Golgi apparatus N. small, membranous structure found in most cells that functions to store and transport proteins manufactured in other parts of the cell. The structure is usually well developed and abundant in cells that produce secretions (e.g., those in endocrine and exocrine glands). Also called Golgi body; Golgi complex.

Golgi cells N. type of nerve cell (neuron) found in the brain and spinal cord.

Golytely N. trade name for a solution containing polyethylene glycol and various electrolytes. It induces diarrhea and is used to cleanse the bowel prior to various procedures (e.g., colonoscopy).

gonad (gō′năd′) N. gland that produces sex cells (gametes). In males the gonads are the testes; in females, the ovaries. Also vital in production of sex hormones (e.g., estrogen, testosterone). ADJ. gonadal

gonadotropin (gō-năd′ə-trō′pĭn) N. hormone that stimulates the function of the gonads. The anterior pituitary gland secretes two gonadotropins: follicle-stimulating hormone and luteinizing hormone; during pregnancy the placenta secretes chorionic gonadotropin, which helps to maintain the pregnancy. Also called gonadotrophin. ADJ. gonadotropic, gonadotrophic

gonococcus (gŏn′ə-kŏk′əs) N. bacterium (*Neisseria gonorrhoeae*) that causes gonorrhea.

gonorrhea (gŏn′ə-rē′ə) N. common sexually transmitted disease caused by the bacterium *Neisseria gonorrhoeae* and transmitted through contact with an infected person or with secretions containing the bacteria. Symptoms include painful urination and burning, itching, and pain around the urethra and in women the vagina, accompanied by a greenish yellow, pus-containing discharge. If untreated, the infection spreads, esp. in women, infecting the reproductive organs, causing inflammation of the liver, and if widespread, leading to septicemia and polyarthritis, with painful lesions in joints and tendons and infection of the conjunctiva of the eye that can lead to blindness. Treatment is by antibiotics. ADJ. gonorrheal

goose bump N. colloquial term for a skin reaction occurring in cold, fright, or stress; the arrector pili contract, causing the hairs of the skin to stand up; also called gooseflesh.

gout (gout) N. disease in which a defect in uric acid metabolism causes the acid and its salts to accumulate in the blood and joints, causing pain and swelling of the joints (esp. the big toe area), accompanied by fever and chills. The disease is more common among men than women and usually has a genetic basis. If untreated, the disease causes destructive tissue changes in the joints and kidneys. Treatment includes a purine-free diet and use of drugs to reduce inflammation and to increase the excretion of uric acid salts or decrease their formation. Also called gouty arthritis.

graafian follicle (grä′fē-ən) N. fully developed, egg-containing sac in the ovary that ruptures during ovulation to release an egg, or ovum. Many primary follicles, each containing an immature ovum, are embedded in the wall of the ovary. Under the influence of follicle-stimulating hormone released by the pituitary, one follicle ripens into a mature graafian follicle containing a mature ovum in the early phase of each menstrual cycle. At ovulation the follicle ruptures and the ovum is released. The collapsed follicle—now the corpus luteum—produces the hormone progesterone and prepares the uterus to receive a fertilized egg; if fertilization does not occur, the corpus luteum is shed in menstruation.

gracilis (grăs′ə-lĭs) N. slender, superficial muscle that runs along the inside of the thigh and functions in movement of the thigh and leg.

gradient N. graded change in the magnitude of a physical quantity or dimension.

graft (grăft) N. tissue or organ that is taken from one site and transplanted to another site on the same person (autograft), as in transplanting thigh skin to the arm to replace badly burned skin, or that is taken from one person and inserted in another, as in a kidney transplant. *See also* TRANSPLANT.

-gram (grăm) suffix indicating something written, drawn, or otherwise recorded, as in electrocardiogram.

Gram's stain (grămz) N. method of chemically staining bacteria that is used as a means of identifying and classifying them. A series of stains and solutions is applied to a bacterium; if it appears violet or blue, it is termed Gram-positive; if pink or red, Gram-negative. Also called Gram's method.

grand mal (grän′mäl′, grănd′ măl′) N.
1. type of seizure during which the patient becomes unconscious, may develop bluish discoloration (cyanosis) of the skin and lips due to oxygen

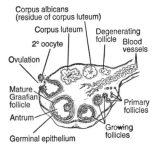

Corpus albicans
(residue of corpus luteum)

Corpus luteum

Degenerating follicle

2° oocyte

Blood vessels

Ovulation

Mature Graafian follicle

Primary follicles

Antrum

Growing follicles

Germinal epithelium

The development of the Graafian follicle, beginning with the primary follicle and continuing with the release of the secondary oocyte, which becomes the mature egg cell (ovum).

lack, and experiences convulsions involving the entire body; also called a generalized seizure.

2. type of epilepsy characterized by recurrent grand mal seizures (*compare* PETIT MAL).

granulation (grăn'yə-lā'shən) N. growth of small projections of tiny blood vessels and connective tissue that form on the surfaces of a wound during the healing process; sometimes called granulation tissue.

granule (grăn'yo͞ol) N. small particle or grain. ADJ. granular

granulocyte (grăn'yə-lō-sīt') N. type of white blood cell characterized by granules in the cytoplasm; it includes the basophil, eosinophil, and neutrophil.

granulocytic leukemia See MYELOCYTIC LEUKEMIA.

granulocytopenia (grăn'yə-lō-sī'tə-pē'nē-ə) See AGRANULOCYTOSIS.

granuloma (grăn'yə-lō'mə) N. mass of nodular granulation tissue resulting from injury, infection, or inflammation. Treatment depends on the cause and probable course of the granuloma.

granuloma inguinale (grăn'yə-lō'mə) (ĭng'gwə-nā'lē) N. sexually transmitted disease caused by the bacterium *Calymmatobacterium granulomatis* and characterized by a pimply rash that develops into ulcers of the skin and subcutaneous tissue of the genital and groin region. Treatment is by antibiotics.

granulomatosis N. condition characterized by the development of widespread granulomas.

graphospasm N. pain in the hand and arm due to prolonged writing; also called writer's cramp.

grass N. street term for marijuana.

Graves's disease (grāvz) See EXOPTHALMIC GOITER.

gravid ADJ. pregnant.

gravid-, -gravida (grăv'ĭd) comb. forms meaning pregnant or a pregnant woman (e.g., secundigravida, a woman pregnant for the second time) (*compare* PARA-).

gravida (grăv'ĭ-də) N.

1. pregnant woman.

2. designation by number of the pregnancy a woman is in, gravida I indicating her first pregnancy, gravida III her third.

gray matter N. gray tissue of the central nervous system, made up primarily of nerve cell bodies and neuroglia cells. It is found in the cerebral cortex and other parts of the brain and forms an H-shaped center of the spinal cord surrounded by lighter, so-called white matter; gray matter in the spinal column functions as the center for spinal reflex activity. (*Compare* WHITE MATTER.)

green monkey disease See MARBURG DISEASE.

greenstick fracture See FRACTURE.

grief (grēf) N. pattern of responses, physical (faster heart and breathing rates, sweating, increased energy reserves, slowed or disturbed digestive processes) and emotional (typically proceeding from disbelief and denial to anger and guilt to final acceptance) to the loss of a loved one or separation from him/her.

grippe (grĭp) See INFLUENZA.

griseofulvin (grĭz′ē-ə-fūl′vĭn) N. generic name for commonly used oral antifungal drug.

groin (groin) N. area where the abdomen and thighs join; also called inguen.

groove (grōōv) N. narrow channel or depression in a structure; for example, the costal groove lodges the blood vessels and nerves between two ribs. *See also* SULCUS.

gross ADJ. visible to the unaided eye, as a gross (vs. microscopic) examination.

gross anatomy N. study of the structure of the body and its parts without the aid of a microscope.

group therapy N. psychotherapy involving several (usually six to eight) persons and a therapist, with the interactions of the group members considered an important part of the therapy.

growth N. increase in size of an organism or any of its parts, as occurs normally in a child or abnormally in a tumor.

growth hormone (GH) N. hormone synthesized and released by the anterior pituitary gland that stimulates the growth of long bones in the limbs and increases protein synthesis and the use of fats for energy. Excessive production results in gigantism or acromegaly; a deficiency, in dwarfism. Also called somatotropin.

growth-hormone-releasing factor (GHRF) N. substance released by the hypothalamus that stimulates the release of growth hormone by the anterior pituitary gland.

GSF *See* GALVANIC SKIN RESPONSE.

GU *See* GENITOURINARY.

guanabenz N. antihypertensive (trade name Wytensin) that reduces blood pressure via its effect on the central nervous system. Adverse effects include dry mouth and drowsiness.

guanine (gwä′nēn′) N. organic compound, one of the bases found in DNA (deoxyribonucleic acid) and RNA (ribonucleic acid).

gubernaculum (gōō′bər-năk′yə-ləm) N., *pl.* gubernacula, structure that guides (e.g., gubernaculum testis, the cord involved in the descent of the testes).

guiac test (gwī-ăk) N. chemical test of stool for blood, especially blood that is not visible to the naked eye (occult blood). If the test is positive, the stool is classified as guiac-positive. Testing stool for occult blood is a routine part of the physical exam in patients over 40 years of age as a screen for colon cancer. A newer kind of stool blood test kit, known as a fecal immunochemical test (FIT), detects a specific portion of a human blood protein. This test is done essentially the same way as conventional guiac test, but it is more specific and reduces the number of false-positive results. Vitamins (e.g., vitamin C) or foods (e.g., red meat) do not affect the FIT. *See* COLON CANCER (*compare* HEMATOCHEZIA).

guided imagery *See* TABLE OF ALTERNATIVE MEDICINE TERMS.

Guillain-Barre syndrome (gē-yăn′bə-rā′) N. form of peripheral polyneuritis marked by pain, weakness, and sometimes paralysis of the limbs that may spread to the trunk of the body.

The cause is unknown; it usually develops 1–3 weeks after a viral infection or immunization. Treatment is supportive, possibly including mechanical ventilation; in most cases symptoms resolve within a few weeks or months. Also called infectious polyneuritis.

gullet (gŭl'ĭt) *See* ESOPHAGUS.

gum *See* GINGIVA.

gumboil N. abscess of the (gum) and tooth root resulting from injury, infection, or dental decay. The gums are usually red, swollen, and painful. Treatment includes antibiotics, special mouthwashes, and sometimes incision and drainage of the abscess.

gumma (gŭm'ə) N. soft tumor—a granuloma—characteristic of the tertiary stage of syphilis and found in the liver, brain, or other tissues.

gustation (gŭ-stā'shən) N. sensation of taste or the process of tasting.

gustatory organ (gŭs'tə-tôr'ē) *See* TASTE BUD.

gut (gŭt) *See* INTESTINE; CATGUT.

gyn-, gyne-, gyneco-, gyno- prefixes indicating a relationship to women or the female sex (e.g., gynopathy, disease of women).

gynecologist (gī'nĭ-kŏl'ə-jĭst) N. a physician who practices gynecology.

gynecology (gī'nĭ-kŏl'ə-jē) N. medical specialty concerned with the health care of women, including function and diseases of the reproductive organs. It combines both medical and surgical concerns and is usually practiced in combination with obstetrics.

gynecomastia (jĭn'ĭ-kō-măs'tē-ə) N. excessive development of the breasts in males, usually the result of hormonal imbalance, liver malfunction, or treatment with various drugs, including steroids and some antihypertensives; may occur transiently in newborns or during puberty.

gyrus (jī'rəs) N., *pl.* gyri, curved portion (convolution) of the surface of the brain, caused by infolding of the cortex.

H

H symbol for the element hydrogen.

H vitamin N. old name for biotin.

habit (hăb′ĭt) N. customary practice or behavior; automatic response or pattern of behavior learned by frequent repetition (*compare* ADDICTION).

habitual abortion *See* ABORTION.

habituation (hə-bĭch′o͞o-ā′shən) N.
1. process of becoming accustomed to something.
2. in pharmacology, dependence on a drug (including alcohol or tobacco) resulting from repeated use but lacking severe physiological signs of addiction or need to increase dosage.
3. in psychology, decrease or loss of response to a particular stimulus after repeated exposure to that stimulus (*compare* ADAPTATION).

habitus (hăb′ĭ-təs) N.
1. general physical build of a person (e.g., an athletic habitus).
2. person's tendency to require or be affected by something, as a disease.

hair (hâr) N. threadlike, keratin-containing appendage of the outer layer of the skin present over most of the body surface except the palms, soles, lips, and a few other small areas. A hair develops inside a tubular hair follicle beneath the skin, with the root of the hair expanded into a bulb. The part above the skin consists of an outer cuticle that covers the cortex, which contains pigment and gives the hair its color, and an inner medulla. A hair may be raised by small arrector pili muscles attached to the follicle. Also called pilus.

hair cells N. specialized hearing receptor cells of the inner ear, located in the organ of Corti within the cochlea. Rod-shaped hair-like processes project from each cell. Sound waves cause movement of fluid within the cochlea, leading to motion of the hairs. Motion results in a change in the hair cells' electrical charge and causes a nerve impulse to be transmitted via the auditory nerve to the brain. The brain converts the impulse to what we perceive of as a sound.

hair follicle N. tubular sheath of cells in the epidermis layer of the skin that surrounds the root of a hair. Sebaceous glands and small arrector pili muscles are associated with hair follicles.

HAIR FOLLICLE

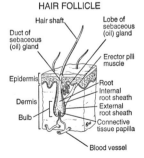

hairy tongue N. dark overgrowth of the papillae (tiny projections) of the tongue that is a side effect of some antibiotics;

it is benign and gradually subsides; also called furry tongue; black tongue.

Halcion N. trade name for the sleeping pill triazolam.

Haldol N. trade name for haloperidol.

half-life N. amount of time needed for a radioactive substance to lose one half of its radioactivity or to decay by one half.

halitosis (hăl'ĭ-tō'sĭs) N. offensive breath; it may result from poor mouth hygiene, diseased teeth or gums, some systemic diseases, the ingestion of certain foods (e.g., garlic, onions), or drugs.

halitus (hăl'ĭ-təs) N. exhaled breath.

hallucination (hə-loo'sə-nā'shən) N. perception of something that is not actually present; it may be visual (seeing objects that are not present), auditory (hearing noises that are not present), olfactory, gustatory, or tactile. Hallucinations are a common symptom of severe mental illness (e.g., schizophrenia); they also occur following injury to the head, in delirium accompanying severe illness, in delirium tremens in toxic states, and from the use of hallucinogens. ADJ. hallucinative, hallucinatory

hallucinogen (hə-loo'sə-nə-jən) N. substance (e.g., LSD—lysergic acid diethylamide, mescaline, phencyclidine—angel dust) that excites the central nervous system, producing hallucinations (false perceptions); mood changes; increases in pulse, blood pressure, and body temperature; dilation of the pupils of the eyes; and other physiological and psychological changes. ADJ. hallucinogenic

hallucinosis (hə-loo'sə-nō'sĭs) N. abnormal mental state in which the patient has almost continual hallucinations.

hallux (hăl'əks) N., *pl.* halluces, great toe; ADJ. hallucal

halogen (hăl'ə-jən) N. any of a family of chemicals, including chlorine, bromine, fluorine, and iodine, used in drugs and disinfectants.

haloperidol (hăl'ō-pĕr'ĭ-dôl; -dōl') N. tranquilizer (trade name Haldol) used in the treatment of psychosis and Gilles de la Tourette syndrome; also sometimes used to treat sleep disorders. Adverse side effects include hypotension and muscular incoordination.

halophil N. microorganism favoring a high-salt environment for growth; also called halophile. ADJ. halophilic

halothane (hăl'ə-thān') N. inhalation anesthetic widely used to produce general anesthesia for many types of surgical procedures; it is most often used in combination with analgesics and muscle relaxants. Among its advantages are its properties of being nonexplosive, nonflammable, and nonirritating to the respiratory passages. Serious potential adverse reactions include hepatitis and permanent liver damage.

hamartia N. defect in development due to abnormal tissue combination. ADJ. hamartial

hamartoma (hăm'är-tō'mə) N. benign tumor consisting of an overgrowth of mature cells that normally occur in the affected part, but often with one element or type predominating.

hamate bone (hā'māt') N. wrist (carpal) bone that projects a hook-shaped (hamate) part on its palmar surface, in line with the fourth and fifth fingers. ADJ. hamate, hammular

Hamman-Rich syndrome N. lung disease characterized by excessive and abnormal fibrosis of the connective tissue of the lung; results in shortness of breath, tachypnea, anorexia, and weight loss; eventually, the patient develops heart failure; although the condition may be improved with corticosteroids, it often results in death.

hammertoe (hăm′ər-tō′) N. condition in which one or more toes (most commonly the second toe) is permanently flexed, giving a clawlike appearance.

hamstring muscle (hăm′strĭng′) N. any of three powerful muscles at the back of the thigh. *See* MAJOR MUSCLES OF THE BODY, in Appendix.

hamstring tendon N. any of the tendons at the back of the knee; they connect the hamstring muscles with the bones of the knee area.

hand N. that part of the upper limb distal to the forearm and extending from the wrist to include the fingers. It contains

HAND AND WRIST BONES

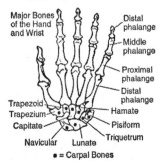

• = Carpal Bones

27 bones, including 8 in the wrist, 5 in the metacarpal region, and 14 in the fingers. Also called manus. *See also* WRIST.

handedness (hăn′dĭd-nĭs) N. preference to use either the left or the right hand for writing and other delicate manipulations. Handedness is thought to be hereditary and is related to cerebral dominance, with left-handedness being associated with dominance of the right hemisphere of the brain and vice versa. Of 100 persons, usually about 67 are right-handed.

handicap (hăn′dē-kăp′) N. impairment or disability resulting in a disadvantage for a given person in performing normal activities of daily living.

hangnail (hăng′nāl′) N. a narrow, loose strip of skin near the base of a fingernail in the region of the cuticle. Tearing the fragment usually produces a painful, easily infected sore.

Hansen's disease (hăn′sənz) *See* LEPROSY.

haploid (hăp′loid′) ADJ. pert. to a cell, specifically a gamete, or mature sex cell, that has half the chromosome number characteristic of the species. Thus, in humans, the sex cells—the ovum (egg) and spermatozoon—each have the haploid chromosome number 23; at fertilization, when the gametes fuse to form a zygote, the zygote has the chromosome number 46, characteristic for humans. (*Compare* DIPLOID.)

haptoglobin (hăp′tə-glō′bĭn) N. protein found in plasma that binds hemoglobin and clears it from wounds; the amount of haptoglobin is increased in certain inflammatory diseases, decreased in hemolytic anemia.

hard palate N. bony portion of the roof of the mouth, bounded on the front and sides by the gums and, in the back, continuous with the soft palate.

hardening of the arteries *See* ARTERIOSCLEROSIS.

harelip (hâr′lĭp′) N. congenital deformity in which there are one or more clefts in the upper lip; it results from failure of the upper jaw and nasal processes to close during embryonic development and is often associated with cleft palate. It can be repaired surgically during infancy.

Hartnup disease (härt′nəp) N. hereditary defect of the metabolism of certain amino acids, characterized by dry, scaly skin lesions, gastrointestinal problems, extreme photosensitivity, and often psychological and mental abnormalities.

Hashimoto's disease (hăsh′ĭ-mō′tōz) N. autoimmune disorder of the thyroid gland, most common in middle-aged women, in which antibodies are produced against thyroid tissue. Symptoms include an enlarged, lumpy thyroid gland. Treatment is by administration of thyroid hormones.

hashish N. drug prepared from the Indian hemp plant *Cannabis sativa* that produces euphoria, distorted perceptions, and sometimes hallucinations. *See also* CANNABIS; MARIJUANA.

haustrum (hô′strəm) N., *pl.* haustra, pouch, esp. in the colon. ADJ. haustral

Haverhill A fever (hāv′rəl, hā′vər-əl) *See* RATBITE FEVER.

Haversian canal (hə-vûr′zhən) N. one of many tiny (about 0.05 millimeter) canals, containing blood vessels, nerve filaments, and connective tissue, found as the central tube in the Haversian systems of bone.

Haversian system N. basic unit of bone, consisting of a central Haversian canal around which bone matrix and bone cells occur.

hay fever N. type of allergic rhinitis, with symptoms of sneezing, runny or stuffy nose, and watery eyes, that occurs seasonally on exposure to pollen. Antihistamines are frequently used to alleviate the symptoms; if the specific allergen can be identified, desensitization may be possible. Also called pollinosis.

HB *See* HEMOGLOBIN.

HCG *See* HUMAN CHORIONIC GONADOTROPIN.

HDL *See* HIGH-DENSITY LIPOPROTEIN.

head (hĕd) N.
1. upper part of the body, esp. that which contains the brain and organs of sight, hearing, taste, and smell.
2. rounded portion of a bone, which fits into a groove in another to form a joint (e.g., the head of the humerus—upper arm bone—fits into the shoulder joint).
3. that part of a muscle that is away from the bone that it moves.

headache (hĕd′āk′) N. pain, ranging from mild to severe, that occurs in the head. There are many causes of headache, and treatment depends on the cause. Also called cephalgia. *See also* HISTAMINE HEADACHE; MIGRAINE;

SINUS HEADACHE; TENSION HEADACHE.

healing N. process of restoring health or normal function or of natural repair of damaged or cut tissue.

healing touch *See* TABLE OF ALTERNATIVE MEDICINE TERMS.

Health Maintenance Organization (HMO) N. system of health care whereby members pay a specified fee entitling them to comprehensive care, often including both in-hospital and outpatient services. Most HMOs limit the choice of physicians and hospitals to either their own institutions and employees or those who have specifically contracted to provide care to member patients. *See* TABLE OF MANAGED CARE TERMS.

hearing (hēr′ĭng) N. sense of receiving and interpreting sounds. Sound waves enter the outer ear, cause vibrations of the eardrum (tympanic membrane) and bones of the middle ear, and are transmitted to the inner ear, from which they are transmitted along the auditory nerve to the brain for interpretation.

hearing aid N. electronic device, usually worn in or near the ear, that intensifies sound; it is used to help some people with hearing impairment.

hearing impairment N. decrease or limitation in sensitivity to sound. *See also* DEAFNESS.

heart (härt) N. muscular, roughly cone-shaped organ that pumps blood throughout the body. Lying behind the sternum between the lungs, it is about the size of a closed fist, about 12 centimeters (5 inches) long, 8 centimeters (3 inches) wide at its broadest upper part, and about 6 centimeters (2¼ inches) thick and weighs about 275–345 grams (10–12 ounces) in males, 225–275 grams (8–10 ounces)

THE HEART IN THE CHEST

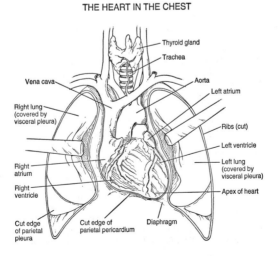

Thyroid gland
Trachea
Vena cava
Aorta
Left atrium
Right lung (covered by visceral pleura)
Ribs (cut)
Left ventricle
Left lung (covered by visceral pleura)
Right atrium
Apex of heart
Right ventricle
Cut edge of parietal pleura
Cut edge of parietal pericardium
Diaphragm

THE HEART

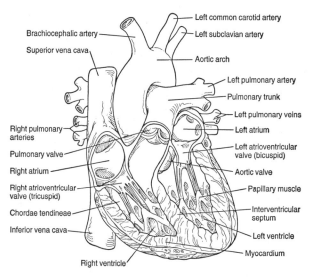

Left common carotid artery

Brachiocephalic artery

Left subclavian artery

Superior vena cava

Aortic arch

Left pulmonary artery

Pulmonary trunk

Left pulmonary veins

Right pulmonary arteries

Left atrium

Pulmonary valve

Left atrioventricular valve (bicuspid)

Right atrium

Aortic valve

Right atrioventricular valve (tricuspid)

Papillary muscle

Chordae tendineae

Interventricular septum

Inferior vena cava

Left ventricle

Right ventricle

Myocardium

in females. Under the outer epicardium membranes, the heart wall—myocardium—consists of cardiac muscle; the innermost layer—the endocardium—is continuous with the lining of the blood vessels. The heart is divided into left and right sides by a septum; each side has an upper atrium (auricle) and lower ventricle. Through coordinated nerve impulses and muscular contractions, initiated in the sinoatrial node of the right atrium, the heart pumps blood throughout the body. Deoxygenated blood, carried to the heart by the vena cava, flows into the right atrium and passes into the right ventricle, from which it flows through pulmonary arteries to the lungs, where it gives up its wastes and becomes freshly oxygenated. The oxygenated blood then passes through the pulmonary veins into the left atrium and from there into the left ventricle. From the left ventricle it is pumped throughout the body via the aorta and its many branches. The heart normally beats about 70 times per minute. It is nourished by coronary blood vessels.

heart attack N. popular term for a disruption of the normal circulation of the heart. *See also* MYOCARDIAL INFARCTION.

heart block N. conduction disorder of the heart whereby electrical impulses are slowed either partially or completely; it may be a congenital condition or the result of a heart disorder, including those caused by medication or poisoning; symptoms may or may not occur, depending on the location of the block and the resultant heart rate.

heart failure N. inability of the heart to pump enough blood to maintain normal body requirements. It may be caused by congenital defects or by any condition (e.g., atherosclerosis of coronary arteries, aortic stenosis, myocardial infarction) that damages or overloads the heart muscle. Symptoms include edema, shortness of breath, and feelings of faintness. Treatment depends on the specific cause of the heart malfunction and on the age and general condition of the patient.

heart massage *See* CARDIAC MASSAGE.

heart murmur N. abnormal heart sound indicating turbulent blood flow, regardless of the cause. Some heart murmurs are benign and of no significance; others are signs of abnormal heart function. Also called cardiac murmur.

heart rate N. number of heart contractions (beats) per minute. A normal adult heart rate is about 60–80 beats per minute; an abnormally rapid heart rate (over 100 beats per minute in an adult) is tachycardia; an abnormally slow rate (below 60 beats per minute in an adult) is bradycardia. A child normally has a heart rate faster than an adult. *See also* PULSE.

heart sound N. any of four distinct sounds produced within the heart during its normal cycle of contraction and relaxation and heard with a stethoscope placed on the chest over the heart. The first sound (a dull, prolonged lub) is caused by closure of the valves between the atria and ventricles and marks the beginning of ventricular contraction; the second (a short sharp dub) occurs with closing of the semilunar valves as the ventricle begins to relax; the third (a weak, dull sound usually not heard except in heart failure) occurs as the ventricles fill with blood during their relaxed phase; the fourth (not usually heard in normal hearts) occurs as the atria contract. Changes in the characteristic sounds usually indicate abnormalities in heart structure or function and are important diagnostic aids.

heart surgery N. any surgical procedure involving the heart.

HEART VALVES

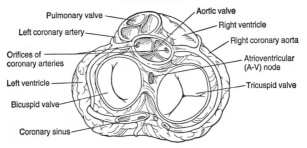

Pulmonary valve

Left coronary artery

Orifices of coronary arteries

Left ventricle

Bicuspid valve

Coronary sinus

Aortic valve

Right ventricle

Right coronary aorta

Atrioventricular (A-V) node

Tricuspid valve

A SUMMARY OF THE HEART VALVES

Valve	Location	Function
Tricuspid valve	Between right atrium and right ventricle	Prevents blood from moving from right ventricle back into right atrium during ventricular contraction
Pulmonary semilunar valves	Between right ventricle and pulmonary artery	Prevents blood from moving back from pulmonary artery into right ventricle during ventricular relaxation
Bicuspid (mitral valve)	Between left atrium and left ventricle	Prevents blood from moving from left ventricle during ventricular contraction
Aortic semilunar valve	Between left ventricle and aorta	Prevents blood from moving back from aorta into ventricle during ventricular relaxation

In closed heart surgery, a small incision is made into the heart; a heart-lung machine is not used. In open-heart surgery, the heart is opened, the chambers of the heart are made visible, and blood is detoured from the operating field through the heart-lung machine.

heart valve N. any of four structures (two semilunar valves [pulmonary valve, aortic valve], the mitral valve, and the tricuspid valve) within the heart that, by closing and opening, control blood flow in the heart and permit flow in only one direction.

heartburn (härt′bŭrn′) N. painful, burning sensation in the chest, below the sternum, resulting from irritation in the esophagus, most often due to backflow of acidic stomach contents into the esophagus. It is often a symptom of hiatus hernia, peptic ulcer, or other disorder. Also called pyrosis.

heart-lung machine N. apparatus, used during heart surgery, that takes over the functions of the heart and lungs temporarily. It includes a pump and a means of oxygenating blood.

heat exhaustion N. condition characterized by dizziness, nausea, weakness, muscle cramps, and pale, cool skin and caused by overexposure to intense heat and depletion of body fluids and electrolytes. It is most common in infants and the elderly. Recovery usually occurs with rest, replacement of water and electrolytes, and removal from the intense heat. Also called heat prostration. (*Compare* HEATSTROKE.)

heat rash N. fine papular inflammation of the skin resulting from heat or high humidity. *See also* MILIARIA.

heatstroke N. severe, sometimes fatal, condition caused by prolonged exposure to intense heat and failure of the body's temperature-regulating capacity. Symptoms include high body temperature, rapid heart beat; red hot, dry skin; confusion;

and possibly convulsions and loss of consciousness. Treatment includes cooling of the body, fluid and electrolyte replacement, and sedation. Also called sunstroke; heat hyperpyrexia. (*Compare* HEAT EXHAUSTION.)

hebephrenia (hē′bə-frē′nē-ə) N. form of schizophrenia marked by severe disintegration of personality. It typically becomes evident during puberty with symptoms of extreme silliness; inappropriate laughter; facial grimaces; talking and gesturing to oneself; withdrawal from contact with others, and delusions and hallucinations. Also called disorganized schizophrenia. ADJ. hebephrenic

Heberden node N. enlargement of a terminal joint of a finger sometimes occurring in osteoarthritis or other degenerative joint disease.

heel N. posterior part of the foot, formed by the calcaneus.

Hegar's sign N. softening of the uterine cervix that occurs in early pregnancy.

Heimlich maneuver (hīm′lĭk; līkh′) N. emergency procedure to help someone who is choking because food or other material is lodged in the trachea. The rescuer should hold the choking person from behind and place one fist, thumb side in, against the victim's abdomen, in the midline immediately above the navel. The other hand should be placed over the fist. Quick upward thrusts are then administered to force the obstruction out of the trachea. A maximum of five thrusts should be tried, but each individual thrust should be delivered with sufficient force as to attempt to clear the air-

way by itself. Vomiting or internal organ damage can result from this maneuver, though the risks are lessened if the rescuer has been properly trained by the American Red Cross or the American Heart Association in cardiopulmonary resuscitation.

heliation N. use of sunlight for treatment.

Helicobacter pylori (*H. pylori*) (hĕl-ĭ-kō-băk-tər pī′lōr-ī) N. spiral-shaped bacterium found in the stomach. Generally acknowledged as the main cause for most peptic ulcers and many cases of chronic gastritis (inflammation of the stomach). This organism can weaken the protective coating of the stomach and duodenum (first part of the small intestines) and allow digestive juices to irritate the sensitive lining of these body parts. Treatment for gastritis or peptic ulcer typically requires antibiotics effective against *H. pylori*. See GASTRITIS; PEPTIC ULCER.

helix (hē′lĭks) N. coil-shaped part; the hereditary material DNA (deoxyribonucleic acid) has a double-helix configuration.

helminth (hĕl′mĭnth′) N. any of various parasitic worms, including flatworms, tapeworms, and roundworms, some of which infest humans causing disease. ADJ. helminthic

helminthiasis (hĕl′mĭn-thī′ə-sĭs) N. infestation of the body with worms that may affect the skin or the intestines or other internal organs.

heloma (hē-lō′mə) N., *pl.* helomata, hard-tissue formation; a corn or callus.

helper T cell (hĕl′pər) *See* T CELL.

hem-, hema-, hemato-, hemo-
prefixes indicating an association with blood (e.g., hemodilution, adding fluid to blood and thus reducing the number of red blood cells per unit of volume).

hemagglutination (hē′mə-gloot′n-ā′shən) N. clumping together of red blood cells. ADJ. hemagglutinative

hemangioma (hē-măn′jē-ō′mə) N., *pl.* hemangiomata, benign tumor consisting of blood vessels. Some occur as birthmarks (strawberry hemangioma), often spontaneously disappearing; others develop later in life, often in the elderly.

hemarthrosis N. bleeding into a joint or joint cavity, causing pain and swelling of the joint area; may result from injury or certain diseases (e.g., hemophilia).

hematemesis (hē′mə-těm′ĭ-sĭs, hē′mə-tə-mē′sĭs) N. vomiting of blood, most often caused by bleeding in the esophagus (e.g., from varicose veins), stomach, or upper intestine (e.g., from an ulcer).

hematin *See* HEME.

hematinic N. drug (e.g., ferrous sulfate or other iron-containing compound) that increases the hemoglobin content of the blood; it is used to treat or prevent iron-deficiency anemia.

hematochezia N. passage of stools containing visible blood. Causes include diverticulosis, colon cancer, and peptic ulcer.

hematocoele N. tumor or swelling caused by leakage of blood from blood vessels, esp. a swelling of the membrane covering the testis.

hematocolpometra N. accumulation of menstrual blood in the vagina because of an imperforate hymen.

hematocrit (hĭ-măt′ə-krĭt′) N. measure of the volume of red blood cells as a percentage of the total blood volume. The normal range is 43–49% in males, 37–43% in females. *See also* BLOOD COUNT; DIFFERENTIAL BLOOD COUNT.

hematocytopenia N. abnormally low number of red blood cells in the blood.

hematogen N. any blood-producing material; also called hematinogen.

hematohidrosis N. secretion of sweat containing blood; also called hematidrosis.

hematologist (hē′mə-tŏl′ə-jĭst) N. specialist in hematology.

hematology (hē′mə-tŏl′ə-jē) N. science of blood and blood-forming tissues, including its functions, diseases, and use in treatment. ADJ. hematologic, hematological

hematoma (hē′mə-tō′mə) N. localized collection of blood, usually clotted, in an organ, space, or tissue due to escape of blood from a blood vessel, often the result of trauma; when the hematoma occurs near the skin surface, it causes discoloration (e.g., a black eye).

hematopoiesis (hē′mə-tō-poi-ē′sĭs) N. process by which blood cells are produced, esp. as occurring in the bone marrow; also called hemopoiesis. ADJ. hematopoietic

hematuria (hē′mə-toŏr′ē-ə) N. presence of blood in the urine, often a symptom of disease in the urinary tract.

heme (hēm) N. red-pigmented, nonprotein, iron-containing part of the hemoglobin molecule of red blood cells; also called hematin.

hemeralopia N. abnormal condition in which bright light causes a blurring of vision; a side effect of some anticonvulsant drugs; also called day blindness.

hemi- comb. form meaning half (e.g., hemifacial, affecting only one side of the face).

hemianopia (hěm′ē-ə-nō′pē-ə) N. blindness to one half of the visual field in one or both eyes; also: hemianopsia. ADJ. hemianopic

hemic ADJ. pert. to blood.

hemicrania *See* MIGRAINE.

hemiplegia (hěm′ĭ-plē′jə) N. paralysis affecting only one side of the body; also called unilateral paralysis. ADJ. hemiplegic

hemisphere (hěm′ĭ-sfēr′) N. half of a ball-like part; in medicine, half of the lateral half of the cerebrum or cerebellum of the brain.

hemochromatosis (hē′mə-krō′mə-tō′sĭs) N. disorder of iron metabolism in which iron accumulates in tissues; it is characterized by bronze pigmentation of the skin, an enlarged and impaired liver, diabetes mellitus, and abnormalities of the pancreas and joints. It may be hereditary (idiopathic, or classic, hemochromatosis) or acquired through iron overload from repeated transfusions or intake of iron-containing compounds. Also called bronzed diabetes; iron-storage disease. (*Compare* HEMOSIDEROSIS.)

hemodialysis (hē′mō-dī-ăl′ĭ-sĭs) N. procedure, used in toxic conditions and renal (kidney) failure, in which wastes and impurities are removed from the blood by a special machine. The blood is shunted to and from a dialyzer where, through diffusion and ultrafiltration, wastes are removed. Popularly known as artificial kidney.

hemodynamics N. study of the forces involved in circulating blood throughout the body; includes the function of the heart and of the blood vessels.

Hemofil N. trade name for human antihemophilic factor, used in the treatment of hemophilia.

hemoglobin (Hb) N. complex compound, containing the nonprotein, iron-containing pigment heme and the protein globin, found in red blood cells (erythrocytes) that transports oxygen to cells throughout the body and carries carbon dioxide away from body cells. In the high oxygen concentration of the lungs, hemoglobin binds with oxygen to form oxyhemoglobin. In the tissues of the body, the oxygen is given off and the hemoglobin combines with carbon dioxide to form carboxyhemoglobin, which is carried back to the lungs. There the carbon dioxide is given off and more oxygen picked up for transport to the body cells. Normal hemoglobin concentration in blood is 13.5–18 grams per deciliter for males, 12–16 grams per deciliter for females.

hemoglobinemia N. presence of excessive hemoglobin in blood plasma.

hemoglobinopathy N. any of a group of inherited disorders characterized by an alteration in the normal structure of hemoglobin. Types of hemoglobinopathies include sickle-cell disease and thalassemia.

hemoglobinuria N. abnormal presence of free hemoglobin in the urine. ADJ. hemoglobinuric

hemolysin N. substance that breaks down or dissolves red blood cells. Hemolysins are found in some bacteria, venom, and foods.

hemolysis N. breakdown of red blood cells and the release of hemoglobin. It occurs normally at the end of the life span of a red blood cell, abnormally in certain antigen-antibody reactions, on exposure to certain bacteria and venoms, in hemodialysis, and in certain other conditions. *See also* HEMOLYTIC ANEMIA.

hemolytic anemia N. disorder in which there is premature destruction of red blood cells. Anemia—abnormally low hemoglobin levels—may or may not be present, depending on the ability of bone marrow to increase red blood cells production. Hemolytic anemia can result from certain infections or inherited disorders of red blood

cells but most often is a response to drugs or toxic substances (e.g., snake venom). (*Compare* APLASTIC ANEMIA.)

hemophilia N. inherited disorder characterized by excessive bleeding and occurring only in males. Several forms of the disease, including hemophilia A and hemophilia B (also called Christmas disease), occur; in all forms one of the blood clotting factors necessary for normal blood coagulation is missing or present in abnormally low amounts. Greater than usual blood loss in dental extractions and simple injuries, and bleeding into joint areas, commonly occur; severe internal hemorrhage is less common. Treatment involves administration of missing blood coagulation factors (clotting factors) in some cases and transfusions to replace lost blood.

hemoptysis (hē-mŏp′tĭ-sĭs) N. coughing up blood from the respiratory tract. The blood is usually frothy, bright red, and mixed with sputum. Uncommonly, it may occur in small amounts in mild upper respiratory infection and bronchitis; profuse bleeding

HEMOGLOBIN

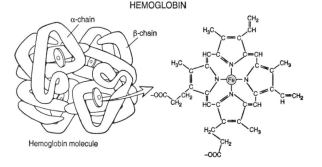

Hemoglobin molecule

usually indicates severe infection or disease of the bronchi or lungs. Heart disease may also result in small amounts of hemoptysis.

hemorrhage (hĕm′ər-ĭj) N. loss of a large amount of blood during a short time, either externally or internally. The bleeding may be from an artery (the blood flows in spurts and is bright red), from a vein (the blood flows slowly and is dark), or from a capillary (the blood oozes). External bleeding may be controlled by pressure and ice on the wound or by a tourniquet applied proximally to the wound; internal bleeding requires prompt medical attention. Loss of large amounts of blood can lead to shock and death. ADJ. hemorrhagic

hemorrhagic fever N. any of several kinds of arbovirus (e.g., transmitted by insects or crustaceans) infection usually occurring in a specific geographic area; symptoms include fever, malaise, and respiratory or gastrointestinal symptoms, followed by capillary hemorrhage.

hemorrhoid (hĕm′ə-roid′) N. swelling of a vein or veins (varicosity) in the lower rectum or anus, either internal, above the anal sphincter, or external, outside the anal sphincter. Frequently associated with constipation, straining to defecate, pregnancy, or prolonged sitting, hemorrhoids are often painful and sometimes bleed with defecation. Treatment includes topical agents to shrink and anesthetize the hemorrhoids, compresses, and, if severe, ligation or surgical excision. Also called piles. ADJ. hemorrhoidal

hemorrhoidectomy (hĕm′ə-roi-dĕk′tə-mē) N. surgical procedure for tying and excising hemorrhoids.

hemosiderosis N. abnormal deposition of an iron-containing compound (hemosiderin) in tissues, often associated with diseases in which there is extensive destruction of red blood cells (e.g., thalassemia) (*compare* HEMOCHROMATOSIS).

hemostasis (hē′mə-stā′sĭs) N. cessation of bleeding, either naturally through the blood coagulation process, mechanically (e.g., with surgical clamps) or chemically (e.g., with drugs). ADJ. hemostatic

hemostat (hē′mə-stăt′) N. pliers-like instrument used to compress blood vessels to stop the bleeding.

hemothorax (hē′mə-thôr′ăks′) N. accumulation of blood in the pleural cavity or pleural space; it is usually the result of injury, sometimes of blood vessel rupture associated with lung disease. The blood must be drained, or impaired lung function and infection may occur.

Henle's loop (hĕn′lēz) N. U-shaped portion of a microscopic kidney tubule in the nephron; site of action of many important drugs, including some diuretics (thus, the term—loop diuretics—for drugs like furosemide).

heparin (hĕp′ər-ĭn) N.
1. chemical produced in certain white blood cells (basophils) and connective tissue cells (mast cells), esp. in the lungs and liver, that inhibits the activity of the thrombin factor in blood coagulation and thus prevents clotting within the blood vessels.
2. drug (heparin sodium) used

as an anticoagulant in the treatment of thromboembolic disorders.

hepat-, hepato- comb. forms indicating an association with the liver (e.g., hepatalgia, pain in the liver).

hepatic (hǐ-păt′ĭk) ADJ. pert. to the liver.

hepatic duct N. tube that carries bile from the liver toward the intestine; it joins with the cystic duct from the gallbladder to form the common bile duct.

hepatic portal system *See* PORTAL SYSTEM.

hepatitis (hĕp′ə-tī′tĭs) N. inflammation of the liver, characterized by jaundice, loss of appetite, abdominal discomfort, an enlarged and abnormally functioning liver, and dark urine. It may be caused by bacterial or viral infection, infestation with parasites, alcohol, drugs, toxins, or transfusions of incompatible blood, or as a complication of another disease (e.g., infectious mononucleosis), and may be mild and brief or prolonged and severe, even life-threatening. Five hepatitis viruses (A, B, C, D, E) have been described, though other variants are likely present.
Hepatitis A is caused by the hepatitis A virus and can be contracted through contaminated water, food, or person to person contact. Though the disease is often mild, prolonged chronic illness may result. There is no treatment, though gamma globulin may be administered prophylactically. Previously called infectious hepatitis.
Hepatitis B is caused by the hepatitis B virus and may be severe, leading to chronic liver damage. Those at greatest risk are intravenous drug abusers, homosexual men, and health care personnel (needle sticks). Infection may be prevented, in many cases, by a series of vaccinations. These vaccinations are now mandatory in many school systems in the United States. Also called serum hepatitis.
Hepatitis C is similar to hepatitis B. It is spread primarily through blood, though sexual transmission has been described. Nearly 50% of victims develop chronic hepatitis. The drug alpha interferon has been helpful in treatment.
Hepatitis D is caused by a defective virus and can only occur when concomitant hepatitis B infection is present. Thus, hepatitis D is prevented by vaccination against hepatitis B. Also called delta agent hepatitis.
Hepatitis E is similar in presentation to hepatitis A; it spreads via contaminated food and water, usually causing only acute infection; there is a 20% mortality rate in pregnant women.

hepatocyte (hĕp′ə-tə-sīt′) N. major functional cell of the liver; inflammation or injury to these cells results in hepatitis.

hepatolenticular degeneration *See* WILSON'S DISEASE.

hepatoma (hĕp′ə-tō′mə) N. primary malignant tumor of the liver, most common in tropical parts of the world, esp. where fungus-produced toxins (aflatoxins) may contaminate food; also sometimes associated with hepatitis or cirrhosis of the liver. Symptoms include an enlarged liver, pain, loss of appetite, weight loss, and the presence of alphafetoprotein in the plasma.

hepatomegaly (hĕp′ə-tə-mĕg′ə-lē) N. abnormal enlargement of the liver, usually a sign of liver disease.

hepatotoxic ADJ. damaging to the liver, e.g., certain drugs or alcohol.

hereditary (hə-rĕd′ĭ-tĕr′ē) ADJ. pert. to transmission from parents to offspring; inherited (e.g., hereditary disorder, a disorder that is passed from parents to offspring).

heredity (hə-rĕd′ĭ-tē) N.
1. process by which specific traits or characteristics are transmitted, through genes, from parents to offspring.
2. total genetic makeup of an individual. ADJ. hereditary

hermaphrodite (hər-măf′rə-dīt′) N. person who has the tissues of both testes and ovaries; true hermaphroditism is rare among humans.

hernia (hûr′nē-ə) N. protrusion of an organ through an abnormal opening in the muscular wall surrounding the organ area. It may be congenital or acquired as a result of injury, muscular weakness, or disease. Common types of hernia include hiatus hernia, inguinal hernia, and umbilical hernia. Also called rupture. ADJ. hernial

herniated disc N. rupture of fibrocartilage of the disc between vertebrae of the spinal column (intervertebral discs), occurring most often in the lumbar region. With the ruptured disc there is a lack of cushioning between the vertebrae above and below and resultant pressure on spinal nerves, causing pain. Also called slipped disc; ruptured intervertebral disc.

heroin (hĕr′ō-ĭn) N. strongly addictive drug made from morphine; it has no medical uses in the United States but is widely abused.

herpangia (hûr′păn-jī′nə) N. viral infection occurring most often in children, characterized by sore throat; papules on the tongue, pharynx, and palate; fever; headache; and pain in the abdomen and extremities. It usually subsides within a short time.

herpes (hûr′pēz) N. any of a group of viruses that cause painful blisterlike eruptions on the skin.
herpes genitalis N. infection, caused by type 2 herpes simplex virus, usually transmitted by sexual contact, and characterized by recurrent attacks of painful eruptions on the skin and mucous membranes of the genital area. Symptoms include fever, malaise, urinary problems, painful coitus, swelling of lymph glands in the inguinal area, and lesions on the glans or foreskin of the penis in males and on the vagina and cervix, sometimes with a discharge from the cervix, in females. Treatment is aimed at relieving symptoms; there is no cure. Also called genital herpes.
herpes simplex N. infection, caused by herpes simplex virus, that usually affects the skin and nervous system, producing small, transient, sometimes painful blisters on the skin and mucous membranes. Herpes simplex 1 (HS1) most commonly affects the facial region, esp. the area near the mouth and nose. Symptoms include tingling and burning, followed by blisterlike eruptions that

dry and crust before healing. Treatment involves keeping the area clean to prevent secondary infection and topical use of drying medications. Also called cold sore.

herpes simplex 2 (HS2) commonly affects the genital region. *See also* HERPES GENITALIS.

herpes zoster N. infection with herpes zoster virus, usually occurring in adults, and characterized by blisterlike eruptions along the course of an inflamed nerve. Symptoms include pain—chronic or intermittent, mild or severe—along the course of the lesions, sometimes with fever, malaise, and headache. Treatment is symptomatic and includes cold compresses and calamine applications on the lesions. Complications, occurring most often in the elderly, include postherpetic neuralgia, which may last for months. Also called shingles.

herpes zoster virus *See* CHICKEN POX.

heterogeneous (hĕt′ər-ə-jē′nē-əs) ADJ. made up of dissimilar or diverse parts or materials, not of the same consistency throughout (*compare* HOMOGENEOUS).

heterogenous (hĕt′ə-rŏj′ə-nəs) ADJ. not from the same source (*compare* HOMOGENOUS).

heterograft (hĕt′ə-rō-grăft′) N. tissue from an individual of one species used as a temporary graft, as in cases of severe burn, on an individual of another species. A heterograft is usually rapidly rejected but provides temporary cover for an injured area, reducing fluid loss. Also called xenograft. (*Compare* HOMOGRAFT.)

heterophil test N. blood test that, when positive, usually indicates infectious mononucleosis.

heteroploidy N. condition of having an abnormal number of chromosomes, either more or less than the number normal for body cells of the species.

heterosexual (hĕt′ə-rō-sĕk′shōō-əl) N. man or woman whose sexual preference is for persons of the opposite sex (*compare* HOMOSEXUAL).

heterozygous ADJ. having two different alleles of a gene at corresponding loci (sites) on homologous chromosomes. A person heterozygous for a given trait inherits one allele from each parent, and the dominant allele usually manifests itself. (*Compare* HOMOZYGOUS.)

hexachlorophene N. topical anti-infective agent used as a disinfectant and antiseptic scrub.

Hexadrol N. trade name for the anti-inflammatory dexamethasone.

hexestrol N. estrogen compound used to treat menstrual irregularities and menopausal symptoms and to prevent pregnancy.

hexobarbital N. short-acting sedative-hypnotic.

Hg symbol for the element mercury.

hiatus (hī-ā′təs) N. normal opening in a membrane or other tissue. ADJ. hiatal

hiatus hernia (hûr′nē-ə) N. protrusion of part of the stomach through the diaphragm. It is a common disorder and in many cases produces no symptoms. Symptoms, when present, include gastroesophageal reflux (heartburn), the flow of acid stomach contents into the esophagus. Also called hiatal hernia; diaphragmatic hernia.

hiccup (hĭk′əp) N. characteristic sound produced by involuntary spasm of the diaphragm and rapid closure of the glottis as air is breathed in. Hiccups sometimes indicate indigestion, too-rapid eating, or alcoholism, but in most cases have no identifiable cause. Also called hiccough, singultus.

hidrosis (hī-drō′sĭs) N. production and secretion of sweat.

hidrotic (hī-drŏt′ĭk) ADJ. pert. to sweat.

high altitude pulmonary edema N. accumulation of edema fluid in the lungs during exposure to high altitudes (usually greater than 9000 ft); in addition to breathing problems, persons also may develop brain edema and experience visual and thinking problems; treatment is removal of the victim to a lower altitude as soon as possible.

high blood pressure See HYPERTENSION.

high density lipoprotein (HDL) N. protein of plasma that contains relatively more protein and less fats; it serves to transport cholesterol and other lipids from plasma to tissues. According to some studies, high HDL levels are associated with lowered risks of cardiovascular disorders.

high-protein diet N. diet rich in plant and animal proteins; used either as a treatment for malnutrition or in an attempt to increase the body's muscle mass.

hilus (hī′ləs) N., pl. hili, depression or small pit in an organ, esp. the entry site for blood vessels and nerves; also called hilum. ADJ. hilar

hindbrain (hīnd′brān′) N. that part of the brain consisting of the cerebellum, pons, and medulla oblongata.

hinge joint (hĭnj) N. freely movable (synovial) joint in which bones are articulated in such a way as to permit extensive motion in one plane. The elbow, knee, and interphalangeall joints are hinge joints. (*Compare* BALL-AND-SOCKET JOINT; GLIDING JOINT; PIVOT JOINT.)

hip (hĭp) N. area of the body formed by the lower part of the torso (pelvis) and the upper part of the thigh.

hip joint N. ball-and-socket joint in which the head of the femur (thigh bone) fits into the acetabulum of the innominate bone of the pelvis. The joint involves several ligaments and permits extensive motion. Also called coxa joint.

hippocampus (hĭp′ə-kăm′pəs) N. structure of the brain, part of the limbic system. ADJ. hippocampal

Hippocratic Oath N. statement, attributed to the ancient Greek physician Hippocrates, that serves as an ethical guide for physicians and is incorporated into the graduation ceremonies at many medical schools.

Hirschsprung's disease N. congenital condition in which the colon does not have a normal nerve network; there is little urge to defecate, feces accumulate, and the colon becomes dilated (megacolon). Symptoms include intermittent diarrhea and constipation, loss of appetite, and distended abdomen. Surgical repair involves joining the normal colon section to the rectum. *See also* MEGACOLON.

hirsutism (hûr′soo-tĭz′əm) N. excessive hairiness, sometimes the result of heredity, endocrine (hormonal) imbalance, disease, or drug intake.

Hismanal N. trade name for the antihistamine drug, astemizole.

hist-, histio-, histo- comb. forms indicating an association with tissue (e.g., histogenesis, tissue development).

histamine (hĭs′tə-mēn′, -mĭn) N. compound found in mast cells and released in allergic responses and inflammatory conditions; it causes small blood vessels to widen, decreases blood pressure, increases gastric secretions, and constricts smooth muscles of the bronchi and uterus. Specific and different receptors are responsible for the gastric effects, which include control over the amount of stomach acid (hydrochloric acid) released. Thus, agents that specifically block these receptor sites (H_2 receptors) have been used in the treatment of peptic ulcers, gastritis, and gastroesophageal reflux.

histamine blocker N. general term for any agent that blocks receptors for the compound histamine; the two receptor sites are referred to as H_1 and H_2. H_1 receptors mediate histamine-associated allergic reactions, dilate blood vessels and are blocked by the classic antihistamines. H_2 receptors mediate the secretion of gastric acid. (*See also* HISTAMINE). H_2 blockers, generally referred to as histamine blockers, include cimeti-

dine, ranitidine, famotidine, and nizatidine.

histamine headache N. headache associated with the release of histamine from cells. Symptoms include sharp pain on one side of the head, runny nose, and watery eyes. Treatment is by antihistamines and agents to constrict dilated arteries. Also called cluster headache. (*Compare* MIGRAINE; TENSION HEADACHE.)

histidine (hĭs′tĭ-dēn′) N. essential (not produced by the body, required in the diet) amino acid.

histiocytic leukemia (hĭs′tē-ə-sĭt′ĭk) (loo-kē′mē-ə) *See* MONOCYTIC LEUKEMIA.

histochemistry N. study of cells and tissues using both microscopic and chemical staining techniques.

histocompatibility (hĭs′tō-kəm-păt′-ə-bĭl′ĭ-tē) N. ability of the cells of one tissue to survive in the presence of cells of another tissue, as in the ability of cells of a transplanted organ to survive in the presence of cells of another organism. A high degree of histocompatibility is necessary for a successful graft or transplant.

histology (hĭ-stŏl′ə-jē) N. science of tissues, including their cellular composition and organization.

histoplasmosis (hĭs′tō-plăz-mō′sĭs) N. infection caused by inhaling spores of the fungus *Histoplasma capsulatum,* most common in the Ohio and Mississippi River valleys; symptoms include fever, malaise, cough, and enlarged lymph nodes. In most cases the disease subsides spontaneously; less often, it progresses to severe infestation of the lungs and death.

HIV N. abbrev. for human immunodeficiency virus, the cause of acquired immunodeficiency syndrome (AIDS); two virus types (HIV-1 and HIV-2) have been identified, though infection with HIV-2 in the United States is infrequent. Nonetheless, blood supplies are typically screened for both. *See* AIDS.

hives (hīvz) *See* URTICARIA.

Hodgkin's disease (hŏj′kĭnz) N. malignant disorder in which there is painless, progressive enlargement of lymphatic tissue. Symptoms include generalized itching, weight loss and loss of appetite, low-grade fever, and night sweats. It occurs more often among males and usually manifests itself between the ages of 15 and 35. Treatment with radiotherapy and/or chemotherapy effects long-term remissions in more than one half of cases and cures in a large percentage of those with localized disease.

holistic medicine (hō-lĭs′tĭk) N. system of medical care based on the concept that a person is an integrated entity, more than the sum of his/her physiological, mental, psychological, and social parts.

homeopathy (hō′mē-ŏp′ə-thē) N. medical system, based on the idea that like cures like, which uses drugs or other substances that would produce in healthy persons the symptoms shown by the sick person (e.g., treating a fever by giving small doses of a drug that raises body temperature) (*compare* ALLOPATHY).

homeostasis (hō′mē-ō-stā′sĭs) N. steady state in the internal environment of the body (e.g., temperature, electrolyte balance, respiration, heart rate) maintained by various feedback and control mechanisms, involving primarily the nervous and endocrine systems. ADJ. homeostatic

homogeneous ADJ. consisting of like parts; having a uniform quality (*compare* HETEROGENEOUS).

homogenous (hə-mŏj′ə-nəs) ADJ. derived from the same source (*compare* HETEROGENOUS).

homograft (hō′mə-grăft′) N. tissue from one person transplanted to another person of the same species but of different genetic makeup. The recipient's immune system must be repressed to prevent rejection of the graft or transplanted organ. (*Compare* HETEROGRAFT.)

homologous (hə-mŏl′ə-gəs) ADJ. corresponding or similar in position, structure, function, or characteristics; derived from an organism of the same species, such as a homologous skin graft or homologous chromosomes.

homosexual (hō′mə-sĕk′shoō-əl) N. man or woman whose sexual preference is for persons of the same sex (*compare* HETEROSEXUAL).

homozygous ADJ. having two identical alleles of a gene at corresponding loci (sites) on homologous chromosomes, the result of having inherited the same allele from each parent. The recessive gene usually manifests itself when homozygous. (*Compare* HETEROZYGOUS.)

homunculus N. dwarf with no deformity or abnormality and

TWO MAIN TYPES OF HORMONES

Type of Hormone	Examples
Steroid	Estrogens, testosterone, aldosterone, cortisol
Nonsteroid	
Amines	Norepinephrine, epinephrine
Peptides	ADH, oxytocin
Proteins	Insulin, somatotropin, prolactin
Glycoproteins	FSH, LH, TSH

all parts of the body proportionate.

hookworm disease (hŏŏk′wûrm′) N. condition, occurring chiefly in the tropics and subtropics, that results from intestinal infestation by hookworms, which most often enter the body by penetrating the skin, esp. that of the feet when walking barefoot in hookworm-infested soil areas. Symptoms include abdominal discomfort, diarrhea, and blood loss sometimes leading to anemia. Treatment is with anthelminthic drugs.

hordeolum N. bacterial (often staphylococcal) infection of a gland at the base of an eyelash, characterized by a pus-filled cyst, redness, pain, and other signs of inflammation. Treatment includes antibiotics and hot compresses. Also called stye.

hormone (hôr′mōn′) N. complex chemical produced and secreted by endocrine (ductless) glands that travels through the bloodstream and controls or regulates the activity of another organ or group of cells—its target organ. (For example, growth hormone released by the pituitary gland controls the growth of long bones of the body.) There are two main types of hormones—steroids (e.g., estrogen, testosterone, aldosterone, cortisol) and nonsteroidal. Secretion of hormones is regulated by feedback mechanisms and neurotransmitters. *See also* ENDOCRINE GLAND; ENDOCRINE SYSTEM. ADJ. hormonal

Horner's syndrome (hôr′nərz) N. group of symptoms—drooping upper eyelid, constricted pupil, absence of facial sweating—occurring as a result of damage to nerves in the cervical (neck) region of the spine.

horny layer *See* STRATUM CORNEUM.

horripilation (hô-rĭp′ə-lā′shən) N. gooseflesh; erection of the hairs on the body in cold or fear.

hospice (hŏs′pĭs) N. program designed to provide care for terminally ill patients and their families. Both home and in-hospital environments are utilized; the goal is to provide physical and emotional support. The hospice team is multidisciplinary in nature, often consisting of physicians, nurses, clergy, social workers, and other professionals.

host (hōst) N.
1. organism in which another, usually parasitic, organism lives.
2. recipient of a transplanted organ or tissue (*compare* DONOR).

hot flash N. transient feeling of warmth experienced by some women during menopause; the frequency and severity of the flashes vary widely.

human bite N. bite to any portion of the body caused by the human mouth and teeth; these bites are highly prone to infection due to the large number of bacteria present in human saliva.

human chorionic gonadotropin (HCG) N. hormone produced by the placenta in early pregnancy that functions to maintain the pregnancy. It can be detected in the urine and serum of pregnant women, and assays for this hormone serve as the basis for pregnancy tests. Some of the newer blood tests may give positive results within days after conception.

human immunodeficiency virus (HIV) N. virus that causes acquired immunodeficiency syndrome (AIDS); two virus types (HIV-1 and HIV-2) have been identified, though infection with HIV-2 in the United States is infrequent. Nonetheless, blood supplies are typically screened for both. See AIDS.

human insulin 70/30 N. See TABLE OF COMMONLY PRESCRIBED DRUGS—GENERIC NAMES.

human insulin regular N. See TABLE OF COMMONLY PRESCRIBED DRUGS—GENERIC NAMES.

human insulin-NPH N. See TABLE OF COMMONLY PRESCRIBED DRUGS—GENERIC NAMES.

humerus (hyoo'mər-əs) N. upper arm bone extending from the shoulder to the elbow. Its head articulates with the scapula (shoulder bone), its body is cylindrical, and its condyle end has depressions for articulations with the ulna and radius of the lower arm at the elbow. ADJ. humeral

humor (hyoo'mər) N. fluids in the body esp. the aqueous humor of the eye. ADJ. humoral

humpback (hŭmp'băk') See KYPHOSIS.

Humulin N. trade name for recombinant human insulin, a newer form of insulin made from recombinant DNA and used in the treatment of diabetes mellitus. It is identical to natural human insulin and is used to treat diabetics who exhibit allergic reactions or resistance to earlier preparations, which are made from beef and pork insulin. For unknown reasons, some patients may tend to have a higher incidence of hypoglycemic reactions when first started on human insulin. See TABLE OF COMMONLY PESCRIBED DRUGS—TRADE NAMES.

hunger (hŭng'gər) N. sensation of needing to eat; may be accompanied by pain in the upper stomach region or weakness, depending on the degree of severity.

Huntington's chorea (hŭn'tĭng-tənz) N. abnormal hereditary condition (autosomal dominant disease) characterized by progressive chorea (involuntary rapid, jerky motions) and mental deterioration, leading to dementia. Symptoms usually first appear in the third or fourth decade of life and progress to death, often within 15 years.

Hurler's syndrome (hûr'lərz) N. hereditary disease (autosomal recessive disease) in which mucopolysaccharides and lipids accumulate in the tissues, causing mental retardation, enlarged liver and spleen, enlarged head (sometimes hydrocephalus), and low forehead; it usually leads to death in childhood from cardiac or pulmonary complications.

hyalin (hī'ə-lĭn) N. clear, glassy material that results from the breakdown of certain tissues.

hyaline cartilage N. most common type of cartilage; the bluish-white elastic cartilage covering the ends of bones, connecting the ribs to the breastbone, and supporting facial structures and the trachea.

hyaline membrane disease N. *See* RESPIRATORY DISTRESS SYNDROME OF THE NEWBORN.

hyaloid membrane N. transparent membrane that surrounds the vitreous humor of the eye and separates it from the retina.

hyaluronic acid N. chemical present in the vitreous humor of the eye, in movable joints, and certain other tissues; it is a cementing and protective substance, forming a gel in intercellular spaces.

hyaluronidase N. enzyme, found in testes, semen, and other tissues, that increases the permeability of connective tissue and the absorption of fluids; injected to increase the absorption of other drugs.

hybrid N. offspring of a cross between two individuals of different species; for example, a mule is a hybrid, the result of mating a male donkey and a female horse. Most hybrids are sterile.

hydantoin N. any of a group of anticonvulsants used in the management of epilepsy. The most widely used hydantoin is phenytoin (diphenylhydantoin, trade name Dilantin).

hydatid (hī'də-tĭd) N. cystlike, usually fluid-filled structure, esp. that which forms around the dog tapeworm *Echinococcus granulosus*. *See also* ECHINOCOCCOSIS.

hydatid disease *See* ECHINOCOCCOSIS.

hydatid mole N. abnormality occurring in pregnancy during which portions of the chorion degenerate, forming grapelike masses throughout the placenta, causing death of the embryo and sometimes leading to a malignancy in the uterus. It occurs in about 1 in 1500 pregnancies in the United States and is much more common in some Far Eastern countries. Early symptoms include extreme nausea, uterine bleeding, and an unusually large uterus. It is important that all molar tissue be removed from the uterus to minimize the risk of developing choriocarcinoma. Also called hydatidiform mole.

hydatidosis *See* ECHINOCOCCOSIS.

Hydergine N. trade name for a fixed-combination drug containing ergot alkaloids.

hydralazine (hī-drăl'ə-zēn') N. drug (trade name Apresoline) that dilates blood vessels and is used, often in combination with a diuretic, in the treatment of hypertension and congestive heart failure. Adverse effects include headache, rapid heart rate, and gastrointestinal disturbances. It may also exacerbate angina in a small number of patients.

hydraminios N. abnormality of pregnancy in which there is an excess of amniotic fluid surrounding the fetus; sometimes associated with toxemia of pregnancy or diabetes mellitus in the mother, multiple pregnancy, or fetal disorder.

hydrarthrosis (hī´drär-thrō´sĭs) N. swelling of a joint because of excess synovial fluid; it most often affects the knee and usually indicates inflammation (colloquially called water on the knee).

hydration (hī-drā´shən) N. process of combining with water, usually reversible; often used medically in reference to the amount of fluid intake and body fluid content—the patient's state of hydration. A patient is well-hydrated if the normal amount if present, dehydrated if the fluid level is low, and over-hydrated if there is excess body fluid.

hydremia (hī-drē´mē-ə) N. excess fluid volume, compared with cell volume of the blood. ADJ. hydremic

hydroa (hī-drō´ə) N. eruption of small, usually very itchy, blisters on skin exposed to sunlight, occurring most often in children.

hydrocarbon (hī-drə-kär´bən) N. organic compound containing only carbon and hydrogen.

hydrocele (hī´drə-sēl´) N. condition in which watery fluid accumulates in a sac, esp. the scrotum (the sac surrounding the testes). The condition may subside spontaneously, or the fluid may be drained.

hydrocephalus (hī´drō-sĕf´ə-ləs) N. abnormal condition in which cerebrospinal fluid accumulates in the ventricles (central spaces) of the brain because of blockage of normal fluid outflow from the brain or failure of fluid to be absorbed into the bloodstream quickly enough. The result is enlargement of the head (esp. in infants and young children) and increased pressure that damages the brain. The condition may be congenital—it is estimated to occur in 1 out of every 500 births—and manifests itself immediately after birth or more slowly during early childhood with abnormally rapid head growth, bulging fontanelles, and small face; if untreated, it progresses to cause lethargy, defective reflexes, seizures, and eventually death. When acquired later in life (e.g., as a result of trauma, brain tumor, or infection), the symptoms are primarily neurological, resulting from pressure on the brain, and include headache, loss of muscular coordination, and visual abnormalities. Treatment usually involves surgical procedures to remove or shunt the excess fluid. The outcome depends on the cause and severity of the condition. Also called hydrocephaly. *See also* MACRO-CEPHALY. ADJ. hydrocephalic

hydrochloric acid N. chemical, secreted in the stomach, that is a major constituent of gastric juice.

hydrochlorothiazide N. diuretic (trade names Esidrix and Hydrodiuril) used in the treatment of hypertension. Adverse effects include electrolyte imbalance. *See* TABLE OF COMMONLY PRESCRIBED DRUGS—GENERIC NAMES.

hydrochlorothiazide/triamterine N. *See* TABLE OF COMMONLY PRESCRIBED DRUGS—GENERIC NAMES.

hydrocodone N. narcotic analgesic, similar to codeine, used in the oral treatment of moderate to severe pain; also used as a cough suppressant; side effects include constipation, nausea, and drowsiness; it may be habit-forming.

hydrocodone w/acetaminophen N. *See* TABLE OF COMMONLY PRESCRIBED DRUGS—GENERIC NAMES.

hydrocortisone (hī′drə-kôr′tĭ-sōn′) (-zōn′) *See* CORTISOL.

Hydrocortone N. trade name for the anti-inflammatory cortisol.

Hydrodiuril N. trade name for the diuretic hydrochlorothiazide.

hydroflumethiazide N. diuretic used to treat hypertension and edema. Adverse effects include electrolyte imbalances.

hydrogen (hī′drə-jən) N. element, a constituent of water and many biological compounds. *See also* TABLE OF IMPORTANT ELEMENTS.

hydrogen bond N. weak chemical bond involving the sharing of an electron with a hydrogen atom that increases the overall stability of a molecule; important in the specificity of base pairing in nucleic acids (DNA, RNA) and in the determination of protein shape. *See also* DEOXYRIBONUCLEIC ACID; RIBONUCLEIC ACID.

hydrogen peroxide (pə-rŏk′sīd′) N. clear liquid compound (H_2O_2) applied in water solution to cleanse wounds and as a mouthwash.

hydrolysis (hī-drŏl′ĭ-sĭs) N. chemical combination of water with a salt to form an acid and a base; dissolution of a bond by reaction with water.

hydromorphone (hī′drō-môr′-fōn′) N. narcotic analgesic used to treat moderate to severe pain. Adverse effects include drowsiness, dizziness, constipation, and the potential for addiction.

hydronephrosis (hī′drō-nə-frō′sĭs) N. distension of the kidney, caused by accumulation of urine that cannot flow out because of an obstruction (e.g., tumor, calculus stone, edema) of the ureter. Symptoms include pain, high fever, and the presence of blood and pus in the urine. Treatment involves removal of the obstruction in the ureter. ADJ. hydronephrotic.

hydrophilic (hī′drə-fĭl′ĭk) ADJ. having a strong affinity for water; tending to dissolve in, attract, hold, mix with, or be wetted by water.

hydrophobia (hī′drə-fō′bē-ə) N.
1. rabies.
2. irrational fear of water.

hydrophobic (hī′drə-fō′bĭk, -fŏb′ ĭk) ADJ. lacking affinity for water; tending not to dissolve in, attract, hold, mix with, or be wetted by water.

Hydropres N. trade name for a fixed-combination drug containing the diuretic hydrochlorothiazide and the antihypertensive reserpine; used to treat hypertension.

hydrops (hī′drŏps′) *See* EDEMA.

hydrotherapy (hī′drə-thĕr′ə-pē) N. use of water to treat disorders; mostly limited to exercises in special pools for rehabilitation of paralyzed patients.

hydrothorax (hī-drə-thôr′ăks′) N. accumulation of fluid in the pleural cavity (the cavity surrounding the lungs).

hydroxyapatite N. combination of calcium phosphate and calcium carbonate in the bones and skeleton; comprises the majority of bone crystals.

hydroxyzine (hī-drŏk'sĭ-zēn') N. minor tranquilizer used to treat anxiety and motion sickness.

hymen (hī'mən) N. fold of tissue at the opening of the vagina that may be absent, thin and pliable, or, rarely, tough and dense, completely occluding the opening. If the vaginal opening is completely closed (imperforate), coitus and the escape of menstrual fluid are impossible.

hyoid bone (hī'oid') N. small, isolated, v-shaped bone that supports the tongue.

hyoscine See SCOPOLAMINE.

hyoscyamine N. drug used to treat excess motility of the gastrointestinal tract.

hyper- prefix meaning, above, beyond, excessive (e.g., hyperacidity, excess acid, as in the stomach).

hyperactivity (hī'pər-ăk-tĭv'ĭ-tē) N. condition characterized by excessive movement and restlessness, seen esp. in children. See ATTENTION DEFICIT, also DISORDER.

hyperadrenalism See CUSHING'S DISEASE.

hyperadrenocorticism (hī'pər-ə-drē'nō-kôr'tĭ-kə-lĭz'əm) See CUSHING'S SYNDROME.

hyperaldosteronism See ALDOSTERONISM.

hyperalimentation (hī'pər-ăl'ə-měn-tā'shən) See TOTAL PARENTERAL NUTRITION.

hyperbaric chamber (hī'pər-băr'ĭk) N. chamber in which the oxygen pressure is higher than in the atmosphere; used to treat carbon monoxide poisoning, diving accidents, burns, infections (particularly gas gangrene), and certain breathing disorders.

hyperbetalipoproteinemia N. genetic disorder of lipid metabolism in which there are abnormally high levels of serum cholesterol and a tendency to develop atherosclerosis and heart disease at an early age. Treatment involves a low-cholesterol diet and sometimes the use of drugs to lower blood lipid levels.

hyperbilirubinemia (hī'pər-bĭl'ĭ-rōō-bə-nē'mē-ə) N. abnormally high amounts of the bile pigment bilirubin in the blood, usually characterized by jaundice, loss of appetite, and malaise. It may occur in liver or biliary tract disease and in diseases in which there is excessive red blood cell destruction (hemolytic anemia), and is common in newborns. See also HYPERBILIRUBINEMIA OF THE NEWBORN.

hyperbilirubinemia of the newborn N. excess of the bile pigment bilirubin in the blood of a newborn, characterized by jaundice. A common disorder, it is usually due to immaturity of the liver, deficiency of enzymes, and normal destruction of fetal red blood cells; in many cases it subsides spontaneously, in other cases is treated by phototherapy (strong light). Severe cases, more often due to an abnormal condition (e.g., erythroblastosis fetalis), produce signs of spleen and liver enlargement, anemia, kernicterus (sometimes leading to mental retardation), and other complications, sometimes leading to death. The mild physiologic condition is also called neonatal hyperbilirubinemia.

hypercalcemia (hī′pər-kăl-sē′ mē-ə) N. abnormally high levels of calcium in the blood, usually the result of excessive bone resorption in hyperparathyroidism, Paget's disease, or other disorders of bone and calcium function; also caused by certain drugs (e.g., thiazides, furosemide, vitamin D, calcium, lithium). Symptoms include muscle pain and weakness, loss of appetite, and, if severe, kidney failure. ADJ. hypercalcemic.

hypercalciuria (hī′pər-kăl′sē-yoŏr′ē-ə) N. abnormally large amounts of calcium in the urine, usually resulting from excess bone resorption (e.g., in osteoporosis, hyperparathyroidism) also called hypercalcinuria. ADJ. hypercalciuric

hypercapnia (hī′pər-kăp′nē-ə) N. excess carbon dioxide in the blood.

hypercholesterolemia (hī′pər-kə-lĕs′tər-ə-lē′mē-ə) N. higher than normal amounts of cholesterol in the blood; the condition is associated with an increased risk of atherosclerosis and cardiovascular disease. A low-cholesterol diet is usually recommended. Some forms of the condition are familial. *See also* FAMILIAL HYPER-CHOLESTEROLEMIA.

hyperdactyly (hī′pər-dăk′tə-lē) *See* POLYDACTYLY.

hyperemesis (hī′pər-ĕm′ĭ-sĭs) N. severe vomiting, esp. hyperemesis gravidarum, an abnormal condition of pregnancy characterized by severe vomiting, weight loss, fluid and electrolyte imbalance, and, if severe, resultant brain, liver, and kidney damage. Treatment is by drugs to arrest vomiting and maintenance of adequate food intake and fluid and electrolyte balance.

hyperemia (hī′pə-rē′mē-ə) N. increased blood in part of the body, caused by inflammatory response or blockage of blood outflow; the skin typically becomes reddened and warm in the affected area. ADJ. hyperemic

hyperglycemia (hī′pər-glī-sē′mē-ə) N. higher than normal amount of glucose in the blood, most often associated with diabetes mellitus but sometimes occurring in other conditions (*compare* HYPOGLYCEMIA)

hyperhidrosis N. excessive perspiration, sometimes caused by strong emotion, heat, hyperthyroidism, or menopausal changes.

hyperinsulinism (hī′pər-ĭn′sə-lə-nĭz′əm) N. excess of the hormone insulin; abnormal production usually is caused by a tumor (insulinoma) or exogenous administration; may result in hypogycemia (when excess insulin lowers the level of sugar in the blood) or accompany certain forms of diabetes mellitus (when the patient becomes resistant to insulin, and the body produces more in an effort to maintain homeostasis).

hyperkalemia (hī′pər-kə-lē′mē-ə) N. higher than normal potassium levels in the blood, with symptoms of nausea, diarrhea, muscle weakness and, if severe, heart abnormalities; occurs in kidney failure and sometimes as an adverse effect following diuretic use.

hyperkinetic syndrome (hī′pər-kə-nĕt′ĭk) *See* ATTENTION DEFICIT DISORDER.

hyperlipoproteinemia (hī′pər-lĭp′ō-prō′tē-nē′mē-ə) N. any of a large group of disorders of lipoprotein and cholesterol metabolism resulting in higher than normal cholesterol and lipoprotein levels in the blood. Some of the disorders are hereditary (e.g., familial hypercholesterolemia) whereas others are acquired.

hypermenorrhea (hī′pər-měn′ə-rē′ə) *See* MENORRHAGIA.

hypermotility N. excessive movement, esp. in the intestines.

hypernatremia (hī′pər-nə-trē′mē-ə) N. higher than normal levels of sodium in the blood, resulting from too-frequent urination, diabetes insipidus, profuse sweating, diarrhea, or other disorder.

hypernea N. deep, rapid breathing that occurs normally after exercise or abnormally with fever, pain, hysteria, or respiratory or cardiac disorder (*compare* DYSPNEA).

hyperopia (hī′pə-rō′pē-ə) N. farsightedness; a condition in which light rays are brought to a focus behind the retina (*compare* MYOPIA).

HYPEROPIA

Normal Eye

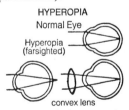

Hyperopia (farsighted)

convex lens

In a normal eye, the image comes to a focus on the retina. In hyperopia, the image comes to a focus behind the retina. The defect can be corrected by convex lenses.

hyperparathyroidism (hī′pər-păr′ə-thī′roi-dĭz′əm) N. condition characterized by excessive secretion of parathyroid hormone from the parathyroid glands due to disease of the parathyroid glands or resulting from another disorder (e.g., too-low blood calcium levels). Higher than normal levels of calcium in the blood result, with effects on many systems of the body, including kidney damage, osteoporosis, gastrointestinal disturbances, muscle weakness, and central nervous system changes leading to personality disturbances, and, if severe, coma. Treatment may involve surgical removal of all or part of the parathyroid glands or correction of any underlying causes.

hyperpigmentation (hī′pər-pĭg′mən-tā′shən) N. unusual darkening of the skin; it may be caused by exposure to the sun, by certain drugs, or by adrenal gland disorder (*compare* HYPOPIGMENTATION).

hyperpituitarism (hī′pər-pĭ-tōō′-ĭ-tə-rĭz′əm) N. overactivity of the pituitary gland, causing excess secretion of all or some of the pituitary hormones, esp. overactivity of the anterior lobe, leading to excess secretion of growth hormone and the disorders acromegaly and gigantism.

hyperplasia (hī′pər-plā′zhə) N. excessive formation of cells (*compare* APLASIA; HYPOPLASIA). ADJ. hyperplastic

hyperpyrexia (hī′pər-pī-rěk′sē-ə) N. extremely elevated body temperature sometimes occurring with acute infections in children or in others during general anesthesia. Treatment is by sponging the body with tepid water and administering antipyretic (fever-reducing) drugs.

hypersensitivity reaction N. inappropriate and excessive response to an allergen. Common allergens are pollen, dust, animal hairs, and certain foods. The degree of the response depends on the nature and amount of the allergen, the way it enters the body, and other factors. Reactions range from mild allergic symptoms such as runny nose and watery eyes to severe systemic reactions leading to anaphylactic shock.

hypersplenism (hī′pər-splĕn′ĭz′-əm) N. condition marked by an enlarged spleen and a decrease in the number of one or more types of blood cells; it is associated with many disorders and treatment depends on the underlying cause.

Hyperstat N. trade name for the vasodilator diazoxide, used to treat severe hypertension.

hypertension (hī′pər-tĕn′shən) N. common disorder, often with no symptoms, in which the blood pressure is persistently above 140/90 mg Hg. Causes of hypertension include adrenal and kidney disorders, toxemia of pregnancy, thyroid disorders, and emotional stress, but in most cases—essential hypertension—the cause is unknown, though obesity, hypercholesterolemia, and high sodium levels are predisposing factors. Symptoms, when present, include headache, palpitations, and easy fatigability. Severe hypertension damages the cardiovascular system and frequently results in heart disorders or cardiovascular accidents. Treatment is by diuretics, vasodilators, central nervous system depressants and inhibitors, and ganglionic blocking agents (beta blockers, e.g., propranolol). Adequate rest and a low-sodium, low-fat diet are also usually advised. Also called high blood pressure. ADJ. hypertensive.

hyperthermia (hī′pər-thûr′mē-ə) N. extremely high body temperature, sometimes induced as a treatment, as in some forms of cancer. *See also* MALIGNANT HYPERTHERMIA.

hyperthyroidism (hī′pər-thī′roi-dĭz′əm) N. overactivity of the thyroid gland due to tumor, overgrowth of the gland, or exophthalmic goiter.

hypertonic (hī′pər-tŏn′ĭk) ADJ. having a higher osmotic pressure than a comparison solution. In reference to muscle tone, having greater than normal tension or relaxation; colloq. stiff. *See* OSMOSIS.

hypertrichosis (hī′pər-trī-kō′sĭs) N. excessive growth of hair; may be due to diseases of the endocrine glands or the ovaries; some drugs (e.g., minoxidil) may result in this condition. *See also* HIRSUTISM.

hypertriglyceridemia (hī′pər-trī-glĭs′ər-ĭ-dē′mē-ə) N. condition resulting in abnormal elevation of the blood triglyceride level.

hypertrophy (hī-pûr′trə-fē) N. increase in the size of an organ or other part, resulting from enlargement of the individual cells (*compare* ATROPHY; HYPERPLASIA). ADJ. hypertrophic

hyperventilation (hī′pər-vĕn′tl-ā′shən) N. ventilation rate in the lungs that is greater than demanded by body needs, the result of too frequent and/or too deep breathing; often associated with emphysema; asthma; hyperthyroidism; central nervous system disorders; increased metabolic needs from fever, infection, or exercise; or acute anxiety or pain. The carbon dioxide level in the blood decreases, and the oxygen level increases. Symptoms include faintness, tingling of the fingers and toes, and, if continued, chest pain and respiratory alkalosis.

hypervitaminosis (hī′pər-vī′tə-mə-nō′sĭs) N. abnormal condition resulting from excessive intake of vitamins. Serious effects may occur when too much vitamin A, D, or K is ingested (*compare* AVITAMINOSIS).

hypervolemia (hi′pər-vŏ-lē′mē-ə) N. increase in the volume of circulating blood. ADJ. hypervolemic

hypesthesia (hĭp′nĭs-thē′zhə) N. lessened sensitivity to touch.

hyphema (hī-fē′mə) N. bleeding into the anterior chamber of the eye, usually the result of injury.

hypnagogue N. agent that tends to induce drowsiness or sleep.

hypnosis (hĭp-nō′sĭs) N. passive, sleeplike state in which perception and memory are altered, and the person is more responsive to suggestion and has more recall than usual; used in psychotherapy and in medicine to induce relaxation and relieve pain. Susceptibility to hypnosis varies widely.

hypnotherapy (hĭp′nō-thĕr′ə-pē) N. use of hypnosis in psychotherapy.

hypo- prefix meaning under, beneath, deficient (e.g., hypoacidity, lower than normal acidity, as in the stomach).

hypoadrenalism (hī′pō-ə-drē′nə-lĭz′əm) *See* ADDISON'S DISEASE.

hypobetalipoproteinemia N. hereditary disorder in which the levels of beta lipoproteins,

lipids, and cholesterol are lower than normal. There are no symptoms, and there is no treatment. (*Compare* HYPERBETALIPROPROTEINEMIA.)

hypocalcemia (hī′pō-kăl-sē′mē-ə) N. abnormally low level of calcium in the blood, due to hypoparathyroidism, vitamin D deficiency, kidney malfunction, or other disorder. Mild hypocalcemia produces few signs; severe cases lead to cardiac arrhythmias and tetany. ADJ. hypocalcemic

hypocapnia (hī′pō-kăp′nē-ə) N. low level of carbon dioxide in the blood.

hypochondriasis N. condition in which a person has excessive concern about his/her health and unrealistic interpretations of real or imagined symptoms, often accompanied by anxiety and depression; also called hypochondria. ADJ. hypochondriacal

hypodermic (hī′pō-dər-mĭk) ADJ. relating to or located below the epidermis. A hypodermic needle is a hollow needle commonly used with a syringe to inject substances into the body. May also be used to take liquid samples from the body, such as taking blood from a vein in venipuncture. *See also* DERMIS; EPIDERMIS; SYRINGE; VENIPUNCTURE.

hypogammaglobulinemia (hī′pō-găm′ə-glŏb′yə-lə-nē′mē-ə) N. lower than normal concentration of gamma globulins (immunoglobulins) in the blood, associated with an increased risk of infection. It may be congenital and transient (as in some infants), congenital and permanent (as in some sex-linked immune disorders), or acquired, as a result of kidney disease, exposure to certain drugs, or other factors. (*Compare* AGAMMAGLOBULINEMIA.)

hypoglossal nerve (hī′pə-glô′səl) N. one of a pair of motor nerves, the twelfth cranial nerves, involved in swallowing and in movements of the tongue.

hypoglycemia (hī′pō-glī-sē′mē-ə) N. lower than normal level of glucose in the blood, usually resulting from administration of too much insulin (in diabetes mellitus), excessive insulin secretion from the pancreas, or poor diet. Symptoms include headache, weakness, anxiety, personality changes, and, if severe and untreated, coma and death. Treatment is by administration of glucose. (*Compare* HYPERGLYCEMIA.) ADJ. hypoglycemic

hypoglycemic agent (hī′pō-glī-cē′mĭk) N. any of a large group of drugs including insulin and glyburide, which decrease the level of glucose in the blood and are used in the treatment of diabetes mellitus.

hypokalemia (hī′pō-kə-lē′mē-ə) N. abnormally low level of potassium in the blood, leading to weakness and heart abnormalities; it may result from diuretic intake, adrenal tumor, starvation, or other disorder. ADJ. hypokalemic

hypolipoproteinemia *See* ABETALIPOPROTEINEMIA; HYPOBETALIPOPROTEINEMIA.

hyponatremia (hī′pō-nə-trē′mē-ə) N. lower than normal concentration of sodium in the blood, caused by dehydration (as from prolonged vomiting or diarrhea), excessive water in the bloodstream, or diuretic intake. ADJ. hyponatremic

hypoparathyroidism (hī′pō-păr′ə-thī′roi-dĭz′əm) N. underactivity of the parathyroid glands, causing a lowering of calcium levels in the blood; symptoms include muscle spasms and nervous system changes, and, if untreated, tetany.

hypophysis (hī-pŏf′ĭ-sĭs) N. pituitary gland. *See also* ANTERIOR PITUITARY GLAND; POSTERIOR PITUITARY GLAND.

hypopigmentation N. unusual lack of skin color, as in albinism and vitiligo (*compare* HYPERPIGMENTATION).

hypoplasia (hī′pō-plā′zhə) N. underdevelopment of an organ due to decrease in the number of cells (*compare* APLASIA; HYPERPLASIA).

hypoplastic dwarf *See* PRIMORDIAL DWARF.

hypopnea (hī-pŏp′nē-ə) N. shallow or slow respiration; it is a normal sign in athletes but an indication of brain disorder in other persons.

hypoproteinemia (hī′pō-prō′tē-nē′mē-ə) N. abnormally low level of protein in the blood, usually with abdominal pain, nausea, diarrhea, and edema. It may be caused by inadequate dietary intake of protein or by intestinal or renal disease.

hyposmia N. lessened sensitivity to smell. ADJ. hyposomic

hypospadias (hī′pō-spā′dē-əs) N. opening of the urethra in an abnormal location on the underside of the penis.

hypotension (hī′pə-tĕn′shən) N. blood pressure that is abnormally low (in adults, usually less than 90 mm systolic); it may result from hemorrhage, excessive fluid loss, heart malfunction, Addison's disease, or other disorder. In some people blood pressure drops when they rise from a horizontal position (orthostatic hypotension). Transient hypotension may cause light-headedness and syncope. Severe hypotension leads to inadequate blood circulation and shock. (*Compare* HYPERTENSION.)

hypothalamus (hī'pō-thăl'ə-məs) N. part of the brain that controls the endocrine system, the autonomic nervous system, and many other body functions (e.g., body temperature, thirst, hunger). ADJ. hypothalmic

hypothermia (hī'pə-thûr'mē-ə) N.
1. condition in which the body temperature is below 35° Celsius (95° Fahrenheit), most often occurring in the elderly or very young who are exposed to excessive cold; symptoms include pallor; slow, shallow respiration; and slow, faint heartbeat.
2. deliberate reduction of body temperature to slow metabolic rate and lower oxygen demands for therapeutic reasons or certain surgical procedures.

hypothrombinemia (hī'pō-thrŏm'bə-nē'mē-ə) N. lower than normal levels of prothrombin (Factor II) in the circulating blood, leading to poor clot formation, long clotting time, and sometimes excessive bleeding. It often results from vitamin K deficiency or anticoagulant therapy.

hypothyroidism (hī'pō-thī'roi-dĭz'əm) N. decreased activity of the thyroid gland. *See also* CRETINISM; MYXEDEMA.

hypotonic ADJ. having a lower osmotic pressure than a comparison solution. *See* OSMOSIS.

In reference to muscle tone, having less than normal tension or relaxation; colloq. floppy.

hypovitaminosis (hī'pō-vī'tə-mə-nō'sĭs) *See* AVITAMINOSIS.

hypovolemic shock N. physical collapse caused by severe blood or fluid loss and circulatory malfunction; symptoms include feeble pulse, rapid heartbeat, clammy skin, and low blood pressure.

hypoxia (hī-pŏk'sē-ə) N. inadequate amounts of available oxygen in the blood. Symptoms include bluish discoloration of the skin (cyanosis), high blood pressure (hypertension), rapid heart rate (tachycardia), mental confusion, and, if severe, irregular breathing and finally respiratory and cardiac failure.

hysterectomy (hĭs'tə-rĕk'tə-mē) N. surgical removal of the uterus, through the abdominal wall or the vagina, done to remove tumors or to treat hemorrhage, severe pelvic inflammatory disease, or a cancerous or precancerous condition. In a total hysterectomy, the uterus and cervix are removed; in a radical hysterectomy or panhysterectomy, the ovaries, oviducts, uterus, cervix, and associated lymph nodes are removed.

hysteria (hĭ-stĕr'ē-ə) N. neurotic disorder marked by abnormal emotional response and often by physical symptoms, as shown in unusual sensory, circulatory, intestinal, or other responses. In severe cases, paralysis of a limb may be a chief symptom.

hystero- comb. form indicating a relationship with the uterus (e.g. hysterocele, protrusion, hernia, of the uterus).

hysterosalpingogram N. X ray of the uterus and Fallopian tubes, usually done to determine whether there is a blockage; useful in diagnosing causes of infertility.

hysteroscopy (hĭs′tə-rŏs′kə-pē) N. visual inspection of the uterus, using an endoscope introduced through the vagina, done to examine the uterine lining, to remove a specimen for analysis, or to excise small polyps.

hysterotomy (hĭs′tə-rŏt′ə-mē) N. surgical incision (cutting) of the uterus, sometimes done as a means of abortion.

Hytrin N. trade name for the antihypertensive terazosin. *See* TABLE OF COMMONLY PRESCRIBED DRUGS—TRADE NAMES.

Hyzaar N. *See* TABLE OF COMMONLY PRESCRIBED DRUGS—TRADE NAMES.

I

I symbol for the element iodine.

-iasis suffix indicating disease-produced, disease-producing characteristics (e.g., elephantiasis).

iatrogenic (ī-ăt′ra-jĕn′ĭk) ADJ. pert. to a condition caused by medical diagnostic procedures, or exposure to medical treatment, facilities, and personnel (e.g., corticosteroid-induced Cushing's syndrome). N. iatrogenesis

ibuprofen (ī′byoo̅-prō′fən) N. nonsteroidal anti-inflammatory agent (trade name Motrin) used in the treatment of arthritis; available in nonprescription strength for relief of mild to moderate pain. Adverse effects include gastrointestinal disturbances and skin irritation. *See* TABLE OF COMMONLY PRESCRIBED DRUGS—GENERIC NAMES.

ichthammol N. thick, black liquid used topically as an anti-infective to treat certain skin diseases.

ichthyosis (ĭk′thē-ō′sĭs) N. any of several congenital diseases in which the skin is dry and scaly, i.e., fishlike.

ICSH *See* LUTEINIZING HORMONE.

ictero- comb. form indicating an association with jaundice (e.g., icterogenic, producing jaundice).

icterus (ĭk′tər-əs) N. *See* JAUNDICE (*See also* HYPERBILIRUBINEMIA; KERNICERUS). ADJ. icteric

icterus neonatorum *See* JAUNDICE OF THE NEWBORN.

ictus (ĭk′təs) N. seizure (e.g., in epilepsy) or sudden attack (e.g., in

cerebrovascular accident). ADJ. ictal, ictic

ICU *See* INTENSIVE CARE UNIT.

id (ĭd) N. in psychoanalysis, the unconscious; unconscious part of one's psyche, the source of instincts and drives, based largely on the tendency to avoid pain and to pursue pleasure (*compare* EGO; SUPEREGO).

ideation (ī′dē-ā′shən) N. process of forming ideas, images, impressions, or concepts. ADJ. ideational

identical twins (ī-dĕn′tĭ-kəl) *See* MONOZYGOTIC TWINS.

identification (ī-dĕn′tə-fĭ-kā′shən) N. in psychology, adoption of the traits and characteristics of another person; it is a normal part of personality development, as in a child identifying with the parent of the same sex.

identity crisis (ī-dĕn′tĭ-tē) N. period of confusion about one's identity and role in society, occurring most often during a transition from one stage of life to another, esp. at adolescence.

idiopathic (ĭd′ē-ə-păth′ĭk) ADJ. of unknown cause (e.g., idiopathic disease, a disease for which no identifiable cause can be determined). N. idiopathy

idiosyncrasy (ĭd′ē-ō-sĭng′krə-sē) N.
1. characteristic or manner unique to an individual or group.
2. peculiar or unusual variation, as in an unusual reaction to a

drug or particular food. ADJ. idiosyncratic

idiot (ĭd'ē-ət) N. obsolete term for a person who is severely mentally retarded (I.Q. under 20) (*compare* IMBECILE; MORON; *see also* MENTAL RETARDATION). N. idiocy

idiot savant (ĭd'ē-ət să-vänt') N. person with severe mental retardation but able to carry out specific, limited intellectual functions (e.g., calculate square roots or calendar dates).

Ig *See* IMMUNOGLOBULIN.

IgA *See* IMMUNOGLOBULIN A.

IgD *See* IMMUNOGLOBULIN D.

IgE *See* IMMUNOGLOBULIN E.

IgG *See* IMMUNOGLOBULIN G.

IgM *See* IMMUNOGLOBULIN M.

ileitis (ĭl'ē-ī'tŭs) N. inflammation of the ileum. *See also* CROHN'S DISEASE.

ileo- comb. form indicating an association with the ileum (e.g., ileocecal, pert. to the ileum and cecum).

ileocecal valve N. valve between the ileum of the small intestine and the cecum of the large intestine that prevents the backflow of material from the large to the small intestine.

ileostomy (ĭl'ē-ŏs'tə-mē) N. surgical formation of an opening of the ileum onto the abdominal wall through which feces pass; performed in cancer of the colon, severe or recurrent Crohn's disease, or ulcerative colitis (*compare* COLOSTOMY).

ileum (ĭl'ē-əm) N. distal portion of the small intestine, starting at its attachment with the jejunum and ending at the cecum, the beginning of the large intestine. ADJ. ileac, ileal

ileus (ĭl'ēəs) N. disturbance in the coordinated contractions of intestinal muscle so that materials do not pass through to the lower bowel; causes include medications, pain, disturbances in electrolyte balance, and peritonitis. *Compare* INTESTINAL OBSTRUCTION.

iliac arteries N. arteries that supply most of the blood for the pelvis and lower extremities. The right and left common iliac arteries are the terminal branches of the abdominal aorta.

iliac veins N. veins that drain blood from the pelvis and lower limbs; the right and left common iliac veins join to form the inferior vena cava.

ilio- comb. form indicating an association with the ilium (e.g., iliococcygeal, pert. to the ilium and coccyx).

ilium (ĭl'ē-əm) N., *pl.* ilia, one of the three bones (the other two being the ischium and pubis) that unite before birth to form the innominate, or hip, bone. ADJ. iliac

illness (ĭl'nĭs) N. impairment of normal physiological function affecting part or all of an organism.

illusion (ĭ-loō'zhən) N. false impression; wrongful interpretation of what has been perceived by the senses (*compare* HALLUCINATION). ADJ. illusional

imagery (ĭm'ĭj-rē) N. in psychiatry, formation of images, concepts, and ideas.

Imavate N. trade name for the antidepressant imipramine.

imbecile (ĭm'bə-sĭl, -səl) N. obsolete term for a person who is moderately mentally retarded (I.Q. 20–49) (*compare* IDIOT;

MORON). *See also* MENTAL RE-TARDATION. ADJ. imbecilic

imbibition (ĭm-bə-bĭsh′ən) N. absorption of fluid by a solid body or gel; drinking.

imbrication N. overlapping arrangement of parts, like tiles on a roof.

Imdur N. *See* TABLE OF COMMONLY PRESCRIBED DRUGS—TRADE NAMES.

imipramine N. antidepressant (trade name Tofranil) used to treat depression. Also used in the treatment of cataplexy which often accompanies narcolepsy. Adverse effects include sedation, gastrointestinal upset, and cardiovascular disturbances.

Imitrex N. *See* TABLE OF COMMONLY PRESCRIBED DRUGS—TRADE NAMES.

immersion N. covering completely with water.

imminent abortion *See* ABORTION.

immiscible (ĭ-mĭs′ə-bəl) ADJ. incapable of mixing, such as oil and water.

immobilization N. medical procedure in which a part of the body, such as a limb, is rendered immovable; for example, a splint may be used to immobilize a sprained wrist.

immune (ĭ-myo͞on′) ADJ. protected from and not susceptible to a disease, esp. an infectious disease.

immune gamma globulin N. immunizing agent, made from pooled human plasma, used to immunize against certain infectious diseases (e.g., measles, poliomyelitis) and to treat immunodeficiencies (e.g., hypogammaglobulinemia). Adverse reactions include pain and inflammation at the injection

site. Also called immune globulin.

immune response N. defense reaction of the body whereby an invading substance—an antigen, such as grafted tissue, a transplanted organ, bacteria, virus, or fungus—is recognized as foreign and antibodies specific against the antigen are produced to neutralize and/or destroy it. There are two basic kinds of immune response: humoral, mediated by B lymphocytes or B cells (chiefly against bacterial invasion), and cell-mediated, involving T cells (chiefly against viral and fungal invasion and transplanted tissue).

immune system N. complex interactions that protect the body from pathogenic organisms and other foreign invaders (e.g., transplanted tissue), including the humoral response, chiefly involving B cells and the production of antibodies, and the cell-mediated response, chiefly involving T cells and the activation of specific leukocytes. The organs involved include the bone marrow, the thymus, and lymphoid tissue.

immunity (ĭ-myo͞o′nĭ-tē) N. state of being not susceptible to a particular disease. Immunity may be natural, or innate, or it may be acquired during life (e.g., as a result of infection or vaccination). *See also* ACQUIRED IMMUNITY; ACTIVE IMMUNITY; PASSIVE IMMUNITY.

immunization (ĭm′yə-nĭ-zā′shən) N. process (e.g., vaccination) by which resistance to an infectious disease is induced or increased.

immunoassay (ĭm′yə-nō-ăs′ā) N. measurement of the amount of a protein by using an antibody

THE IMMUNE SYSTEM

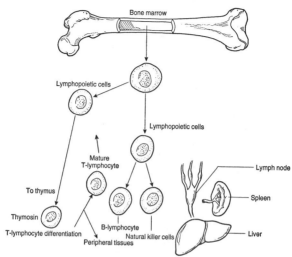

that binds specifically to that protein.

immunocompetent (ĭm′yə-nō-kŏm′pĭ-tənt) ADJ. possessing the normal ability (immune system) to respond to infection or tissue damage.

immunocompromised (ĭm′yə-nō-kŏm′prə-mīzd) ADJ. lacking the normal ability (immune system) to respond to infection or tissue damage. Many factors, ranging from drugs to viral infection (e.g., HIV, AIDS) may affect the immune system adversely.

immunodeficiency (ĭm′yə-nō-dĭ-fīsh′ən-sē) N. abnormal condition in which some part of the body's immune system is inadequate, and consequently resistance to infectious disease is decreased. Immunodeficiency may be congenital or acquired. *See also* ACQUIRED IMMUNE DEFICIENCY SYNDROME; AGAM-

MAGLOBULINEMIA; HYPOGAMMA-GLOBULINEMIZA.

immunogen (ĭm′yə-nəjən, -jĕn′) N. organism or substance that provokes an immune response; an antigen. ADJ. immunogenic

immunoglobulin (Ig) (ĭm′yə-nō-glŏb′yə-lĭn) N. any of the five classes of structurally distinct antibodies, produced in lymph tissue in response to the invasion of a foreign substance. The five major kinds are immunoglobulin A, D, E, G, and M. Also called immune serum globulin. *See also* ANTIBODY; ANTIGEN.

immunoglobulin A (IgA) N. one of the five classes of immunoglobulins. One of the most common immunoglobulins, it is present in body secretions and is the chief antibody in the mucous membranes of the gastrointestinal and respiratory tract and in saliva and tears.

immunoglobulin D (IgD) N. one of the five classes of immunoglobulins; it is present in small amounts in serum and is thought to function in certain allergic responses.

immunoglobulin E (IgE) N. one of the five classes of immunoglobulins; it is present primarily in the skin and mucous membranes and is believed to function in response to environmental antigens and to play a role in allergic reactions characterized by skin eruptions.

immunoglobulin G (IgG) N. one of the five classes of immunoglobulins; widespread in the body, it is the main antibody defense against most bacterial invasions and other antigens.

immunoglobulin M (IgM) N. one of the five classes of immunoglobulins; a large molecule, it is found in blood and is involved in combating blood infections and in triggering immunoglobulin G production.

immunologist (ĭm′yə-nŏl′ə-jĭst) N. specialist in immunology.

immunology (ĭm′yə-nŏl′ə-jē) N. study of the body's response to foreign invasion (e.g., bacteria, virus, fungus, transplanted tissue). ADJ. immunologic; immunological

immunosuppression (ĭm′yə-nō-sə-prĕsh′ən) N.
1. lowering of the body's normal immune response to the invasion of foreign material. It may be deliberate, as in the administration of drugs to decrease the immune response to prevent rejection of transplanted organs, or incidental, resulting from chemotherapy or radiotherapy in cancer treatment.
2. abnormal condition in which the body's normal immune responses are inadequate. *See also* IMMUNODEFICIENCY; ACQUIRED IMMUNE DEFICIENCY SYNDROME. ADJ. immunosuppressed

immunosuppressive ADJ. pert. to a substance that lowers the body's normal immune response.

impacted tooth (ĭm-păk′tĭd) N. tooth, usually a wisdom tooth, so firmly wedged in the socket that it cannot break through the gum.

impaction N. cramping or tight wedging of materials or parts in a limited space, esp. feces lodged in the lower colon. *Also see* IMPACTED TOOTH.

impairment (ĭm-pâr′mənt) N. injury, functional loss, or weakened state (e.g., hearing impairment). Typically, impairment is a medical determination, based on a standardized set of normal physical examination findings. Disability, on the other hand, encompasses legal and functional performance aspects.

impedance N. opposition to the flow of electric current or sound waves.

imperforate (ĭm-pûr′fər-ĭt) ADJ. lacking an opening; for example, an imperforate hymen completely closes the vagina and prevents the outflow of menstrual blood. *See also* IMPERFORATE ANUS.

imperforate anus N. any of several congenital defects in which there is partial or complete obstruction of the anal opening due to a developmental defect. Treatment is by surgery.

impermeable (ĭm-pûr′mē-ə-bəl) ADJ. not allowing fluid to pass through, as with a membrane.

impetigo (ĭm′pĕ-tī′gō) N. bacterial (usually streptococcal and/or staphylococcal) infection of the skin, common in children and very contagious, in which localized skin redness develops into fluid-containing small blisters that gradually crust and erode. Treatment is by topical and sometimes oral antibiotics, careful washing, and steps to prevent the spread of the infection.

implant (ĭm-plănt′) V. to attach a part or tissue to a host (e.g., to insert a tooth). N. tissue or part inserted into a host for repair of a damaged part (e.g., a blood vessel graft) or for therapeutic reasons (e.g., pacemaker inserted in the chest).

implantation (ĭm′plăn-tā′shən) N. placing and attaching an organ part or cell into a new place, esp. the attachment and penetration of the fertilized egg (blastocyst) into the wall of the uterus during early prenatal development.

impotence (ĭm′pə-təns) N.
1. weakness.
2. inability of the male to achieve erection of the penis or, less commonly, to ejaculate. Impotence may be organic, due to disease (e.g., diabetes mellitus) or ingestion of certain drugs, or psychogenic. Also called impotency. Erectile dysfunction (ED) is a total inability to achieve erection, an inconsistent ability to do so, or a tendency to sustain only brief erections. The word "impotence" may also be used to describe other problems that interfere with sexual intercourse and reproduction, such as lack of sexual desire and problems with ejaculation or orgasm. Using the term "erectile dysfunction" makes it clear that those other problems are not involved. ADJ. impotent. *See also* PENILE IMPLANT (*compare* ERECTILE DYSFUNCTION; STERILITY).

impregnate (ĭm-prĕg′nāt) V.
1. to inseminate and make pregnant.
2. to saturate with substance. N. impregnation

impression (ĭm-prĕsh′ən) N. mold of a part of the body from which a replacement can be made, esp. in dentistry, the mold of the mouth from which dentures are made.

impulse (ĭm′pŭls′) N.
1. sudden urge to do something.
2. electrochemical changes in the membrane of a nerve through which a signal is transmitted.

Imuran trade name for the immunosuppressive drug azathioprine.

in situ ADJ./ADV. in its natural place or place of origin (e.g., carcinoma in situ, a cancer that has not spread).

in utero ADJ./ADV. within the uterus.

in vitro ADJ./ADV. literally, in glass, outside the living organism and in an artificial environment, as within a test tube or other laboratory apparatus (*compare* IN VIVO).

in vivo ADJ./ADV. in the living organism (*compare* IN VITRO).

inactivation N. loss of activity, rendering inert by any means; in biochemistry, often refers to inactivation of an enzyme in a chemical reaction either deliberately by medication or pathologically by illness.

inactive colon N. lack of normal tone in the large intestine, resulting in decreased contractions and propulsive movements, delay in the normal passage of material through the intestine to the anus, often an enlargement of the colon, and constipation. It may be congenital (e.g., Hirschsprung's disease) or acquired (e.g., through inadequate food and fluid intake, faulty elimination habits, intake of certain drugs, certain diseases). Treatment includes efforts to establish regular elimination habits, use of stool softeners and agents to increase fecal bulk, and a diet containing adequate bulk and fluids. *See also* MEGACOLON.

inanition (ĭn'ə-nĭsh'ən) N. condition of exhaustion and weakness caused by inadequate nutrition, resulting from malnutrition, starvation, or disease.

inborn (ĭn'bôrn') ADJ. present at birth, either as a result of heredity or acquired during intrauterine life (e.g., certain developmental abnormalities). *See also* CONGENITAL ANOMALY; INBORN ERROR OF METABOLISM.

inborn error of metabolism N. any of a number of diseases, including galactosemia, phenylketonuria, and Tay-Sachs disease, in which an inherited defect—usually missing or inadequate levels of a specific enzyme—produces an abnormality in metabolism.

inbreeding (ĭn'brē-dĭng) N. production of offspring by the mating of closely related persons (or other animals or plants).

incest (ĭn'sĕst') N. sexual intercourse between persons closely related, usually so closely (e.g.,

father and daughter) that legal marriage would be impossible. ADJ. incestuous

incidence N. number of times an event occurs in a given period of time, as the number of times a given disease occurs during a year (*compare* PREVALENCE).

incision (ĭn-sĭzh'ən) N. slit or opening made by cutting, as with a scalpel.

incisor (ĭn-sī'zər) N. any of eight front teeth, four in each jaw, flanked by the canines, used for cutting and tearing food.

incisure (ĭn-sī'zhər) N. in anatomy, notch or small hollow.

inclusion (ĭn-kloo'zhən) N. small body found within another, as inclusions in the cytoplasm of a cell.

incoherent ADJ. disordered; lacking logical connection or orderly continuity; unable to express oneself in an intelligible manner. N. incoherence

incompatibility (ĭn'kəm-păt'ə-bĭl'ĭ-tē) N.
1. condition in which two substances (organisms, tissues, drugs) cannot exist together (e.g., one drug cancels or alters the therapeutic effect of another drug given at the same time).
2. in immunology, degree to which the body's immune system will reject or otherwise react to foreign material, such as transfused blood or transplanted tissue. (When a person's tissues cannot be transplanted to another, the term is histoincompatibility.) ADJ. incompatible

incompetence (ĭn-kŏm'pĭ-təns) N. inability of an organ or part to function normally (e.g., valvular incompetence, inability of a valve to close an opening completely). ADJ. incompetent

incompetent cervix (ĭn-kŏm′pĭ-tənt) N. in obstetrics, condition in which the opening of the cervix of the uterus becomes dilated (without labor) before term often causing miscarriage or premature birth. Treatment is by surgical suturing.

incompetent patient N. person who is mentally unable to make his or her own medical decisions, as well as to realize the possible consequences of these decisions; incompetent patients may have a legal guardian or durable power of attorney to assist in the management of their affairs.

incomplete abortion (ĭn′kəm-plēt′) See ABORTION.

incomplete fracture See FRACTURE.

incontinence (ĭn-kŏn′tə-nəns) N. inability to control urination and/or defecation. (See also ENURESIS). Causes may be physical (e.g., diabetes, spinal cord injury, Alzheimer's disease) or emotional. ADJ. incontinent

incoordination (ĭn′kō-ôr′dn-ā′shən) N. inability to produce controlled, harmonious muscular movement.

incubation period (ĭn′kyə-bā′shən) N. time between exposure to a disease-causing organism and the appearance of the symptoms of the disease (e.g., the 2- to 3-week interval between exposure to the chicken pox organism and the appearance of symptoms).

incubator (ĭn′kyə-bā′tər) n.
1. special transparent device that provides a controlled environment (e.g., a particular temperature) for a premature or low-birth-weight infant.
2. laboratory device for the cultivation of eggs or microorganisms.

incurable (ĭn-kyōōr′ə-bəl) ADJ. being such that a cure is currently impossible within the realm of known medical practice.

incus (ĭng′kəs) N. one of three small bones in the middle ear (the others are the malleus and stapes); also called anvil.

indapamide (ĭn-dăp′ə-mīd′) N. diuretic (trade name Lozol) used in the treatment of hypertension. Adverse effects are mild and include headache, dizziness, fatigue, and weakness.

Inderal N. trade name for the cardiac drug propranolol. See TABLE OF COMMONLY PRESCRIBED DRUGS—TRADE NAMES.

index case (ĭn′dĕks′) N. first, or model, case of a disease, as contrasted with subsequent cases.

index finger N. forefinger; finger between the thumb and middle finger.

indication (ĭn′dĭ-kā′shən) N. in medicine, reason to prescribe a drug or perform a procedure; for example, the presence of a bacterial infection is an indication for the use of a specific antibiotic. v. indicate

indicator (ĭn′dĭ-kā′tər) N. substance (e.g., paper, tablet, tape) used to test for a particular reaction because of a predictable, easy-to-detect change; for example, litmus paper turns pink on exposure to an acid.

indigenous ADJ. occurring naturally or native to a particular environment (e.g., the gastrointestinal tract) or geographic region.

indigestion (ĭn′dĭ-jĕs′chən) N. symptom complex consisting of nonspecific abdominal distress ostensibly due to incomplete or abnormal breakdown of food; may include nausea, pain, heartburn, belching, gas, or diarrhea. Also called dyspepsia. Sometimes, a heart attack may mimic symptoms of indigestion. *See* DYSPEPSIA.

Indocin N. trade name for the nonsteroidal anti-inflammatory agent indomethacin.

indolent (ĭn′də-lənt) ADJ.
1. slow in growth or development (e.g., a tumor).
2. inactive, sluggish, slow to heal (e.g., indolent ulcer).

indomethacin (ĭn′dō-mĕth′ə-sĭn) N. nonsteroidal anti-inflammatory agent (trade name Indocin) used to treat arthritis and certain other inflammatory conditions. Adverse effects include peptic ulcer, gastrointestinal disturbances, dizziness, and tinnitus.

induce (ĭn-dōōs′, -dyōōs′) V. to start, cause, or stimulate the beginning of an activity (e.g., to induce anesthesia or to induce labor).

induced abortion (ĭn-dōōst′, -dyōōst′) *See* ABORTION.

induction of labor (ĭn-dŭk′shən) N. in obstetrics, artificial starting of the childbirth process by puncturing the amniotic sac surrounding the fetus or by administering a drug (oxytocin) to stimulate contractions of the muscles of the uterus. Labor may be induced to speed childbirth in cases of maternal or fetal distress, or electively (e.g., to avert the possibility of a woman delivering outside of a hospital).

induration (ĭn-də-rā′shən) N. hardening of a tissue or part, esp. the skin due to edema, inflammation, or other abnormality. ADJ. indurated

industrial disease (ĭn-dŭs′trē-əl) *See* OCCUPATIONAL DISEASE.

inebriation (ĭn-ē′brē-ā′shən) N. state of being drunk on ethyl alcohol; intoxicated.

inelastic ADJ. not flexible; unable to stretch; remaining the same length and tension.

inert (ĭn-ûrt′) ADJ.
1. not moving.
2. in pharmacology, not active, used, for example, as a binder or flavoring agent in a drug.
3. in chemistry, not taking part in a chemical reaction or acting as a catalyst.

inertia (ĭ-nûr′shə) N. state of inactivity or sluggishness (e.g., uterine inertia, in which the contraction of the muscular wall of the uterus is inadequate).

infant (ĭn′fənt) N. a child from birth to 1 year (some extend the range to 2 years). ADJ. infantile

infant death *See* SUDDEN INFANT DEATH SYNDROME.

infant feeding *See* DEMAND FEEDING; BREAST FEEDING.

infant mortality rate N. number of deaths of infants under 1 year of age per 1,000 live births in a given geographic region or institution in a given period (usually 1 year).

infantile paralysis (ĭn′fən-tīl′, -tĭl) (pə-răl′ĭ-sĭs) *See* POLIOMYELITIS.

infantilism (ĭn′fən-tl-ĭz′əm) N. condition in which childhood characteristics (mental and/or physical) continue into adulthood.

infarct (ĭn′färkt′, ĭn-färkt′) N. area of dead tissue resulting from diminished or stopped blood flow to the tissue area.

infarction (ĭn-färk′shən) N. formation of dead tissue as a result of diminished or stopped blood flow to the tissue area. *See also* MYOCARDIAL INFARCTION.

infect (ĭn-fĕkt′) V. to transmit a disease-causing organism.

infection (ĭn-fĕk′shən) N.
1. invasion of disease-producing microorganisms into a body, where they may multiply, causing a disease.
2. disease caused by disease-producing microorganisms (e.g., certain bacteria). (*Compare* INFESTATION; CONTAGION.)

infectious (ĭn-fĕk′shəs) ADJ.
1. caused by an infection.
2. capable of producing an infection.

infectious disease N. disease caused by a pathogenic agent, such as a bacterium or virus. The disease may or may not be contagious. (*Compare* COMMUNICABLE DISEASE.)

infectious hepatitis *See* VIRAL HEPATITIS.

infectious mononucleosis (mŏn′ō-nōō′klē-ō′sĭs) N. acute infection, caused by the Epstein-Barr herpes virus and most common among young people; it is not highly contagious. Symptoms include fever, swollen lymph glands, sore throat, enlarged spleen and liver, abnormal liver function, fatigue, and malaise. Treatment is symptomatic, including bed rest to prevent spleen rupture or other spleen or liver complications. One attack usually confers immunity. Also called glandular fever; kissing disease.

infectious polyneuritis (pŏl′ē-nōō-rī′tĭs) *See* GUILLAIN-BARRÉ SYNDROME.

inferior (ĭn-fēr′ē-ər) ADJ. in anatomy, below or lower than a given reference point; the knee is inferior to the hip.

inferior vena cava N. large vein that returns deoxygenated blood to the heart from the body below the diaphragm. It is formed by junction of the common iliac veins in the lower back region and travels upward along the vertebral column, pierces the diaphragm, and empties into the right atrium of the heart (*compare* SUPERIOR VENA CAVA).

infertility (ĭn′fər-tĭl′ĭ-tē) N. condition of being unable to bear young—in a woman, an inability to conceive, in a male, an inability to impregnate. Female infertility may be due to a defective ovum, an ovulation disorder, a blockage of the Fallopian tubes, a uterine disorder, or a hormonal imbalance; in a male, infertility may be due to a lower-than-normal number of sperm produced or to sperm with abnormal shape or motility. Many cases of infertility can be corrected through surgery, drugs, or other medical procedures.

infestation N. presence, and usually the growth and increase, of parasites or other organisms on the skin (e.g., ringworm infestation) or within the body, usually producing signs of disease (*compare* INFECTION). V. infest

infiltration (ĭn′fĭl-trā′shən) N. process where something passes into and is deposited within a cell, tissue, or organ. Prior to suturing a laceration, local anesthetic is infiltrated into the skin surrounding the borders to prevent discomfort. Various tumors may infiltrate (spread into or within) the lung, liver, or brain.

inflammation (ĭn′flə-mā′shən) N. response of the tissues of the body to irritation or injury, characterized by pain, swelling, redness, and heat. The severity, specific characteristics, and duration of the inflammation depend on the cause, the particular area of the body affected, and the health of the person. ADJ. inflamed; inflammatory

inflammatory bowel disease *See* CROHN'S DISEASE; ULCERATIVE COLITIS.

influenza (ĭn′flōō-ĕn′zə) N. acute, contagious, virus-caused infection of the respiratory tract; symptoms usually begin suddenly and include fever, sore throat, cough, muscle aches, headache, fatigue, and malaise, and often signs of the common cold (watery eyes, runny nose). Treatment is symptomatic and includes rest, pain relievers, and fever reducers, and increased fluid intake. The disease usually subsides within a week; complications (e.g., bacterial pneumonia) usually affect only the very young, the old, or those weakened by another abnormal condition. Several strains of the virus have been identified, and new strains emerge at intervals, often named for the geographic region in which they are first discovered (e.g., Asian flu). Medications are now available which, if given early, may reduce the severity of illness. Also called flu; grippe.

informed consent (ĭn-fôrmd′) N. permission obtained from a patient for the performance of a particular procedure or test, after being told fully the risks, options, and expected results.

Informed consent, usually in a signed statement, is generally required before any invasive procedure (e.g., surgery or diagnostic procedures in which instruments are inserted into the body), before admission to any experimental or research study, and in certain other situations. The legal standard for informed consent varies from state to state. Most states have the "reasonable patient" standard, meaning that the health care provider must tell the patient what the reasonable lay patient would want to know. A few states use the "reasonable provider" standard, meaning that the health care provider is only required to tell the patient what the provider feels is important for the patient know to make an informed decision.

infra- comb. form meaning situated below, occurring below (e.g., infraclavicular, below the clavicle).

infrared therapy N. use of infrared radiation (e.g., in hot water bottles, heating pads, or incandescent lights) to relieve pain and increase blood circulation to a particular area of the body.

infundibulum (ĭn′fən-dĭb′yə-ləm) N., *pl.* infundibula, funnel-shaped part, esp. the part of the brain (the hypophyseal stalk) that connects to the hypothalamus and pituitary gland. ADJ. infundibular

infusion (ĭn-fyōō′zhən) N.
1. introduction of a substance (e.g., fluid, drug, electrolyte) directly into a vein or between tissues, often by gravitational force (*compare* INJECTION).
2. substance introduced into the body by infusion.

ingesta (ĭn-jĕs′tə) N. solid and liquid materials taken into the mouth.

ingestion (ĭn-jĕs′chən) N. the act of putting food and other material into the mouth. V. ingest. ADJ. ingestive

ingrown hair (ĭn′grōn′) N. hair that does not emerge from the follicle but remains embedded in the skin, usually causing inflammation.

ingrown toenail N. toenail whose free ends grow into, or become pressed into, the skin, causing inflammation and sometimes secondary infection.

inguinal (ĭng′gwə-nəl) ADJ. pert. to the groin (e.g., inguinal hernia).

inguinal hernia N. hernia in which a loop of the intestine enters the inguinal canal and in males, sometimes fills the scrotum; the most common type of hernia, it is usually treated surgically.

INH See ISONIAZID.

inhalation (ĭn′hə-lā′shən) N. act of breathing in, whereby air or other gas or vapor (e.g., anesthetic gas) is taken into the lungs. V. inhale

inhalation anesthesia (ăn′ĭs-thē′zhə) N. general anesthesia achieved by inhalation of an anesthetic gas or volatile liquid; widely used inhalation anesthetics include cyclopropane, halothane, enflurane, and isoflurane.

inhalation therapy N. treatment in which oxygen, water, or a drug is introduced into the respiratory tract with inhaled air. It may be used to provide oxygen or to administer drugs to liquefy mucus or dilate the bronchial passageways.

inherent ADJ. inborn, innate (*compare* ACQUIRED; INDIGENOUS).

inheritance (ĭn-hĕr′ĭ-təns) N. acquisition of characteristics and conditions by transmission (of genetic material) from parents to offspring; the total genetic makeup of an individual.

inherited disorder See GENETIC DISEASE.

inhibition (ĭn′hə-bĭsh′ən) N. slowing or stopping of an otherwise normal response (e.g., the restriction of a specific impulse drive, or activity); in psychology, evidence shown by a person's actions that he/she is restraining a display of an instinctual drive (e.g., averting any encounter with sexual activity).

inion N. bump that protrudes at the back of the head.

injection (ĭn-jĕk′shən) N.
1. act of putting a liquid into the body forcefully by means of a syringe; the fluid may be injected into a vein (intravenous), muscle (intramuscular), under the skin (subcutaneous), or into the skin (intradermal) (*compare* INFUSION).
2. substance inserted into the body by force.

injury (ĭn′jə-rē) N. wound or damage to a part of the body.

innate (ĭ-nāt′, ĭn′āt′) ADJ.
1. inborn, hereditary, or congenital.
2. pert. to an essential characteristic of someone or something.

innate immunity See NATURAL IMMUNITY.

innervate (ĭ-nûr′vāt′) V. provide nerve fibers to an organ or body region; for example, the median nerve innervates part of the hand.

innervation (ĭn'ər-vā'shən) N. distribution and action of nerve fibers to an organ or body region.

innocuous ADJ. harmless.

innominate artery N. artery arising from the arch of the aorta that divides into the right subclavian artery and the right common carotid artery, supplying blood to the right side of the head and neck and the right shoulder and arm. *See* MAJOR ARTERIES AND VEINS OF THE BODY, in Appendix.

innominate bone N. hip bone, formed by the fusion of the ilium, ischium, and pubis. The innominate bone, together with the sacrum and coccyx, forms the pelvis.

inoculation (ĭ-nŏk'yə-lā'shən) N. process of deliberately injecting a substance into the body to produce or increase immunity to the disease associated with the substance; it may be done by placing a drop of the substance on the skin and scratching the skin in that area, by puncturing the skin, or by intradermal, subcutaneous, or intramuscular injection. V. inoculate

inoculum (ĭ-nŏk'yə-ləm) N. substance (a live, weakened, or killed virus; a toxin; or an immune serum) introduced into the body to produce or increase immunity to a specific disease; also called inoculant.

inotropic ADJ. influencing the force of contraction of a muscle. Positive inotropic agents, such as digitalis drugs, improve contraction of the heart muscle. Disease states, such as congestive heart failure, lead to a decreased inotropic state of the heart causing impairment of effective muscle contraction.

insanity N.
1. legal term meaning the inability to distinguish right from wrong, an inability to control one's life, or to act in a socially acceptable manner.
2. colloquial term for severe mental illness.

insemination N. introduction of semen into the vagina, either during coitus or through other techniques. *See also* ARTIFICIAL INSEMINATION.

insertion N. anatomical term for the point of attachment of the movable end of a muscle, typically to bone. More generally, means placement of something, such as insertion of a breathing tube into the trachea.

insidious ADJ. pert. to gradual, subtle, or hard-to-discern development, as in a disease (e.g., glaucoma) that develops without early symptoms (*compare* ACUTE).

insoluble ADJ. incapable of dissolving in solution.

insomnia N. condition characterized by difficulty in falling asleep or staying asleep or by seriously disturbed sleep (e.g., frequent short awakenings). It may result from a variety of psychological and physical causes; treatment depends on the cause and condition of the person. (*Compare* NARCOLEPSY.)

inspiration N. act of drawing air into the lungs. Contraction of the diaphragm causes the lungs to expand and air to flow in.

instinct N. complex, unlearned pattern of response and behavior that is specific to a particular species and released by certain environmental stimuli (e.g., sucking, in a newborn infant). ADJ. instinctive

insufflation N. blowing of a material (e.g., gas or powder) into a tube, cavity, or organ of the body to allow visual examination, to determine if an obstruction is present, or to introduce a drug (e.g., introduction of gas into the Fallopian tubes to determine whether or not they are open, Rubin test).

insulin N.
1. hormone secreted by the beta cells of the islets of Langerhans of the pancreas; it regulates the metabolism of glucose and, secondarily, intermediary processes in the metabolism of carbohydrates and fats. Inadequate insulin levels lead to too-high glucose levels and other disturbances of metabolism, often associated with diabetes mellitus.
2. drug made from the natural hormones and used to treat diabetes mellitus.

insulin shock N. abnormal physiological state in which the blood glucose level is too low (hypoglycemia); it may be caused by an overdose of insulin, decreased food intake, or excess exercise. Symptoms include sweating, trembling, nervousness, irritability, and pallor; if not corrected, it can lead to convulsions and death. Treatment requires the administration of glucose. (*Compare* DIABETIC COMA; KETOACIDOSIS.)

Intal N. trade name for the inhaled powder cromolyn, used in the treatment of chronic asthma.

integration N. organization, unification, and use of experiences, insights, and reactions into a functional whole with coordinated thinking, feeling and acting. V. integrate

integrin N. receptor on the cell membrane that binds with various proteins and chemicals as a form of cell-to-cell communication.

integument *See* SKIN. ADJ. integumentary

integumentary system N. skin and its appendages: nails, hair, sebaceous glands.

intellect N. capacity to know, perceive, and understand, in contrast to the capacity for emotion.

THE INTEGUMENTARY SYSTEM

Organ	Primary Functions
Epidermis	Protects underlying tissues
Dermis	Nourishes epidermis, provides strength
Hair follicles Hairs Sebaceous glands	Produce hair Provide sensation and some protection for the head Secrete lipid coating that lubricates hair shaft
Sweat glands	Produce perspiration for evaporative cooling
Nails	Protect and stiffen distal tips of digits
Sensory receptors	Provide sensations of touch, pressure, temperature, and pain
Superfacial fascia	Stores fat

intellectualization N. in psychiatry, defense mechanism in which reasoning is used to block emotional conflict and stress.

intelligence N. ability to learn, to understand, to apply experience, and to make judgments. *See also* INTELLIGENCE QUOTIENT.

intelligence quotient (IQ) N. numerical expression of a person's intellectual level measured against the statistical average for his/her age or as mental age (measured by standardized tests) as ratio of chronological age. Virtually all intelligence tests are designed so that the average IQ in the population is about 100.

intensive care unit (ICU) N. hospital unit in which patients with life-threatening conditions are provided with constant care and close monitoring that often involves the use of sophisticated machines to care for and maintain the patient.

inter- prefix meaning between (e.g., intercellular, between cells).

intercellular space N. area between cells of a tissue, organ, or organism.

intercourse *See* COITUS.

interferon N. protein produced by cells that induces immunity to viral infection. Various types of this substance are being used to attempt to fight cancer.

intern N. physician (graduate of a medical school) in the first postgraduate year, learning under the supervision of more experienced physicians in a hospital; sometimes called a first-year resident.

internal (ĭn-tûr′nəl) ADJ. within, inside (e.g., internal organs, organs inside the body).

internal injury N. wound or damage to a part of the body not normally visible on the surface of the skin; for example, a person involved in a motor vehicle accident may rupture his spleen and bleed internally without any signs of injury visible on the back or abdomen.

internal medicine N. that branch of medicine concerned with the function of internal organs and the diagnosis and treatment of disorders affecting these organs.

internalization (ĭn-tûr′nə-lĭ-zā′shən) N. unconscious process of adopting and absorbing the beliefs, values, and attitudes of another or of the society to which the person belongs.

interneuron N. neuron whose sole purpose is to connect other neurons to facilitate communication between them, esp. between sensory and motor neurons; important in reflex arcs and in blocking out extraneous stimuli to the brain (helps people maintain attention). *See also* REFLEX ARC.

internist (ĭn-tûr′nĭst) N. specialist in internal medicine.

interoceptor (ĭn′tər-ō-sĕp′tər) N. sensory nerve ending inside the body that responds to stimuli within the body (e.g., digestion, blood pressure).

interpersonal therapy N. short-term form of psychotherapy for depression that focuses on the patient's disturbed personal relationships that both cause and exacerbate the depression. Short term usually involves up to 20 sessions (usually weekly meetings, 1 hour per session) and maintains a focus on one or two key issues that seem to be most closely related to the depression. Although depression may not be caused by interpersonal events, it usually has an interpersonal component—it affects relationships and roles in those relationships. Interpersonal therapy was developed to address these issues. Data have shown that this form of therapy is equally as effective in the short-term treatment of depression as antidepressant medication therapy, though it also works well in conjunction with medications. *See also* DEPRESSION.

intersex N. person who has the characteristics of both sexes or who has external genitalia that are ambiguous or not appropriate to the normal male or female. *See also* HERMAPHRODITE; PSEUDOHERMAPHRODITISM.

interstice (ĭn-tûr′stĭs) N. space in a tissue or between parts of the body. ADJ. interstitial

interstitial cell-stimulating hormone (ICSH) (ĭn′tər-stĭsh′əl) *See* LUTEINIZING HORMONE.

interstitial fluid N. part of the extracellular fluid; fluid found between cells of the body that helps to provide a large part of the fluid environment of the body.

interstitial plasma cell pneumonia *See* PNEUMOCYTOSIS.

interstitial pneumonia N. chronic inflammation of the lungs, characterized by progressive dyspnea, fever, and bluish discoloration of the skin (cyanosis). It may be caused by a hypersensitivity reaction to a particular drug or by an autoimmune disorder. Treatment is symptomatic, but the disease often progresses to pulmonary or heart failure. (*Compare* BRONCHOPNEUMONIA.)

intertrigo (ĭn′tər-trī′gō′) N. irritation of two skin surfaces that are in contact, as in the armpits, under the breasts, or between the thighs. Prevention involves weight reduction, keeping the surfaces clean and dry, and applying antifungal preparations if needed.

interval (ĭn′tər-vəl) N. space between parts or time between events (e.g., the Q-T interval in the activity of the ventricles of the heart).

intervertebral (ĭn′tər-vûr′tə-brəl) ADJ. pert. to the space between two vertebrae, as the intervertebral discs.

intervertebral disc N. fibrocartilaginous disc found between all of the vertebrae of the spinal column, except the first two (the axis and the atlas).

intestinal bypass (ĭn-tĕs′tə-nəl) N. surgical procedure, used in the treatment of obesity, in which a large part of the small intestine is bypassed so that food is not absorbed there and weight is lost.

intestinal flora N. microorganisms (e.g., *Escherichia coli*) normally present in the intestinal tract and essential to its normal function.

intestinal flu N. inflammation of the stomach and intestine caused by a virus; symptoms include abdominal discomfort, nausea, vomiting, and diarrhea. *See also* GASTROENTERITIS.

intestinal juice N. secretions of glands lining the intestine.

intestinal obstruction N. blockage in the intestine that results in failure of the contents of the intestine to pass through to the lower bowel; it may be due to tumor, adhesions, hernia, narrowing from Crohn's disease or ulcerative colitis, or other cause. Symptoms include pain, abdominal distension, constipation, and vomiting of fecal matter. Treatment includes taking nothing by mouth, evacuation of the contents of the stomach, intravenous fluids, and possibly, surgical removal of the obstruction. *Compare* ILEUS.

intestine (ĭn-tĕs′tĭn) N. that part of the alimentary canal extending from the pyloric opening of the stomach to the anus. It is divided into two major parts: the small intestine (made up of the duodenum, jejunum, and ileum), where most digestion and absorption of food occurs; and the large intestine (consisting of the cecum; appendix; ascending, transverse and descending colon; and the rectum), where water is absorbed from material passing from the small intestine. Waves of muscular contractions—peristalsis—propel material through the intestine. ADJ. intestinal

intima (ĭn′tə-mə) N. innermost lining of a part, esp. of a blood vessels. ADJ. intimal

intoxication (ĭn-tŏk′sĭ-kā′shən) N. state of being poisoned or inebriated because of ingestion of excessive alcohol, another drug, or a toxic substance. ADJ. intoxicated

intra- prefix meaning within (e.g., intra-abdominal, within the abdomen).

intracellular (ĭn′trə-sĕl′yə-lər) ADJ. within a cell.

intracellular fluid N. fluid, usually containing dissolved solutes, contained within cell membranes (*compare* EXTRACELLULAR FLUID; INTERSTITIAL FLUID).

intracerebral ADJ. within the brain.

intracranial (ĭn′trə-krā′nē-əl) ADJ. within the cranium.

intracranial aneurysm (ăn′yə-rĭz′əm) N. aneurysm of a cranial artery. Symptoms include headache, stiff neck, nausea, and sometimes loss of consciousness; rupture of the aneurysm is a serious, often fatal, condition.

intractable (ĭn-trăk′tə-bəl) ADJ. not readily responsive to treatment; not easily cured or treated.

intracutaneous, intradermal (ĭn′trə-kyōō-tā′nē-əs) (ĭn′trə-dûr′məl) ADJ. within the skin (e.g., an intradermal injection).

intradermal test (ĭn′trə-dûr′məl) N. procedure used in allergy testing in which a small amount of the suspected allergen is injected within the skin. Wheal formation and reddening of the skin within 30 minutes of the injection indicate a positive result. Also called subcutaneous test. (*Compare* PATCH TEST; SCRATCH TEST.)

intramuscular (ĭn′trə-mŭs′kyə-lər) ADJ. within a muscle (e.g., an intramuscular injection.)

intraocular lens (ĭn′trə-ŏk′yə-lər) N. artificial lens implanted into the eye after surgical cataract removal to replace the cataract-damaged natural lens.

intraocular pressure N. internal pressure of the eye regulated by resistance to the outward flow of aqueous humor. *See also* GLAUCOMA.

intraosseous N. injection technique in which a needle is percutaneously placed into the bone marrow cavity of either the tibia or the femur; because the bone marrow cavity directly feeds into the venous blood circulation, fast infusion of both medications and fluids is possible; intraosseous infusion is the technique of choice in pediatric patients when an intravenous line cannot be started within one minute.

intrauterine device (IUD) (ĭn′trə-yōō′tər-ĭn) N. contraceptive device, consisting of a bent plastic or metal (a coil, loop, or other shape) inserted through the vagina into the uterus, where it functions to prevent pregnancy. Complications of IUD use include infection, undetected expulsion, perforation of the uterus, bleeding, and pain. *See also* CONTRACEPTION.

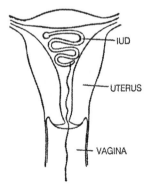

An IUD after insertion into the uterus.

intravasation (ĭn-trăv′ə-sā′shən) N. entry of a foreign substance into a blood vessel.

intravenous (ĭn′trə-vē′nəs) ADJ. into or within a vein.

intravenous feeding (IV) N. administration of nutrients through a vein.

intravenous injection N. hypodermic injection into a vein to instill a fluid, withdraw blood, or begin a blood transfusion or intravenous feeding.

intravenous pyelography (IVP) (pī′ə-lŏg′rə-fē) N. radiological technique for examining the structures of the urinary system to detect tumors, cysts, stones, or structural or functional abnormalities. A contrast medium is injected intravenously, and a series of X rays traces the clearance of the medium by the urinary system.

intrinsic factor (ĭn-trĭn′zĭk, -sĭk) N. substance secreted by the mucous membranes of the stomach that is essential for absorption of vitamin B_{12}; lack of intrinsic factor leads to deficiency of vitamin B_{12} and resultant pernicious anemia.

introitus (ĭn-trō′ĭ-təs) N. entrance or opening to a hollow organ or hollow tube (e.g., the introitus of the vagina).

Intropin N. trade name for dopamine.

introversion (ĭn′trə-vûr′zhən, -shən) N. tendency to turn one's interests inward toward the self (*compare* EXTROVERSION).

intubation N. placement of a tube into an opening, esp. insertion of a breathing tube into the trachea to allow passage of oxygen or anesthetic gas.

intumescence (ĭn′tōō-mĕs′əns) N. swelling or increase in volume. ADJ. intumescent

intussusception (ĭn′tə-sə-sĕp′shən) N. infolding of one part of the intestine into the lumen of another part, causing an obstruction. Symptoms include abdominal pain and bloody stool. Treatment is by surgery.

invagination (ĭn-vaj′ə-nā′shən) N. condition in which one part of an organ folds into or becomes telescoped into another part of the organ, as in the intestine, sometimes causing an obstruction.

invasive (ĭn-vā′sĭv) ADJ. marked by a tendency to spread, esp. into healthy tissue, such as invasive cancer. In reference to medical procedures, one in which a body cavity is entered, such as with a needle.

inversion (ĭn-vûr′zhən, -shən) N. abnormal condition in which an organ is turned inward or inside out (e.g., the uterus after childbirth when its upper part is pulled into the cervical canal).

involuntary (ĭn-vŏl′ən-tĕr′ē) ADJ. done without conscious thought or control of the will.

involuntary muscle *See* SMOOTH MUSCLE.

involution (ĭn′və-lōō′shən) N. decrease in the size of an organ, as in the return of the uterus to its normal size after childbirth. V. involute.

iodine (ī′ə-dīn′) N. nonmetallic element that is an essential nutrient (in small amounts) and is used in antiseptics, in radioisotope scanning procedures, and in certain treatments of thyroid cancer. *See also* TABLE OF IMPORTANT ELEMENTS.

iodopsin (ī′ə-dŏp′sĭn) N. photosensitive chemical in the cones of the retina that plays a part in color vision.

ion (ī′ən, ī′ŏn′) N. electrically charged particle. Many ions play an integral role in the maintenance of normal body function.

ionic bond *See* BONDING.

ipecac (ĭp′ĭ-kăk′) N. drug used to induce vomiting in some types of poisoning and drug overdose. Adverse effects include gastrointestinal irritation and prolonged vomiting.

ipratropium bromide (ĭp′rə-trō′pē-əm) N. inhaled bronchodilator (trade name Atrovent), similar to atropine, that is effective in the long-term treatment of chronic obstructive pulmonary disease. Although it has been used also to treat asthma, it does not seem to work as well in this disease. *See* TABLE OF COMMONLY PRESCRIBED DRUGS —GENERIC NAMES.

IPV *See* SALK VACCINE.

IQ *See* INTELLIGENCE QUOTIENT.

iridectomy (ĭr′ĭ-dĕk′tə-mē) N. surgical removal of part of the iris of the eye, usually performed to remove a foreign body or tumor or to enhance drainage of aqueous humor in cases of glaucoma.

iridocyclitis (ĭr′ĭ-dō-sī-klī′tĭs) N. inflammation of the iris and ciliary body of the eye.

iridokeratitis N. inflammation of the iris and cornea of the eye.

iridoncus (ĭr′ĭ-dŏng′kəs) N. swelling of the iris of the eye.

iridotomy (ĭr′ĭ-dŏt′ə-mē) N. surgical procedure in which an incision is made in the iris to enlarge the pupil or to treat glaucoma.

iris (ī′rĭs) N. circular, colored part of the eye suspended in the aqueous humor and perforated by the pupil. ADJ. iritic

iritis (ī-rī′tĭs) N. inflammation of the iris, causing tearing, pain, and decreased visual sharpness.

iron (ī′ərn) N. metallic element essential for hemoglobin synthesis in the body and used in various drugs. *See also* TABLE OF IMPORTANT ELEMENTS.

iron-deficiency anemia N. type of anemia caused by lack of adequate iron to synthesize hemoglobin. Symptoms include fatigue, pallor, and weakness.

iron lung N. large, cylindrical device formerly used as a means of providing artificial respiration for victims of disease (esp. poliomyelitis). The patient's body, from the neck down, was placed into the chamber, and vacuum suction used to facilitate breathing.

iron-storage disease *See* HEMO-CHROMATOSIS.

irradiation (ĭ-rā′dē-ā′shən) N. exposure to heat, light, X ray, or other form of radiant energy for diagnostic or therapeutic purposes.

irreducible (ĭr′ĭ-dŏō′sə-bəl) ADJ. not able to be returned to normal, as an irreducible hernia.

irreversible ADJ. impossible to reverse or to be reversed; unchangeable, permanent with no significant chance of improvement, as in irreversible brain damage from a stroke.

irrigation N. washing out of a body part or a wound with water or a medicated solution.

irritable bowel syndrome (ĭr′ĭ-tə-bəl) N. condition characterized by recurrent abdominal pain, usually crampy in nature, and diarrhea, often alternating with periods of constipation. Occurring most often in young adults, it has no known organic cause and is often associated with emotional stress. Also called spastic colon; mucous colitis. (*Compare* CROHN'S DISEASE; ULCERATIVE COLITIS.)

irritant N. stimulus, often physical, that causes irritation or inflammation.

ischemia (ĭ-skē′mē-ə) N. decreased blood supply to a given body part, sometimes resulting from vasoconstriction, thrombosis, or embolism (*See also* INFARCT). ADJ. ischemic

ischium (ĭs′kē-əm) N., *pl.* ischia, one of the three parts of the hip (innominate bone), the other two being the ilium and pubis. ADJ. ischiatic

islands of Langerhans (ī′lənd) (läng′ər-häns′) N. cell clusters within the pancreas that form the endocrine part of the organ, secreting hormones important in controlling sugar metabolism. Beta cells secrete insulin, alpha cells secrete glucagon, and other cells secrete pancreatic juices. Also called islets of Langerhans.

-ism suffix indicating a condition of or theory of (e.g., hyperthyroidism).

Ismo N. trade name for the oral nitroglycerine-like preparation, isosorbide mononitrate.

iso- comb. form indicating equality or sameness (e.g., isomorphous, of the same form).

isoagglutination (ī′sō-ə-glŏŌt′n-ā′shən) N. process in which antibodies (isoagglutinins) occurring naturally in blood cause clumping of red blood cells of a different group, carrying a corresponding antigen (isoagglutinogen) but of the same species.

isoantibody (ī'sō-ăn'tĭ-bŏd'ē) N. antibody that occurs naturally against foreign tissues of a person of the same species.

isograft (ī'sə-grăft) N. graft taken from another individual or animal of the same genotype (genetic information) as the recipient; sometimes called autograft.

isolation (ī'sə-lā'shən) N.
1. process of separating one thing from all others like it.
2. separation of a patient from others, e.g., to prevent the spread of an infectious disease.
3. in surgery, separation of a structure from surrounding structures.

isomer (ī'sə-mər) N. one of two or more chemical substances that have the same molecular formula but different chemical and physical properties and different arrangements of the atoms in the molecule.

isometric exercises (ī'sə-mĕt'rĭk) N. exercises that increase muscle tension by applying pressure against stable resistance, as in pressing hands together; also called isometrics (*compare* ISOTONIC EXERCISES).

isoniazid (INH) (ī'sə-nī'ə-zĭd) N. drug used to treat tuberculosis. Adverse effects include disturbances of peripheral nerve function, liver toxicity, rashes, and fever.

isoproterenol N. drug (trade name Isuprel) used to treat bronchial asthma and to stimulate the heart. Adverse effects include hypotension and abnormalities of cardiac rhythm.

Isoptin N. trade name for the calcium channel blocker verapamil.

Isordil N. trade name for the cardiac drug isosorbide.

isosorbide dinitrate N. drug (trade name Isordil) used to treat angina pectoris and congestive heart failure. Adverse effects include hypotension, dizziness, and headache.

isosorbide mononitrate N. oral nitroglycerine-like drug; acts as a vasodilator and is used in the treatment of angina. *See* TABLE OF COMMONLY PRESCRIBED DRUGS—GENERIC NAMES.

isotonic (ī'sə-tŏn'ĭk) ADJ. of equal pressure or concentration, esp. in a solution. *See* OSMOSIS.

isotonic exercises N. form of exercise in which the muscle contracts and there is movement; joint mobility and muscle strength are improved (*compare* ISOMETRIC EXERCISES).

isotope (ī'sə-tōp') N. one of two or more forms of an element having the same atomic number and the same or nearly the same properties but differing in atomic mass (because of difference in number of neutrons in the nucleus); for example, deuterium is an isotope of hydrogen. *See also* RADIOISOTOPE.

isradipine N. oral calcium channel blocker (trade name DynaCirc) used in the treatment of hypertension.

isthmus (ĭs'məs) N. narrow connecting part, as the band of tissue connecting the lobes of the thyroid gland.

Isuprel N. trade name for the cardiac stimulant, isoproterenol.

itch (ĭch) N. annoying sensation on the skin that impels the person to scratch the site (*compare* PRURITUS; SCABIES; TINEA).

-itis suffix meaning inflammation (e.g., neuritis, nerve inflammation).

IUD *See* INTRAUTERINE DEVICE.

IV *See* INTRAVENOUS FEEDING.

IVP *See* INTRAVENOUS PYELOGRA-
PHY.

J

jacket N. covering, as of plaster of Paris, leather, or other material, placed over the torso to provide support or help correct a deformity.

Jacksonian epilepsy (jăk-sō′nē-ən ĕp′ə-lĕp′sē) N. type of epilepsy characterized by recurrent motor seizure episodes that typically start as a twitching or convulsive movement of a small group of muscles and then spread to other muscles on the same side of the body as, for example, twitching of the fingers of one hand spreading to muscles of the hand, forearm, and arm. The affected person usually remains conscious during the attack.

Jacquemier's sign N. bluish or purplish coloration of the mucous membrane lining of the vagina that occurs in early pregnancy.

jactitation (jăk′tĭ-tā′shən) N. tossing, twitching, and jerking movements of a person with a severe illness.

Jakob-Creutzfeldt disease (yä′kôp-kroits′fĕlt) *See* CREUTZFELDT-JAKOB DISEASE.

jamais vu (zham′ā-voō) N. sensation of being strange or unfamiliar with a person or surroundings that actually are familiar. It can occur in normal persons but is most often associated with certain types of epilepsy. (*Compare* DÉJÀ VU.)

jargon (jär′gən) N. characteristic language of an occupational group; specialized technical terminology characteristic of a particular subject; colloq. lingo.

Jarvik heart N. type of artificial heart used, with variable success, in recent human implantations.

JARVIK ARTIFICIAL HEART

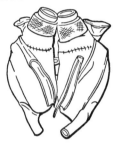

jaundice (jôn′dĭs) N. yellowing of the skin and whites (sclerae) of the eyes, caused by an accumulation of the bile pigment bilirubin in the blood. Jaundice is a symptom of several disorders: (1) most commonly, obstruction (e.g., by a gallstone) of the ducts that carry bile to the intestine; (2) disease of the liver due to infection (e.g., hepatitis), alcoholism, poisons, or other factor; and (3) anemia, in which there is excessive destruction of red blood cells. Also called icterus. (*See also* KERNICTERUS; HYPERBILIRUBINEMIA.) ADJ. jaundiced

jaundice of the newborn N. physiological jaundice occurring in some infants in the first few weeks of life and caused by destruction of excess hemoglobin in red blood cells; it usually disappears spontaneously; also called physiological jaundice of the newborn; icterus neonatorum.

jaw N. bones that form the framework of the mouth and serve for the attachment of teeth. The upper jaw bone is the maxilla; the lower jaw bone, the mandible.

jejune (jə-jōō′n) ADJ. lacking in nutritive value.

jejunitis (jə-jōō′nī′tĭs) N. inflammation of the jejunum.

jejuno- (jə-jōō′nō) comb. form indicating an association with the jejunum (e.g., jejunostomy, surgical creation of an opening between the jejunum and the anterior abdominal wall, sometimes made to allow artificial feeding).

jejunoileitis (jə-jōō′nō-īl′ē-ī′tĭs) N. inflammation of both the jejunum and ileum of the small intestine.

jejunum (jə-jōō′nəm) N. that part of the small intestine between the duodenum and the ileum; in humans, it is about 2.4 meters (8 feet) long. ADJ. jejunal

jerk N. sudden movement; a muscle reflex. Efforts to elicit certain jerks (e.g., the knee jerk) are used to help diagnose specific nerve transmission disorders.

jet lag N. condition marked by fatigue, sleep disturbances, and sluggish body functions, caused by a disruption of the body's normal circadian (daily) rhythm resulting from travel through several time zones.

jock itch colloquial term for tinea cruris.

joint N. point where two or more bones meet. A joint may be immovable (fibrous), as those of the skull; slightly movable (cartilaginous), as those connecting the vertebrae; or freely movable (synovial), as those of the elbow and knee. Also called articulation.

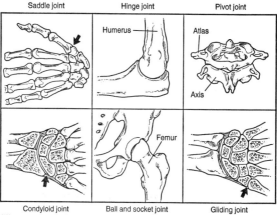

Six different types of freely movable joints.

JOINT MOVEMENTS AND ANTAGONISTIC
(OPPOSING) MOVEMENTS

Action	Antagonistic Action
Flexion: the decreasing of the angle between two bones	Extension: the increasing of the angle between two bones
Abduction: the movement of a body part away from a midline	Adduction: the movement of a body part toward a midline
Medial rotation: the turning of a bone on its own axis toward the midline of the body	Lateral rotation: the turning of a bone on its own axis away from the midline of the body
Supination: the placing of the palm of the hand in the anatomical position	Pronation: the placing of the palm of the hand away from the anatomical position
Elevation: the raising of a body part	Depression: the lowering of a body part
Protraction: the thrusting forward of a body part	Retraction: the withdrawal of a body part
Dorsiflexion: the bending of the foot toward the shin	Plantar flexion: the bending of the foot away from the shin
Inversion: the rotation of the sole of the foot inward	Eversion: the rotation of the sole of the foot outward

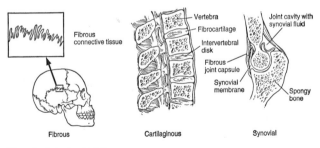

Three basic types of joints.

jugular (jŭg′yə-lər) ADJ. pert. to the throat or neck.

jugular veins N. any of several veins in the neck that drain blood from the head and empty into larger veins leading to the heart.

juice N. any of several liquids of the body. It may be normal (e.g., gastric juice, pancreatic juice) or abnormal (e.g., cancer juice, milklike substance found in certain cancerous growths). Also called succus.

jumentous ADJ. smelling strongly like an animal, as, e.g., urine in certain diseases.

junction N. point where two parts come together (e.g., neuromuscular junction, point where a nerve and muscle come together).

juvenile (jōō′və-nīl′) ADJ. occurring in someone under the age of 18; pertaining to youth or childhood.

juvenile diabetes (jōō′və-nīl′ dī′ə-bē′tĭs) *See* DIABETES MELLITUS.

juvenile rheumatoid arthritis (rōō′mă-toyd âr-thrī′tĭs) *See* STILL'S DISEASE.

juxta- (jŭk′stə) comb. form indicating proximity, nearness (e.g., juxtaspinal, near the spine).

juxtaposition (jŭk′stə-pə-zĭsh′ən) N. side-by-side position.

K

K
1. symbol for the element potassium.
2. abbreviation for the Kelvin temperature scale.

K vitamin N. fat-soluble vitamin essential for blood coagulation and important in certain energy-transfer reactions. Rich sources include green leafy vegetables, egg yolk, yogurt, and fish-liver oils. *See also* VITAMIN; TABLE OF VITAMINS.

Kakke disease *See* BERI-BERI.

kala-azar (kä'lə-ə-zär') N. visceral form of leishmaniasis. Occurring mainly in warm regions of Asia, Africa, Central and South America, and parts of the Mediterranean area, it is caused by the protozoan *Leishmania donovani*, transmitted by the bite of a sand fly. Symptoms include anemia, enlarged spleen and liver, fever, and loss of weight. Treatment includes antimony preparations, blood transfusions, and rest. Also called Assam fever; dumdum fever.

kalemia (kā-lē'mē-ə) N. presence of potassium in the blood.

kaliuresis N. loss of potassium in the urine; also called kaluresis. ADJ. kaliuretic, kaluretic

kallikrein (kǎl'-ĭ-krēn') N. plasma, urine, and body tissue enzyme that is normally inactive; when activated, causes significant vasodilation; may contribute to low blood pressure (hypotension) and shock.

kaolin (kā'ə-lə-n) N. aluminum-and silicon-containing product used internally, often with pectin, in the trade-name product Kaopectate, as an adsorbent to treat diarrhea and externally as a dusting powder, or, in an ointment base, as a poultice.

Kaopectate N. trade name for a fixed-combination antidiarrheal containing the adsorbent kaolin and the emollient pectin.

Kaposi's sarcoma (kə-pō'sēz sär-kō'mə́) N. malignant neoplasm that starts as soft purplish or brownish spots on the feet and then spreads from the skin to the lymph nodes and internal organs. Until the early 1980s it occurred almost exclusively among older Jewish, Italian, and black men, but after that time it increased in incidence and is now one of the common manifestations of acquired immune deficiency syndrome (AIDS).

karyo- (kǎr'ē-ō) comb. form indicating an association with a nucleus (e.g., karyogamy, fusion of cell nuclei, as in fertilization).

karyokinesis (kǎr'ē-ō-kə-nē'sĭs) N. division of the cell nucleus during mitosis and meiosis.

karyolymph (kǎr'ē-ə-lĭmf') N. clear fluid of the cell nucleus in which the nucleolus, chromatin, and other structures are dispersed.

karyolysis (kǎr'ē-ŏl'ĭ-sĭs) N. breakdown of the cell nucleus. ADJ. karyolytic

karyon (kǎr'ē-ŏn) N. cell nucleus

karyoplasm (kǎr'ē-ə-plǎz'əm) *See* NUCLEOPLASM.

karyotype (kăr′ē-ə-tīp′) N.
1. appearance of the chromosomal makeup of a cell, including the number, arrangement, size, and structure of the chromosomes as determined by a photomicrograph taken during mitosis.
2. diagrammatic representation of the chromosomal makeup of a cell arranged according to a given classification system. ADJ. karyotypic

karyotyping N. process of analyzing and classifying the chromosomes of a cell and preparing a karyotype diagram; used in the diagnosis of certain chromosomal abnormalities (e.g., Down's syndrome).

Kawasaki disease N. acute illness, primarily in children, characterized by a rash, swollen lymph glands, fever, inflammation of the mucous membranes of the mouth, and a strawberry tongue; joint pain, pneumonia, meningitis, cardiac abnormalities, and aneurysms develop in some cases. The cause is unknown, and diagnosis is difficult based on the exclusion of all other known diseases. Treatment is largely symptomatic. Also called mucocutaneous lymph node syndrome.

Kayser-Fleischer ring (kī′zər-flī′shər) N. pigmented ring at the outer edge of the cornea of the eye that is a sign of Wilson's disease.

K-Dur-20 N. *See* TABLE OF COMMONLY PRESCRIBED DRUGS—TRADE NAMES.

Keflex N. trade name for the cephalosporin-family antibiotic cephalexin. *See* TABLE OF COMMONLY PRESCRIBED DRUGS—TRADE NAMES.

Keflin N. trade name for the cephalosporin-family antibiotic cephalexin.

Male and female karyotypes.

Keftab N. tablet preparation of the oral cephalosporin antibiotic cephalexin.

Kegel exercises N. regimen of exercises for women designed to improve the ability to retain urine and to increase the muscular contractility of the vagina; sometimes advised to help overcome weakness of the pubococcygeus muscles that may occur after childbirth. The exercises involve the squeezing, pulling-up action required to stop the stream of urine when voiding. Also called pubococcygeus exercises.

keloid (kē′loid′) N. overgrowth of collagenous scar tissue at the site of a wound on the skin. The lesion is generally rounded and raised, often with clawlike margins; it may flatten and become less noticeable with time or it may be treated by cryosurgery, corticosteroid injections, surgery, or other means.

Kelvin (kĕl′vĭn) ADJ. pert. to a temperature scale used in science in which 0 Kelvin (absolute zero) is equivalent to 273.16 Celsius.

Kenalog N. trade name for the glucocorticoid triamcinolone.

kerat-, kerato- comb. form indicating a relationship to the cornea of the eye (e.g., keratectomy, removal of part of the cornea), or to horny cells or horny tissue, esp. of the skin (e.g., keratolysis, loosening of the horny layer of the outer skin).

keratalgia N. pain in the cornea.

keratectasia N. bulging or protrusion of the cornea of the eye.

keratin (kĕr′ə-tĭn) N. protein that forms horny tissues such as the nails and is also found in the outer skin and hair. ADJ. keratic

keratinization (kĕr′ə-tn-ĭ-zā′shən) N. process by which cells become horny because of the deposit of keratin in them; it occurs in outer layers of the skin and associated structures (e.g., nails and hair).

keratinocyte (kə-răt′n-ə-sīt′) N. cell in the skin that synthesizes keratin.

keratitis (kĕr′ə-tī′tĭs) N. inflammation of the cornea that produces watery, painful eyes and blurred vision; it may be caused by irritation, as from exposure to dust or certain vapors, or by infection.

keratoacanthoma (kĕr′ə-tō-ăk′ən-thō′mə) N. keratin-containing skin nodule, most often occurring on the face, hands, or arms; it usually disappears spontaneously, often leaving a scar.

keratocoele N. hernia of the cornea.

keratoconjunctivitis (kĕr′ə-tō-kən-jŭngk′-tə-vī′tĭs) N. inflammation of the cornea and conjunctiva, tissues lining the eyelids and covering the front of the eyeball.

keratoconus (kĕr′ə-tō-kō′nəs) N. cone-shaped protrusion of the cornea; it may be treated by special contact lenses or by epikeratophakia.

keratoderma (kĕr′ə-tō-dûr′mə) N. any surface growth or covering that appears horny.

keratoiritis N. inflammation of the cornea and the iris.

keratomalacia (kĕr′ə-tō-mə-lā′shē-ə) N. softening, drying, and ulceration of the cornea, usually resulting from severe vitamin A deficiency in the diet or from a disease that impairs vitamin A absorption or storage in the body (e.g., cystic fibrosis; sprue).

keratomycosis N. fungus infection of the cornea.

keratonosis N. general term for any abnormal condition of the outer skin.

keratonosus N. general term for a disease of the cornea.

keratopathy (kĕr′ə-tŏp′ə-thē) N. any disease of the cornea without inflammation.

keratoplasty (kĕr′ə-tō-plăs′tē) N. surgical procedure in which diseased tissue of all or part of the cornea of the eye is replaced by healthy corneal tissue from a donor; corneal graft.

keratorhexis (kĕr′ə-tō-rĕk′sĭs) N. tear or break in the cornea.

keratoscleritis (kĕr′ə-tō-sklə-rī′tĭs) N. inflammation of the cornea and sclera.

keratoscopy (kĕr′ə-tŏs′kə-pē) N. examination of the cornea to detect abnormal curvature; a special instrument, called a keratoscope, is used to study light reflected from the front surface of the cornea.

keratosis (kĕr′ə-tō′sĭs) N., *pl.* keratoses, skin condition characterized by an overgrowth of horny skin layers. ADJ. keratotic

  actinic keratosis N. overgrowth of outer skin layers caused by long-term overexposure to the sun.

  keratosis follicularis N. uncommon hereditary disorder characterized by dark, sometimes purulent (containing pus) crusted patches. Treatment includes vitamin A orally and topically and sometimes corticosteroids.

  seborrheic keratosis N. condition marked by well-circumscribed wartlike lesions that are often itchy and covered with a greasy crust and occur most often on the face, neck, upper chest, and upper back. Treatment is by curettage, cryotherapy, or electrodesiccation.

kerion (kēr′ē-ŏn′) N. pustule-covered swelling that oozes fluid, caused by *Tinea capitas*, fungus infection of the scalp.

kernicterus (kûr-nĭk′tər-əs) N. abnormal accumulation of the bile pigment bilirubin (hyperbilirubinemia) in the brain and other nerve tissue, causing yellow staining and damage to the involved tissues. In newborns it may cause mental retardation and sensory and motor disturbances. *See also* HYPERBILIRUBINEMIA OF THE NEWBORN.

Kernig's sign (kûr′nĭgz) N. symptom of meningitis in which the patient is unable to extend the leg at the knee, when the thighs are held at right angles to the body, because of stiffness of the hamstring muscles.

keroid ADJ. hornlike or cornea-like.

Ketalar N. trade name for the general anesthetic ketamine hydrochloride.

ketamine hydrochloride (kē′tə-mēn′ hī′drə-klôr′īd′) N. nonbarbiturate general anesthetic (trade name Ketalar) that does not cause complete muscle relaxation and is used mainly for brief, minor surgical procedures and for pediatric and geriatric patients. On emergence from anesthesia, hallucinations, delirium, and other psychological signs may occur; increased blood pressure and intracranial pressure are also sometimes found.

ketoacidosis (kē'tō-ăs'ĭ-do'sĭs) N. acidosis with an accumulation of ketone bodies, occurring primarily as a complication of uncontrolled diabetes mellitus. It is characterized by a fruity breath odor, nausea and vomiting, shortness of breath, mental confusion, and, if untreated, coma (diabetic coma). Treatment includes the administration of insulin and fluids and the correction of electrolyte imbalance. (*Compare* INSULIN SHOCK.) ADJ. ketoacidotic

ketoaciduria (kē'tō-ăs'ĭ-dŏo'rē-ə) *See* KETONURIA.

ketone (kē'tōn') N. any of a group of organic chemicals derived by oxidation of alcohol and containing a carbon-oxygen group. Among the ketones are acetone and acetoacetic acid.

ketone bodies N. products (acetone, B-hydroxybutyric acid, and acetoacetic acid) of the breakdown of fats in the body. Excessive fat metabolism and production of ketone bodies lead to their excretion in urine, as in uncontrolled diabetes mellitus.

ketonemia (kē'tə-nē'mē-ə) N. abnormally high levels of ketone bodies in the blood, as in uncontrolled diabetes mellitus.

ketonuria (kē'tə-nŏor'ē-ə) N. excessive amounts of ketone bodies in the urine; it is usually the result of uncontrolled diabetes mellitus, starvation, or metabolic disorder affecting fat metabolism; also called ketoaciduria.

ketoprofen N. nonsteroidal anti-inflammatory agent (trade name Orudis) used in the treatment of osteoarthritis, rheumatoid arthritis, and other inflammatory conditions. Adverse effects include gastrointestinal bleeding and nausea.

ketorolac tromethamine N. nonsteroidal, anti-inflammatory agent (trade name Toradol) used either orally or parenterally to treat moderate to severe pain. Potential side effects include gastritis, intestinal bleeding, exacerbation of asthma, and hyperkalemia.

ketosis (kē-tō'sĭs) N. abnormal accumulation of ketones in the body, resulting from inadequate intake or metabolism of carbohydrates and increased fatty acid metabolism, leading to the formation of ketone bodies. Ketosis occurs most often in starvation and uncontrolled diabetes mellitus. It is characterized by a fruity breath odor and the presence of ketone bodies in the urine; if untreated, it can lead to ketoacidosis, coma, and death.

kidney N. either of two bean-shaped excretory organs that filter wastes (esp. urea) from the blood and excrete them and water in urine and help to regulate the water, electrolyte, and pH balance of the body. The kidneys are located in the dorsal part of the abdominal cavity, one on each side of the vertebral

URINARY SYSTEM

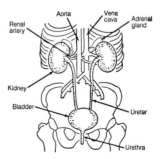

STRUCTURE OF THE KIDNEY

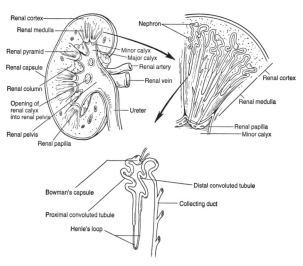

column. Each kidney, about 11 centimeters (4.5 inches) long, 6 centimeters (2.5 inches) wide and 2.5 centimeters (1 inch) thick, consists of an outer cortex and inner medulla and contains one million or more filtering units, called nephrons. Blood passes through tufts of capillaries (glomeruli) in the nephrons, where it is filtered; the filtrate then passes through renal tubules, where some substances (e.g., sugar, some salts) are selectively reabsorbed, into collecting ducts. The final product—known as urine—passes out of the kidney through tubes known as ureters and is carried to the bladder. The function of the kidney is controlled by hormones, esp. the antidiuretic hormone produced by the pituitary gland. The kidney is subject to inflammation, infection, the formation of stones (urinary calculi), and other disorders.

kidney failure *See* RENAL FAILURE.

kidney stone *See* URINARY CALCULUS.

kilo- prefix meaning one thousand of a given unit (e.g., kilogram, 1,000 grams).

kinanesthesia (kĭn'ăn-ĭs-thē'zhə) N. inability to sense movement.

kine-, kinesio- comb. forms indicating an association with movement, esp. body movement and muscle action (e.g., kinesalgia, pain from muscle action).

kinematics N. study of motion, including flexion, abduction, and adduction; it is important in orthopedics and rehabilitation medicine (*compare* KINETICS).

kinesiology (kə-nē'sē-ŏl'ə-jē) N. study of muscular activity and the anatomy, physiology, and mechanics of the movement of the body and its parts.

kinesthesia (kĭn'ĭs-thē'zhə) N. perception of body position and movement. ADJ. kinesthetic

kinetics (kə-nĕt'ĭks) N. study of motion, including the forces producing and modifying motion (*compare* KINEMATICS).

kinetosis N. illness or abnormality caused by movement (e.g., airsickness, carsickness).

kinin (kī'nĭn) N. group of large protein molecules that influence the contraction of smooth muscle. The result may be low blood pressure, pain, or changes in normal blood flow.

kissing disease *See* INFECTIOUS MONONUCLEOSIS.

klebsiella (klĕb'zē-ĕl'ə) N. gram-negative bacteria, some of which cause respiratory infections (e.g., bronchitis, pneumonia) and infections affecting other parts of the body.

kleptomania (klĕp'tə-mā'nē-ə) N. compulsion to steal. The objects are usually taken, not for their monetary value or need, but for their symbolic meaning associated with some emotional conflict; they are often returned or hidden. Treatment usually involves psychotherapy to uncover the underlying emotional problems.

Klinefelter's syndrome (klīn'fĕl' tərz) N. defect in which at least one extra X chromosome (XXY) is present in a male (normally XY) and that is characterized by small testes, enlarged breasts, long legs, decreased or absent sperm production, and mental retardation. Persons with more than one extra X (e.g., XXXY) usually show marked physical and mental abnormalities.

Klonopin N. *See* TABLE OF COMMONLY PRESCRIBED DRUGS—TRADE NAMES.

K-lor, Klorvess, K-lyte/Cl N. trade names for a potassium chloride solution used to treat electrolyte imbalances.

Klor-Con N. *See* TABLE OF COMMONLY PRESCRIBED DRUGS—TRADE NAMES.

knee N. joint complex, fronted by the kneecap (patella), at which the thighbone (femur) and lower leg connect. It includes joints at which the femur and tibia (a lower leg bone) meet, a joint where the femur and patella meet, and numerous ligaments and bursae.

knee joint N. hinged joint made up of three articulations: two at which the femur (thighbone) and tibia (a lower leg bone) meet and one at which the femur and patella (kneecap) meet.

KNEE JOINT

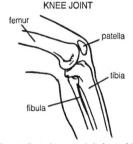

femur
patella
tibia
fibula

The patella, or kneecap, is in front of the articulation of the femur with the lower leg bones—the tibia and fibula.

kneecap *See* PATELLA.

knee-jerk reflex N. *See* PATELLAR REFLEX.

knock-knee N. condition in which the legs are curved inward so that the knees are close together and the ankles far apart as the person stands or walks; also called genu valgum.

knuckle N. joints of the fingers, esp. the joints where the fingers attach to the main part of the hand.

koilonychia N. condition in which the nails are thin and concave (spoon-shaped), sometimes associated with iron-deficiency anemia.

Koplik's spots N. small red spots with bluish white centers found on the mucous membrane of the mouth and tongue and characteristic of measles, usually appearing 1 or 2 days before the measles rash.

Korsakoff's psychosis (syndrome) (kôr′sə-kôfs′) N. condition, occurring most often in chronic alcoholics, marked by disorientation, impaired memory, and other mental abnormalities. It is thought to be due to degenerative changes in the thalamus of the brain caused by vitamin B deficiency associated with excessive alcohol intake. Treatment includes adequate nutrition and the administration of vitamins, esp. B complex vitamins. (*Compare* WERNICKE'S ENCEPHALOPATHY.)

kraurosis (krô-rō′sĭs) N. drying, thickening, and shriveling of the skin, esp. that of the external genitalia of a woman (kraurosis vulvae).

Krebs cycle (krĕbz) N. complex sequence of enzyme-catalyzed reactions occurring in cells, through which sugars, fatty acids, and amino acids are broken down to produce carbon dioxide and high-energy electrons linked to coenzymes. The electrons carried by the coenzymes then enter the electron transport system, which generates a large quantity of adenosine triphosphate (ATP). Also called Krebs citric acid cycle; tricarboxylic acid (TCA) cycle. *See also* ELECTRON TRANSPORT SYSTEM.

Kupffer's cells (ko͝op′fər) N. specialized cells found in the liver that destroy bacteria, foreign proteins, and worn-out blood cells.

kuru (ko͝or′o͞o) N. progressive disease of the central nervous system characterized by tremors and increasing lack of coordination and leading to paralysis and death, usually within a year after the onset of symptoms. The disease, known only among the Fore people of New Guinea, is thought to be caused by a prion, an abnormal form of a normal protein known as a cellular prion protein, and to have been transmitted through cannibalistic practices in which the diseased brain tissue of the dead was eaten or wiped on the body; with the abandonment of cannibalism the disease has now virtually disappeared. *See also* CREUTZFELDT-JAKOB DISEASE; PRION.

kwashiorkor (kwä′shē-ôr′kôr′) N. disease, primarily of children, caused by a severe protein deficiency; it is characterized by retarded growth, changes in skin and hair coloring, loss of appetite, diarrhea, anemia, degenerative changes in the liver, edema, and signs of multiple vitamin deficiencies.

Kwell N. trade name for a drug, available in lotion and shampoo form, used to kill lice and itch mites.

kyphosis (kī-fō′sĭs) N. abnormality of the vertebral column in which there is increased convex curvature in the upper spine, giving a hunchback or humped back appearance. Mild cases are often self-limiting and asymptomatic; severe or progressive cases may cause back pain and are sometimes treated with special back braces. Also called humpback. (*Compare* LORDOSIS; SCOLIOSIS.) ADJ. kyphotic

L

labetalol (lə-bĕt′ə-lôl′) N. oral/parenteral antihypertensive (trade names Trandate and Normodyne) that blocks receptors (alpha and beta) of the sympathetic nervous system, leading to a decrease in blood pressure. Although the drug is usually well tolerated, excessive hypotension can occur after intravenous administration.

labia majora (mə-jôr′ə) N., *sing.* labium majus, two long folds of skin that form the outer and larger lips of the external female genitalia, one on each side of the vaginal opening outside the labia minora; in some women the outer surface of the labia majora is covered with pubic hair.

labia minora (mə-nôr′ə) N., *sing.* labium minus, two folds of skin that form the inner smaller lips of the female genitalia, extending from the clitoris backwards on each side of the vaginal opening, inside the labia majora.

labile ADJ. unstable; tending to change. N. lability

labio- comb. form indicating an association with the lips or liplike structures (e.g., labiodental, pert. to the lips and teeth).

labium (lā′bē-əm) N., *pl.* labia, liplike edge or liplike structure, esp. the structures (labia majora and labia minora) enclosing the vulva. ADJ. labial

labor N. process by which a baby is born and the placenta is expelled from the uterus. Labor has three stages: the first, or stage of dilation, characterized by contractions of the uterine wall and dilatation of the opening of the cervix; the second, or stage of expulsion, during which the baby is born; and the third, or afterbirth stage, in which the placenta is expelled. The average duration of labor is about 13 hours in first pregnancies (12 hours in first stage, 1 hour in second, few minutes in third) and about 8 hours in subsequent pregnancies. *See also* BRAXTON-HICKS CONTRACTIONS.

labor coach N. person (often the father) who assists a woman in labor by providing emotional support and encouragement to use breathing, concentration, and exercise techniques learned in childbirth-preparation classes; also called monitrice. *See also* BRADLEY METHOD OF CHILDBIRTH; LAMAZE METHOD OF CHILDBIRTH.

labor pain N. discomfort and pain caused by contractions of the uterus.

labrum (lā′brəm) N., *pl.* labra, lip edge or liplike structure (e.g., labrum glenoidule, cartilage of the glenoid cavity in the shoulder).

labyrinth (lăb′ə-rĭnth′) N. intricate communicating channels of the inner ear where the sense of equilibrium originates. The bony labyrinth is a space in the temporal bone containing the semicircular canals, vestibule, and cochlea. Movement of the

LABYRINTH

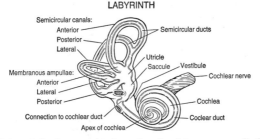

Semicircular canals:
Anterior
Posterior
Lateral
Membranous ampullae:
Anterior
Lateral
Posterior
Connection to cochlear duct
Apex of cochlea
Semicircular ducts
Utricle
Saccule Vestibule
Cochlear nerve
Cochlea
Coclear duct

endolymph in the semicircular canals stimulates hair cells in the ampullae, and the stimulations are sent to the brain, which sends impulses to the muscles to adjust body movements. ADJ. labyrinthine

labyrinthitis (lăb′ə-rĭn-thī′tĭs) N. inflammation of the inner ear; it usually produces vertigo, loss of balance, and vomiting; also called otitis interna.

laceration (lăs′ə-rā′shən) N. wound with a jagged edge, resulting from a tearing or scraping action. V. lacerate

lacrimal (lăk′rə-məl) ADJ. pert. to tears.

lacrimal apparatus N. structures that secrete and drain tears from the eye. Tears produced in the lacrimal gland drain through small openings at the corner of the eye into special ducts that pass into the nasal cavity.

LACRIMAL APPARATUS

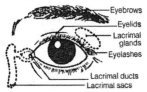

Eyebrows
Eyelids
Lacrimal glands
Eyelashes
Lacrimal ducts
Lacrimal sacs

From the lacrimal glands, tears drain through the lacrimal ducts and lacrimal sacs into the nasal passageways.

lacrimal bone N. small, fragile facial bone located at the inner part of the orbital cavity.

lacrimal gland N. either of two oval-shaped structures (exocrine glands) located on the upper outer side of the eye that secrete tears that moisten the conjunctiva of the eye.

lacrimal sac N. either of two oval-shaped dilated ends of the nasolacrimal duct that fill with tears secreted by the lacrimal glands.

lacrimation (lăk′rə-mā′shən) N. 1. normal continuous secretion of tears by the lacrimal glands. 2. copious tear production, as in weeping.

lactalbumin (lăk′tăl-byo͞o′mĭn) N. protein found in milk.

lactase N. enzyme secreted by glands in the small intestine that converts lactose (milk sugar) into simpler sugars.

lactase deficiency N. abnormality in which a deficiency in the amount of the enzyme lactase results in an inability to digest lactose (milk sugar). It is usually congenital, more common in people of Asian and African heritage, but may also result from gastrectomy, disease of the small intestine, or certain other disorders. *See also* LACTOSE INTOLERANCE.

lactation (lăk-tā′shən) N.
1. synthesis and secretion of milk by the mammary glands of the breast.
2. time during which an infant or child is nourished with breast milk. ADJ. lactational

lacteal (lăk′tē-əl) N. lymph channel in the villi of the small intestine that absorbs digested fat (chyle).

lactic ADJ. pert. to milk.

lactic acid N.
1. chemical formed by the process of glycolysis; during strenuous exercise it may accumulate in muscle cells.
2. acid formed by the action of certain bacteria on milk and milk products.

lactiferous (lăk-tĭf′ər-əs) ADJ. pert. to a structure that produces and/or conveys milk, as the lactiferous ducts of the breast.

lactiferous duct N. any of several ducts that transport milk from the lobes of the breast to the nipple.

lactifuge N. agent that reduces milk secretion (e.g., a drug given to suppress milk production in a woman who is not breast feeding).

lactogen N. drug or other substance that enhances milk production. ADJ. lactogenic

lactogenic hormone (lăk′tə-jĕn′ĭk) See PROLACTIN.

lactose (lăk′tōs) N. sugar (made up of glucose and galactose) found only in milk; it is split into its constituent sugars by the enzyme lactase.

lactose intolerance N. disorder, due to a defect or deficiency of the enzyme lactase, resulting in an inability to digest lactose and symptoms of bloating, flatulence, abdominal discomfort, nausea, and diarrhea on ingestion of milk and milk products. See also LACTASE DEFICIENCY.

lactosuria N. presence of milk in the urine, occurring during pregnancy or lactation.

lacuna (lə-kyōō′nə) N., pl. lacunae, small hollow or cavity in or between body parts, esp. a cartilage-filled depression in bone. ADJ. lacunar

laetrile (lā′ĭ-trĭl′) N. chemical (amygdalin), derived from the seeds of apricots, plums, and some other fruits, that, when taken into the body, causes cyanide production. It has been publicized as a treatment for cancer, but there is no evidence that it is therapeutic.

lagophthalmos (lăg′ŏf-thăl′mŏs′) N. abnormal condition in which an eye cannot be closed completely, because of disorder of the cornea or neurological or muscular disorder.

lal-, lalio-, lalo- comb. forms indicating a relationship with speech (e.g., lalopathy, a speech disorder).

lallation N.
1. unintelligible speechlike utterances, as the babbling of an infant.
2. speech disorder in which the sound "l" is used in place of other sounds, esp. "r," or is mispronounced (compare LAMBDACISM).

Lamarckism N. theory of evolution, postulated by Jean Baptiste Lamarck in the 19th century, that holds that adaptations to environmental conditions lead to structural changes in organisms, through the increased use or disuse of certain parts, and that these acquired characteristics are then transmitted to the offspring. ADJ. Lamarckian

Lamaze method of childbirth (lə-mäz′) N. method of psycho-physical preparation for child-birth, developed by the French obstetrician Fernand Lamaze in the 1950s, that is now the most widely used method of natural childbirth. In classes during pregnancy and in practice ses-sions at home, the pregnant woman, usually with the help of a coach (called a monitrice), learns the physiology of preg-nancy and childbirth and tech-niques of relaxation, concentra-tion, and breathing, and exercises certain muscles to promote con-trol during labor and childbirth. (*Compare* BRADLEY METHOD OF CHILDBIRTH; READ METHOD OF CHILDBIRTH.)

lambdacism N. speech disorder marked by incorrect or exces-sive pronunciation of the sound "l" or substitution of the sound "r" for "l" (*compare* LALLATION).

lamella (lə-mĕl′ə) N., *pl.* lamel-lae, any platelike part, as a bone. ADJ. lamellar

lamina (lăm′ə-nə) N., *pl.* lami-nae, thin membrane or platelike structure, as the two parts of a vertebra that join to hold the spinous process of the vertebra over the spinal cord. ADJ. lam-inar

laminectomy (lăm′ə-nĕk′tə-mē) N. surgical procedure in which the bony arches (laminae) of one or more vertebrae are chipped or removed to relieve pressure on the spinal cord, to remove tumors, or to treat disorders in-volving the vertebral column (e.g., ruptured intervertebral disk).

lance v. to pierce, open, or cut into, as a boil for drainage.

lancinating ADJ. cutting, sharp, knifelike, as in lancinating pain.

landmark N. recognizable ana-tomic structure used as a refer-ence point to measure or describe physical findings or other anatomic structures.

Lanoxin N. trade name for the car-diac drug digoxin. *See* TABLE OF COMMONLY PRESCRIBED DRUGS—TRADE NAMES.

lansoprazole N. *See* TABLE OF COMMONLY PRESCRIBED DRUGS —GENERIC NAMES.

lanugo (lə-noō′gō) N. fine, downy hair covering a fetus; it is nor-mally shed during the ninth month of gestation but may be present on newborns, esp. pre-mature newborns.

laparo- comb. form indicating an association with the abdomen, loin, or flank (e.g., laparocele, a hernia through the abdomen).

laparoscopy (lăp′ə-rŏs′kə-pē) N. examination of the abdominal cavity, esp. the ovaries and Fal-lopian tubes, through a laparo-scope (a type of endoscope) introduced through a small in-cision in the abdominal wall; also used in women as a steril-ization procedure in which the fallopian tubes are ligated.

laparotomy (lăp′ə-rŏt′ə-mē) N. any surgical procedure in which an incision is made into the abdominal wall, often done for exploration (e.g., to examine abdominal organs).

large intestine N. that portion of the digestive tract containing the cecum; appendix; ascend-ing, transverse, and descending colons; and the rectum.

Larodopa N. trade name for lev-odopa.

LARGE INTESTINE

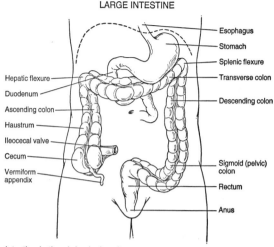

Large intestine in the abdominal cavity.

Larotid N. trade name for the antibacterial amoxicillin.

larva (lär-və) N. the early form or first stage of an insect during its development. *pl.* larvae

laryngectomy (lăr′ən-jĕk′tə-mē) N. surgical removal of all or part of the larynx, usually performed to treat carcinoma of the larynx. After a laryngectomy a person must learn esophageal speech or use artificial means for speaking.

laryngismus (lăr′ĭn-jĭz′məs) N. spasm of the larynx caused by sudden contraction of the laryngeal muscles, often marked by sudden and noisy indrawing of breath, sometimes associated with croup or irritation of the larynx (e.g., from inhaled anesthetic or a foreign body).

laryngitis (lăr′ĭn-jī′tĭs) N. inflammation of the mucous membrane of the larynx and swelling of the vocal cords, characterized by loss or hoarseness of voice, cough, and sometimes difficult breathing. It may be acute, caused by bacterial or viral infection or irritation (e.g., from irritating fumes); or chronic, from excessive use of the voice, excessive smoking, or long-term exposure to irritants. Treatment depends on the cause, but usually includes rest of the voice, a moist atmosphere, and the avoidance of irritants. (In young children spasm of the larynx and difficulty in breathing may result.)

laryngo- comb. form indicating an association with the larynx (e.g., laryngostenosis, narrowing of the larynx).

laryngopharyngeal ADJ. pert. to the larynx and pharynx.

laryngopharyngitis (lə-rĭng′gō-făr ĭn-jī′tĭs) N. inflammation of the larynx and pharynx.

LARYNX

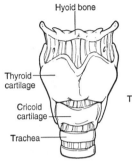

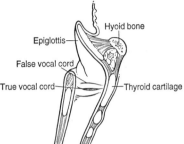

laryngoscope (lə-rĭng'gə-skōp') N. instrument for examining the larynx.

laryngospasm (lə-rĭng'gə-spăz'əm) N. closure of the larynx that blocks the passage of air to the lungs; usually associated with severe allergic reaction or severe laryngeal inflammation, esp. in young children.

laryngotracheobronchitis (lə-rĭng'gō-trā'kē-ō-brŏn-kī'tĭs) N. inflammation of the larynx, trachea, and bronchial passageways; it may be caused by bacterial or viral infection and is characterized by hoarseness, difficulty in breathing, and cough. Treatment depends on the cause; it may include steam inhalation, cough suppressants, and antibiotics, if indicated.

larynx (lăr'ĭngks) N. organ that contains the vocal cords and is responsible for sound production; it is part of the air passageway connecting the pharynx and the trachea, and it produces a bump—the Adam's apple—in front of the neck, also called voice box. ADJ. laryngeal

laser N. acronym for Light Amplification by Stimulated Emission of Radiation; an instrument that produces a very thin beam of light—of one wavelength—with radiation intense enough to be used surgically to destroy tissue or to separate parts.

Lasix N. trade name for the diuretic furosemide. *See* TABLE OF COMMONLY PRESCRIBED DRUGS—TRADE NAMES.

lassa fever (lăs'ə) N. highly contagious viral disease, largely confined to central West Africa; it is characterized by fever, inflammation of the pharynx, difficulty in swallowing, and bruises, frequently with the complication of renal failure leading to cardiac failure and death.

latanoprost N. *See* TABLE OF COMMONLY PRESCRIBED DRUGS—GENERIC NAMES.

latency phase (lāt'n-sē) N. in psychoanalytic theory, the fourth stage in a person's development, generally between the ages of 6 and puberty, during which the sex drive is not active, but is sublimated into other activities (*compare*

ORAL PHASE; ANAL PHASE; PHALLIC PHASE; GENITAL PHASE).

latent (lāt′nt) ADJ. dormant; existing as a potential (e.g., latent diabetes, mild disorder of carbohydrate metabolism occurring only when stress loads of glucose are given).

latent schizophrenia (skĭt′sə-frē′nē-ə) N. form of schizophrenia characterized by mild symptoms and/or a preexisting tendency to the disease in its usual form; also called borderline schizophrenia.

lateral ADJ. pert. to a side; away from the center plane, as the cheeks are lateral to the nose.

latero- comb. form indicating an association with the side of something (e.g., lateroabdominal, at or toward the side of the abdomen).

laughing gas *See* NITROUS OXIDE.

lavage (lăv′ĭj) N. process of washing out an organ, esp. the stomach (gastric lavage), bladder, or paranasal sinuses. *See also* IRRIGATION.

law N. in science, reliable principle, standard, relationship, or observation; a fact. *See also* ALL-OR-NONE-LAW.

laxation N. bowel movement.

laxative N. agent that promotes evacuation of the bowel, esp. fluid evacuation, by stimulating peristalsis (e.g., senna, aloe products); by increasing the bulk or fluidity of the feces (e.g., magnesium sulfate, magnesium hydroxide); or by lubricating the intestinal wall (e.g., mineral oil); also called cathartic; purgative.

layer N. thin, sheet-like structure composed of a single thickness, often of cells.

LDL N. abbrev. for low density lipoprotein.

L-Dopa *See* LEVODOPA.

LE *See* SYSTEMIC LUPUS ERYTHEMATOSUS.

lead N.
1. metallic element. (*See also* TABLE OF IMPORTANT ELEMENTS; LEAD POISONING.)
2. connection attached to the body to record electrical activity, as in an electrocardiograph or electroencephalograph.

lead poisoning N. toxic condition caused by inhaling or ingesting lead or lead compounds (e.g., in some paints). Acute poisoning causes gastrointestinal disturbances, mental disturbances, and paralysis of the extremities, sometimes followed by convulsions and collapse. Chronic poisoning causes irritability, anorexia and anemia, and often progresses to produce acute symptoms. Treatment is by chelation. Also called plumbism.

leaflet N. thin triangular flap of a heart valve, such as a mitral valve leaflet.

learning disability N. any of several abnormal conditions of children and adults who, although having at least average intelligence, have difficulty in learning specific skills, e.g., reading (dyslexia) or writing (dysgraphia) or have other problems associated with normal learning procedures. It may result from psychological or organic causes or from slow development of motor skills, but in many cases the cause is unknown. *See also* ATTENTION DEFICIT DISORDER.

Leboyer method of childbirth N. approach to childbirth, formulated by the French obstetrician

Charles Leboyer, that aims to minimize the trauma of birth and to provide as gentle and pleasant an introduction to life outside the uterus as possible for the newborn. Delivery typically occurs in a quiet, dimly lit room; the infant's head is not pulled, the infant is not overstimulated in any way, and immediate maternal-infant bonding is encouraged. (*Compare* BRADLEY METHOD OF CHILDBIRTH; LAMAZE METHOD OF CHILDBIRTH; READ METHOD OF CHILDBIRTH; *see also* NATURAL CHILDBIRTH.)

lecithin (lĕs'ə-thĭn) N. any of a group of phospholipids essential for the metabolism of fats; a deficiency leads to liver and kidney disorders, high serum cholesterol levels, and atherosclerosis. Rich food sources include egg yolk, corn, and soybeans. Lecithins are also used in the processing of foods, drugs, and cosmetics.

leech (lēch) N. worm, some species of which are parasitic, sucking blood from humans and other animals. Leeches were once commonly used in medicine for blood-letting.

left atrioventricular valve (ā'trē-ō-vĕn-trĭk'-yə-lər) *See* MITRAL VALVE.

left-handedness N. tendency to prefer use of the left hand in performing tasks (e.g., writing, grasping, throwing); also called sinistrality.

leg N. supporting limb; in humans either of the lower extremities, including the femur, patella, tibia, and fibula bones; specifically, the lower leg, from the ankle to the knee and including the tibia and fibula.

Legionnaire's disease (lē'jə-nârz') N. acute pneumonia caused by the bacterium *Legionella pneumophilia;* symptoms include muscle pain, fever, cough, chills, and chest pain. Treatment is by erythromycin.

leio- comb. form indicating an association with smoothness (e.g., leiodermia, smooth, glossy skin).

leiomyoma (lī'ō-mī-ō'mə) N. benign tumor of smooth muscle, most often occurring in the uterus (leiomyofibroma) or digestive tract.

leiomyosarcoma N. malignant tumor of smooth muscle, occurring most often in the bladder, prostate, uterus, or digestive tract.

Leishmaniasis (lēsh'mə-nī'ə-sĭs) N. infection, most common in warm climates, with protozoa of the genus Leishmania; it occurs in two forms: visceral (*see also* KALA-AZAR) and cutaneous, affecting skin tissues (*see also* ORIENTAL SORE). Treatment often involves the use of antibiotic agents.

lens N.
1. in anatomy, transparent crystalline structure of the eye, behind the pupil, that helps to focus light onto the retina. (In a cataract, the lens becomes cloudy.)
2. transparent material—glass or plastic—that is ground and shaped to refract light in a certain way; used in eyeglasses, contact lenses, microscopes, and cameras. *See also* CONTACT LENS; LENS IMPLANT.

lens implant N. artificial clear plastic lens implanted in the eye, usually when the natural lens has been removed because of a cataract but sometimes to treat other eye abnormalities.

Lente insulin N. trade name for an insulin preparation used in the treatment of diabetes mellitus.

lentigo (lĕn-tī′gō) N., *pl.* lentigines, brown, roundish flat spot on the skin, often the result of exposure to the sun.

leontiasis N. condition in which a person has a somewhat lionlike facial expression or head structure; occurs in some diseases (e.g., leprosy).

leper N. person who has leprosy.

leprosy (lĕp′rə-sē) N. chronic, communicable disease, caused by *Mycobacterium leprae,* that is widespread throughout the world, chiefly in tropical and subtropical regions. In tuberculoid leprosy, tumorlike changes occur in the skin and cutaneous nerves; in the more serious and progressive lepromatous leprosy, lesions spread over much of the body with widespread nerve involvement affecting many systems of the body. Treatment usually involves the use of sulfones (esp. dapsone); a vaccine with promising results is also being used. Also called Hansen's disease. ADJ. leprous

-lepsia, -lepsis, -lepsy comb. forms indicating an association with seizures (e.g., epilepsy).

leptin N. protein hormone produced by adipose (fat) tissue. Its concentration in the body provides the brain with a rough indication of the body's fat mass for the purposes of regulating appetite and metabolism. Binds to brain receptors, resulting in suppression of anabolic circuits and activation of catabolic circuits, causing decreased food intake and increased energy expenditure. Frank deficiencies in leptin secretion are a rare cause of human obesity. Blood concentrations of leptin are usually increased in obese humans, suggesting that they are in some way insensitive to it, rather than suffering from leptin deficiency. Thus, exogenous administration of leptin as a weight-loss technique have generally failed. Leptin also plays a role in female puberty, which will not usually occur until an adequate body mass is present. This may explain why very low body fat in human females is often associated with cessation of menstrual cycles. *See also* ANABOLISM; CATABOLISM.

lepto- comb. form meaning thin, narrow, fragile (e.g., leptocephaly, abnormally narrow head).

leptomeninges (lĕp′tō-mə-nĭn′jēz) N. arachnoid membrane and pia mater, the inner two of the three layers covering the brain and spinal cord. *See also* MENINGES.

leptomeningitis (lĕp′tō-mĕn′ĭn-jī′tĭs) N. inflammation of the leptomeninges.

leptons N. one of the two groups of matter particles. There are six types of leptons, all exist in pairs, each pair consisting of an electrically charged particle and a neutrino. The best-known pair is the electron and the electron neutrino. Leptons are subject to the electromagnetic and weak interactions. *See also* ATOM (*compare* QUARK).

leptospirosis (lĕp′tō-spī-rō′sĭs) N. infection caused by the spirochete *Leptospira interrogans,* transmitted to humans from infected animals (esp. dogs and rats), often from their urine. Symptoms include chills, fever, muscle pain, and jaundice. Treatment is by antibiotics, and most cases are mild, but severe cases (Weil's disease) can cause liver and kidney damage.

leresis N. talkativeness, rambling speech, esp. in the aged.

lesbian (lĕz′bē-ən) N. female homosexual; female whose sexual preference is for other women.

lesbianism (lĕz′bē-ə-nĭz′əm) N. sexual preference by a woman for other women.

Lescol N. *See* TABLE OF COMMONLY PRESCRIBED DRUGS—TRADE NAMES.

lesion (lē′zhən) N. general term for any visible, local abnormality of tissue (e.g., an injury, wound, boil, sore, rash).

let-down N. sensation in the breasts of nursing women as the milk flows into the ducts of the breast, as when the infant begins to suck or when the mother prepares to nurse; also called milk-ejection reflex.

lethal ((lē′thəl) ADJ. pert. to or causing death.

lethal dose N. amount of a drug that will cause death.

lethal gene N. any gene that produces an effect that causes the death of the organism at any stage, from fertilized egg to advanced age. The gene that causes Huntington's chorea is an example of a lethal gene.

lethargy (lĕth′ər-jē) N. state of sluggishness, apathy, unresponsiveness; found in certain diseases (e.g., sleeping sickness).

leucine (loō′sēn′) N. amino acid, obtained by the digestion of proteins, that is essential for growth.

leukemia (loō-kē′mē-ə) N. one of the major types of cancer, malignant neoplasm of blood-forming tissues, characterized by abnormalities of the bone marrow, spleen, lymph nodes, and liver and by rapid and uncontrolled proliferation of abnormal numbers and forms of leukocytes (white blood cells). Leukemia may be acute, rapidly progressing from signs of fatigue and weight loss to extreme weakness, repeated infections, and fever, or it may be chronic, progressing slowly over a period of years. Leukemia is usually classified according to the type of white blood cell that is proliferating abnormally. Treatment involves chemotherapy, blood transfusions, antibiotics to control infections, and, sometimes, bone

THE THREE TYPES OF BLOOD CELLS

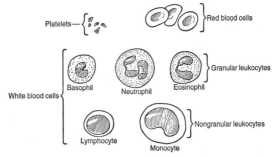

Platelets—

Red blood cells

White blood cells

Basophil Neutrophil Eosinophil } Granular leukocytes

Lymphocyte Monocyte } Nongranular leukocytes

MICROSCOPIC APPEARANCE OF LEUKOCYTES
AFTER WRIGHT'S STAINING

Leukocytes	Appearance
Granulocytes	
Neutrophils	Fine, light-blue cytoplasmic granules; 3- to 5-lobed nucleus
Eosinophils	Bright-red cytoplasmic granules; 2-lobed nucleus
Basophils	Large, dark purplish-blue cytoplasmic granules; irregular nucleus; often S-shaped
Agranulocytes	
Lymphocytes	Thin layer of nongranular, blue cytoplasm; large, bright purple nucleus
Monocytes	Thick layer of nongranular cytoplasm; large horseshoe- or kidney-shaped, purple nuclei

marrow transplants. Also called cancer of the blood. (*See also* ACUTE MYELOCYTIC LEUKEMIA; ACUTE LYMPHOID LEUKEMIA; CHRONIC LYMPHOCYTIC LEUKEMIA; CHRONIC MYELOCYTIC LEUKEMIA.) ADJ. leukemic

Leukeran N. trade name for the antineoplastic chlorambucil.

leuko- comb. form indicating an association with white blood cells (e.g., leukopoiesis, development of white blood cells).

leukocyte (loo'kə-sīt') N. white blood cell (WBC). There are five types of leukocytes: three granulocytes with granules in the cytoplasm—neutrophils, basophils, and eosiniphils—and two agranulocytes, lacking granules in the cytoplasm—lymphocytes and monocytes. An important part of the body's defense mechanism, leukocytes phagocytose (engulf and digest) bacteria and fungi and function in allergic reactions and the response to cellular injury. Also called white blood cell; white corpuscle.

leukocytosis (loo'kə-sī-tō'-sĭs) N. abnormal increase in the number of leukocytes in the blood; it frequently occurs as a result of infection, esp. bacterial infection; a very large increase occurs in leukemia (*compare* LEUKOPENIA).

leukoderma (loo'kə-dûr'mə) N. loss of skin pigment in a localized area (*compare* VITILIGO).

leukoencephalitis (loo'kō-ĕn-sĕf'ə-lī'tĭs) N. inflammation of the white matter of the brain.

leukoma (loo-kō'mə) N. white opacity in the cornea of the eye, most often the result of corneal inflammation or ulceration but sometimes congenital; also called leucoma.

leukonychia (loo'kō-nĭk'ē-ə) N. white discoloration of the nails; it may result from trauma, certain systemic disorders, or unknown causes.

leukopenia (loo'kə-pē'nē-ə) N. abnormal decrease in the number of leukocytes in the blood, to fewer than 5,000 per cubic millimeter; it may affect one type or all types of white blood cells. Leukopenia may occur as an adverse drug reaction or as a result of radiation exposure, poisoning, or other abnormal condition (e.g., aplastic anemia). (*Compare* LEUKOCYTOSIS.) ADJ. leukopenic

leukoplakia (loō'kə-plā'kē-ə) N. thickened, white patches on mucous membranes, esp. those of the mouth region and genitalia; they can become malignant (*compare* LICHEN PLANUS).

leukopoiesis (loō'kō-poi-ē'sĭs) N. normal development and production of white blood cells (leukocytes) by the bone marrow.

leukorrhea N. whitish discharge from the vagina; it occurs normally, varying in amount during different phases of the menstrual cycle and during pregnancy, lactation, and after menopause. A large increase in amount or a change in color or odor usually indicates infection in the reproductive tract.

leukotomy (loō-kŏt'ə-mē) *See* lobotomy.

leukotrichia (loō'kə-trĭk'ē-ə) N. condition of having white hair.

Levaquin N. *See* TABLE OF COMMONLY PRESCRIBED DRUGS—TRADE NAMES.

levator (lə-vā'tər) N.
1. muscle that lifts or raises a structure (e.g., levator scapulae, which lifts the shoulder blade).
2. surgical instrument used to lift depressed bone fragments in a fracture.

levo- comb. form meaning left (e.g. levorotation, turning to the left) (*compare* DEXTRO-).

levodopa (L-Dopa) (lē'və-dō'pə) N. drug (trade names include Bendopa, Brocadopa, and Larodopa) used to treat parkinsonism. Adverse effects include anorexia, gastrointestinal disturbances, and movement disorders.

levofloxacin N. *See* TABLE OF COMMONLY PRESCRIBED DRUGS—GENERIC NAMES.

levothyroxine N. *See* TABLE OF COMMONLY PRESCRIBED DRUGS—GENERIC NAMES.

Levoxyl N. *See* TABLE OF COMMONLY PRESCRIBED DRUGS—TRADE NAMES.

levulose (lĕv'yə-lōs') *See* FRUCTOSE.

Leydig cells (lī'dĭg) N. cells in the testes that secrete the hormone testosterone.

LGV *See* LYMPHOGRANULOMA VENEREUM.

LH *See* LUTEINIZING HORMONE.

Li symbol for the element lithium.

libido (lĭ-bē'dō) N. sexual drive; in psychoanalytic theory, one of the major drives that is a source of energy.

Librax N. trade name for a fixed-combination drug containing the sedative chlordiazepoxide (Librium) and the anticholinergic clidinium, used to treat gastrointestinal spasm and discomfort.

Libritabs, Librium (lĭb'rē-əm) N. trade names for the antianxiety agent chlordiazepoxide.

lichen (lī'kən) N. any of several skin disorders characterized by thickened, hardened lesions grouped closely together.

lichen planus (lī'kən plā'nəs) N. skin disorder characterized by small, flat, purplish, usually itchy papules, occurring most often on the wrists, forearms, and thighs (*compare* LEUKOPLAKIA).

lichenification (lī-kĕn'ə-fĭ-kā'shən) N. thickening and hardening of skin, often resulting from scratching or irritation.

lidocaine (lī′də-kān′) N. local anesthetic agent (trade name Xylocaine) used topically on the skin and mucous membranes and parenterally to treat cardiac arrhythmia. Adverse effects from systemic use include cardiac arrest and central nervous system disturbances; from topical use, hypersensitivity reactions.

Lidosporin N. trade name for a fixed-combination drug containing the antibacterial polymyxin and the local anesthetic lidocaine, used to treat ear infections.

lien (lī′ən) *See* SPLEEN.

lieno- comb. form indicating an association with the spleen (e.g., lienocele, rupture of the spleen).

ligament (līg′ə-mənt) N. shiny, usually whitish, band of fibrous connective tissue that binds joints together and connects bones and cartilage (*compare* TENDON).

ligand N.
1. molecule or chemical bound to another chemical group or molecule; following a chemical reaction, the ligand typically emerges unchanged chemically.
2. general term for any molecule that binds any receptor anywhere in the body, leading to any biological effect. *See also* SIGNAL TRANSDUCTION.

ligation (lī-gā′shən) N. tying a blood vessel or duct with silk thread, wire, or other filament to prevent bleeding (e.g., during surgery) or to prevent passage of material through a duct (e.g., to prevent fertilization from occurring in the fallopian tube). *See also* TUBAL LIGATION.

ligature (līg′ə-chŏŏr′) N. filament (catgut), thread (silk), or wire (chromic) used to encircle a part to close it off (as a blood vessel) or to fasten or tie the part.

light adaptation N. reflex changes in the eye to allow vision in increased light (e.g., in normal light after being in the dark or in very bright light after being in normal light); it involves a contraction of the pupil so that less light enters (*compare* DARK ADAPTATION).

light diet N. diet consisting of easily digested foods, with avoidance of highly seasoned and fried foods, suitable for convalescent and bedridden persons.

light reflex *See* PUPILLARY REFLEX.

lightening N. descent of the uterus into the pelvic cavity occurring in late pregnancy; it leaves more room in the upper abdomen and changes the profile of the pregnant woman's abdomen. The fetus is said to have dropped.

limb N. extremity of the body; arm or leg.

limbic system (līm′bĭk) N. group of structures in the brain, including the hippocampus, cingulate gyrus, and amygdala, that is connected to and normally controlled by other parts of the brain (e.g., hypothalamus); the system is associated with emotions and feelings, such as anger, fear, and sexual arousal, but little is known about its function.

limbus (līm′bəs) N., *pl.* limbi, outer edge or border of a part (e.g., limbus corneae, edge where the cornea and sclera of the eye join). ADJ. limbal, limbic

line N., *pl.* lineae,
1. elongated mark or stripe on the body.

2. origin of an organism or cell (as in cell line); also called linea.

lingua (lĭng'gwə) N. *See* TONGUE. *pl.* linguae, ADJ. lingual

lingual (lĭng'gwəl) ADJ. pert. to the tongue (e.g., lingual artery, artery that supplies the tongue and surrounding area).

lingula N. tonguelike part, esp. lingula cerebelli, thin forward projection of the cerebellum of the brain.

linguo- comb. form indicating an association with the tongue (e.g., linguogingival, pert. to the tongue and gingiva).

liniment (lĭn'ə-mənt) N. preparation (usually containing an alcohol or oil) applied to the skin to relieve muscular discomfort.

linked genes N. genes located close together on the same chromosome that tend to be transmitted as a unit.

lip N.
1. soft external structures that form the top and bottom borders of the mouth cavity.
2. liplike enclosures of the vulva. *See* LABIA MAJORA, LABIA MINORA.
3. any liplike border of an organ or groove.

lipase (lĭp'ās') N. any of several enzymes, secreted in the digestive tract, that catalyze the breakdown of fats.

lipemia (lĭ-pē'mē-ə) N. abnormally high amount of fat in the blood.

lipid N. any of a group of greasy organic compounds, including fatty acids, waxes, phospholipids, and steroids. Lipids are stored in the body and serve as energy reserves.

lipidosis (lĭp'ĭ-dō'sĭs) N. any of several disorders of fat metabolism in which abnormal levels of certain lipids accumulate in the body. Among the disorders are Gaucher's disease, Niemann-Pick disease, and Tay-Sachs disease.

Lipitor N. *See* TABLE OF COMMONLY PRESCRIBED DRUGS—TRADE NAMES.

lipo- comb. form indicating an association with fats or lipids (e.g., lipopexia, accumulation of fat in body tissues).

lipofuscin (lĭp'ō-fŭs'ĭn) N. insoluble fatty pigment present in cardiac and smooth muscle cells; represents indigestible portions of cells that have been phagocytosed as a part of normal aging. Sometimes called the aging pigment, it has no direct harmful effects on the cell.

lipolysis (lĭ-pŏl'ĭ-sĭs) N. breakdown of fat by biochemical or physical means.

lipoma (lĭ-pō'mə) N. benign tumor consisting of fat cells; also called adipose tumor. ADJ. lipomatous

lipomatosis (lĭ-pō'mə-tō'sĭs) N. condition in which fat accumulates in tumorlike masses (lipomas) in the body.

lipophilic ADJ. having an affinity for fat; absorbing or easily dissolving in fat.

lipoprotein N. protein combined with a lipid; lipoproteins are found in blood plasma and lymph and transport lipids in the body.

liposarcoma (lĭp'ō-sär-kō'mə) N. malignant tumor of fat cells.

liposome (lĭp'ə-sōm') N. sealed shell formed when certain fatty substances are in a water-based solution. As it forms, the liposome traps part of the solution in the shell. Liposomes may be filled with a number of different substances and used to transport medications to specific organs.

liquefaction (lĭk´wǝ-făk´shǝn) N. conversion of solid tissue into a liquid or semi-liquid form; may be associated with normal cell turnover or tissue loss due to injury or disease.

liquid diet N. diet consisting of foods that can be served in liquid or strained form, plus custards, puddings, and similar foods. It is prescribed after certain types of surgery and in some infectious and inflammatory conditions.

liquor N. solution consisting of a medication dissolved in water; alcoholic beverage.

lisinopril N. one of a class of drugs that block the formation of angiotensin, leading to vasodilation. Sold under the trade names Prinivil and Zestril, it is used in the treatment of hypertension and congestive heart failure. Adverse effects include dizziness, headache, fatigue, and diarrhea. *See* TABLE OF COMMONLY PRESCRIBED DRUGS—GENERIC NAMES.

lisinopril/hydrochlorothiazide N. *See* TABLE OF COMMONLY PRESCRIBED DRUGS—GENERIC NAMES.

listeriosis N. infectious disease, caused by the bacterium *Listeria monocytogenes,* common in many animals and occasionally transmitted to humans, esp. newborns or immunosuppressed persons. In humans, it causes a dark red rash, enlargement of the spleen and liver, endocardi-

tis, fever, malaise, and other abnormalities, frequently progressing to meningitis and encephalitis. Treatment is by antibiotics.

Lithane N. trade name for a lithium preparation used to treat some forms of depression and bipolar disorder.

lithiasis (lĭ-thī´ǝ-sĭs) N. formation of stones (calculi) in an internal organ (e.g., the gallbladder or kidney) (*See also* CHOLELITHIASIS; URINARY CALCULUS). ADJ. lithiasic

lithium (lĭth´ē-ǝm) N. metallic element. *See also* TABLE OF IMPORTANT ELEMENTS, LITHIUM CARBONATE.

lithium carbonate N. drug (trade names Lithane and Eskalith) used to treat manic episodes of bipolar (manic-depressive) disorder. Adverse effects include kidney damage, salt and water retention, and sometimes disturbances in mental and muscular functioning.

Lithonate N. trade name for lithium carbonate.

lithotomy (lĭ-thŏt´ǝ-mē) N. surgical removal of a stone (calculus) esp. from the urinary tract.

lithotomy position N. position in which the person lies on his/her back with knees bent, thighs spread and rotated outward; used for a vaginal or rectal examination.

lithuresis (lĭth´yōo-rē´sĭs) N. passing of small stones or small pieces of a stone with the urine.

live birth N. birth of an infant who exhibits any sign of life (e.g., respiration, movement of voluntary muscle, heartbeat), independent of the length of gestation. A live birth may not

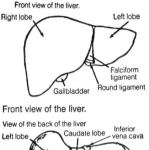

Front view of the liver.

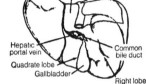

View of the back of the liver.

its release into the intestinal tract; it synthesizes substances involved in blood clotting (e.g., fibrinogen); it produces plasma proteins; it synthesizes vitamin A; it detoxifies poisonous substances; and it breaks down worn-out erythrocytes (red blood cells). ADJ. hepatic

liver abscess (ăb′sĕs′) N. localized accumulation of pus in the liver; often due to amebiasis.

liver cancer N. malignant neoplastic disease of the liver occurring most often as a metastasis from another cancer. Primary liver cancer is common in parts of Africa and Asia, where it is often associated with aflatoxins (toxins produced by certain strains of the fungus Aspergillus), but it is rare in the United States, often associated, when it does occur, with cirrhosis of the liver. Symptoms include loss of appetite, weakness, bloating, jaundice, and enlarged, tender liver and mild upper abdominal discomfort. The lesions often metastasize through the portal and lymphatic systems. Treatment depends on the nature and extent of the neoplasm; it may involve removal of a primary tumor and/or chemotherapy.

be viable (capable of surviving).

livedo (lǐ-vē′dō) N. a discolored area on the skin.

liver N. largest and one of the most complex organs of the body, located in the upper right part of the abdominal cavity. The liver weighs about 1 pound (1.6 kg) in males, a little less in females; is dark reddish brown, soft, and solid; is divided into four lobes; and is supplied by two blood systems, the hepatic artery, bringing freshly oxygenated blood to the liver, and the hepatic portal vein (part of the portal blood system), carrying nutrients from the stomach and intestines to the liver. The liver has numerous functions: it is a site of protein, carbohydrate, and fat metabolism; it helps regulate the level of blood sugar, converting excess glucose into glycogen and storing it; it secretes bile, which is stored in the gallbladder before

living will N. written advance directive whereby a mentally competent patient directs his or her physician in the provision of future medical care if he or she becomes terminally ill and incapable of making decisions; in most states, living wills are legally enforceable.

Lo/Ovral N. trade name for an oral contraceptive containing estradiol and norgestrel.

lobar pneumonia (lō′bər nŏo-mōn′yə) N. severe, bacterial (often streptococcal) infection of one or more lobes of the lung; it is characterized by fever; cough; rapid, shallow breathing; cyanosis; inflammation of the membrane lining of the lung; nausea and vomiting; and, if untreated, consolidation (solidification) of lung tissue. Treatment is by antibiotics. (*Compare* BRONCHOPNEUMONIA; INTERSTITIAL PNEUMONIA.)

lobe N. rounded part of an organ, separated from other parts of the organ by connective tissue or fissures; the brain, liver, and lungs are divided into lobes.

lobectomy (lō-běk′tə-mē) N. surgical procedure in which a lobe of the lung is removed; performed to treat intractable tuberculosis or bronchiectasis or to remove a malignant tumor.

lobotomy (lə-bŏt′ə-mē) N. surgical procedure in which certain nerve fibers in the frontal lobe of the brain are severed (usually by a wire inserted through the eye socket) to prevent transmission of various impulses. Once commonly used to treat certain mental illness, it is now rarely performed because it has many undesirable effects. Also called leukotomy.

lobule (lŏb′yōōl) N. small lobe or part of a lobe. ADJ. lobular

local ADJ. pert. to a small circumscribed area.

local anesthesia (ăn′ĭs-thē′zhə) N. administration of a local anesthetic agent to induce loss of sensation in a small area of the body. It may be applied topically, as in spraying on the skin before removing a small lesion, or it may be injected subcutaneously (beneath the skin). Brief dental and surgical operations are the most common indications for use. (*Compare* GENERAL ANESTHESIA; REGIONAL ANESTHESIA; TOPICAL ANESTHESIA.)

local anesthetic (ăn′ĭs-thět′ĭk) N. agent that reduces or eliminates sensation, esp. pain, in a limited area of the body by blocking the transmission of nerve impulses in the area.

localization N. limiting of a condition, effect, or finding to a given area or part. V. localize, ADJ. localized

lochia (lō′kē-ə) N. discharge from the vagina after childbirth. The discharge gradually decreases in amount and changes in color (from red to yellowish to gray-white) during the 6 weeks following childbirth.

lockjaw N. common term for tetanus, during the late stages.

locomotion N. mobility; self-propelled movement.

loculus (lŏk′yə-ləs) N., *pl.* loculi, small cavity or space. ADJ. locular, loculate

locus (lō′kəs) N., *pl.* loci, specific site, esp. the location of a gene on its chromosome.

locus of infection N. specific site in the body where an infection originates.

Lodine N. trade name for the nonsteroidal anti-inflammatory agent, etodolac.

Loestrin N. trade name for an oral contraceptive containing estradiol and norethindrone.

logo- comb. form indicating an association with words (e.g., logomania, talking excessively).

logorrhea (lŏg′ə-rē′ə) N. rapid flow of words, often incoherent, associated with some mental disorders.

loin N. region of the back and side of the body between the lowest rib and the pelvis, also called lumbus.

lomefloxacin HCl N. oral antibiotic (trade name Maxaquin) used once daily to treat bronchitis and urinary tract infection caused by Gram-negative organisms; adverse effects include photosensitivity reactions.

Lomotil N. trade name for a fixed-combination antidiarrheal.

lomustine N. antineoplastic, known as CeeNU, used in the treatment of several types of cancer. Adverse effects include nausea, vomiting, and bone marrow depression.

long-acting ADJ. pert. to a drug or other agent that has prolonged effect because of slow release of its active principle or continued absorption over an extended period (*compare* SHORT-ACTING).

Loniten N. trade name for the vasodilator minoxidil.

loop N.
1. band that forms a circle or U-shaped curve (e.g., loop of Henle, a U-shaped part of the inner kidney).
2. colloquial term for a type of intrauterine device.

Lopid N. trade name for the drug gemfibrozil. *See* TABLE OF COMMONLY PRESCRIBED DRUGS—TRADE NAMES.

Lopressor N. trade name for the beta blocker metoprolol. *See* TABLE OF COMMONLY PRESCRIBED DRUGS—TRADE NAMES.

Lorabid N. trade name for the oral antibiotic, loracarbef. *See* TABLE OF COMMONLY PRESCRIBED DRUGS—TRADE NAMES.

loracarbef N. oral synthetic antibiotic (trade name Lorabid), distantly related to the cephalosporins; used in the treatment of mild to moderate respiratory, skin, and urinary tract infections. *See* TABLE OF COMMONLY PRESCRIBED DRUGS—GENERIC NAMES.

loratadine N. *See* TABLE OF COMMONLY PRESCRIBED DRUGS—GENERIC NAMES.

loratidine/pseudoephedrine N. *See* TABLE OF COMMONLY PRESCRIBED DRUGS—GENERIC NAMES.

lorazepam N. (trade name Ativan) benzodiazepine tranquilizer used to treat anxiety, tension, and some forms of insomnia. Adverse effects include drowsiness and, after prolonged or high-dosage use, withdrawal symptoms. *See* TABLE OF COMMONLY PRESCRIBED DRUGS—GENERIC NAMES.

lordosis (lôr-dō′sĭs) N.
1. normal curvature of the cervical (neck) and lumbar spine, seen from the side as an anterior concavity.
2. increased degree of inward curvature (*compare* KYPHOSIS; SCOLIOSIS).

losartan N. *See* TABLE OF COMMONLY PRESCRIBED DRUGS—GENERIC NAMES.

losartan/hydrochlorothiazide N. *See* TABLE OF COMMONLY PRESCRIBED DRUGS—GENERIC NAMES.

Lotensin N. *See* TABLE OF COMMONLY PRESCRIBED DRUGS—TRADE NAMES.

lotion N. liquid applied externally to treat a skin disorder or to protect the skin.

Lotrel N. *See* TABLE OF COMMONLY PRESCRIBED DRUGS—TRADE NAMES.

Lotrisone N. *See* TABLE OF COMMONLY PRESCRIBED DRUGS—TRADE NAMES.

Lou Gehrig's disease (lōō′gĕr′ĭgz) *See* AMYOTROPHIC LATERAL SCLEROSIS.

lovastatin (lō′və-stăt′n) N. oral agent (trade name Mevacor) indicated for the reduction of elevated blood cholesterol levels (hypercholesterolemia) when the response to diet has been inadequate. Adverse effects include liver abnormalities and muscle aches. *See* TABLE OF COMMONLY PRESCRIBED DRUGS—TRADE NAMES.

low density lipoprotein (LDL) N. plasma protein that is relatively rich in fat. It facilitates deposition of cholesterol in the walls of arteries, and may contribute to atherosclerosis; studies suggest that increased LDL levels are associated with an increased incidence of coronary artery disease.

low-birth-weight infant N. infant born weighing less than 2,500 grams regardless of gestational age. These babies are at risk for developing lack of oxygen during labor, and low blood sugar and slow growth and development after birth.

lower respiratory tract (rĕs′pər-ə-tôr′ē) *See* RESPIRATORY TRACT.

low-fat diet N. diet containing limited amounts of fat; omitting cream, fried foods, and foods prepared in oil, gravy, and butter; and stressing high-carbohydrate foods. It is used in some gallbladder conditions and other disorders.

low-sodium diet N. diet that limits the intake of sodium chloride (salt); it is often used in treatment of hypertension, edema, kidney or liver disease, and certain other disorders. Foods such as bacon, frankfurters, salted butter, ham, sausage, cheese and many canned or frozen foods are prohibited. Also called low-salt diet.

loxapine N. tranquilizer (trade name Loxitane) used to treat schizophrenia. Adverse effects include low blood pressure, liver toxicity, and hypersensitivity reactions.

Loxitane N. trade name for the tranquilizer loxapine.

Lozal N. trade name for the diuretic indapamide.

LSD *See* LYSERGIC ACID DIETHYLAMIDE.

lucid ADJ. clear, understandable (e.g., a lucid statement). N. lucidity

lumbago (lŭm-bā′gō) N. pain in the lumbar region of the back, usually caused by muscle strain, arthritis, vascular insufficiency, or ruptured intervertebral disc.

lumbar ADJ. pert. to that part of the back between the ribs and the pelvis.

lumbar nerves N. five pairs of spinal nerves arising from the lumbar portion of the spinal cord.

lumbar plexus N. network of nerves formed by the ventral divisions of some of the lumbar nerves; it is located inside the posterior abdominal wall and supplies the caudal (lower) part of the abdominal wall, the front of the thigh, and part of the middle leg.

lumbar puncture N. insertion of a hollow needle into the subarachnoid space of the lumbar region of the spinal cord for diagnostic (e.g., to obtain a sample of cerebrospinal fluid for analysis) or therapeutic (e.g., to remove blood or pus or inject a drug) purposes. Adverse effects of the procedure include headache, nausea, and infection. Also called spinal tap; spinal puncture.

lumbo- comb. form indicating an association with the lumbar region of the spinal column, the small of the back (e.g., lumbocostal, pert. to the loins and ribs).

lumbosacral ADJ. pert. to the loins (small-of-the-back area) and sacrum (the back part of the pelvis between the hips).

lumbosacral plexus N. network of nerves formed by the ventral divisions of the lumbar, sacral, and coccygeal nerves; it supplies the lower limbs, perineum, and coccygeal area.

lumbus *See* LOIN.

lumen (loo′mən) N., *pl.* lumina, cavity, canal, or channel within an organ or tube; the space inside a structure. ADJ. lumenal

Luminal N. trade name for the anticonvulsant and sedative phenobarbital.

luminescence (loo′mə-nĕs′əns) N. production of light without the production of heat; light not due to incandescence or thermal sources; occurs at low temperatures.

LUNGS

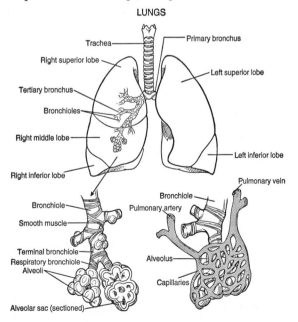

lumpectomy (lŭm-pĕk′tə-mē) N. surgical removal of a tumor without removal of much surrounding tissue or nearby lymph nodes; performed in some cases of breast cancer and other tumors.

lumpy jaw *See* ACTINOMYCOSIS.

lunate bone N. one of the carpal (wrist) bones.

lung N. either of a pair of highly elastic, spongy organs in the chest that are the main organs of respiration, inhaling air from which oxygen is taken and exhaling carbon dioxide. The lungs are composed of lobes, the right lung with three, the left with two. The lobes are divided into lobules, each of which contains blood vessels, lymphatics, nerves, and ducts connecting the alveoli, or air spaces, where the actual oxygen-carbon dioxide exchange takes place.

lung cancer N. one of the most common types of cancer; the incidence has rapidly been increasing in women. Predisposing factors include smoking and exposure to asbestos, vinyl chloride, coal products, and other industrial and chemical products. Symptoms include cough, difficulty in breathing, blood-tinged sputum, and repeated infections. Treatment depends on the type, site, and extent of the cancer and may include surgery, chemotherapy, and/or radiotherapy.

lupus (loō′pəs) *See* SYSTEMIC LUPUS ERYTHEMATOSUS; LUPUS VULGARIS.

lupus vulgaris (loō′pəs vŭl-gâr′ĭs) N. rare form of tuberculosis characterized by skin ulcers that heal slowly and leave deep scars.

luteal phase (loō′tē-əl) *See* SECRETORY PHASE.

luteinizing hormone (LH) N. hormone synthesized and released by the pituitary gland in response to estradiol. The release of LH matures the egg and weakens the wall of the follicle in the ovary. This process leads to ovulation—release of the mature egg. *See also* FOLLICLE-STIMULATING HORMONE.

luteotropin (loō′tē-ə-trō′pĭn) *See* PROLACTIN.

luxation N. misalignment, displacement, or dislocation of an organ or joint. *See also* SUBLUXATION.

Lyme arthritis (līm är-thrī′tĭs) N. acute inflammatory disease, thought to be caused by a tick-borne bacterium, that affects one or more joints (esp. the knees and other large joints), causing heat, swelling, and skin redness, often accompanied by chills, fever, and malaise. Cardiac abnormalities and neurologic complications sometimes occur. Preventive measures include wearing protective clothing (long-sleeved shirt, and pants tucked into boots) in wooded areas and examination of the body for ticks after possible exposure. Treatment is by pain relievers (e.g., aspirin), antibiotics (tetracycline, penicillin), and sometimes corticosteroids.

lymph N. thin fluid that bathes the tissues of the body, circulates through lymph vessels, is filtered in lymph nodes, and enters the blood system through the thoracic duct at the junction of the subclavian vein and jugular vein. It contains chyle and leukocytes (mostly lymphocytes), but otherwise is similar to plasma. ADJ. lymphatic, lymphoid, lymphous

LYMPH NODE

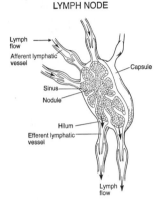

lymph node N. any of the small structures that filter lymph and contain lymphocytes. Lymph nodes are concentrated in several areas of the body, such as the armpit, groin, and neck. Also called lymph gland.

lymph-, lympho- comb. forms indicating an association with lymph (e.g., lymphadenopathy, any disease of the lymph system).

lymphadenitis (lĭm-făd′n-ī′tĭs) N. inflammation of the lymph nodes; it usually occurs as a result of systemic neoplastic disease, bacterial infection, or inflammatory condition.

lymphadenopathy (lĭm-făd′n-ŏp-ə-thē) N. swelling of lymph glands, or nodes; often termed "swollen glands" Swollen, firm, and possibly tender lymph nodes are commonly found in the groin, armpits, and neck. The cause may range from an acute (short-lasting) infection like flu to lymphoma (cancer of the lymph nodes) and human immunodeficiency virus (HIV) infection.

lymphangiectasis (lĭm-făn′jē-ĕk′tə-sĭs) N. dilatation of lymph vessels; also called lymphangiectasia.

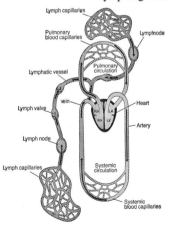

The lymphatic system as it relates to the circulatory system.

PRINCIPAL ORGANS OF THE LYMPHATIC SYSTEM

Organ	Primary Function
Lymphatic vessels	Carry lymph from peripheral tissues to the veins of the cardiovascular system
Lymph nodes	Monitor the composition of lymph; site of cells that engulf pathogens; immune response
Spleen	Monitors circulating blood; site of cells that engulf pathogens; site of cells that regulate the immune response
Thymus	Controls development and maintenance of T-lymphocytes

lymphangioma (lĭm-făn′jē-ō′mə) N. benign tumor made up of dilated lymph vessels.

lymphangitis (lĭm′făn-jī′tĭs) N. inflammation of a lymph vessel that usually results from infection, causing red streaks extending from the infected area, accompanied by fever, headache, and muscle pain. Treatment is by antibiotics.

lymphatic system (lĭm-făt′ĭk) N. network of capillaries, vessels, ducts, nodes, and organs that help to maintain the fluid environment of the body and to protect the body by producing lymph and conveying it around the body. Lymphatic capillaries unite to form lymph vessels, which have numerous valves to control lymph flow and nodes to filter it. The lymphatic vessels lead to two large vessels: the thoracic duct and right lymphatic duct, both in the neck, from which the lymph drains into the bloodstream. Specialized lymph organs include the spleen, thymus, and tonsils. ADJ. lymphatic

lymphedema (lĭm′fĭ-dē′mə) N. accumulation of lymph in tissues, leading to swelling; it occurs most often in the legs. It can be congenital or result from lymph vessel obstruction from tumor or inflammation.

lymphocyte (lĭm′fə-sīt′) N. agranulocyte leukocyte (white blood cell) that normally makes up about 25% of the total white blood cell count but increases in the presence of infection. Lymphocytes occur in two forms: B cells, the chief agents of the humoral immune system, which recognize specific antigens and produce antibodies against them; and T cells, the agents of the cell-mediated immune system, which secrete immunologically active compounds and assist B cells in their function.

lymphocytopenia (lĭm′fō-sī′tə-pē′nē-ə) N. lower-than-normal number of lymphocytes in the blood circulation, because of malignancy, nutritional deficiency, blood disorder, infection, or certain other conditions; also called lymphopenia.

lymphogranuloma venereum (LGV) (lĭm′fō-grăn′yə-lō′mə) N. infectious disease, caused by the bacterium *Chlamydia trachomatis* and transmitted by sexual contact. It is characterized by genital lesions and swelling of lymph nodes in the groin area, headache, fever, and malaise. Treatment is by antibiotics, usually tetracyclines. Also called lymphopathia venereum.

lymphokine (lĭm′fə-kīn′) N. any of a number of proteins released by lymphocytes (e.g., interleukin, interferon).

lymphoma (lĭm-fō′mə) N. neoplasm of lymph tissue, usually malignant, one of four major types of cancer. Lymphomas differ widely in the types of cells affected and the prognosis; general characteristics include enlarged lymph nodes, weakness, fever, weight loss, and malaise, followed by enlargement of the spleen and liver. Types of lymphomas include Burkitt's lymphoma and Hodgkin's disease. Treatment is usually by chemotherapy and radiotherapy. ADJ. lymphomatoid

lymphopoiesis (lĭm′fō-poi-ē′sĭs) N. production of lymphocytes, occurring mainly in the bone marrow, lymph nodes, spleen, and thymus.

lymphuria N. presence of lymph in the urine.

lyophilization (lī-ŏf′ə-lĭ-zā′shən) N. freeze-drying; process of rapidly freezing a substance, then dehydrating it in a high vacuum.

lysergic acid diethylamide (LSD) (lī-sûr′jĭk) N. hallucinogen drug that produces illusions, hallucinations, distorted perceptions, feelings of panic, depression, or paranoia, and widespread physical symptoms (e.g., increased body temperature and blood pressure, dilation of the pupils, muscle weakness). Psychological dependence may occur. The drug is not used therapeutically but is a drug of abuse. Treat-

ment of LSD intoxication involves attempts to calm the person and the use of tranquilizers and barbiturates. Colloquial term: acid.

lysine (lī′sēn′) N. essential amino acid, needed for growth in children.

lysine intolerance N. disorder in which a lack of or defect in certain enzymes produces inability to utilize the amino acid lysine, resulting in weakness, vomiting, and coma. Treatment is by limiting lysine content in the diet. (*Compare* LYSINEMIA.)

lysinemia (lī′sə-nē′mē-ə) N. inborn error of metabolism in which a defect in or lack of enzymes leads to inability to metabolize the amino acid lysine; it is characterized by muscle weakness and mental retardation. Treatment is by limiting the intake of lysine in the diet. (*Compare* LYSINE INTOLERANCE.)

lysis (lī′sĭs) N. destruction or breakdown of one substance (e.g., a cell or microorganism) by a specific agent.

lysogenic (lī′sə-jĕn′ĭk) ADJ. producing lysis.

lysosome (lī′sə-sōm′) N. organelle found in the cytoplasm of most cells, esp. leukocytes and kidney and liver cells, which contains enzymes that function in digestive processes within cells.

lysozyme (lī′sə-zīm′) N. enzyme, found in tears, saliva, sweat, and certain other substances, that functions in the destruction of the cell walls of certain bacteria; also called muramidase.

M

macerate V. to soften something, as an organ or part. N. maceration, ADJ. macerative

macr-, macro- comb. forms indicating abnormally large size (e.g., macroblepharia, oversized eyelids).

macrencephaly (măk′rĕn-sĕf′ə-lē) N. abnormally large brain. ADJ. macroencephalic

Macrobid N. *See* TABLE OF COMMONLY PRESCRIBED DRUGS—TRADE NAMES.

macrocephaly (măk′rō-sĕf′ə-lē) N. abnormality (usually but not always congenital) characterized by an abnormally large head and brain, usually resulting in mental and growth retardation. It differs from hydrocephalus in that the overgrowth is symmetrical, and there is no increased intracranial pressure. (*Compare* MICROCEPHALY.)

macrocyte (măk′rə-sīt′) N. abnormally large erythrocyte (red blood cell) occurring in megaloblastic anemia. ADJ. macrocytic

macrocytic anemia (măk′rə-sīt′ĭk) N. blood disorder, often caused by deficiency of folic acid and vitamin B₁₂, in which red blood cell production is impaired and abnormally large and fragile red blood cells are present.

Macrodantin N. trade name for the antibacterial nitrofurantoin.

macroglobulinemia N. increased levels of high molecular weight proteins (macroglobulins) in the blood; though small amounts of macroglobulins are normally present, increased levels are abnormal and may be due to a number of disease states (e.g., multiple myeloma, lupus, liver cirrhosis).

macroglossia N. congenital disorder characterized by an abnormally large tongue, seen in Down's syndrome and certain other disorders.

macrophage (măk′rə-fāj′) N. large scavenger cell (phagocyte) that engulfs and digests invading microorganisms and cell debris. Some are fixed (e.g., in connective tissues, liver, and spleen); others circulate in the blood.

macula (măk′yə-lə) N., *pl.* maculae, small, pigmented spot, such as a freckle, that is different from surrounding tissue. ADJ. macular, maculated

macula lutea (măk′yə-lə loō′tē-ə) N., small yellow spot on the retina where vision is most acute.

macule N. small blemish or discoloration that is not raised above the skin surface (e.g., freckle) (*compare* PAPULE). ADJ. macular

mad cow disease *See* BOVINE SPONGIFORM ENCEPHALOPATHY.

magnesium (măg-nē′zē-əm) N. metallic element essential to normal body functioning. *See also* TABLE OF IMPORTANT ELEMENTS.

magnesium sulfate N. salt of magnesium used orally to treat constipation and heartburn and parenterally to prevent seizures, esp. in preeclampsia. Also used in the treatment of cardiac arrythmias and in myocardial infarction.

major affective disorder N. any of a group of psychotic disorders not caused by an organic disorder and characterized by persistent disturbances of mood and thought processes and inappropriate emotional responses, as occur in some forms of bipolar disorder.

major surgery N. any surgical procedure that requires general anesthesia or assistance in respiration (*compare* MINOR SURGERY).

mala N. cheek or cheek bone.

malabsorption N. abnormal absorption of nutrients from the digestive tract, occurring in malnutrition, celiac disease, sprue, and other disorders that impair normal absorption. *See also* MALABSORPTION SYNDROME.

malabsorption syndrome N. complex of symptoms, including loss of appetite, bloating, weight loss, muscle pain, and stools with high fat content, that result from abnormal intestinal absorption and occur in celiac disease, sprue, cystic fibrosis, and certain other disorders.

malacia (mə-lā′shē-ə) N. state of abnormal softening or sponginess (e.g., osteomalacia). ADJ. malacic

malaise (mă-lāz′) N. vague feeling of weakness or illness, often an early sign of illness.

malaria (mə-lâr′ē-ə) N. serious infectious illness characterized by recurrent episodes of chills, fever, headache, anemia, muscle ache, and enlarged spleen. It is caused by *Plasmodium protozoa* transmitted from human to human through the bite of an infected Anopheles mosquito or through blood transfusions or infected hypodermic needles; it is largely confined to tropical and subtropical areas. Treatment is by chloroquine or, in resistant cases, a combination of quinine, sulfonamides, and other drugs. Prevention includes removal of swampy areas where Anopheles mosquitos breed, the use of insecticides and mosquito netting, and the use of antimalarial drugs when travelling in areas where malaria is prevalent.

malathion poisoning N. toxic condition caused by ingestion or inhalation of the insecticide malathion; it is characterized by vomiting, nausea, abdominal cramps, weakness, breathing difficulties, and confusion. Treatment includes atropine, gastric lavage, respiratory assistance, cathartics, and oxygen.

male ADJ. pert. to the sex that produces sperm to fertilize the female's eggs for the production of children (*compare* FEMALE). N. man or boy.

malformation N. abnormal shape or structure; deformity; in medicine, often refers to a congenital problem.

malfunction N. failure to function normally for any reason.

malignant (mə-lĭg′nənt) ADJ. harmful; tending to cause death; worsening or progressing, esp. a cancer that is invasive and metastatic (spreading); *compare* BENIGN.

malignant hypertension N. most lethal form of hypertension, characterized by very elevated blood pressure that produces damage in the inner linings of the blood vessels and the heart, spleen, kidneys, and brain, often leading to death. It may occur without a discoverable organic cause (essential hypertension) or it may be due to or associated with a variety of diseases (secondary hypertension).

malignant hyperthermia (MH) N. hereditary condition (autosomal dominant disease) in which very high body temperatures and muscle rigidity occur when the person is exposed to certain anesthetics (e.g., halothane, methoxyflurane). Treatment includes cooling, administration of oxygen, and intravenous administration of the drug dantrolene.

malignant neoplasm (mə-lĭg′nənt nē′ə-plăz′əm) N. tumor that tends to grow and spread to other body parts; also called malignant tumor.

malignant neuroma (mə-lĭg′nənt noō-rō′mə) *See* NEUROSARCOMA.

malingering N. deliberate feigning of the symptoms of a disease to achieve some desired end; pretending illness. V. malinger

malleable ADJ. capable of being shaped, bent, or drawn out, esp. by pressure.

malleolus (mə-lē′ə-ləs) N., *pl.* malleoli, bumplike projection on a bone, as on the inner and outer sides of the ankle. ADJ. malleolar

malleus (măl′ē-əs) N. one of the three small bones of the middle ear (the others are the incus and the stapes), connecting the tympanic membrane to the incus.

malnutrition N. state of poor nutrition, resulting from an insufficient, excessive, or unbalanced diet or from impaired ability to absorb and assimilate foods.

malocclusion (măl′ə-kloō′zhən) N. a condition in which the teeth of the opposing jaws do not contact or mesh normally; it is often corrected by orthodontics.

Malphigian corpuscle (kôr′pə-səl) N. any of a number of small bodies in the cortex of the kidney that contain a Bowman's capsule and glomerulus.

malpractice N. negligent or incorrect performance of professional duties; in medicine, the term refers specifically to care rendered patients by health-care providers and institutions. Generally, four prerequisites are necessary to establish a valid claim for medical malpractice: (1) a provider-patient relationship existed; (2) negligent care was rendered; (3) the patient suffered damage or harm; and (4) the damage or harm done to the patient was a direct result of the negligent care. In recent years the increase in the number of malpractice suits and the huge amounts sometimes awarded to plaintiffs have led to a steep rise in insurance premiums for physicians, nurses, and hospitals and ultimately to greater costs for medical care to the public.

Malta fever *See* BRUCELLOSIS.

mamm-, mammo- comb. forms indicating an association with the breast or milk-secreting glands (e.g., mammogenesis, formation and development of the milk-giving glands).

mamma N., *pl.* mammae, breast; milk-giving gland in the female. ADJ. mammary

mammary glands (măm′ə-rē) N. milk-secreting glands of the female breast.

mammogram (măm′ə-grăm′) N. X-ray film of the soft tissue of the breast.

mammography (mă-mŏg′rə-fē) N. procedure in which the soft tissues of the breast are x-rayed to detect benign or malignant tumors. Periodic mammography is generally recommended for women thought at high risk for breast cancer and in certain other situations. (*Compare* MAMMOTHERMOGRAPHY.)

mammothermography N. diagnostic procedure in which infrared sensors are used to detect warm and cold areas (thermography) of the breast as a means of diagnosing tumors (*compare* MAMMOGRAPHY).

managed care organization N. health insurance plan that relies on a gatekeeper to coordinate the utilization and delivery of medical services. *See* TABLE OF MANAGED CARE TERMS.

Mandelamine N. trade name for the antibacterial methenamine.

mandible (măn′də-bəl) N. large bone making up the lower jaw, consisting of a horizontal part, a horseshoe-shaped body, and two perpendicular branches that connect to the body. The mandible contains sockets for the 16 lower teeth and grooves and attachments for the facial artery and various muscles. (*Compare* MAXILLA.)

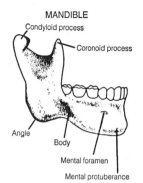

MANDIBLE

Lateral view of the mandible, or lower jaw.

Mandol N. trade name for the cephalosporin antibiotic cefamandole nafate.

maneuver (mə-noō′vər) N. manipulation; movement of parts or a change of position, usually done by use of the hands (e.g., manipulation of a fetus to aid delivery); also refers to a particular set of actions performed as part of a physical examination (e.g., a Valsalva maneuver consists of bearing down while holding the breath).

manganese (măng′gə-nēz′) N. metallic element important in trace amounts in metabolism. *See also* TABLE OF IMPORTANT ELEMENTS.

mania (mā′nē-ə) N. mood disorder, occurring in bipolar disorder, delirium, and certain major affective disorders, in which the person tends to respond excessively, with abnormal amounts of motion, overtalkativeness, elation, hyperactivity, and sometimes violent and destructive behavior. ADJ. maniacal, manic.

manic-depressive N. person whose mental state periodically swings from mania to depression. *See also* BIPOLAR DISORDER.

manic-depressive psychosis (sī-kō'sĭs) *See* BIPOLAR DISORDER.

manipulation (mə-nĭp'yə-lā'shən) N. skillful use of hands to reduce a fracture; to diagnose, as in palpation; or to perform other diagnostic or therapuetic maneuvers (e.g., move a fetus before birth).

mannitol (măn'ĭ-tôl') N. diuretic, sometimes known under the trade name Osmitrol, used to promote the excretion of urine, to decrease abnormally high pressure in the eye or cranium, or to test kidney function. Adverse effects include heart abnormalities, edema of the lungs, headache, and vomiting.

Manoplax N. trade name for the vasodilator, flosequinan.

Mantoux test (măn'tōō') N. skin test to determine past or present infection with tuberculosis. A protein derivative of tubercle bacillus is injected intradermally; a hardened red area appearing 1–3 days after injection signifies a positive reaction and past or present exposure to the tubercle bacillus. *See also* TUBERCULIN TEST.

manubrium (mə-nōō'brē-əm) N., *pl.* manubria, part of the sternum (breastbone) nearest the head.

manus (mā'nəs) *See* HAND.

MAO *See* MONOAMINE OXIDASE.

MAO inhibitor *See* MONOAMINE OXIDASE INHIBITOR.

maple syrup urine disease N. inherited disorder of metabolism in which the enzyme necessary for the breakdown of amino acids lysine, leucine, and isoleucine is lacking and the person has hyperreflexia (overactive reflexes) and urine with a characteristic maple syrup odor. Treatment includes a diet low in these amino acids; untreated, the disorder leads to mental retardation and often death in early childhood.

mapping N. in genetics, process of locating genes on a chromosome; also called chromosome mapping.

maprotiline (mə-prōt'l-ēn') N. antidepressant (trade name Ludiomil). Adverse effects include sedation and gastrointestinal, cardiac, and neurological disturbances.

marasmus (mə-răz'məs) N. extreme malnutrition, emaciation, and wasting, esp. in a young child; it usually results from inadequate protein and calorie intake but may also result from malabsorption, metabolic disorders, repeated vomiting and diarrhea, or certain infectious diseases. Symptoms include wasting of subcutaneous tissue and muscle and often a pallid appearance and subnormal body temperature. Treatment includes reestablishment of fluid and electrolyte balance and gradual introduction of foods.

marble bone disease *See* OSTEOPETROSIS.

Marburg disease (mär'bûrg') N. viral disease of vervet (green) monkeys transmitted to humans by contact with the infected animal, esp. blood or tissues used in laboratory studies. In humans it causes a serious and often fatal illness characterized by fever, rash, headache, vomiting, diarrhea, and gastrointestinal hemorrhage. There is no treatment, but antiserum and measures to reduce blood loss are sometimes effective. Also called green monkey disease; Marburg-Ebola disease.

marcoglobulin N. high molecular weight protein normally found in the blood in small amounts; increased in various disease states (e.g., multiple myeloma, lupus, liver cirrhosis), resulting in marcoglobulinemia.

Marfan's syndrome (mär′fănz sĭn′drōm′) N. inherited abnormality (autosomal dominant disorder) characterized by elongation of bones, esp. of the arms, legs, fingers, and toes; joint hypermobility, and abnormalities of the eyes (e.g., dislocation of the lens) and circulatory system (e.g., fiber fragmentation in the aorta, leading to aneurysm). There is no specific treatment.

Marie-Strumpell disease See ANKYLOSING SPONDYLITIS.

marijuana (măr′ə-wä′nə) N. drug, made from dried leaves of the *Cannabis sativa* plant, which, when smoked, provides a sense of euphoria often accompanied by changes in mood, perception, memory, and fine motor skills. The drug has been used to help relieve the nausea associated with cancer chemotherapy. Street names include pot, grass, and weed.

marrow (măr′ō) See BONE MARROW.

Marseilles fever N. disease, common around the Mediterranean area and in India, caused by a rickettsia (*Rickettsia conorii*) transmitted by the brown dog tick (*Rhipicephalus sanguineus*). It is characterized by chills, fever, a black-crusted ulcer at the side of the tick bite, and a rash. Also called boutonneuse fever; Indian tick fever; Kenya fever.

marsupialize V. to form a pouch surgically, as in treatment of a cyst by opening it, draining it, and suturing the edges to adjacent tissues.

masculinization (măs′kyə-lə-nĭ-zā′shən) N. abnormal development of male secondary sexual characteristics (e.g., excess body and facial hair, deeper voice) by a female, usually as the result of hormonal treatment or malfunction of the adrenal glands. *See also* VIRILIZATION.

mask V. to conceal or obscure something, as the masking of one disease by the symptoms of another. N.
1. a masklike appearance, as sometimes occurs during pregnancy. *See* CHLOASMA.
2. cover worn over the nose and mouth to prevent inhalation of toxic or irritating substances or to deliver oxygen or anesthetic gas.

mask of pregnancy *See* CHLOASMA.

masochism (măs′ə-kĭz′əm) N. sexual pleasure derived from receiving mental, emotional, or physical abuse (*compare* SADISM). ADJ. masochistic

massage (mə-säzh′) N. manipulation of the soft tissues of the body through rubbing, stroking, kneading, or gripping to improve muscle tone, relax the person, or improve circulation. *See also* CARDIAC MASSAGE; EFFLEURAGE.

mast cell N. large connective tissue cell that contains histamine, heparin, serotonin, and bradykinin, which are released in response to injury, inflammation, or allergic reaction.

mastalgia N. pain in the breast.

mastectomy (mă-stĕk′tə-mē) N. surgical removal of one or both breasts to remove a malignant tumor. A mastectomy is sometimes followed by reconstructive surgery which may include use of the patient's own tissue to form a breast or the insertion of an implant containing silicon gel, a saline solution, or both under a flap of skin and muscle at the site where the breast was removed. *See also* LUMPECTOMY.

modified radical mastectomy N. removal of a breast with the underlying pectoralis minor muscle and some adjacent lymph nodes (the major chest muscle—the pectoralis major—is not removed).

radical mastectomy N. removal of a breast, underlying chest muscles (both pectoralis major and pectoralis minor), lymph nodes in the armpit area, and fat and other tissues in the surrounding area.

simple mastectomy N. removal of a breast, with the underlying chest muscles and adjacent lymph nodes and tissues left intact.

mastication N. chewing and grinding food with the teeth.

mastitis (mă-stī′tĭs) N. inflammation of the breast, usually due to bacterial (streptococcal or staphylococcal) infection; it is most common in the first 2 months of lactation and is accompanied by pain, swelling, fever, malaise, and swelling of the lymph nodes in the armpit area. Treatment includes antibiotics, analgesics, and rest; nursing can usually continue. A rare chronic form sometimes occurs in association with severe tuberculosis. *See also* FIBROCYSTIC DISEASE OF THE BREAST.

mastocytosis N. variety of rare disorders in which there is an abnormal proliferation of mast cells throughout the body and skin. Stroking or firm touching of the skin causes the mast cells to release histamine and other substances, leading to hives and itching. Organ infiltration may result in life threatening problems, such as respiratory or cardiac dysfunction.

mastoid (măs′toid) ADJ. breastlike in shape or appearance, esp. the bump (mastoid process of the temporal bone) behind the ear. ADJ. mastoidal

mastoidectomy (măs′toi-dĕk′tə-mē) N. surgical removal of part of the mastoid portion of the temporal bone, done to treat chronic otitis media or mastoiditis, when antibiotics are not effective.

mastoiditis (măs′toi-dī′tĭs) N. infection of the mastoid bones, usually resulting from middle ear infection; it is most common in children and is characterized by pain, fever, earache, and malaise. Treatment is by antibiotics; some residual hearing loss sometimes occurs.

masturbation (măs′tər-bā′shən) N. manipulation and stimulation of one's own genitals to achieve sexual pleasure, usually orgasm. It is practiced by most people at some point in their lives.

materia medica N. study of the origins, preparation, uses, and effects of drugs and other substances used therapeutically in medicine.

maternal ADJ. pert. to a mother.

maternal-infant bonding *See* BONDING.

matrix (mā′trĭks) N. substance of an organ or tissue in which other specialized structures are embedded (e.g., the ground substance of connective tissue).

maturation (măch′ə-rā′shən) N. process of obtaining full development, as in the development of mature ova and spermatozoa, or the development of physical, mental, and emotional abilities during childhood and adolescence.

Maxaquin *See* LOMEFLOXACIN HCL.

maxilla (măk-sĭl′ə) N., *pl.* maxillae, one of a pair of large bones that form the upper jaw. It consists of a pyramidal body and four processes; contains sockets for the 16 upper teeth; and forms part of the structure of the orbits, nasal cavity, and roof of the mouth. (*Compare* MANDIBLE.) ADJ. maxillary

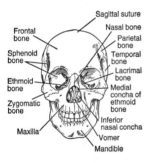

Frontal bone
Sphenoid bone
Ethmoid bone
Zygomatic bone
Maxilla
Sagittal suture
Nasal bone
Parietal bone
Temporal bone
Lacrimal bone
Medial concha of ethmoid bone
Inferior nasal concha
Vomer
Mandible

maxillary artery (măk′sə-lĕr′ē) N. either of two branches of the external carotid arteries that arise near the parotid gland and divide into branches supplying the deep parts of the face. *See* MAJOR ARTERIES AND VEINS OF THE BODY, in Appendix.

maxillary sinus N. one of a pair of air cells forming a cavity in the maxilla; the mucous membrane lining is continuous with that of the nasal cavity.

maxillo- comb. form indicating an association with the maxilla, or upper jaw (e.g., maxillofacial, pert. to the lower jaw and face).

Maxzide N. trade name for antihypertensive that consists of a fixed combination of the diuretics triamterene and hydrochlorothiazide.

McArdle's disease N. inherited disease in which larger than normal amounts of glycogen accumulate in skeletal muscle, causing muscle cramping and weakness after exercise.

McBurney's point (mək-bûr′nēz) N. point of maximum sensitivity in acute appendicitis; it lies one-third of the way on a line drawn from the projection of the right hip to the umbilicus.

measles (mē′zəlz) N. acute, contagious, viral disease, occurring primarily in children who have not been immunized and involving the respiratory tract and a spreading rash. Highly contagious, measles is spread by direct contact with droplets from the nose, mouth, or throat of infected persons, often in the prodromal (earliest) stage. After an incubation period of about 2 weeks, fever, malaise, cough, loss of appetite, and photophobia develop, followed by characteristic blue-centered, small red spots on the membranes of the tongue and mouth (Koplik's spots). Two or 3 days later the characteristic rash appears, starting as pinkish spots in the head region and spreading to a red maculopapular rash over the trunk and extremities. Fever to 103° Fahrenheit (39.5° Celsius) or higher and inflammation of the pharynx and trachea occur.

About 5 days later the lesions flatten, become brownish and fade, and the fever subsides. Treatment includes pain relievers, fever reducers, rest, and lotions (e.g., calamine) to soothe the skin and relieve itching. Complications include otitis media, pneumonia, laryngitis, and occasionally encephalitis. One attack provides life-long immunity. Prevention is by immunization with live measles vaccine, usually done when the child is 1–1½ years old; or, in those unvaccinated and exposed to the disease, passive immunization with immunoglobulin. Also called morbilli.

meatus (mē-ā′təs) N. opening or tunnel through any part of the body (e.g., acoustic meatus, leading from the external ear to the tympanic membrane).

Mebaral N. trade name for the anticonvulsant and sedative mephobarbital.

mebendazole N. anthelmintic used to treat pinworm, roundworm, and hookworm infestations. Adverse effects include gastrointestinal disturbances.

mechanical ventilation N. use of an artificial ventilator (breathing machine) to assist a patient's breathing.

mechanism N. process that occurs during a reaction, injury, or development of disease. In trauma, the mechanism of injury refers to items such as where a car was hit, whether the driver was restrained, if the driver hit the windshield.

Meckel's diverticulum (měk′əlz dī′vûr-tĭk′yə-ləm) N. congenital sac protruding from the ileum (last part of the small intestine), caused by incomplete closure of the yolk sac; it occurs in about 2% of the population. It usually produces no symptoms but may cause signs of appendicitis, intestinal obstruction, or bleeding in children. Treatment is by surgery, done if symptoms are present and/or to avoid obstruction or inflammation of the area.

meclizine (měk′lĭ-zēn′) N. antihistamine (trade name Antivert) used to treat and prevent motion sickness. Adverse

MCBURNEY'S POINT

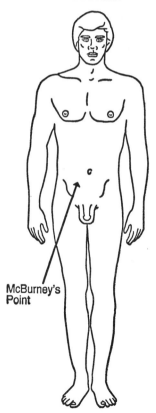

McBurney's Point

effects include drowsiness, skin rash, dry mouth, and rapid heartbeat.

meclofenamate N. nonsteroidal anti-inflammatory agent (trade name Meclomen) used to treat rheumatoid arthritis and osteoarthritis. Adverse effects include dizziness and gastrointestinal disturbances; the drug also interacts with many other drugs.

meconium (mĭ-kō'nē-əm) N. first stools of newborn, which are thick, sticky, greenish to black, and composed of bile pigments, gland secretions, amniotic fluid, and other intrauterine debris. The presence of meconium in the amniotic fluid usually indicates fetal distress.

medi-, medio- comb. forms indicating a relationship to the middle, midline, or middle plane (e.g., mediodorsal, pert. to the middle and back).

medial (mē'dē-əl) ADJ. situated toward the midline of the body or the central part of an organ or tissue; also called mesial.

MediAlert ID N. form of identification, worn usually either as a necklace or wrist bracelet, indicating that the wearer has a medical condition (e.g., penicillin allergy, heart disease).

mediastinum (mē'dē-ə-stī'nəm) N. space in the chest cavity between the lungs that contains the heart, aorta, esophagus, trachea, and thymus.

Medicaid (mĕd'ĭ-kād') N. federally and state-funded program of health care for needy persons, regardless of age. Five basic services are provided: in-patient hospital, outpatient hospital, laboratory and X ray, skilled nursing home, and physician. In each state, income and assets criteria determine eligibility.

medical examiner N. physician, usually a pathologist, with specific training in death investigation. The coroner and medical examiner may be one individual, or the medical examiner may work for the coroner's office. Compare CORONER.

Medicare N. federally administered system of health insurance, available to persons aged 65 and over, whether working or retired. Part A, Hospital Insurance, provides some protection against the costs of hospitalization, certain related inpatient institutional care, and home care. Part B, Supplementary Medical Insurance, in return for payment of a monthly fee that is adjusted annually, covers part of physicians' and surgeons' fees and certain other services (e.g., X ray and laboratory tests, radiotherapy, and medical equipment used at home, such as an oxygen tent or wheelchair). Although Medicare is unquestionably helpful, many elderly persons consider it advisable to have private health insurance as well.

medication N.
1. drug or other substance used to treat an illness.
2. administration of a medicine.

medicine N.
1. drug or other substance used to treat an illness.
2. art and science of diagnosing, treating, and preventing illness and maintaining good health.
3. that area of medical science concerned with the diagnosis and treatment of disease, as distinct from surgery.

medico- (mĕd'ĭ-kō') comb. form indicating a relationship to medicine (e.g., medicodental, pert. to both medicine and dentistry).

medicolegal (měd′ĭ-kō-lē′gəl) ADJ. pert. to medicine and law, esp. to topics such as malpractice, patient consent for operations, and patient information.

Mediterranean anemia *See* THALASSEMIA.

Mediterranean fever *See* BRUCELLOSIS.

medium N.
1. substance through which something moves or acts. A contrast medium, for example, has a density different from body tissues and when used with X ray or similar technique allows visual comparison of structures.
2. substance (e.g., agar) used as food for microorganisms; a culture medium.

medroxyprogesterone N. progestin compound (trade name Provera) used to treat menstrual disorders. See TABLE OF COMMONLY PRESCRIBED DRUGS —GENERIC NAMES.

medulla (mĭ-dŭl′ə) N., *pl.* medullae, innermost part of an organ or structure, as in the adrenal medulla (*compare* CORTEX). ADJ. medullary

medulla oblongata (mĭ-dŭl′ə ŏb′lŏng-gă′tə) N. lowest part of the brain stem, an extension in the skull of the upper end of the spinal cord; it is the most vital part of the brain, containing centers controlling respiration, heart and blood vessel function, and other activities as well as pathways for impulses entering and leaving the skull. Injury to the medulla oblongata is often fatal.

medullary (měd′l-ĕr′ē) ADJ.
1. pert. to the medulla oblongata.
2. pert. to bone marrow.

3. pert. to the central nervous system.

Mefoxin N. trade name for the cephalosporin antibacterial cefoxitin.

mega-, megalo- comb. forms meaning great, huge, large (e.g., megacardia, abnormally large heart; megalocyte, abnormally large red blood cell).

megacolon (měg′ə-kō′lən) N. abnormal enlargement of the colon due to an accumulation of impacted feces. It may be congenital (Hirschsprung's disease); acquired (as in chronic refusal to defecate, esp. in children); or toxic, a complication of ulcerative colitis. Treatment is by surgery, esp. for congenital and toxic forms, and by enemas and laxatives.

megakaryocyte (měg′ə-kăr′ē-ə-sīt′) N. large bone marrow cell that gives rise to platelets.

megaloblast (měg′ə-lō-blăst′) N. large, abnormal red blood cell that contains a nucleus; often found in pernicious anemia.

megaloblastic anemia (ə-nē′mē-ə) N. blood disorder in which large, immature and dysfunctional red blood cells circulate; associated with pernicious anemia and folic acid deficiency.

megalomania (měg′ə-lō-mā′nē-ə) N. abnormal state of mind in which the person has delusions of grandeur and believes himself/herself to be of great power, importance, or achievement.

-megaly comb. form indicating enlargement (e.g., dactylomegaly, enlargement of the fingers or toes).

megavitamin therapy N. theory that the intake of very large doses of vitamins—much above recommended daily doses—will prevent or cure many physical and psychological disorders.

megestrol N. progestational compound used to treat endometrial cancer.

megrim *See* MIGRAINE.

meibomian cyst (mī-bō′mē-ən) *See* CHALAZION.

meiosis (mī-ō′sĭs) N. type of cell division that produces daughter cells with the haploid chromosome number. It occurs during the production of mature sperm and ova; the diploid chromosome number characteristic of the species is restored at fertilization. Meiosis consists of two consecutive divisions, each divided into four phases. Also called reduction division. *See also* DIPLOID; HAPLOID (*compare* MITOSIS). ADJ. meiotic

melancholia (měl′ən-kō′lē-ə) N. extreme sadness, extreme depression. *See also* BIPOLAR DISORDER; DEPRESSION.

melanin (měl′ə-nĭn) N. dark brown to black pigment that occurs in skin, hair, and parts of the eye.

melanocyte (měl′ə-nō-sīt′) N. melanin producing cell found throughout the basal layer of the epidermis and controlled by melanocyte-stimulating hormone.

melanocyte-stimulating hormone (MSH) N. hormone, secreted by the anterior pituitary gland, that controls the intensity of pigmentation in melanocytes.

melanoderma (měl′ə-nō-dûr′mə) N. abnormal darkening of the skin caused by increased melanin deposits.

melanoma (měl′ə-nō′mə) N. any of several malignant neoplasms, primarily of the skin, consisting of melanocytes. Most melanomas develop from a pigmented nevus (mole); any change in color or shape of such a mark suggests melanoma. The incidence of melanoma has increased 93% since 1980. Ultra-

MEIOSIS
(reduction division)

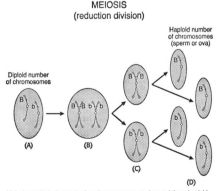

Meiosis results in the production of sperm or ova, each containing a haploid (half [26]) number of chromosomes (D). Diploid cells containing the total number of chromosomes ([46] A) transiently double their chromosome complement (B). Two successive meiotic divisions produce two diploid (C), then four haploid cells (sperm or ova, D).

CELL MEMBRANE

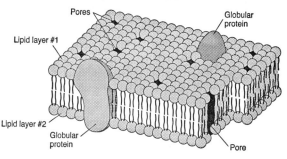

violet radiation exposure (e.g., from the sun or tanning salons) is believed to be a primary cause. Prognosis depends on the location, depth, and size of the lesion, and on the general health of the patient.

melanosome (měl′ə-nō-sōm′) N. melanin pigment granule produced by melanocytes that gives color to the skin and hair.

melasma (mə-lăz′mə) *See* CHLO-ASMA.

melatonin (měl′ə-tō′nĭn) N. only hormone secreted by the pineal gland; its function in humans is unknown.

melena (mə-lē′nə) N. abnormal dark, tarry stool, containing blood, usually from gastrointestinal bleeding.

melioidosis N. uncommon and serious, often fatal, infectious disease caused by the bacterium *Pseudomonas pseudomallei*, occurring mostly in China and Southeast Asia, and characterized by pneumonia, lung abscesses, and septicemia. Treatment is by antibacterials (e.g., chloramphenicol, tetracycline).

Mellaril N. trade name for the tranquilizer thioridazine.

melphalan N. antineoplastic drug (trade name Alkeran) used to treat multiple myeloma and certain other malignancies. Adverse effects include bone marrow depression, nausea, and vomiting.

membrane N. thin layer of tissue that covers an organ or lines a cavity or part (e.g., the pleura is a membrane enclosing the lung). It consists of two lipid layers in which globular proteins float. Membranes may be mucous, serous, or synovial. ADJ. membranous

membranous labyrinth (měm′brə-nəs lăb′ə-rĭnth′) N. network of membranous semicircular ducts, containing the fluid endolymph, that are suspended within the bony semicircular canals of the inner ear and function in the maintenance of balance.

memory N. ability to retain and recall into consciousness previously experienced ideas and sensations and learned information. The retention and recall are associated with specific chemical changes in the brain and can be affected by organic brain disorders and various psychological disorders. In general, memory is classified as recent or long-term.

menarche (mən-är′kē) N. first menstruation, usually occurring between the ages of 9 and 16. ADJ. menarchal, menarcheal

Mendelism (mĕn′dl-ĭz′əm) N. theory of inheritance based on Mendel's laws.

Mendel's laws N. basic principles of inheritance, developed in the 19th century by the Austrian monk Gregor Mendel on the basis of breeding experiments, which form the basis of the modern understanding of heredity. According to the laws, each characteristic of a person is determined by a pair of units now known as genes. One unit (allele) of each pair is contributed by each parent, carried in the gamete (egg or sperm). At fertilization the alleles combine to form a unit that determines the characteristic in the offspring. Some units are dominant over others called recessives; some interact in other ways. These basic principles formed the foundation on which subsequent biochemical studies of genes and chromosomes were made, leading to the development of modern genetics.

Meniere's disease (mān-yârz′) N. disease of the inner ear, characterized by recurrent episodes of dizziness, progressive hearing loss (usually unilateral), and tinnitus (ringing in the ears), often accompanied by nausea and vomiting. The cause is unknown, but the disease sometimes follows middle ear infection or injury to the head. Treatment is symptomatic, including the use of antihistamines.

meninges N. three connective tissue membranes that protect and enclose the brain and spinal cord. The outer layer is tough, thick dura mater; the middle layer is the delicate, spiderweb-like arachnoid; and the inner layer is the highly vascularized pia mater. The inner two layers are collectively called leptomeninges; the cerebrospinal fluid circulates between them.

MENINGES

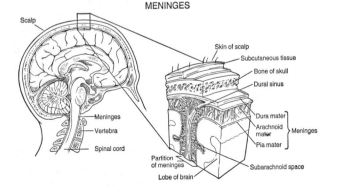

Scalp

Skin of scalp
Subcutaneous tissue
Bone of skull
Dural sinus

Meninges
Vertebra
Spinal cord

Dura mater
Arachnoid mater } Meninges
Pia mater

Partition of meninges
Lobe of brain
Subarachnoid space

meningioma (mə-nĭn′jē-ō′mə) N. usually slow-growing tumor arising from the membranes enclosing the brain and spinal cord (meninges); symptoms arise from pressure on underlying nerve tissue. Some tumors are malignant. Treatment is by surgery if the tumor is accessible.

meningism (mə-nĭn′jĭz′əm) N. symptoms (e.g., stiff neck) that mimic those of meningitis but in which there is no inflammation of the meninges; occurs most often in children.

meningitis (mĕn′ĭn-jī′tĭs) N. inflammation of the meninges, most commonly due to bacterial infection, but sometimes caused by viral or fungal infection, spreading tuberculosis, neoplasm, or chemical irritation. Symptoms include headache, stiff neck, fever, nausea, vomiting, and intolerance to light and sound, often followed by convulsions and delirium. Treatment depends on the cause; bacterial meningitis is treated by antibiotics. Viral meningitis is usually self-limited, but fungal or other forms may be more difficult to treat.

meningo- comb. form indicating an association with the meninges (e.g., meningoarteritis, inflammation of the arteries of the meninges).

meningocele N. congenital sac-like protrusion of either the cerebral (brain) or the spinal meninges, containing cerebrospinal fluid but no nerve tissue. Treatment is by surgery. (*Compare* MYELOMENINGOCELE.)

meniscectomy (mĕn′ĭ-sĕk′tə-mē) N. surgical removal of crescent-shaped cartilage (meniscus) of the knee, done when torn carti-

lage in the knee joint area causes chronic pain or difficulty in movement.

meniscus (mə-nĭs′kəs) N. crescent-shaped cartilage found in joints, particularly the knee; often torn in sports injuries (e.g., torn lateral or medial meniscus). Also refers to the curved upper surface of a liquid in a closed space, such as a fluid meniscus in a test tube.

menopause (mĕn′ə-pôz) N. cessation of menstruation, usually occurring naturally between the ages of 45 and 55. The term is also used to refer to that stage of a woman's life during which gradual hormonal changes, sometimes accompanied by vasomotor symptoms, such as hot flashes, and other signs (e.g., dryness of vaginal membranes and palpitations), lead to the cessation of menstrual periods. The production of gonadotropins from the pituitary and estrogens from the ovaries gradually decrease; ovulation ceases; and menstrual periods stop. The periods may become scanty and irregular in occurrence, or there may be episodes of heavy bleeding or abrupt cessation. Emotional disturbances may result from hormonal imbalances during the period, but many of the symptoms once believed due to menopause cannot be reliably attributed to it. Women from different ethnic and or cultural groups report different menopausal symptoms. In one study, hot flashes occurred in about 30% of Caucasians and 45% of African Americans. Hispanic women tended to complain of urine leakage, vaginal dryness, and heart pounding. Japanese and Chinese women experienced far fewer menopausal symptoms, except for forgetfulness. Also called **climacteric** and, colloquially, **change of life.** ADJ. **menopausal**

menorrhagia N. abnormally heavy or prolonged menstrual periods; it occurs occasionally in many women; sometimes caused by benign uterine tumors, but if chronic, it may lead to anemia; also called **hypermenorrhea** (*compare* OLIGOMENORRHEA).

menostasis N. condition in which menstrual products cannot leave the uterus or vagina, because of narrowing or closure of the normal openings. ADJ. **menostatic**

menses (mĕn′sēz) N. flow of blood and other material from the uterus during menstruation.

menstrual cycle N. recurring cycle, beginning at menarche and ending at menopause, in which the endometrial lining of the uterus proliferates in preparation for pregnancy and, if pregnancy does not occur, is shed at menstruation. The menstrual cycle is under the control of female reproductive hormones and is necessary for reproduction to occur. In the average woman, about 30 milliliters of blood is lost during menstruation. Because of this blood loss, women have higher dietary requirements for iron than do males to prevent iron deficiency. The menstrual cycle is divided into three phases— the menstrual phase, the proliferative phase, and the secretory phase. During each, the hormonal milieu differs, as do anatomic changes within both the uterus and in the ovaries. The average menstrual cycle is 28 days—the first day of menstrual flow is considered day one of the cycle. The length of the cycle varies greatly among women. The proliferative phase (sometimes called the follicular phase) follows menstruation. During this time (average 8 days), the pituitary gland produces follicle-stimulating hormone (FSH) that promotes the growth of a graafian follicle (egg sac; also called a follicle) within the ovary. The ovum (egg) matures in the follicle during the proliferative phase. FSH also stimulates the ovary

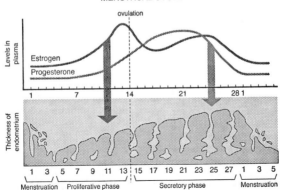

MENSTRUAL CYCLE

to produce estrogen (predominantly in the form of estradiol), causing endometrial tissue to build up and line the inside of the uterus. The mature ovum bursts from the follicle (ovulation or the ovulatory phase) about 2 weeks prior to the next menstrual cycle. The sexually mature female releases one egg (or occasionally two) at the time of ovulation. The ovum then travels from the ovary down the fallopian tube, and into the uterus. The follicle then becomes known as the corpus luteum. The secretory phase (sometimes called the luteal phase) follows—after ovulation and formation of the corpus luteum, luteinizing hormone (LH) released by the pituitary gland causes the corpus luteum to grow and to secrete progesterone. Progesterone makes the endometrial lining stronger and spongy in texture. It also stimulates glands in the endometrium that produce uterine fluid to support embryonic development if fertilization occurs. If pregnancy does not occur, the levels of progesterone and estrogen peak about a week after ovulation and then begin to drop. The flow of blood to the endometrium decreases, and its upper portion is broken down and shed during menstruation. At the same time, the corpus luteum withers. Once menstruation occurs, the cycle begins anew. *See also* ESTROGEN; FOLLICLE-STIMULATING HORMONE; IRON-DEFICIENCY ANEMIA; LUTEINIZING HORMONE; MENSTRUAL FLOW; MENSTRUAL PHASE; MENSTRUATION; PROGESTRONE.

menstrual flow N. flow of blood and other material from the uterus at roughly monthly intervals during a woman's reproductive years. The average blood loss in the flow is about 30 milliliters, but the amount varies greatly among women.

menstrual phase N. that phase of the menstrual cycle during which the lining of the uterus is shed. The first day of the menstrual flow is considered day 1 of the menstrual cycle.

menstruation (měn′strōō-ā′shən) N. discharge of blood and uterine material from the vagina at intervals of about a month during a woman's reproductive years; also called catamenia. (*See also* MENSES; MENSTRUAL CYCLE). ADJ. menstrual

mental ADJ.
1. pert. to the mind.
2. pert. to the chin.

mental age N. age at which a person functions intellectually, determined by standardized tests (*compare* CHRONOLOGICAL AGE; DEVELOPMENTAL AGE).

mental block N. imprecise term indicating failure of the mind to properly interpret, understand, or use particular concepts or information.

mental disorder N. any disorder of the mind, such as disturbance of perceptions, memory, emotional equilibrium, thought, or behavior; it may be genetic, congenital, or acquired as a result of physical, psychological, chemical, or social factors; also called mental illness.

mental retardation N. disorder characterized by below-average intellectual capability with defects in the ability to learn and adapt. More males than females are affected. It may be genetic, congenital, biological, or psychosocial. On standardized intelligence tests with the average intelligence quotient

(IQ) set at 90–110, mental retardation is generally classified as borderline with IQ 71–84; mild with IQ 50–70; moderate with IQ 35–49; severe with IQ 20–34; and profound with IQ below 20.

mentation N. any mental activity.

mento- comb. form indicating an association with the chin (e.g., mentolabial, pert. to the chin and lip).

mentum N. chin.

meperidine N. narcotic analgesic (trade name Demerol) commonly used to treat moderate to severe pain. Adverse effects include drowsiness, gastrointestinal disturbances, circulatory and respiratory depression, and the potential for addiction.

meprobamate (mĕp′rō-băm′āt′) N. sedative and tranquilizer (trade names include Equanil, Miltown, and Meprin) used to treat anxiety and muscle tension. Adverse effects include drowsiness, ataxia, allergic reactions, and interaction with other drugs acting on the central nervous system.

Mepron N. trade name for the antibiotic atovaquone.

meralgia (mə-răl′jē-ə) N. pain in the thigh.

mercaptopurine (mər-kăp′tō-pyoor′ēn) N. antineoplastic and immunosuppressive drug (trade name Purinethol) used in the treatment of acute lymphocytic leukemia and certain other neoplasms. Adverse effects include nausea, vomiting, and bone marrow depression.

mercury N. toxic metallic element sometimes used in ointments. *See also* TABLE OF IMPORTANT ELEMENTS.

mercury poisoning N. toxic condition caused by the ingestion or inhalation of mercury or mercury-containing products (e.g., fungicides and certain pigments); contamination of waters with industrial wastes containing mercury has led to contaminated fish and seafood in some areas. Acute poisoning causes a metallic taste in the mouth, gastrointestinal symptoms (e.g., vomiting, diarrhea), and kidney disturbances that may lead to death. Chronic poisoning, resulting from exposure to small amounts of mercury over a long period, causes irritability, slurred speech, staggering gait, and teeth and gum disorders. Treatment includes gastric lavage. *See also* MINAMATA DISEASE.

mercy killing *See* EUTHANASIA.

meromelia (mĕr′ō-mē′lē-ə) N. congenital absence of any part of a limb including phocomelia and adactyly (*compare* AMELIA).

merozoite (mĕr′ə-zō′īt) N. stage in the life cycle of the malaria parasite and of certain other parasites.

mescaline N. psychoactive alkaloid derived from a cactus (*Lophophora williamsii*) that produces euphoria, hallucinations, anxiety, heart palpitations, and other signs of excitement. It is used by some American Indian tribes to produce feelings of ecstasy during ceremonies, and as a street drug. Also called peyote.

mesencephalon (mĕz′ĕn-sĕf′ə-lŏn′) N. *See* MIDBRAIN.

mesenchyme (mĕz′ən-kīm′) N. embryonic tissue that forms connective tissue, blood, and

smooth muscles. ADJ. mesen-
chymal

mesentery (mĕz′ən-tĕr′ē) N. fold
of peritoneum that holds abdominal organs (e.g., stomach, parts
of the small intestine, spleen)
to the posterior wall of the abdomen. ADJ. mesenteric

mesial *See* MEDIAL.

mesocolon (mĕz′ə-kō′lən) N. fold
of peritoneum that holds the
lower parts of the colon to the
inside of the abdominal wall.
ADJ. mesocolic

mesoderm (mĕz′ə-dûrm′) N. in
the embryo, middle germ cell
layer from which muscle, bone,
cartilage, blood, vascular and
lymph tissue, and other tissues
develop. (The other two cell
layers are the inner endoderm
and the outer ectoderm.)

mesomorph (mĕz′ə-môrf′) N.
person with well-developed
skeletal and muscular structure,
intermediate between the ectomorph and endomorph. ADJ.
mesomorphic

mesosalpinx N. free end of the
broad ligament within which
the Fallopian tubes lie.

mesothelioma (mĕz′ə-thē′lē-ō′
mə) N. rare, malignant tumor of
the mesothelial lining of the
pleura or peritoneum, usually
associated with exposure to
asbestos.

messenger RNA (mRNA) N.
form of ribonucleic acid (RNA)
that transmits information from
deoxyribonucleic acid (DNA)
in the nucleus to the ribosome
sites of protein synthesis in the
cell. *See also* TRANSFER RNA.

metabolic rate N. amount of energy expended in a given period.

metabolism N. combined chemical and physical process that
takes place in the body, involves the distribution of nutrients, and results in growth,
energy production, elimination
of wastes, and other body functions. There are two basic
phases of metabolism: anabolism, the constructive phase,
during which small molecules
resulting from the digestive
process are built up into complex compounds that form the
tissues and organs of the body;
and catabolism, the destructive
phase, during which larger
molecules are broken down into
simpler substances with the
release of energy. ADJ. metabolic

metabolite N. substance taking
part in metabolism, either a
product of a metabolic process
or a substance necessary for a
metabolic process.

metacarpus (mĕt′ə-kär′pəs) N.
any of the five bones of the
hand between the wrist (carpus)
and the finger (phalanges); they
are usually numbered I through
V, starting on the thumb side.
ADJ. metacarpal

metamorphopsia N. vision defect
in which objects appear distorted; it is usually due to a
defect in the retina.

metamorphosis (mĕt′ə-môr′fə-
sĭs) N. change in shape or structure, esp. a change from one
distinct form to another (e.g., in
insects from larva to pupa to
adult).

metaphase (mĕt′ə-fāz′) N. stage
in mitosis and meiosis during
which chromosomes become
aligned along the equatorial
plane of the spindle in preparation for separation and distribution to the daughter cells.

metaphysis (mĭ-tăf′ĭ-sĭs) N., *pl.*
metaphyses, growing portion of
a long bone, between the diaphysis (shaft) and epiphyses
(ends). ADJ. metaphyseal

metaplasia (mĕt′ə-plā′zhə) N.
conversion of a normal tissue
into an abnormal form; typically
noted on microscopic examination by changes in cell shape
and structure. Cervical metaplasia is an abnormal and sometimes precancerous change
noted in cervical cells obtained
during a Pap smear.

metaproterenol (mĕt′ə-prō-tĕr′-
ə-nôl) N. bronchodilator (trade
name Alupent), available in
oral and inhalant forms, and
used to treat asthma, emphysema, and other lung conditions. Adverse effects include
tachycardia and shakiness.

metastasis (mə-tăs′tə-sĭs) N.
spread of a tumor from its site
of origin to distant sites, usually through the bloodstream,
the lymphatic system, or across
a cavity such as that contained
in the peritoneum. V. metastasize, ADJ. metastatic

metatarsus (mĕt′ə-tär′səs) N. any
of the five bones of the foot,
between the ankle (tarsus) and
the toes (phalanges); they are
usually numbered I to V, starting on the medial (great toe)
side. ADJ. metatarsal

metencephalon (mĕt′ĕn-sĕf′ə-
lŏn′) N. part of the brain, including the pons and the cerebellum.

meteortropism N. effects of climate on biological occurrences
(e.g., angina, joint pains).

metformin N. *See* TABLE OF COM-
MONLY PRESCRIBED DRUGS—
GENERIC NAMES.

methadone (mĕth′ə-dōn′) N. synthetic narcotic pain reliever used
to treat opiate- (esp. heroin-)
addicted persons and sometimes to relieve severe pain.
Adverse effects include drowsiness, gastrointestinal disturbances, respiratory and circulatory
depression, and the potential
for addiction.

methamphetamine (mĕth′ăm-
fĕt′ə-mēn′) N. central nervous
system stimulant used to treat
narcolepsy and certain other
disorders. Adverse effects include central nervous system
excitation, increase in blood
pressure, nausea, and the potential for drug dependence.

methanol N. methyl alcohol;
wood alcohol; colorless, flammable liquid used as a solvent
for ethyl alcohol. Highly toxic
if ingested, methanol can cause
blindness, kidney failure, and
death.

methapyrilene N. antihistamine
used in the treatment of rhinitis,
dermatitis, pruritus, and other
allergic responses. Adverse effects include drowsiness, dry
mouth, skin rash, rapid heartbeat, and hypersensitivity reactions.

methaqualone (mĕth′ə-kwā′lōn′)
N. sedative-hypnotic (trade
name Quaalude), used as a street drug.
Adverse effects include loss of
inhibition, gastrointestinal disturbances, and drug dependence.
No longer available through
legitimate sources, it is used
now only as an illegal drug of
abuse.

metharbital N. anticonvulsant
(trade name Gemonil) used to
treat epilepsy. Adverse effects
include ataxia, irritability, and
gastric distress.

methenamine (mə-thē′nə-mĕn′) N. antibacterial contained in many products (e.g., Urotone) used to treat urinary tract infections. Adverse effects include rashes and gastrointestinal distress.

methicillin (mĕth′ĭ-sĭl′ĭn) N. antibiotic of the penicillin family that is not rendered inactive by the penicillinase enzyme released by certain bacteria; it is used to treat certain staphylococcal infections. Adverse effects include allergic reactions, kidney disturbance, and occasionally inflammation or phlebitis at the side of injection.

methionine (mə-thī′ə-nēn′) N. essential (not produced by the body, required in the diet) amino acid.

methocarbamol N. skeletal muscle relaxant (trade name Robaxin) used to treat spasms of skeletal muscles. Adverse effects include low blood pressure, dizziness, drowsiness, and nausea.

methodology N. principles and procedures used in scientific research or other endeavor.

methotrexate N. antineoplastic drug used to treat certain cancers. Adverse effects include mouth sores, digestive upsets, bone marrow depression, and rashes.

methyclothiazide N. diuretic and antihypertensive (trade name Enduron) used to treat high blood pressure. Adverse effects include electrolyte imbalance and hypersensitivity reactions.

methyl salicylate N. oil of wintergreen; a liquid used as a counterirritant and pain reliever, applied externally for minor muscle and joint pain.

Adverse effects include skin reactions.

methyl testosterone (tĕs-tŏs′tə-rōn′) N. androgen preparation (trade names Estratest and Metandren) used to treat testosterone deficiency and female breast cancer and to stimulate growth and weight gain. Adverse effects include edema, masculinization, and jaundice.

methyldopa (mĕth′əl-dō′pə) N. antihypertensive (trade names Aldomet and, when combined with a diuretic, Aldoril) used to treat high blood pressure. Adverse effects include sedation, dry mouth, and liver and blood abnormalities.

methylene blue N. crystalline powder, used in kidney function tests, as a urinary antiseptic, and in the treatment of cyanide poisoning and certain other disorders.

methylphenidate (mĕth′əl-fĕn′ĭ-dāt′) N. central nervous system stimulant (trade name Ritalin) used to treat attention deficit disorder and narcolepsy. Adverse effects include loss of appetite, insomnia, nervousness, and allergic reactions.

methyprylon N. sedative hypnotic (trade name Noludar) used to treat sleep disorders. Adverse effects include dizziness, gastrointestinal disturbances, headache, paradoxical excitement, and the possibility of dependence.

methysergide N. vasoconstrictor (trade name Sansert) used to treat migraine. This drug is used only when other attempts to treat severe and frequent migraine are unsuccessful, because of serious potential adverse effects, including pulmonary and cardiac abnormalities, blood disorders, and pains in various parts of the body.

metoprolol N. oral/parenteral beta blocker (trade name Lopressor) used in the treatment of hypertension, angina, arrhythmias, and acute myocardial infarction. Adverse effects include depression, exacerbation of congestive heart failure or asthma, and acrocyanosis. See TABLE OF COMMONLY PRESCRIBED DRUGS—GENERIC NAMES.

metralgia N. pain in the uterus.

metritis (mǐ-trī'tǐs) N. inflammation of the uterus. *See also* ENDOMETRITIS.

metroptosis N. prolapse of the uterus; downward displacement of the uterus, with the neck (cervix) sometimes protruding from the vagina. It most often occurs in women who have had children. Treatment is by surgery.

metrorrhagia (mē'trə-rā'jē-ə) N. bleeding from the uterus other than that of menstruation, usually indicative of uterine disease (e.g., cervical cancer).

Mevacor N. trade name for lovastatin. See TABLE OF COMMONLY PRESCRIBED DRUGS—TRADE NAMES.

mexiletine N. antiarrhythmic (trade name Mexitil) indicated for the treatment of ventricular arrhythmias. Side effects include nausea, vomiting, and dizziness.

Mexitil N. trade name for the antiarrhythmic mexiletine.

Mg symbol for the element magnesium.

MH *See* MALIGNANT HYPERTHERMIA.

MI *See* MYOCARDIAL INFARCTION.

Miacalcin N. *See* TABLE OF COMMONLY PRESCRIBED DRUGS—TRADE NAMES.

micelle N. aggregate of molecules in a colloidal solution, such as a detergent.

micr-, micro- comb. forms indicating smallness (e.g. microblepharon, abnormally small eyelids).

microbe (mī'krōb') N. small organism, visible only with a microscope (*see also* MICROORGANISM). ADJ. microbic, microbial

microbiology (mī'krō-bī-ŏl'ə-jē) N. that branch of biology concerned with the study of microorganisms, including bacteria, viruses, rickettsiae, fungi, and protozoa.

microbrachia N. defect in development characterized by abnormally small arms.

microcephaly (mī'krō-sĕf'ə-lē) N. congenital abnormality in which the head is abnormally small and the brain is underdeveloped, resulting in some degree of mental retardation (*compare* MACROCEPHALY); also called microcephalus. ADJ. microcephalic

microcytosis N. blood disorder characterized by abnormally small erythrocytes (red blood cells), often associated with iron-deficiency anemia.

microdactyly N. abnormality characterized by unusually small fingers and toes.

microfilament N. microscopic tube or filament within or between cells.

microglia (mī-krŏg'lē-ə) N. small cells of the central nervous system that act as phagocytes, collecting waste products of nerve tissue.

microgram N. metric unit of weight measure equal to one-millionth of a gram. Abbrev. μ or mcg.

Micro-K N. trade name for an oral form of potassium chloride.

micrometer N. metric distance measure equal to one-millionth of a meter.

Micronase N. trade name for the oral antidiabetic glyburide. *See* TABLE OF COMMONLY PRESCRIBED DRUGS—TRADE NAMES.

micronutrient N. compound, such as a vitamin or mineral (e.g., riboflavin, zinc, copper, iodine), needed only in small amounts for normal body function.

microorganism N. very small organism, usually visible only with a microscope; included among microorganisms are bacteria, viruses, rickettsiae, fungi, and protozoa.

microphage (mī′krə-fāj′) N. neutrophil (type of white blood cell) that can ingest small things (e.g., bacteria) (*compare* MACROPHAGE).

microphallus N. abnormally small penis; also called micropenis.

microphthalmos (mī-krŏf-thăl′mŏs′) N. developmental defect characterized by abnormal smallness of one or both eyes.

microscope (mī′krə-skōp′) N. instrument for producing a magnified image of an object that may be so small as to be invisible to the naked eye. There are several types of microscopes, including the light microscope, which uses light as the source of radiation and a combination of lenses to magnify and focus the object; and the electron microscope, in which a beam of electrons is used to scan and produce an image of the object.

microscopic (mī′krə-skŏp′ĭk) ADJ. 1. pert. to a microscope. 2. very small, visible only when magnified and illuminated by a microscope.

microscopic anatomy N. study of the microscopic structure of tissues and organs; included are histology and cytology (*compare* GROSS ANATOMY).

microscopy (mī-krŏs′kə-pē) N. use of a microscope to view objects. ADJ. microscopic

microsomia (mī′krə-sō′mē-ə) N. condition of having an abnormally small and undeveloped, but structurally normal, body.

microsurgery (mī′krō-sûr′jə-rē) N. that branch of surgery performed using special operating microscopes and miniaturized precision instruments to perform delicate and intricate procedures on very small structures and structures not previously accessible to surgery, such as parts of the eye, brain, and spinal cord, and to reattach amputated digits and limbs, requiring suturing of very small nerves and blood vessels.

microtubule (mī′krō-tōō′byōōl) N. hollow, elongated tubular structure within a cell; serves a number of functions, including support of the cell and transfer of chemical messengers within and between cells.

microvillus (mī′krō-vĭl′əs) N. microscopic fold on the surface of a cell membrane; increases the cells surface area significantly. Found in several areas of the body, esp. the small intestine, where microvilli absorb nutrients.

micturition (mĭk′chə-rĭsh′ən) *See* URINATION.

micturition reflex N. normal response to increased pressure in the bladder, with relaxation of the urethral sphincter allowing passage of urine from the body.

midazolam (mĭ-dăz′ə-lăm′) N. injectable benzodiazepine drug (trade name Versed) useful for sedation and reducing painful sensations, esp. during procedures that may be somewhat uncomfortable. Adverse effects include respiratory depression and amnesia. *See also* VALIUM.

midbrain N. part of the brain stem, joining the hindbrain and forebrain, and serving as passageway for impulses to higher brain centers; also called mesencephalon.

middle ear N. that part of the ear consisting of air-filled space in the temporal bone and extending from the tympanic membrane, which separates it from the external ear, to the inner ear. It contains three small bones (the malleus, incus, and stapes) that transmit sound vibrations from the tympanic membrane to the inner ear. The middle ear is connected to the pharynx through the Eustachian tube.

midwife N. person who assists women in labor and childbirth.

Mifepristone N. trade name for the abortion-producing drug RU 486.

migraine (mī′grān′) N. recurring vascular headache, occurring more frequently in women. The cause is unknown, but the pain is associated with dilation of blood vessels. Allergic reactions, menstruation, alcohol, or relaxation after a period of stress often triggers attacks. A typical attack, which may last from several hours to several days, starts with an episode of visual disturbances (e.g., aura or flashing lights), numbness, tingling, vertigo, or other sensations, followed by the onset of severe, usually unilateral pain, sometimes accompanied by nausea, vomiting, photophobia, irritability, and fatigue. Ergotamine preparations that constrict cranial arteries are helpful if taken at the onset of an attack; aspirin does not usually provide relief. Also called megrim; hemicrania. *See also* HISTAMINE HEADACHE; TENSION HEADACHE.

migration N. movement from one location to another; during development various structures migrate from a central location to their final anatomic position (e.g., the testicles are formed in the abdominal cavity and migrate into the scrotal sac).

milia N. minute white cysts of epidermis caused by obstruction of hair follicles and sweat glands; also called whiteheads.

milia neonatorum N. normal skin condition of newborns characterized by minute epidermal cysts on the face and sometimes trunk that disappear spontaneously within a few weeks.

miliaria (mĭl′ē-âr′ē-ə) N. minute vesicles and papules, often surrounded by a reddened area, caused by obstruction of sweat glands during high heat and humidity; itching may result; also called prickly heat.

miliary tuberculosis (mĭl′ē-ĕr′ē tōō-bûr′kyə-lō′sĭs) *See* TUBERCULOSIS.

milk N. fluid secreted by mammary glands (breasts), usually the first food of newborn mammals. Humans also consume the milk of cows and certain other mammals (e.g., goats, yak). Milk contains carbohydrates (lactose), protein (casein), fat, the minerals calcium and phosphorus, and vitamins A, riboflavin, niacin, thiamine, and, when fortified, D.

milk intolerance N. condition caused by a lack of or defect in an enzyme that renders a person unable to digest milk sugar (lactose). *See also* LACTASE DEFICIENCY; LACTOSE INTOLERANCE.

milk of magnesia N. laxative and antacid, containing magnesium hydroxide; it is used to treat constipation and acid indigestion.

milk sugar *See* LACTOSE.

milk tooth *See* DECIDUOUS TOOTH.

milk-ejection reflex *See* LETDOWN.

millimole N. one-thousandth of a mole; abbr. mM.

milrinone N. intravenous drug (trade name Primacor) used to treat severe congestive heart failure; side effects include hypotension and, rarely, cardiac arrhythmias.

Miltown N. trade name for the sedative meprobamate.

Minamata disease (mĭn′ə-mä′tə) N. form of mercury poisoning that occurred among people eating fish from mercury-contaminated waters of Minamata Bay, off Japan, in the 1950s. It is characterized by severe neurological degeneration with symptoms of paresthesia of mouth and limbs, tunnel vision, difficulties with concentration and muscular coordination, weakness, and emotional instability, progressing with continued exposure resulting in damage to the gastrointestinal tract and kidneys, coma, and in some cases death. *See also* MERCURY POISONING.

mind-body medicine *See* TABLE OF ALTERNATIVE MEDICINE TERMS.

mineral N. in nutrition, inorganic substance, such as copper, zinc, or magnesium needed in small amounts by the body for normal growth and function.

mineral deficiency N. lack of a mineral essential to normal nutrition and metabolism; it may be due to a lack of the mineral in the diet or to inability to absorb the mineral. The symptoms of a mineral deficiency vary, depending on the functions of the specific mineral in maintaining the health of the body. Treatment of a deficiency is by adding the element to the diet or correcting the cause of its malabsorption, if possible.

mineral oil N. laxative and stool softener used to treat constipation. Adverse effects include possible laxative dependence, fat-soluble vitamin deficiency, and abdominal cramps.

mineralocorticoid (mĭn′ər-ə-lō-kôr′tĭ-koid′) N. any of several hormones secreted by the adrenal cortex, the most important of which is aldosterone, which functions to maintain normal blood volume and salt and fluid balance in the body.

minimal brain dysfunction (MBD) *See* ATTENTION DEFICIT DISORDER.

Minipress N. trade name for the antihypertensive prazosin.

Minocin N. trade name for the antibacterial minocycline.

minocycline N. tetracycline antibiotic (trade name Minocin) used to treat a wide variety of bacterial and rickettsial infections. Adverse effects include gastrointestinal disturbances, allergic reactions, vertigo (which may be incapacitating), and (in children) discoloration of the teeth.

minor surgery N. any surgical procedure that does not require general anesthesia or respiratory assistance (*compare* MAJOR SURGERY).

minoxidil N. vasodilator used to treat severe and difficult-to-control hypertension. Adverse effects include rapid heartbeat, salt and water retention, gastrointestinal upsets, and hirsutism. Hirsutism is so predictable, in fact, that a liquid form of minoxidil is also marketed, under the trade name Rogaine, as an antibaldness treatment. (Note the two trade names: Loniten for high blood pressure; Rogaine for baldness.)

miosis (mī-ō′sĭs) N.
1. contraction of the sphincter muscle of the iris causing the pupil to become smaller; it may be caused by an increase in light or by certain drugs (*compare* MYDRIASIS).
2. abnormal constriction of the sphincter muscle of the iris, causing abnormally small pupils. ADJ. miotic

miotic ADJ. pert. to or causing constriction of the pupil of the eye, as a miotic drug (e.g., pilocarpine).

mirage N. optical illusion caused by the refraction of light through layers of air of different temperatures.

miscarriage *See* ABORTION, SPONTANEOUS.

miscible (mĭs′ə-bəl) ADJ. capable of mixing with.

mite N. any of a group of small arachnids (relative of spiders and ticks), some of which cause local skin irritation and itching in humans.

Mithracin N. trade name for the antineoplastic mithramycin.

mithramycin N. antineoplastic (trade name Mithracin) used to treat cancer of the testes. Adverse effects include blood-clotting disorders, gastrointestinal upsets, and mouth inflammation.

mitochondrion (mī′tə-kŏn′drē-ən) N. self-replicating organelle found in the cytoplasm of cells, where it functions in cellular metabolism and respiration, providing the cell's major source of energy.

mitogen N. substance that triggers mitosis.

mitomycin (mī′tə-mī′sĭn) N. antineoplastic used to treat certain malignancies. Adverse effects include bone marrow depression and gastrointestinal disturbances.

mitosis (mī-tō′sĭs) N. type of cell division in which a cell divides into two genetically identical daughter cells; it is the way in which new body cells are produced for growth. Division of the cell nucleus takes place in four stages, and the resulting daughter cells have the same number of chromosomes as the parent cell (*compare* MEIOSIS).

mitral valve (mī′trəl) N. one of four valves of the heart; it is situated between the left atrium and left ventricle and allows blood to flow from the left atrium to the left ventricle and prevents backflow. It consists of two flaps or cusps. Also called bicuspid valve; left atrioventricular valve. (*Compare* SEMILUNAR VALVE; TRICUSPID VALVE.)

mitral valve prolapse (prō-laps) N. disorder in which the mitral valve cusps (leaflets) bulge into the left atrium when the left ventricle contracts, sometimes allowing leakage (regurgitation) of small amounts of blood into the atrium. The cause is unknown. Most cases result in little, if any, hemodynamically significant (i.e., causing clinical symptoms or changes in the vital signs) valvular incompetence. There appears to be a familial predisposition but the exact genetic defect is unknown. Most people with mitral valve prolapse have no symptoms. Others have chest pain, a rapid pulse, palpitations (awareness of heartbeats), migraine headaches, fatigue, and dizziness. In some, blood pressure may fall below normal with standing (called orthostatic hypotension). Rarely, syncope or cardiac arrest may occur. Experts believe that abnormalities in the autonomic nervous system are responsible for the symptoms. There is a characteristic clicking sound heard during cardiac auscultation. Termed a "midsystolic

HUMAN MITOSIS

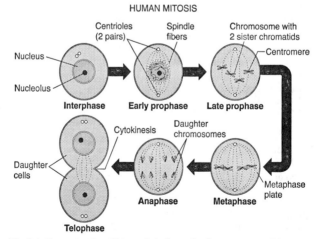

Mitosis is the process by which a cell duplicates its chromosomes and then separates the duplicated genome into two identical halves. It is generally followed immediately by cytokinesis, which divides the cytoplasm and cell membrane. This results in two identical daughter cells with a roughly equal distribution of organelles and other cellular components.

click," this sound is present in most patients. For this reason, the condition was once termed "click-murmur syndrome." A murmur may also be present. Patients with murmurs are at risk for development of bacterial endocarditis, especially following dental work—these individuals require antibiotic prophylaxis prior to the procedure. Echocardiography is useful in demonstrating the underlying prolapse. A group of drugs, the beta blockers, are effective in suppressing most symptoms. In severe cases (e.g., syncope, history of cardiac arrest) an automated implantable cardioverter-defibrillator (AICD) is required. *See also* AUTONOMIC NERVOUS SYSTEM; AUTOMATED IMPLANTABLE CARDIOVERTER-DEFIBRILLATOR; BETA BLOCKERS; ENDOCARDITIS; MITRAL VALVE.

mitral valve stenosis (mī′trəl stə-nō′sĭs) N. obstruction or narrowing of the mitral valve due to scarring from recurrent rheumatic fever; it causes reduced cardiac output, leading to breathlessness, fatigue, and cyanosis. Treatment is by surgery.

mittelschmerz (mĭt′l-shmûrts′) N. pain in the area of the ovary, occurring at the time of ovulation, usually midway in the menstrual cycle.

Mn symbol for the element manganese.

Modicon N. trade name for an oral contraceptive containing estradiol and norethindrone.

modified radical mastectomy (mă-stĕk′tə-mē) *See* MASTECTOMY.

Moeller's glossitis (glô-sī′tĭs) N. chronic burning and pain of the tongue and sensitivity to spicy and hot foods.

moiety (moi′ĭ-tē) N. one of two approximately equal parts.

molar (mō′lər) N. tooth, located in the back of the mouth, used for grinding food. There are usually three molars on each side of the jaw. The first two are present in most individuals while the backmost (wisdom tooth) may or may not break through the gum line.

molar pregnancy *See* HYDATID MOLE.

mole N.
1. small often slightly raised dark blemish on the skin caused by a high concentration of melanin.
2. in chemistry, amount of a given substance having a mass numerically equal to its molecular or atomic weight.

molecule N. in chemistry, the combination of two or more atoms that form a particular chemical or compound.

molecular genetics N. that branch of genetics concerned with the chemical structure, functions, and replications of the molecules—deoxyribonucleic acid (DNA) and ribonucleic acid (RNA)—involved in the transmission of hereditary information.

molluscum (mə-lŭs′kəm) N. skin disease characterized by soft round masses.

molluscum contagiosum N. virus disease of the skin characterized by white, rounded swellings that may resolve spontaneously or may be removed through surgery or other techniques. It is transmitted from person to person, occurring most often in children and adults with impaired immune function.

Mongolian spot N. benign dark spot on the lower back and buttocks of some newborns, usually disappearing during early childhood.

mongolism *See* DOWN'S SYNDROME.

monilia *See* CANDIDA. ADJ. monilial

moniliasis *See* CANDIDIASIS.

Monistat N. trade name for the antifungal miconazole.

monitrice *See* LABOR COACH.

monoamine oxidase (MAO) (mŏn'ō-ăm'ēn) N. enzyme, found in most tissues, esp. the liver and nervous system, that catalyzes the oxidation of many body compounds, including epinephrine, norepinephrine, and serotonin.

monoamine oxidase (MAO) inhibitor N. any of a group of drugs used to treat depression. Adverse effects include dry mouth, drowsiness, and constipation. The drugs interact with many other drugs and with foods (e.g., cheeses, red wine, beer, and yogurt) containing tyramine (an amino acid), sometimes causing an acute hypertensive episode with headache and palpitations.

monoblast N. large, immature monocyte, normally found in the bone marrow but present in the blood in certain diseases, esp. monocytic leukemia.

monoblastic leukemia (lōō-kē'mē-ə) *See* MONOCYTIC LEUKEMIA.

monoclonal (mŏn'ə-klō'nəl) ADJ. arising from similar cell types or lines. Often used regarding antibodies that arise from a single cellular source in the body. Compare to polyclonal, arising from multiple cell types or lines.

monoclonal antibody N. antibody produced from a special cell (hybridoma) that is very specific for a particular location in the body. Monoclonal antibodies are used in many areas of medicine for diagnostic tests and are being tested experimentally as anticancer agents.

monocyte (mŏn'ə-sīt') N. type of granular leukocyte (white blood cell) that functions in the ingestion of bacteria and other foreign particles.

monocytic leukemia (mŏn'ə-sīt'ĭk lōō-kē'mē-ə) N. malignancy of the blood-forming tissues characterized by proliferation of monocytes and monoblasts. Symptoms include anorexia, fatigue, fever, weight loss, enlarged spleen, bleeding gums, and anemia. There are two forms: Schilling's leukemia and Naegeli's leukemia. Also called monoblastic leukemia; histiocytic leukemia.

monocytosis (mŏn'ə-sī-tō'sĭs) N. increase in the number of monocytes in the blood, occurring in some infections and in monocytic leukemia.

mononeuropathy (mŏn'ō-nōō-rŏp'ə-thē) N. any disorder affecting a single nerve trunk, as in nerve compression from a fractured bone. *See also* MULTIPLE MONONEUROPATHY.

mononuclear (mŏn'ō-nōō'klē-ər) N. containing one nucleus; often in reference to a type of white blood cell (monocyte). An abnormal elevation in blood mononuclear cells (monocytosis) occurs during the viral infection mononucleosis.

mononucleosis (mŏn′ō-noō′klē-ō′sĭs) *See* INFECTIOUS MONONU-CLEOSIS.

monoplegia (mŏn′ə-plē′jē-ə) N. paralysis of one limb.

Monopril N. *See* TABLE OF COMMONLY PRESCRIBED DRUGS—TRADE NAMES.

monorchism (mŏn-ôr′kĭz′əm) N. condition in which only one testicle has descended into the scrotum; also called monorchidism. *See also* CRYPTORCHIDISM.

monosaccharide (mŏn′ə-săk′ə-rīd′) N. simple sugar that cannot be dissolved by hydrolysis, such as glucose.

monosomy N. chromosomal abnormality characterized by the absence of one chromosome from the normal diploid number for the species (e.g., 45 in humans, instead of the normal complement of 46) (*compare* TRISOMY) (*See also* TURNER'S SYNDROME).

monovalent ADJ. having a single electron available to chemically combine with another substance; common monovalent cations (carry a positive electrical charge) in the body include sodium (Na^+) and potassium (K^+).

monozygotic twins N. twins developing from a single fertilized egg that splits in half at an early stage of cleavage and develops into two complete fetuses. Monozygotic twins are always of the same sex, have the same genetic makeup, and closely resemble each other in all characteristics. About one-third of all twins are monozygous; such twinning is not hereditary and occurs in all races. Also called identical twins. (*Compare* DIZYGOTIC TWINS; SIAMESE TWINS.)

mons N. rounded eminence, esp. mons pubis, the mound of fatty tissue overlying the pubic symphysis.

monster N. medical term for a grossly malformed, usually non-viable, fetus.

Montgomery's tubercle (toō′bər-kəl) N. any of several sebaceous glands on the areolae of the breast that lubricate and protect the breast during breast-feeding.

moon face N. rounded, puffy face occurring in people treated with large doses of corticosteroids.

morbid (môr′bĭd) ADJ. diseased, abnormal.

morbidity (mōr-bĭd′ĭ-tē) N. 1. state of being diseased. 2. ratio of persons who are diseased to those who are well in a given community.

morbilli (môr-bĭl′ī) *See* MEASLES.

morbilliform ADJ. describing a rash that resembles that of measles.

moribund (môr′ə-bŭnd′) ADJ. dying

morning sickness N. nausea and vomiting that is a common occurrence in pregnancy, usually occurring in the morning but sometimes at other times during the day; it often disappears after the first 3 or 4 months of pregnancy. Symptomatic relief is often provided by not allowing the stomach to be empty and eating small, frequent meals. *See also* HYPEREMESIS GRAVIDARUM.

morning-after pill N. large dose of an estrogen given orally, within 24–72 hours after sexual intercourse to prevent conception; it is most commonly used after rape or incest. The morning-after pill is sometimes prescribed for women when their initial birth control fails (i.e., a condom breaks). Adverse effects include severe nausea and vomiting, blood clot formation, and harmful effects on the fetus if pregnancy is not prevented.

Moro's reflex (môr′ōz) N. normal reflex of a young infant, elicited by a sudden loud noise, in which the baby flexes the legs and outstretches the arms, often with a cry; also called startle reflex.

moron (môr′ŏn′) N. obsolete term for a retarded person with an IQ between 50 and 70 (*compare* IDIOT; IMBECILE; *see also* MENTAL RETARDATION).

morphea (môr-fē′ə) N. localized form of scleroderma, consisting of patches of rigid, dry, smooth skin.

morphine (môr′fēn′) N. narcotic analgesic used to relieve pain. Adverse effects include respiratory depression, cardiovascular abnormalities, and the potential for dependence.

morphogenesis (môr′fō-jĕn′ĭ-sĭs) N. development of the form and structure of an organism. ADJ. morphogenetic

mortality rate (môr-tăl′ĭ-tē) N. death rate; number of deaths per unit of population (e.g., per 100, 10,000, or 1,000,000) in a specific region, age group, or other group.

morula (môr′yə-lə) N. stage in human embryonic development between the zygote and the blastocyst, consisting of a solid spherical mass of cells.

mosaicism (mō-zā′ĭ-sĭz′əm) N. condition in which an organism contains two or more cell populations that differ in genetic makeup.

motility (mō-tĭl′ĭ-tē) N. ability to move spontaneously and independently.

motion sickness N. condition characterized by headache, nausea, vomiting, and malaise, caused by motion, as in a car, boat, or aircraft. Kinds of motion sickness are air sickness, car sickness, and seasickness. Prevention and treatment are by antihistamines (Dramamine), transdermal scopolamine, and motion sickness bands.

motion sickness bands N. elastic bands with a central protruding button, worn on both wrists, that provide acupressure over a nerve point thought to reduce motion sickness; these bands have been used in the British merchant marine for years, and are becoming more widely distributed in the United States; limited evidence suggests that the bands may also help some patients with nausea and vomiting during pregnancy.

motion sickness patch *See* SCOPOLAMINE PATCH.

motor aphasia (ə-fā′zhə) N. inability to utter remembered words, due to lesion in the Broca speech area of the cerebrum, most commonly the result of a cerebrovascular accident (stroke).

motor area N. part of the cerebral cortex associated with the function of voluntary muscles.

motor end plate N. band of terminal fibers of a motor nerve that merges with the fibers of a voluntary muscle, allowing the impulse to be transmitted from the nerve to the muscle.

motor nerve N. nerve that conducts impulses from the brain or spinal cord to muscles or organs of the body (*compare* SENSORY NERVE).

motor neuron (noŏor′ŏn′) N. nerve cell that comprises the pathway between the brain or spinal cord and an effector organ a muscle or gland.

motor neuron disease N. any of several diseases, often familial, characterized by loss of muscle mass, increasing paralysis, and other signs of impaired muscular function.

motor seizure (sē′zhər) N. transitory disturbance in neuron function in a localized motor area of the cerebral cortex. The manifestations depend on the specific motor area affected. *See also* FOCAL SEIZURE.

motor sense N. perception allowing a person to undertake deliberate and purposeful movement.

Motrin N. trade name for the anti-inflammatory ibuprofen. *See* TABLE OF COMMONLY PRESCRIBED DRUGS—TRADE NAMES.

mountain fever *See* ROCKY MOUNTAIN SPOTTED FEVER.

mountain sickness *See* ALTITUDE SICKNESS.

mouth N.
1. oval cavity of the face, bounded by the lips and containing the gums, teeth and tongue, which is the anterior end of the digestive tube. In the mouth food is broken apart by the teeth and tongue and mixed with saliva, as the first step in the digestive process.
2. *see* ORIFICE. ADJ. oral

mouth-to-mouth resuscitation (rĭ-sŭs′ĭ-tā′shən) *See* CARDIOPULMONARY RESUSCITATION.

moxibustion N. form of traditional Chinese medicine in which dried and powdered leaves of *Artemesia vulgaris* are burned either on or in proximity to the skin. The purpose is to affect movement of a person's energy or "qi" through a specific healing channel in the body. Often used in combination with acupuncture.

MRI N. abbrev. for magnetic resonance imaging, another term for nuclear magnetic resonance (NMR) scanning.

mRNA *See* MESSENGER RNA.

MSH *See* MELANOCYTE-STIMULATING HORMONE.

mucin (myōō′sĭn) N. chief ingredient of mucus; lubricant protecting body surfaces.

mucocutaneous ADJ. pert. to the mucous membrane and the skin.

mucocutaneous lymph node syndrome *See* KAWASAKI DISEASE.

mucopolysaccharide (myōō′kō-pŏl′ē-săk′ə-rīd′) N. any of a group of complex carbohydrates that are structural parts of connective tissue.

mucopolysaccharidosis (myōō′-kō-pŏl′ē-săk′ə-rĭ-dō′sĭs) N. any of a group of genetic disorders, including Hurler's syndrome, in which greater than normal levels of mucopolysaccharides accumulate in the tissue. Skeletal deformity, mental retardation, and shortened life expectancy characterize the diseases, which can be detected through amniocentesis.

mucopurulent ADJ. of a combination of mucus and pus.

mucosa (myŏo-kō′sə) N. mucus-membrane or moist tissue layer lining all body cavities or passages that communicate with the exterior; the oral mucosa lines the mouth while the intestinal mucosa lines the gastrointestinal tract.

mucous colitis (myŏo′kəs kə-lī′tĭs) *See* IRRITABLE BOWEL SYNDROME.

mucous membrane N. thin sheet of tissue that covers or lines parts of the body; it consists of a layer of epithelium overlying thicker connective tissue. It protects underlying organs, secretes mucus, and absorbs water and solutes. Also called mucosa.

mucous plug N. in obstetrics, collection of thick mucus, often streaked with blood, that is expelled from the cervix of the uterus just before labor begins or during the early stages of labor. Also used to describe an accumulation of mucus that blocks a bronchus, esp. during an asthma attack.

mucoviscidosis *See* CYSTIC FIBROSIS.

mucus N. viscous secretions of mucous membranes and glands, containing mucin, water, white blood cells, and salts. ADJ. mucous

Müllerian ducts (myŏo-lēr′ē-ən) N. embryonic tubes from which develop the female reproductive organs (oviducts, uterus, vagina).

multicellular (mŭl′tē-sĕl′yə-lər) N. having many cells.

multifactorial (mŭl′tĭ-făk-tôr′ē-əl) ADJ. pert. to a disease or condition resulting from the interaction of many factors, esp. many genes.

multigravida (mŭl′tĭ-grăv′ĭ-də) N. woman who has been pregnant more than once; recorded as gravida II (second pregnancy), gravida III (third pregnancy). Sometimes abbr. as grav I, grav II, G I, G II, etc.

multiple chemical sensitivity syndrome N. syndrome in which multiple symptoms reportedly occur with low-level chemical exposure. Common symptoms include fatigue, difficulty concentrating, depressed mood, memory loss, weakness, dizziness, headaches, heat intolerance, and arthralgias. Agents suspected of causing chemical sensitivity include gasoline, kerosene, natural gas, pesticides, solvents, new carpet and other renovation materials, adhesives and glues, fiberglass, carbonless copy paper, fabric softener, formaldehyde and glutaraldehyde, carpet shampoos (lauryl sulfate) and other cleaning agents, isocyanates, combustion products (poorly vented gas heaters, overheated batteries), and medications (dinitrochlorobenzene for warts, intranasally packed neosynephrine, prolonged antibiotics, and general anesthesia with petrochemicals). The patient should be encouraged to work and to socialize despite the symptoms. The major disability is often the isolation and withdrawal experienced as the patient seeks to avoid chemical exposures. Yet there is no evidence that such avoidance is effective or that continued exposure leads to any adverse biologic effects.

multiple mononeuropathy (mŏn′ō-nŏo-rŏp′ə-thē) N. condition in which there is impaired function of several individual nerves; it may result from uremia, diabetes mellitus, or other disorders.

multiple myeloma (mī′ə-lō′mə) N. malignant neoplasm of bone marrow, causing bone pain and fractures, skeletal deformities, anemia, weight loss, and pulmonary and kidney complications.

multiple personality N. disorder characterized by the presence of two or more distinct personalities in the same person, any of which may dominate at a given time ranging from a few minutes to years, with transitions from one to the other personality usually occurring quickly and at a time of stress. Each personality is complex, possesses developed behavioral patterns and mental and emotional processes, and may or may not be known to the other. Clear-cut examples are rare, but various symptoms appear in some schizophrenics, esp. among young women. Treatment is by psychoactive drugs and long-term psychotherapy.

multiple sclerosis (sklə-rō′sĭs) N. progressive disease in which nerve fibers of the brain and spinal cord lose their myelin cover. It begins usually in early adulthood and progresses slowly with periods of remission and exacerbation. Early symptoms of abnormal sensations in the face or extremities, weakness, and visual disturbances (e.g., double vision) progress to ataxia, abnormal reflexes, tremors, difficulty in urination, emotional instability, and difficulty in walking, leading to increasing disability. There is no specific treatment; corticosteroids and other drugs are used to treat symptoms. Also called disseminated multiple sclerosis.

multivalent ADJ. having the ability to combine with more than two univalent elements or compounds.

mumps N. acute viral disease characterized by swelling of the parotid glands; it is most likely to affect nonimmunized children but may occur at any age, sometimes producing severe illness in adults. After early symptoms of fever, malaise, headache, and low-grade fever, earache, parotid gland swelling, and fever to 104° Fahrenheit (40° Celsius) occur, sometimes with salivary gland enlargement and, in post-pubertal males, swelling and tenderness of the testes. Complications include meningitis, arthritis, and nephritis. Treatment includes rest and drugs to relieve pain and reduce fever. Prevention is by immunization with attenuated live-virus vaccine, routinely given at 15 months of age.

Munchausen's syndrome (mŭn′ chou′zənz) N. condition in which a person presents himself/herself repeatedly, often to multiple hospitals, with what appears to be an acute illness. The complaints are often realistic and somewhat dramatic in nature, but no clinical evidence of disease is ever found.

mupirocin N. antibiotic ointment (trade name Bactroban) effective in the treatment of the skin infection, impetigo. *See* TABLE OF COMMONLY PRESCRIBED DRUGS—GENERIC NAMES.

muramidase (myo͞o-răm′ĭ-dās′) *See* LYSOZYME.

murine typhus (myo͝or′īn′ tīfəs) N. acute infection caused by *Rickettsia typhi*, transmitted by the bite of an infected flea and characterized by chills, fever, headache, muscle aches, and a dull red rash. Treatment is by chloramphenicol or tetracycline. Also called endemic typhus; rat typhus; urban typhus. (*Compare* ROCKY MOUNTAIN SPOTTED FEVER.)

murmur (mûr′mər) N. short, usually soft sound, esp. an abnormal one of the heart or circulation.

muscarinic ADJ. pert. to the effects of the neurotransmitter acetylcholine on nerves of the parasympathetic nervous system.

muscle N. type of contractile tissue, composed of fibers that can contract, causing movement of parts and organs. There are three basic kinds of muscle: skeletal muscle, which is striated in appearance, controls voluntary movement, responds quickly to neural stimulation, and is paralyzed if innervation is lost; smooth muscle, which is not striped in appearance, comprises the musculature of all visceral organs, responds slowly to stimulation, and controls involuntary movement; and cardiac muscle, which is striped in appearance, but does not respond as quickly as skeletal muscle and continues to contract if it loses its neural stimuli. ADJ. muscular. *See* MAJOR MUSCLES OF THE BODY in Appendix.

muscle relaxant N. drug that reduces the contractility of muscle fibers by blocking the transmission of nerve impulses at neuromuscular junctions, by increasing the time between contractions of fibers, by decreasing the excitability of the motor end plate, by interfering with nerve synapses in the central nervous system, or by interfering with calcium release from muscle or by other actions; the drugs are used in the treatment of muscle spasm and as adjuncts to anesthesia for certain surgical procedures.

muscular dystrophy (mŭs′kyə-lər dĭs′trə-fē) N. any of a group of hereditary diseases of the muscular system characterized by weakness and wasting of groups of skeletal muscles, leading to increasing disability. The various forms differ in age of onset, rate of progression, and mode of genetic transmission; the most common is Duchenne's muscular dystrophy.

Duchenne's muscular dystrophy N. most common of the muscular dystrophies (approximately 50%), it is a sex-linked recessive disease (affecting only males) with symptoms first appearing around the age of 4. Progressive wasting of leg and pelvic muscles produces a waddling gait and abnormal

MUSCLE TYPES

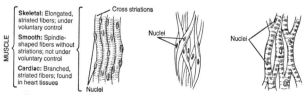

Skeletal: Elongated, striated fibers; under voluntary control
Smooth: Spindle-shaped fibers without striations; not under voluntary control
Cardiac: Branched, striated fibers; found in heart tissues

MUSCLE

Cross striations

Nuclei

Nuclei

Nuclei

SELECTED BODY LOCATIONS AND THEIR MUSCLES

Location	Muscles	Function
Neck	Sternocleidomastoid	Flexes head
Back	Trapezius	Extends upper arm
	Latissimus dorsi	Extends upper arm
Abdominal wall	External oblique	Compresses abdomen
Shoulder	Deltoid	Abducts upper arm
	Pectoralis major	Abducts upper arm
	Serratus anterior	Abducts shoulder
Upper arm	Biceps brachii	Flexes forearm
	Triceps brachii	Extends forearm
	Brachialis	Flexes forearm
Forearm	Brachioradialis	Flexes forearm
	Pronator teres	Pronates, flexes arm
Buttocks	Gluteus maximus	Extends thigh
	Gluteus minimus	Abducts thigh
	Gluteus medius	Abducts thigh
Thigh		
Anterior surface	Quadriceps femoris group:	
	Rectus femoris	Flexes thigh
	Vastus lateralis	Extends leg
	Vastus medialis	Extends leg
	Vastus intermedius	Extends leg
Medial surface	Gracilis	Adducts thigh
	Adductor group (brevis, longus, magnus)	
Posterior surface	Hamstring group	All flex leg
	Biceps femoris	
	Semitendinosus	
	Semimembranosus	
Leg		
Anterior surface	Tibialis anterior	Adducts foot
Posterior surface	Gastrocnemius	Extends foot
	Soleus	Extends foot
Pelvic floor	Levator ani	Forms pelvic floor
	Levator coccygeus	Forms pelvic floor

curvature of the spine, progressing to inability to walk and confinement to a wheelchair (usually by age 12), often accompanied by progressive weakening of cardiac muscle. There is no specific treatment and death, usually from heart disorders, often results by age 20. Also called pseudohypertrophic dystrophy.

limb-girdle muscular dystrophy N. form of muscular

A COMPARISON OF THREE TYPES OF MUSCLE TISSUE

Characteristic	Skeletal Muscle	Smooth Muscle	Cardiac Muscle
Location	Attached to skeleton	Walls of stomach, intestines, etc.	Walls of heart
Type of control	Voluntary	Involuntary	Involuntary
Shape of fibers	Elongated, cylindrical, blunt ends	Elongated, spindle-shaped, pointed ends	Elongated, cylindrical fibers that branch
Striations	Present	Absent	Present
Number of nuclei per fiber	Many	One	One or two
Position of nuclei	Peripheral	Central	Central
Speed of contraction	Most rapid	Slowest	Intermediate
Ability to remain contracted	Least	Greatest	Intermediate

dystrophy (autosomal recessive disease) characterized by progressive muscular weakness beginning in either the shoulder or pelvic girdle.

musculo- comb. form indicating an association with muscles (e.g., musculocutaneous, pert. to muscles and skin).

musculoskeletal (mŭs′kyə-lō-skĕl′ĭ-tl) ADJ. pert. to muscles and skeleton.

musculoskeletal system N. network of bones, muscles, joints, and associated tissues (e.g., ligaments and tendons) of the body involved in the maintenance of body form and movement.

mushroom poisoning N. toxic condition caused by the ingestion of certain species of mushrooms, esp. Amanita species. Symptoms include tearing, salivation, abdominal cramps, diarrhea, difficulty in breathing, and, in severe cases, liver and kidney damage, convulsions, coma, and sometimes death. Treatment depends on the species of mushroom eaten.

mutagen (myōō′tə-jən) N. agent, physical or environmental, that induces a genetic mutation or increases the mutation rate. ADJ. mutagenic

mutagenesis (myōō′tə-jĕn′ĭ-sĭs) N. induction of a mutation, or change, in a gene.

Mutamycin N. trade name for the antineoplastic mitomycin.

mutant gene (myōōt′nt) N. gene that has changed, affecting the normal transmission and expression of a trait.

mutation (myōō-tā′shən) N. change in the genetic structure; it may occur spontaneously or be induced (e.g., by radiation or certain mutagenic chemicals).

mutism (myōō′tĭz′əm) N. inability or refusal to speak. It may be innate, the result of being deaf-mute from birth; acquired through brain damage (aphasia); or caused by severe psychological disorder or trauma.

muton (myōō'tŏn') N. smallest unit of the hereditary material deoxyribonucleic acid (DNA) in which a change can produce a mutation.

my-, myo- comb. forms indicating an association with muscle (e.g., myovascular, pert. to muscles and blood circulation).

myalgia (mī-ăl'jē-ə) N. diffuse muscle pain, occurring in many infectious (e.g., influenza, measles, rheumatic fever, toxoplasmosis) and other disorders (e.g., fibromyositis, Guillain-Barré syndrome, muscle tumor), and sometimes as the result of certain drugs.

myasthenia (mī'əs-thē'nē-ə) N. abnormal muscle weakness, the result of disease, as in myasthenia gravis, or inadequate blood circulation to a given area.

myasthenia gravis N. disease characterized by chronic fatigability and weakness of muscles, esp. in the face and neck region, but also affecting the muscles of the trunk and limbs. Onset is gradual, usually with drooping eyelids and facial muscle weakness, and the course of the disease is variable, sometimes mild with many remissions, in other cases progressing to affect the respiratory system. It is caused by deficiency of acetylcholine at the neuromuscular junctions. Treatment involves rest, restricted physical activity, and the use of anticholinesterase drugs (neostigmine).

myc-, mycet-, myco- comb. forms indicating an association with fungus (e.g., mycetogenic, caused by a fungus).

Mycolog N. trade name for a topical fixed-combination drug containing two antibacterials (gramicidin and neomycin), an antifungal (nystatin), and a glucocorticoid; it is used to treat skin and mucous membrane infections and irritations.

mycology N. the study of fungi and fungus-caused diseases.

mycoplasma (mī'kō-plăz'mə) N. group of very small organisms, the smallest free-living organisms known, some of which produce disease in humans (e.g., *Mycoplasma pneumoniae*); also called pleuropneumonia-like organism (PPLO).

mycoplasma pneumonia (mī'kō-plăz'mə nōō-mōn'yə) N. contagious disease, primarily of children and young adults, caused by *Mycoplasma pneumoniae* and characterized by cough, fever, and other signs of upper respiratory tract infection. Treatment is by erythromycin or tetracyclines.

mycosis (mī-kō'sĭs) N. any fungus-caused disease.

Mycostatin N. trade name for the antifungal nystatin.

mydriasis (mĭ-drī'ə-sĭs) N. dilation of the pupil of the eye, caused by muscle action pulling the iris outward and enlarging the pupil; it occurs in response to a decrease in light or the action of certain drugs (*compare* MIOSIS).

mydriatic N. drug (e.g., atropine) that causes the pupil of the eye to dilate; used to aid examination of the eye and to treat certain eye disorders.

myelatelia N. any developmental defect of the spinal cord.

myelin (mī′ə-lĭn) N. complex material, containing phospholipids and proteins, that forms a sheath around the axons of certain nerve fibers, called myelinated (or medullated) nerve fibers. The myelin is produced by Schwann cells along the axon. Myelinated nerve fibers conduct impulses more rapidly than do unmyelinated fibers.

myelin sheath (mī′ə-lĭn shēth) N. segmented, fatty covering composed of myelin that covers the axons of some nerve fibers.

myelinated (mī′ə-lə-nā′tĭd) ADJ. having a myelin sheath.

myelinization (mī′ə-lə-nĭ-zā′shən) N. development of a myelin sheath around a nerve fiber.

myelitis (mī′ə-lī′tĭs) N. inflammation of the spinal cord.

myeloblast (mī′ə-lə-blăst′) N. precursor of the granulocytic leukocytes (eosinophils, basophils, and neutrophils) that normally occurs in bone marrow but increases in number in peripheral circulation in certain diseases, esp. myeloblastic leukemia.

myeloblastic leukemia (loo-kē′mē-ə) N. malignant neoplasm of the blood-forming tissues characterized by numerous myeloblasts in the circulating blood.

myelocele N. saclike protrusion of the spinal cord through a congenital defect in the vertebral column. *See also* MYELOMENINGOCELE.

myelocystocele N. protrusion of a cyst containing spinal cord material through a developmental defect in the vertebral column. *See also* MYLEOMENINGOCELE.

myelocyte (mī′ə-lə-sīt′) N. immature granulocytic leukocyte (eosinophil, basophil, or neutrophil) normally found in bone marrow and present in the circulating blood in certain diseases esp. myelocytic leukemia.

myelocytic leukemia (mī′ə-lə-sīt′ĭk loo-kē′mē-ə) N. a malignant neoplasm of blood-forming tissues characterized by proliferation of myelocytes and their presence in circulating blood; also called granulocytic leukemia.

myelogram (mī′ə-lə-grăm′) N. X ray of the spinal cord, spinal nerve roots, and subarachnoid space.

myelography (mī′ə-lŏg′rə-fē) N. X-ray procedure in which the spinal cord and subarachnoid space are photographed (myelogram) after injection of a contrast medium into the subarachnoid space; it is used to examine the spinal cord and detect possible lesions.

myeloid (mī′ə-loid′) ADJ.
1. pert. to bone marrow.
2. pert. to the spinal cord.

myeloid leukemia (mī′ə-loid′ loo-kē′mē-ə) *See* ACUTE MYELOCYTIC LEUKEMIA; CHRONIC MYELOCYTIC LEUKEMIA.

myeloma (mī′ə-lō′mə) N. bone-destroying malignant neoplasm of bone marrow tissue that occurs most often in the vertebrae, ribs, pelvis, and skull bones; symptoms include spontaneous bone fractures and bone pain. It may develop in several areas simultaneously (multiple myeloma). Treatment of local lesions is by radiotherapy.

myelomalacia N. softening of the spinal cord, often due to inadequate blood supply.

myelomeningocele N. congenital defect of the central nervous system in which a sac containing a part of the spinal cord and its meninges and cerebrospinal fluid protrudes through an opening in the vertebral column; it is due to a failure of the neural tube to close during embryonic development or to its reopening after closure. It most commonly occurs in the lower thoracic, lumbar, or sacral areas. The extent of neurological dysfunction depends on the location of the anomaly and the amount of spinal tissue involved; lower extremity paralysis and bladder and anal sphincter problems are common, frequently accompanied by hydrocephalus and mental retardation. Immediate treatment includes the prevention of infection and assessment of the probable extent of neurological damage to determine whether surgery to correct the defect is indicated. (*Compare* MENINGOCELE.)

myesthesia (mī'ĭs-thē'zhə) N. perception of sensation (e.g., touch, pressure) by a muscle.

myiasis (mī¯'ə-sĭs) N. infection or infestation with the larvae of flies, most often through a wound or other opening.

myocardial infarction (MI) (ĭn-färk'shən) N. heart attack; death of an area of heart muscle due to interruption of its blood supply through occlusion of the coronary arteries usually by an acute thrombus. This completely occludes the arterial lumen which was previously narrowed by atherosclerosis. Typical symptoms include crushing, viselike pain in the chest that may radiate to the arm, esp. the left arm, neck, or jaw region; shortness of breath;

faintness; anxiety; and an ashen or sweaty appearance. Irregularities of heart rhythm, demonstrable on an electrocardiogram, may be present. The blood pressure may be high or low. Treatment involves oxygen, treatment of pain, and close monitoring to guard against complications such as arrhythmias, heart failure, and cardiac arrest. Prognosis depends on the extent of heart damage, but most patients are able to return to normal life with modifications in their diet, stress levels, and sometimes activity. Sometimes called coronary.

myocardiopathy N. any disease of the heart muscle. *See also* CARDIOMYOPATHY.

myocarditis (mī'ō-kär-dī'tĭs) N. inflammation of the myocardium (heart muscle); it may be caused by viral, bacterial, or fungal infection, or by rheumatic fever, or occur as a complication of another disease. Treatment depends on the cause.

myocardium (mī'ō-kär'dē-əm) N. thick, muscular middle layer of the heart wall, composed almost entirely of cardiac muscle (the other layers being the outer epicardium and inner endocardium). ADJ. myocardial

Myochrysine N. trade name for a gold preparation sometimes used to treat arthritis.

myoclonus (mī-ŏk'lə-nəs) N. sudden spasm of muscles, occurring in some forms of epilepsy and in certain progressive neurological disorders. ADJ. myoclonic

myofibril (mī'ə-fī'brəl) N. one of many contractile filaments that make up a fiber of a striated muscle.

myogenic (mī'ə-jĕn'ĭk) ADJ. originating in muscle.

myoglobin (mī'ə-glō'bĭn) N. iron-containing pigment responsible for the red color of muscle and its ability to store oxygen.

myoglobinuria (mī'ə-glō'bə-nŏŏr'ē-ə) N. presence of myoglobin in the urine.

myogram (mī'ə-grăm') N. recording of muscle activity. *See also* ELECTROMYOGRAM.

myology (mī-ŏl'ə-jē) N. science or study of the structure and function of muscles.

myoma (mī-ō'mə) N. benign muscle tumor, esp. one of the uterine muscle.

myometritis N. inflammation or infection of the myometrium.

myometrium (mī'ō-me'trē-əm) N. muscular layer of the uterine wall, surrounding the endometrium; it is made up of smooth muscle that has small, spontaneous contractions during certain phases of the menstrual cycle and during pregnancy in response to the hormones estrogen, progesterone, and oxytocin.

myonecrosis (mī'ō-nə-krō'sĭs) N. death of muscle cell fibers, sometimes seen in infections of deep wounds.

myoneural junction (mī'ə-nŏŏr'əl) *See* NEUROMUSCULAR JUNCTION.

myopathy (mī-ŏp'ə-thē) N. any disease of the muscles not caused by nerve dysfunction; symptoms depend on the specific disease but generally include muscle weakness and wasting. ADJ. myopathic

myope N. person who has myopia.

myopia (mī-ō'pē-ə) N. nearsightedness; defect in vision caused by elongation of the eyeball or an error in refraction so that the image comes to a focus in front of the retina; it can be corrected by concave lenses (*compare* HYPEROPIA).

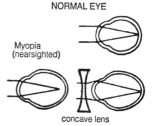

NORMAL EYE

Myopia (nearsighted)

concave lens

In the normal eye, the image comes to a focus on the retina. In myopia, the image comes to a focus in front of the retina. The defect can be corrected by concave lenses.

myorrhexis N. breaking apart of a muscle.

myosarcoma (mī'ō-sär-kō'mə) N. malignant tumor of muscle tissue.

myosin (mī'ə-sĭn) N. protein in muscle that, along with actin, makes up the contractile elements of muscles. *See* TROPONIN, SARCOMERE.

myositis (mī'ə-sī'tĭs) N. inflammation of muscle tissue, usually voluntary muscle, most often caused by infection, parasite infestation, trauma, or degenerative muscle diseases. *See also* POLYMYOSITIS.

myositis ossificans N. rare, inherited disease in which muscle tissue is replaced by bone, leading to stiffness and impaired mobility.

myositis trichinosa *See* TRICHINOSIS.

myotomy (mī-ŏt′ə-mē) N. surgical division of a muscle.

myotonia (mī′ə-tō′nē-ə) N. condition in which a muscle or group of muscles has abnormally prolonged contractions, not readily relaxing after contraction. ADJ. myotonic

   myotonia atrophica *See* MUSCULAR DYSTROPHY, MYOTONIC.

   myotonia congenita N. rare and mild form of myotonia usually manifested only by muscle stiffness; also called Thomsen's disease.

   myotonic muscular dystrophy N. severe form of muscular dystrophy characterized by drooping eyelids, facial weakness, difficulty with speech, and weakness of the hands and feet spreading to arms, shoulders, legs and hips; also called myotonia atrophica; Steinert's disease.

myringa (mə-rĭng′gə) *See* TYMPANIC MEMBRANE.

myringectomy (mĭr′ĭn-jĕk′tə-mē) N. surgical removal of the tympanic membrane.

myringitis (mĭr′ĭn-jī′tĭs) N. inflammation of the tympanic membrane.

myringo- comb. form indicating a relationship with the tympanic membrane (e.g., myringomycosis, fungal infection of the eardrum).

myringoplasty (mə-rĭng′gə-plăs′tē) N. surgical repair of perforations of the tympanic membrane with a tissue graft to help correct hearing loss.

myringotomy (mĭr′ĭng-gŏt′ə-mē) N. surgical incision into the tympanic membrane to relieve pressure and release pus from the middle ear.

myx-, myxo- comb. forms indicating association with mucus (e.g., myxadenitis, mucus gland inflammation).

myxedema (mĭk′sĭ-dē′mə) N. syndrome caused by deficiency of thyroid hormone in adults (hypothyroidism), including cold intolerance, fatigue, sluggishness, skin coarsening, weight gain, mental dullness, and in women menstrual irregularities.

myxoma (mĭk-sō′mə) N. usually benign jellylike tumor of connective tissue that may grow to large size. Symptoms depend on the location of the tumor and result from pressure on or interference with the function of an adjacent or underlying organ.

myxovirus (mĭk′sə-vī′rəs) N. any of a group of medium-sized ribonucleic acid (RNA) viruses, including those that cause mumps and influenza.

N

N symbol for the element nitrogen.

Na symbol for the element sodium.

nabothian cyst N. usually benign cyst that forms in the Nabothian glands of the cervix of the uterus.

nabothian gland N. one of many small, mucus-secreting glands of the cervix of the uterus.

nabumetone N. *See* TABLE OF COMMONLY PRESCRIBED DRUGS —GENERIC NAMES.

nadolol N. beta blocking agent used to treat hypertension and angina. Adverse effects include cardiac arrhythmias, gastrointestinal disturbances, and allergic reactions.

Naegele's rule N. method for calculating expected delivery date. Three months are subtracted from the first day of the last menstrual period and seven days added to that date.

nafcillin N. antibiotic (trade name Nafcil) used to treat infections caused by penicillin-resistant strains of staphylococci. Adverse effects include allergic reactions and gastrointestinal upsets.

nail N. flattened, horny structure, made of keratin from epidermis, at the end of each finger and toe. Each nail is composed of a root, body, and free edge. The root fits into a groove in the skin and is closely molded to the skin of the finger or toe with the nail fold overlying the root. The body of the nail lies over the nail bed; the white crescent-

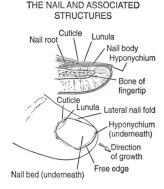

THE NAIL AND ASSOCIATED STRUCTURES

shaped structure at the base of the body is the lunula. Nails grow longer as cells in the stratum germinativum of the root proliferate. Also called unguis.

Naldecon N. trade name for a fixed-combination drug, containing two decongestants (phenylpropanolamine and phenylephrine) and two antihistamines (chlorpheniramine and phenyltoloxamine); used to treat cough and nasal congestion associated with the common cold, bronchitis, influenza, and similar diseases.

Nalfon N. trade name for anti-inflammatory fenoprofen.

nalidixic acid (nā′lĭ-dĭk′sĭk) N. antibiotic (trade name NegGram) used to treat certain infections of the urinary tract. Adverse effects include neurological and gastrointestinal disturbances, and the possibility of seizures, convulsions, and increased intracranial pressure.

naltrexone N. oral agent that antagonizes the actions of opiates, used to aid former drug addicts in remaining opiate-free in their day-to-day activities. It should not be used without a physician's directions. *See also* NARCOTIC ANTAGONIST.

nandrolone N. androgen (trade names Durabolin and Kabolin) used to treat testosterone deficiency, breast cancer in women, and osteoporosis; it also stimulates growth and weight gain. Adverse effects include liver toxicity, electrolyte imbalance, and endocrine disturbances.

nanism (nā'nĭz'əm) N. abnormal smallness, dwarfism.

nano- comb. form indicating extreme smallness (e.g., nanocephaly, an abnormally small head).

nanophthalmos N. condition in which one or both eyes are abnormally small, but other eye defects are not present.

nanus (nā'nəs) N. a dwarf. *See also* HOMUNCULUS; PITUITARY DWARF; PRIMORDIAL DWARF.

nape (nāp, năp) N. back of the neck.

napex N. area just below the bump (occiput) at the back of the head.

naphazoline N. vasoconstrictor (trade names Privine and 4-Way) used in eyedrops and nasal sprays to treat eye irritation and nasal congestion. Adverse effects arise from systemic absorption and include sedation and cardiovascular effects.

naphthalene poisoning N. toxic condition caused by ingestion or inhalation of naphthalene and related compounds, commonly found in mothballs and

some agricultural insecticides; symptoms include nausea, vomiting, abdominal pain, muscle spasm, and convulsions.

naprapathy N. system of medicine based on the idea that many diseases are due to displacement of connective tissues (e.g., ligaments, tendons) and that manipulation of these tissues will bring relief (*compare* CHIROPRACTIC; OSTEOPATHY).

naproxen (nə-prŏk'sən) N. nonsteroidal anti-inflammatory agent (trade names Naprosyn and Anaprox) used in the treatment of arthritis, musculoskeletal inflammation, and moderate pain. Adverse effects include headache, dizziness, gastrointestinal disturbances, and skin eruptions; the drug interacts with many others.

narcissism (när'sĭ-sĭz'əm) N. abnormal interest in oneself, esp. one's body; self-love; in psychoanalytic theory, sexual self-interest, normal in young children but abnormal in adults. ADJ. narcissistic

narcissistic personality N. personality characterized by excessive self-love and self-absorption, unrealistic views about one's own attributes, and little regard for others.

narcolepsy (när'kə-lĕp'sē) N. syndrome characterized by an uncontrollable desire to sleep, sudden sleep attacks lasting from a few minutes to a few hours, episodes of momentary loss of muscle tone (cataplexy), and occasionally visual hallucinations before sleep. The condition usually begins in adolescence and lasts for life; no organic cause is known. Stimulant drugs are sometimes used to prevent attacks. (*Compare* INSOMNIA.) ADJ. narcoleptic

narcoleptic (när′kə-lĕp′tĭk) N.
 1. substance that produces an
 uncontrollable desire to sleep.
 2. person with narcolepsy.

narcosis (när-kō′sĭs) N. state of
 stupor caused by narcotic
 drugs.

narcotic (när-kŏt′ĭk) N. drug,
 derived from opium or produced synthetically, that relieves
 pain, induces euphoria and other
 mood changes, decreases respiration and peristalsis, constricts
 the pupils, and produces sleep.
 Narcotic drugs are addictive,
 producing drug addiction after
 repeated use. Narcotic drugs
 used for pain relief include
 morphine, meperidine (Demerol), and codeine; heroin and
 other narcotics are common
 street drugs. *See also* DRUG AD-
 DICTION.

narcotic antagonist (ăn-tăg′ə-
 nĭst) N. drug (e.g., naloxone)
 used to counter the effects of
 narcotics, esp. respiratory
 depression.

Nardil N. trade name for the antidepressant phenelzine.

nares (nâr′ēz) N. openings in the
 nose that allow the passage of
 air into the pharynx. The paired
 anterior openings are the anterior nares, or nostrils; the paired
 posterior openings at the back
 of the nasal cavity leading to
 the nasopharynx are the posterior nares.

Nasacort N. trade name for an
 inhaled form of the corticosteroid, triamcinolone; used in
 treatment of asthma.

nasal (nā′zəl) ADJ. pert. to the
 nose or nasal cavity.

nasal cavity N. either of the pair
 of cavities that open on the face
 to allow the passage of air into
 the pharynx.

nasal decongestant N. drug that
 provides temporary relief of
 nasal symptoms associated
 with the common cold, rhinitis,
 and upper respiratory infections. Most contain an antihistamine and vasoconstrictor, and
 many are sold without prescription. *See also* DECONGES-
 TANT.

nasal flaring N. dilation of the
 nostrils during inspiration; a
 sign of respiratory distress, particularly in small children and
 infants.

NASAL CAVITY

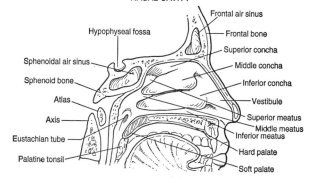

nasal septum (nā'zəl sĕp'təm) N. mucous-membrane-covered bone and cartilage partition dividing the nostrils.

nasal sinus (nā'zəl sī'nəs) N. any of numerous cavities in the skull lined with a mucous membrane continuous with the nasal membrane; among the nasal sinuses are the frontal sinuses, ethmoid sinuses, and maxillary sinuses.

nascent ADJ. just born; beginning to exist.

nasion N. depression at the bridge of the nose that indicates the point where the frontal and nasal bones of the skull meet.

naso- comb. form indicating a relationship with the nose (e.g., nasolacrinal, pert. to the nose and lacrimal apparatus).

nasogastric feeding N. process of delivering nutrients in liquid form through a tube passed into the stomach through the nose; used when the person can digest food but cannot eat (e.g., in some cases of mouth or throat surgery).

nasogastric tube N. tube passed into the stomach through the nose used to aspirate stomach contents and secretions or to facilitate nasogastric feeding.

nasolacrimal duct (nā'zō-lăk'rə-məl) N. duct that carries tears from the lacrimal sac to the nasal cavity.

nasopharynx (nā'zō-făr'ĭngks) N. region of the throat behind the nose, extending from the posterior nares to the soft palate region and containing the pharyngeal tonsils (*compare* OROPHARYNX). ADJ. nasopharyngeal

nasotracheal tube (nā'zō-trā'kē-əl) N. tube inserted into the trachea through the nose and pharynx; it is used to deliver oxygen and respiratory therapy.

natal (nāt'l) ADJ.
1. pert. to birth.
2. pert. to the buttocks (nates).

nates *See* BUTTOCKS.

National Practitioner Data Bank N. database, maintained by the Department of Health and Human Services, that serves as a national source of information on health care practitioners (e.g., physicians, dentists, physician assistants). The data bank includes information on payments made as a result of a malpractice claim, adverse license actions, and actions taken regarding clinical privileges at hospitals. Under present law, hospitals must query the data bank regarding current medical staff members every two years. This information is not available to the general public and can be released only to an attorney of a medical malpractice plaintiff if the hospital has failed to make the proper inquiry on a staff member.

natriuresis (nā'trə-yoŏ-rē'sĭs) N. excretion of abnormally large amounts of sodium in the urine, usually the result of diuretic drug intake or certain metabolic disorders. ADJ. natriuretic

natriuretic N. compound, often a drug, that increases the excretion of sodium in the urine; most diuretics are potent natriuretics, resulting in loss of sodium and water in the urine, often with a mild to moderate decrease in the patient's blood pressure or swelling (edema), if present.

natural childbirth N. labor and childbirth with little or no medical intervention and the mother given minimal or no drugs to relieve pain or aid the birth process. It is considered the safest for the baby, but certain conditions (e.g., inadequate birth canal, fetal distress, illness in the mother) may make it impossible. *See also* BRADLEY METHOD OF CHILDBIRTH; LAMAZE METHOD OF CHILDBIRTH; READ METHOD OF CHILDBIRTH.

natural family planning N. any of several methods of family planning that do not involve the use of drugs (e.g., oral contraceptives), devices (e.g., diaphragm or intrauterine device), or surgical intervention (sterilization). In natural family planning methods several ways are used to determine the time of ovulation and thus the fertile period in a woman's menstrual cycle and that information is used to increase or decrease the chances of conception by avoiding or engaging in coitus at the fertile time. *See also* BASAL BODY TEMPERATURE METHOD OF FAMILY PLANNING; CALENDAR METHOD OF FAMILY PLANNING; OVULATION METHOD OF FAMILY PLANNING; RHYTHM METHOD OF FAMILY PLANNING; CONTRACEPTION.

natural immunity (ĭ-myoō′nĭ-tē) N. stage of being innately resistant or insusceptible to a particular disease; also called innate immunity.

natural selection N. natural process by which the organisms best suited to a particular environment by virtue of their adaptations tend to survive and propagate offspring with their characteristics, whereas those less well adapted have less chance for survival and propagation.

naturopathy (nā′chə-rŏp′ə-thē) *See* TABLE OF ALTERNATIVE MEDICINE TERMS.

nausea (nô′zē-ə) N. feeling that one is going to vomit; it occurs in motion sickness, in early pregnancy, at times of extreme stress, and in many illnesses (e.g., gallbladder disease, gastrointestinal viral infections).

Navane N. trade name for the tranquilizer thiothixene, used in treatment of certain psychotic disorders.

navel (nā′vəl) *See* UMBILICUS.

navicular (nə-vĭk′yə-lər) N. largest of the proximal row of wrist bones on the thumb side; it is boat-shaped and often fractured in young adults. The usual cause is a fall on the outstretched hand, or some type of twisting, violent motion involving the wrist (e.g., kickback from the starting handle of a motor or pulling from a horse's rope). Navicular fractures may be difficult to see on X rays. Also called scaphoid bone. A similarly named bone is found in the foot at the base of the great toe. Navicular fractures, even when properly treated, may result in death of the broken bone (avascular necrosis) due to its perilous blood supply.

nearsightedness (nēr′sī′tĭd-nĭs) *See* MYOPIA.

Nebcin N. trade name for the antibiotic tobramycin.

nebula (nĕb′yə-lə) N. a faint opacity or scar on the cornea; it seldom interferes with vision.

neck N.
1. area of the body between the head and the trunk.
2. constricted section of a body

organ, as the neck of the femur (thighbone).

necro- comb. form indicating an association with death (e.g., necrogenic, causing death).

necrobiosis lipoidica (nĕk′rō-bī-ō′sĭs lĭ-poi′dĭ-kə) N. a skin disease, occurring most often in people with diabetes mellitus, esp. women, in which there is degeneration of skin structure and the development of thin, shiny patches on the skin, esp. in the mid and lower shins.

necrology (nə-krŏl′ə-jē) N. study of death.

necrolysis (nĕ-krŏl′ĭ-sĭs) N. disintegration of dead tissue.

necrophilia (nĕk′rə-fĭl′ē-ə) N. morbid liking or desire for dead bodies, esp. the desire to have sexual contact with a dead body.

necropsy (nĕk′rŏp′sē) *See* AUTOPSY.

necrosis (nə-krō′sĭs) N. death of some or all of the cells in a tissue; usually caused by disease, inadequate blood supply to the tissue, or injury. ADJ. necrotic

necrotizing enteritis (ĕn′tə-rī′tĭs) N. acute inflammation of the small and large intestine caused by infection with the bacterium *Clostridium perfringens;* it is characterized by bloody diarrhea, severe abdominal pain, and vomiting.

necrotizing enterocolitis (NEC) (ĕn-tə-rō-kō-lī′tĭs) N. acute inflammatory condition of the intestine, occurring in premature or low-birth-weight infants; believed due to a defect or immaturity of natural defenses, microorganisms normally present in the gastrointestinal tract producing infection. Symptoms include abdominal distension, decreased bowel sounds, vomiting, bloody diarrhea, lethargy, poor feeding, and often low body temperature. Necrosis of intestinal tissue due to inadequate blood supply, hyperbilirubinemia, edema, abdominal tenderness, and other abnormalities may follow, sometimes leading to perforation of the gastrointestinal lining, peritonitis, respiratory failure, and death. Treatment depends on the severity of the disease but includes nasogastric feeding, antibiotics, and, if perforation of the intestinal wall occurs, surgery.

necrotizing fasciitis (făsh′ē-ī′tĭs) N. severe inflammation and infection, usually by bacteria, of the tissue surrounding the hip or back muscles; is usually severe and may be fatal. Treatment involves prompt recognition, antibiotics, and, often, surgery.

needle biopsy (bī′ŏp′sē) N. removal of a segment of tissue for microscopic analysis by inserting a hollow needle through the skin or external surface of an organ and twisting it around to obtain a sample of underlying cells.

needle sickness N. unusual reaction to acupuncture consisting of nausea and dizziness; relieved by removing the needles.

nefazodone N. *See* TABLE OF COMMONLY PRESCRIBED DRUGS—GENERIC NAMES.

negativism (nĕg′ə-tĭ-vĭz′əm) N. pattern of behavior characterized by opposition, resistance to suggestion, unwillingness to cooperate, and a tendency to act in a contrary way; it may be passive, as in a rigid, immobile position; or active, with belligerent acts.

Neggram N. trade name for antibiotic nalidixic acid.

nemato- comb. form indicating a relationship with nematodes (e.g., nematocide, agent that kills nematodes) or with thread (e.g., nematoid, like a thread).

nematode (nĕm′ə-tōd′) N. any of a large group (phylum Nematoda) of unsegmented worms, tapered at both ends, including roundworms, pinworms, and hookworms; many species infest humans, producing disease.

Nembutal (nĕm′byə-tôl′) N. trade name for the barbiturate pentobarbital.

neo- prefix meaning new (e.g., neoblastic, pert. to a new tissue).

Neobiotic N. trade name for the antibiotic neomycin.

neologism (nē-ŏl′ə-jĭz′əm) N. in psychiatry, invention of a new word that has meaning only to the person who coined it; it is normal in early childhood, but usually a sign of mental illness (e.g. schizophrenia) in an adult.

neomycin (nē′ə-mī′sĭn) N. antibiotic drug (trade name Neobiotic) used orally to treat intestinal infections and topically to treat eye and skin infections. Adverse effects include gastrointestinal upsets, danger of superinfection, and, with prolonged use, damage to ears and kidneys.

neonatal (nē′ō-nāt′l) ADJ. pert. to a neonate or to the first month of life.

neonatal death N. death of a liveborn infant within the first 28 days of life.

neonatal hyperbilirubinemia (hī-pər-bĭl-ĭ-rōō-bə-nē′mē-ə) *See* HYPERBILIRUBINEMIA OF THE NEWBORN.

neonatal intensive care unit (NICU) N. hospital unit designed with special equipment and devices for the care of the seriously ill, premature, or very-low-birth-weight newborn.

neonatal mortality (môr-tăl′ĭ-tē) N. number of infant deaths during the first 28 days of life, per unit of population (e.g., per 1,000 live births) in a given institution, geographic area, or period of time.

neonatal period N. first 28 days of life.

neonate (nē′ə-nāt′) N. infant from birth to 4 weeks (28 days) of life. ADJ. neonatal

neonatology (nē′ō-nā-tŏl′ə-jē) N. that branch of medicine concerned with the newborn, specifically the diagnosis and treatment of neonates.

neoplasia (nē′ō-plā′zhə) N. new and abnormal development of a cell; it may be benign or malignant. ADJ. neoplastic

neoplasm (nē′ə-plăz′əm) N. any abnormal growth of new tissue, benign or malignant. *See also* TUMOR.

Neosporin N. trade name for a fixed-combination topical drug containing the antibiotics polymixin, neomycin, and bacitracin, used in ointment form for skin irritations and minor skin infections and in eyedrop form for minor eye infections.

neostigmine (nē′ō-stĭg′mēn) N. cholinergic drug used to treat myasthenia gravis. Adverse effects include intestinal pain and cramping, excess salivation, and respiratory depression.

nephr-, nephro- comb. forms indicating an association with the kidneys (e.g., nephropathy, any disorder of the kidney).

nephralgia (nə-frăl′jē-ə) N. pain in the kidney, usually felt in the loin.

nephrectomy (nə-frĕk′tə-mē) N. surgical removal of a kidney, performed to remove a tumor, drain an abscess, or treat other kidney disorder.

nephritis (nə-frī′tĭs) N. inflammation of the kidney. *See also* GLOMERULONEPHRITIS.

nephroangiosclerosis N. death of cells of the kidney arterioles associated with hypertension; symptoms include, in addition to high blood pressure, headache, blurred vision, and often an enlarged heart; if hypertension cannot be controlled, it can lead to kidney failure and heart failure; also called nephrosclerosis. *See also* MALIGNANT HYPERTENSION.

nephroblastoma *See* WILMS'S TUMOR.

nephrocalcinosis N. condition in which calcium deposits form in the kidney, often at the site of previous inflammation and leading to diminished kidney function, infection, and blood in the urine; it may be associated with excess calcium in the blood or kidney malfunction.

nephrogenic diabetes insipidus N. unusual form of diabetes insipidus caused by lack of response to normal levels of antidiuretic hormone (ADH) by the kidney, leading to excessive production of dilute urine and extreme thirst.

nephrolith N. calculus (stone) formed in the kidney.

nephrolithiasis (nĕf′rō-lĭ-thī′ə-sĭs) N. disorder characterized by the presence of stones in the kidney. There may be no symptoms, or pain and blood in the urine may occur. If urinary blockage, severe pain, or infection occurs, surgical removal of the stones and/or kidney is indicated. *See also* URINARY CALCULUS.

nephrology (nə-frŏl′ə-jē) N. study of the kidney, its development, anatomy, and physiology, and the diagnosis and treatment of disorders affecting it.

nephron (nĕf′rŏn) N. structural and functional unit of the kidney; there are more than one million nephrons in each kidney. Each nephron consists of a renal corpuscle, containing a glomerulus enclosed in Bowman's capsule; renal tubules; and the loop of Henle. Urine forms as a result of filtration of the blood in Bowman's capsule, as well as absorption and secretion of materials (e.g., water, sodium, potassium) by the renal tubules.

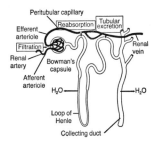

A simplified view of activity at the nephron.

nephroptosis N. abnormal downward placement of the kidney.

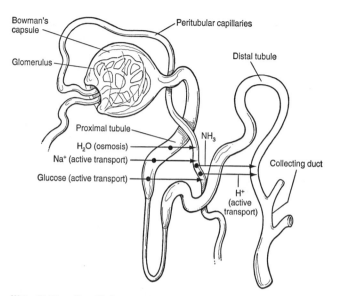

Water (H_2O), sodium (Na^+), ammonia (NH_3), and hydrogen (H^+) move between the various tubules of the nephron (proximal, distal, and collecting tubule) and the surrounding peritubular capillaries, as indicated by arrows. The specific activities of each at particular locations in the nephron are summarized in the table below.

PHYSIOLOGY OF THE NEPHRON

Nephron Structure	Physiology
Glomerulus	Filtration of blood plasma; removal of water and solutes with exception of proteins
Proximal tubules	Reabsorption of sodium ions, other ions, glucose, and amino acids by active transport; reabsorption of chloride ions by diffusion; reabsorption of water by osmosis
Loop of Henle Descending limb	Reabsorption of sodium ions by diffusion
Ascending limb	Reabsorption of sodium chloride by active transport
Distal collecting tubules	Reabsorption of selective ions by active transport; reabsorption of water by osmosis under influence of ADH; secretion of ammonia, certain ions, drugs, hormones, and other substances

nephrosis (nə-frō'sĭs) N. disease of the kidney, esp. a degenerative, non-inflammatory disease.

nephrotic syndrome (nə-frŏt'ĭk sĭn'drōm) N. abnormal condition, marked by edema, the presence of large amounts of protein in the urine, and lower than normal levels of albumin in the blood. Often accompanied by nausea, weakness, and loss of appetite, it is usually associated with disease of the glomerulus (glomerulonephritis) or occurs as a complication of many systemic diseases (e.g., multiple myeloma, diabetes mellitus, systemic lupus erythematosus).

nephrotomy (nə-frŏt'ə-mē) N. incision into the kidney, usually performed to remove a stone.

nephrotoxic ADJ. toxic to a kidney, as some drugs.

nerve N. one or more bundles of fibers that connect the brain and spinal cord (central nervous system) with the rest of the body. Sensory nerves transmit afferent impulses from the sense organs and other organs of the body to the brain and spinal cord. Motor nerves transmit efferent impulses from the brain and spinal cord to the glands, muscles, and other organs of the body. A nerve consists of an epineurium enclosing bundles (fasciculi) of fibers; each fasciculus contains microscopic nerve fibers, each enclosed in a neurolemmal sheath. *See also* NERVOUS SYSTEM; NEURON.

nerve block anesthesia (ăn'ĭs-thē'zhə) *See* CONDUCTION ANESTHESIA.

nerve compression N. harmful pressure on a nerve, causing nerve damage and muscle weakness; nerves over rigid prominences are particularly vulnerable. Rest and alternation of any causal activities often heals the damage. (*Compare* NERVE ENTRAPMENT.)

nerve entrapment N. abnormal condition in which a nerve is subjected to repeated or long-term compression, resulting in nerve damage, often with symptoms of pain and muscle weakness. It most commonly involves nerves located near joints subject to inflammation or swelling, as in arthritis or pregnancy. Carpal tunnel syndrome is a type of nerve entrapment. (*Compare* NERVE COMPRESSION.)

nerve regeneration N. process whereby all or part of a nerve, usually of the peripheral nervous system, replaces damaged or missing portions with normal tissue. Typically, nerve regeneration is a slow process; most peripheral nerves grow at a rate of one millimeter or so every thirty days.

nervous breakdown N. colloquial term for a mental condition that disrupts normal functioning.

nervous system N. extensive network of cells, specialized to conduct information in the form of impulses, that controls, regulates, and coordinates all functions of the body. There are three main divisions: the central nervous system, made up of the brain and spinal cord; the peripheral nervous system, which includes the cranial nerves, spinal nerves; and the autonomic nervous system. The basic unit of the nervous system is the neuron, or nerve cell.

network N. interconnected or intersecting configuration, system of people, or components. Anatomically, the interconnecting

NERVOUS SYSTEM

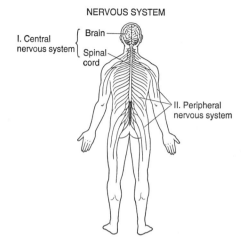

I. Central nervous system { Brain
Spinal cord

II. Peripheral nervous system

nerves of the body form a network, as do the blood vessels. In managed care, the patient receives care from a network of health care providers within the plan. Providers who are not members of the plan are said to be out-of-network.

neur-, neuro- comb. forms indicating an association with a nerve or the nervous system (e.g., neuroblast, a cell in the embryo that develops into a nerve cell).

neural (noŏr′əl) ADJ. pert. to nerves or the nervous system.

neural tube N. in the embryo, a tube of ectodermal tissue from which the brain and spinal cord develop.

neural tube defect N. any of a group of congenital defects involving the brain and spinal cord and resulting from failure of the neural tube to close normally during embryonic development or occasionally from a reopening of the tube after it has closed. The defects range from total absence of the skull to protrusions of the brain material to more common protrusions of spinal cord material (with or without meninges) through an incomplete closure of the vertebral column (e.g., meningocele, myelomeningocele, spina bifida). The amount and extent of mental impairment, neurological dysfunction, and other abnormalities depend on the location and site of the defect. In some cases surgical intervention is undertaken. Many neural tube defects can be determined before birth through analysis of amniotic fluid (e.g., an elevated level of alpha fetoprotein usually indicates a neural tube defect).

neuralgia (noō-răl′jə) N. severe, often burning, pain along the course of a nerve.

neurasthenia (noŏr′əs-thē′nē-ə) N. condition characterized by many physical and psychological symptoms, including fatigue, intolerance to noise, and irritability; it is associated with depression and other abnormal psychological conditions, severe stress, and occasionally organic disease. ADJ. neurasthenic

neurectomy (noŏ-rĕk′tə-mē) N. surgical removal of all or part of a nerve.

neurilemma (noŏ′rə-lĕm′ə) N. thin membranous sheath enclosing a nerve fiber; also called neurolemma

neurilemoma (noŏr′ə-lə-mō′mə) *See* NEUROFIBROMA.

neurinoma (noŏr′ə-nō′mə) N. tumor, usually benign, of the sheath surrounding a nerve.

neuritis (noŏ-rī′tĭs) N. inflammation of a nerve, producing pain, loss of sensation, defective reflexes, and muscular atrophy. It can result from many causes. *See also* RETROBULBAR NEURITIS.

neuroanatomy N. study of the structure, both gross and microscopic, of the nervous system.

neuroblast (noŏr′ə-blăst′) N. embryonic cell that develops into a neuron.

neuroblastoma (noŏr′ō-blă-stō′mə) N. malignant tumor containing embryonic nerve cells; it most commonly develops in the adrenal medulla in children, but may arise in any part of the sympathetic nervous system. Neuroblastomas typically metastasize quickly, spreading to the lymph nodes, liver, lungs, and other organs.

neurodermatitis (noŏr′ō-dûr′mə-tī′tĭs) N. skin disease in which localized areas, esp. the forearm, back of the neck, or outer part of the ankle, itch persistently and become thickened because of constant scratching. The cause is unknown.

neuroendocrine ADJ. pert. to the endocrine and nervous systems, esp. as they function together to control the activities of the body.

neuroepithelioma N. a neoplasm of the neuroepithelium.

neuroepithelium N. epithelium associated with special sense organs and containing sensory nerve endings; it is found in the retina, inner ear, nasal cavity, and taste buds. ADJ. neuroepithelial

neurofibroma (noŏr′ō-fī-brō′mə) N. tumor of the fibrous covering of a peripheral nerve.

neurofibromatosis (noŏr′ō-fī-brō′mə-tō′sĭs) N. congenital disease (autosomal dominant disease) characterized by numerous neurofibromas, by cafe-au-lait spots on the skin, and often by developmental abnormalities of bone, muscle, and internal organs; also called von Recklinghausen's disease.

neurogenesis (noŏr′ə-jĕn′ĭ-sĭs) N. development of nerve tissue.

neurogenic (noŏr′ə-jĕn′ĭk) ADJ. 1. arising in nervous tissue. 2. caused by nervous stimulation.

neurogenic bladder N. urinary bladder that functions abnormally because of a nervous system lesion. *See also* FLACCID BLADDER; SPASTIC BLADDER.

neuroglia (noŏ-rŏg′lē-ə) N. type of cell, including astrocytes, microglia, and oligodendroglia, found in the nervous system; neuroglia serve as support and nourishment for the neurons, the cells involved in nerve im-

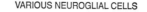

VARIOUS NEUROGLIAL CELLS

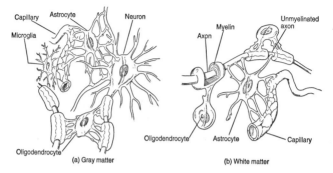

(a) Gray matter

(b) White matter

pulse transmission (compare neuron).

neurohormone (nŏŏr'ō-hôr'mōn) N. hormone secreted by nerve endings (e.g., vasopressin, released from nerve endings in the hypothalamus and released into the bloodstream from the posterior pituitary gland).

neurohumor N. chemical transmitted by a neuron and essential for the activity of adjacent neurons, muscles, or other organs. Important neurohumors are acetylcholine, serotonin, dopamine, and epinephrine. ADJ. neurohumoral. Also called neurotransmitters.

neurohypophysis (nŏŏr'ō-hī-pŏf'ĭ-sĭs) N. *See* POSTERIOR PITUITARY GLAND. ADJ. neurohypophyseal

neurolemma *See* NEURILEMMA.

neurolepsis N. altered state of consciousness marked by indifference to the surroundings; quiescence.

neuroleptic (nŏŏr'ə-lĕp'tĭk) N. drug that produces neurolepsis.

neurologist N. physician who specializes in neurology.

neurology (nŏŏ-rŏl'ə-jē) N. that branch of medicine concerned with the structure, function, and diseases of the nervous system. ADJ. neurologic

neuroma (nŏŏ-rō'mə) N. neoplasm consisting chiefly of neurons and nerve fibers.

neuromuscular (nŏŏr'ō-mŭs'kyə-lər) ADJ. pert. to the nerves and muscles.

neuromuscular blocking agent N. substance that interferes with the transmission or reception of impulses from motor neurons to skeletal muscles; used to induce muscle relaxation during surgery and in the treatment of tetanus, poliomyelitis, and certain other disorders.

neuromuscular junction N. area of contact between a nerve fiber and the muscle it supplies. A neurotransmitter passes across the small gap (synapse) between the motor end plate of the motor nerve and the muscle, triggering contraction of the

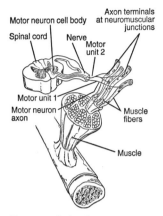

Neuromuscular junction.

muscle. Also called myoneural junction.

neuron (no͝or'ŏn') N. a nerve cell; the basic structural and functional unit of the nervous system, neurons are specialized to carry information in the form of electrochemical impulses from one part of the body to another. Each neuron is composed of a cell body containing a nucleus and one or more processes: dendrites that carry impulses toward the cell body and

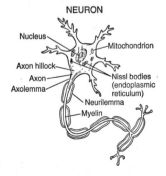

axons that carry impulses away from the cell body. Sensory neurons transmit impulses from sense organs to the brain and spinal cord; motor neurons transmit impulses from the brain and spinal cord to muscles and glands. ADJ. neuronal

Neurontin N. *See* TABLE OF COMMONLY PRESCRIBED DRUGS—TRADE NAMES.

neuropathy (no͝o-rŏp'ə-thē) N. any abnormal condition of the peripheral nerves. ADJ. neuropathic

neurosarcoma N. malignant neoplasm made up of nerve tissue, fibrous tissue, and connective tissue, also called malignant neuroma.

neurosis (no͝o-rō'sĭs) N. inefficient way of thinking or behaving, that may be manifested by depression, anxiety, defense mechanisms, compulsion, phobias, or obsessions and that produces psychological pain or discomfort. The perception of reality is usually not impaired, and behavior remains within socially accepted limits. (*Compare* PSYCHOSIS.)

neurosurgery (no͝or'ō-sûr'jə-rē) N. any surgery involving the brain, spinal cord, or peripheral nerves.

neurosyphilis (no͝or'ō-sĭf'ə-lĭs) N. infection of the central nervous system by the organism causing syphilis.

neurotoxic ADJ. poisonous or harmful to nerves and nerve cells.

neurotoxin (no͝or'ə-tŏk'sĭn) N. toxin, found in the venom of certain snakes, in some fish, shellfish, and bacteria, and in certain other organisms, that is toxic to nervous tissue.

neurotransmitter (noŏr′ō-trăns′mĭt-ər) N. chemical that affects or modifies the transmission of an impulse across a synapse between nerves or between a nerve and a muscle. Important neurotransmitters are acetylcholine, dopamine, gamma-aminobutyric acid, serotonin, and norepinephrine.

neutrino (noō′-trē-nō) N. lepton with no electric charge. Neutrinos participate only in weak and gravitational interactions and are therefore very difficult to detect. There are three known types of neutrinos, all of which have very little mass. *See also* LEPTON.

neutron N. small atomic particle similar in mass to a proton but without an electrical charge.

neutropenia (noō′trə-pē′nē-ə) N. abnormal decrease in the number of neutrophils (a type of white blood cell) in the blood; it is associated with infection, rheumatoid arthritis, leukemia, and certain vitamin deficiencies.

neutrophil (noō′trə-fĭl′) N. granular leukocyte (white blood cell). Neutrophils are phagocytes engulfing bacteria and cellular debris. An increase in the number of neutrophils occurs in acute infections, certain malignant neoplastic diseases, and some other disorders.

nevus (nē′vəs) N. congenital discoloration of the skin; a birthmark or mole. *See also* PORTWINE STAIN; STRAWBERRY HEMANGIOMA.

COMMON NEUROTRANSMITTERS

Neurotransmitter	Location	Actions
Acetylcholine	Neuromuscular junctions, autonomic nervous system, and brain	Excites muscles, decreases heart rate, and relays various signals in the autonomic nervous system and the brain
Norepinephrine	Sympathetic nervous system and brain	Regulates activity of visceral organs and some brain functions
Dopamine	Brain	Involved in control of certain motor functions
Serotonin	Brain and spinal cord	May be involved in mental functions, circadian rhythms, and sleep and wakefulness
Gamma-aminobutyric acid	Brain and spinal cord	Inhibits various neurons
Glycine	Spinal cord	Inhibits various neurons

newborn N. infant recently born; a neonate.

nexus N. connection or link.

NGU *See* NONGONOCOCCAL URETHRITIS.

niacin (nī′ə-sĭn) N. vitamin of the B-complex group, essential for normal function of the nervous system and gastrointestinal tract. Rich sources are meats, fish, eggs, nuts, and wheat germ. Symptoms of deficiency include fatigue, muscle weakness, loss of appetite, mouth sores, nausea, vomiting, and depression; severe deficiency leads to pellagra (*see also* TABLE OF VITAMINS). Niacin is used therapeutically in the treatment of hypercholesterolemia. Also called nicotinic acid.

nicotine (nĭk′ə-tēn′) N. poisonous alkaloid found in tobacco, thought responsible for the dependence of regular smokers on tobacco. In small doses nicotine stimulates the nervous system, causing an increase in pulse rate, a rise in blood pressure, and a decrease in appetite. In large doses, it is a depressant, slowing the heartbeat and leading to respiratory depression.

nicotine patch N. patch, typically worn over the arm or chest, that contains doses of nicotine for transdermal administration (trade name Nicotrol); it relieves nicotine withdrawal symptoms and is offered to smokers who wish to eradicate the habit; side effects include insomnia, redness, and burning at the application site.

nicotine poisoning N. toxic condition caused by the ingestion or inhalation of large amounts of nicotine. Nicotine poisoning is characterized at first by nervous system stimulation, followed by depression, leading,

if untreated, to respiratory failure.

nicotinic acid *See* NIACIN.

Nicotrol N. trade name for the transdermal nicotine patch.

NICU *See* NEONATAL INTENSIVE CARE UNIT.

nidation (nī-dā′shən) N. implantation of the conceptus in the endometrial layer of the uterus.

nidus N. point of origin of a disease.

Niemann-Pick disease (nē′män′) N. inherited disease of lipid metabolism, in which phospholipids accumulate in the bone marrow, spleen, and lymph nodes. Symptoms, which begin in early childhood, include an enlarged spleen and liver, anemia, and progressive mental and physical deterioration, usually leading to death within a few years. The disease is largely confined to people of Jewish descent.

nifedipine (nī-fĕd′ə-pēn′) N. drug (trade name Procardia) of the calcium channel blocker class useful in the treatment of hypertension, angina, heart failure, and migraine. Experimentally, this agent has been used in patients with central nervous system problems as well. Adverse effects include fluid retention, nausea, and tachycardia. Excess hypotension may occur when nifedipine is used for severe hypertension, especially in combination with nitroglycerin. *See* TABLE OF COMMONLY PRESCRIBED DRUGS—GENERIC NAMES.

night blindness N. abnormal reduction in vision in darkness, due to deficiency of vitamin A or to retinal disorder; also called nyctalopia.

night terror N. episode, most often occurring in young children, in which the person awakens in terror with a panicky scream, feelings of fear and anxiety, and total inability to recall any dream or incident provoking the feelings, and typically does not recall the event the next morning (*compare* NIGHTMARE).

nightmare N. dream that arouses feelings of fear, terror, panic, or anxiety (*compare* NIGHT TERROR).

nihilism (nī′ə-lĭz′əm) N. in psychiatry, a delusion that certain things or everything, including the self, does not exist; associated with some forms of schizophrenia.

nipple N. small, pigmented structure that projects from the breast and is surrounded by the pigmented areola. In women the nipple contains the openings of the lactiferous ducts, which transport milk from the milk-producing glands in the breast.

nipple discharge N. spontaneous release of material from the nipple; it may be normal, as in the release of colostrum during pregnancy; or it may be a sign of endocrine or infectious disease or neoplasm.

nipple shield N. rubber or plastic device to protect the nipples of nursing women, esp. cracked or sore nipples, and to allow them to heal.

nitric oxide N. gas normally produced in the body and present in expired air; in blood vessels, it plays a major role in vasodilation. Administration of the drug nitroglycerine increases the nitric oxide level; this leads to dilation of the coronary arteries and increased blood flow to the heart. Certain anti-impotence drugs (e.g., Viagra) exert their effect via a similar mechanism. Recent research suggests that increased levels of exhaled nitric oxide may be an early sign of bronchospasm in asthma.

Nitro-Dur II N. trade name for a transdermal patch preparation of nitroglycerin used in the treatment of angina, congestive heart failure, and myocardial infarction. Concomitant administration with Viagra may be fatal. *See* NITRIC OXIDE.

nitrofurantoin (nī′trō-fyoō-răn′tō-ĭn) N. antibiotic (trade name Macrodantin) used to treat urinary tract infections. Adverse effects include gastrointestinal disturbances, fever, and hypersensitivity reactions. *See* TABLE OF COMMONLY PRESCRIBED DRUGS—GENERIC NAMES.

nitrogen (nī′trə-jən) N. nonmetallic element that is a component of all protein and many organic compounds. Nitrogen compounds are essential parts of all organisms, present in nucleic acids, proteins, and other biologically important compounds. *See also* TABLE OF IMPORTANT ELEMENTS.

nitroglycerin (nī′trō-glĭs′ər-ĭn) N. coronary vasodilator used in the treatment of angina pectoris. Adverse effects include headache, flushing, and low blood pressure. Concomitant administration with Viagra may be fatal. *See* NITRIC OXIDE; TABLE OF COMMONLY PRESCRIBED DRUGS—GENERIC NAMES.

Nitrong N. trade name for extended-release oral tablets of nitroglycerin. Concomitant administration with Viagra may be fatal. *See* NITRIC OXIDE.

Nitrospan, Nitrostat N. trade names for nitroglycerin. Concomitant administration with Viagra may be fatal. *See* NITRIC OXIDE; TABLE OF COMMONLY PRESCRIBED DRUGS—TRADE NAMES.

nitrous oxide (nī′trəs) N. gas used as an anesthetic. Nitrous oxide produces light anesthesia and is used in minor surgery, childbirth, and dentistry, but not alone for major surgery. In small doses it sometimes produces exhilaration and is called laughing gas.

nizatidine (nĭ-zăt′ĭ-dēn′) N. oral histamine blocker (trade name Axid) used in the treatment of peptic ulcer disease. *See* TABLE OF COMMONLY PRESCRIBED DRUGS—GENERIC NAMES.

NMR *See* NUCLEAR MAGNETIC RESONANCE.

nociception N. perception by nerves of injury or pain.

nocturia (nŏk-tŏor′ē-ə) N. excessive urination at night; it may be due to excessive fluid intake before bedtime, to renal disorder, or, in older men, to prostatic disease (*compare* ENURESIS); also called nycturia.

nocturnal emission (nŏk-tûr′nəl) N. involuntary emission of semen during sleep, usually associated with an erotic dream; colloquial: wet dream.

node N.
1. small rounded knot of tissue.
2. a lymph node.

node of Ranvier (rän′vyā) N. gap, occurring at regular intervals, in the myelin sheath of a nerve; the action potential signals "jump" along the axon, from node to node, rather than propagating smoothly, as they do in axons that lack a myelin sheath. This process speeds up the rate of signal conduction in myelinated nerves.

NODE OF RANVIER

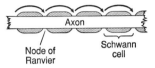

Curved arrows indicate action potential "jumping" along the axon from node to node.

nodule (nŏj′ool) N. small node.

Nolvadex N. *See* TABLE OF COMMONLY PRESCRIBED DRUGS—TRADE NAMES.

noma (nō′mə) N. acute ulceration of mucous membranes of the mouth or genitals, most often seen in undernourished children; it often leads to destruction of underlying bone and connective tissue.

nondisjunction N. failure of homologous pairs of chromosomes to separate during the processes of nuclear division, resulting in an abnormal number of chromosomes in the daughter cells.

nongonococcal urethritis (NGU) (nŏn′gŏn-ə-kŏk′əl yŏor′ĭ-thrī′tĭs) N. infectious disease of the urethra, usually caused by the *Chlamydia trachomatis* parasite and sexually transmitted. Symptoms are painful urination and discharge from the penis in males, and erosion of the cervix in females. A fetus passing through the birth canal of an infected mother may develop infection of the nasopharnyx and eyes. Treatment is by tetracyclines or erythromycin.

noninvasive (nŏn′ĭn-vā′sĭv) ADJ. in medicine, pert. to a diagnostic or therapeutic technique that does not involve puncturing the skin or entering the body cavity or an organ.

nonmyelinated ADJ. nervous system structures not encased by myelin; may be normal, as in parts of the brain and spinal cord, or abnormal. Loss of myelin occurs in several disease states, including multiple sclerosis; these are referred to as demyelinating diseases.

nonpolar ADJ. molecules that lack an affinity for water (hydrophobic) because of the absence of opposite charges (poles) on either end.

nonrapid eye movement (NREM) N. period of sleep representing about 75% of normal sleep time during which dreaming and rapid eye muscle contractions do not occur. NREM sleep periods alternate with short REM (dreaming) sleep periods during normal sleep. Most NREM sleep occurs in four stages: stage 1, characterized by theta rhythm; stage 2, characterized by distinctive sleep patterns; stages 3 and 4, characterized by delta rhythm. (*Compare* RAPID EYE MOVEMENT.) *See also* SLEEP.

nonspecific urethritis (NSU) (nŏn'spĭ-sĭf'ĭk yŏŏr'ĭ-thrī'tĭs) N. inflammation of the urethra not known to be caused by a specific organism. There are often no symptoms in women; in men, urethral discharge. NSU is most likely sexually transmitted.

nonsteroidal anti-inflammatory agent N. large class of drugs which, by various mechanisms, inhibit the process of inflammation in the body; by definition, these drugs are not related to the corticosteroids, which also have an anti-inflammatory effect; side effects commonly include stomach irritation and intestinal bleeding.

nonthrombocytopenic purpura *See* PURPURA.

nonviable (nŏn-vī'ə-bəl) ADJ. incapable of life or living. Often used in reference to a fetus that has died in utero or to tissues that have been damaged, such as in a burn injury.

Noonan's syndrome (nōō'nənz sĭn'drōm') N. disorder, occurring only in males, characterized by short stature, lowset ears, and often decreased fertility.

norepinephrine (nôr'ĕp-ə-nĕf'rĭn) N.
1. hormone secreted by the adrenal medulla and a neurotransmitter released at nerve endings. It constricts small blood vessels, raises blood pressure, slows heart rate, increases the rate of breathing, and relaxes the smooth muscles of the intestinal tract.
2. drug used to treat low blood pressure.

norethindrone (nôr-ĕth'ĭn-drōn') N. progestin compound used in oral contraceptives and in the treatment of endometriosis and abnormal uterine bleeding. Adverse effects include gastrointestinal upsets, breast changes, and irregular uterine bleeding.

norgestrel N. progestin used in oral contraceptives.

Norinyl N. trade name for an oral contraceptive containing norethindrone and mestranol.

Norlestrin N. trade name for an oral contraceptive containing estradiol and norethindrone.

Norlutin N. trade name for norethindrone.

normal dwarf *See* PRIMORDIAL DWARF.

Normodyne N. trade name for the antihypertensive labetolol.

normotensive (nôr′mō-tĕn′sĭv) ADJ. pert. to the condition of having normal blood pressure (*compare* HYPERTENSIVE; HYPOTENSIVE).

nortriptyline (nôr-trĭp′tə-lēn′) N. antidepressant. Adverse effects include sedation, gastrointestinal, cardiovascular, and neurological reactions, and the possibility of drug interaction if taken with other drugs.

Norvasc N. trade name for the oral calcium blocker amlodipine besylate. *See* TABLE OF COMMONLY PRESCRIBED DRUGS—TRADE NAMES.

nose N. structure on the face that serves as a passageway for air into and out of the lungs and as an organ of smell.

nosebleed *See* EPISTAXIS.

noso- comb. form indicating an association with disease (e.g.,

nosology, classifying of diseases).

nosocomial (nŏs′ə-kō′mē-əl) N. ADJ. pert. to a hospital.

nosocomial infection N. infection acquired during a hospital stay.

nostrils *See* NARES.

notch N. small indentation, as on a bone (e.g., mandibular notch, the depression in the middle of the lower jawbone).

notochord (nō′tə-kôrd′) N. rodlike structure in the embryo that in humans and other vertebrates is replaced by the vertebral column.

notomelus N. congenital abnormality in which one or more accessory limbs are attached to the back.

nourish (nŭr′ĭsh) V. to supply foods and nutrients to maintain life. N. nourishment

Novocain (nō′və-kān′) N. trade name for the local anesthetic procaine.

NOSE

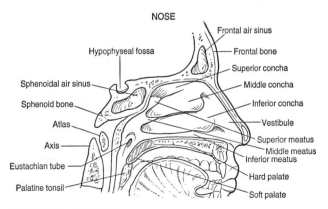

Internal portions of the nose.

noxious (nŏk′shəs) ADJ. harmful, toxic; having adverse effects on living things.

NREM *See* NONRAPID EYE MOVEMENT.

NSAIA N. abbrev. for non-steroidal anti-inflammatory agent.

nucha (noō′kə) N. nape, or back of the neck. ADJ. nuchal

nuchal cord N. condition in which the umbilical cord is wrapped around the neck of the baby as it is being born. It most cases it can be slipped over the child's head or cut without harm to the child.

nucle-, nucleo- comb. forms indicating a relationship to a nucleus (e.g., nucleosis, production of an abnormal number of cell nuclei).

nuclear (noō′klē-ər) ADJ. pert. to a nucleus.

nuclear magnetic resonance (NMR, MRI) (noō′klē-ər rĕz′ə-nəns) N. diagnostic technique in which an electromagnetic field stimulates atomic nuclei within the patient's body, causing those nuclei to release energy that is recorded with sensitive receivers. The technique is much more accurate than X-ray films for showing soft structures and, in some cases, bleeding.

nucleic acid (noō-klē′ĭk) N. compound composed of nucleotides, each of which is made up of a phosphate group, a ribose or deoxyribose sugar, and a purine or pyrimidine base. Nucleic acids are involved in the determination of hereditary characteristics and in energy storage. *See also* DEOXYRIBONUCLEIC ACID; RIBONUCLEIC ACID.

nucleolus (noō-klē′ə-ləs) N. small structure, composed mostly of ribonucleic acid, found in the nucleus of cells and involved in the formation of ribosomes.

nucleoplasm (noō′klē-ə-plăz′əm) N. protoplasm of the nucleus (*compare* CYTOPLASM).

nucleotide (noō′klē-ə-tīd′) N. compound containing a base (a purine or pyrimidine), a sugar, and a phosphate group. Nucleic acids [e.g., deoxyribonucleic acid (DNA) and ribonucleic acid (RNA)] are composed of chains of linked nucleotides.

nucleus (noō′klē-əs) N.
1. usually spherical structure, enclosed in a membrane (the nuclear membrane), and contained within a cell, that controls the cell and its functions. It contains the genetic information for the maintenance, growth, and reproduction of the organism.
2. group of cells, esp. in the central nervous system, having a distinct function (e.g., the auditory center in the brain).
3. in chemistry, the center of an atom.

nullipara (nə-lĭp′ər-ə) N. woman who has never given birth to a viable infant. ADJ. nulliparous

numbness N. partial or total lack of sensation in a part of the body, often accompanied by tingling. Minor nerve damage or more serious nerve injury or dysfunction may cause it.

nurse N. person educated and licensed in the practice of nursing. Includes data collection, diagnosis, planning, treatment, and evaluation within the context of the patient's response to the problem, rather than just the problem itself. Nurses may be generalists or specialize and are ethically and legally accountable for both their actions and actions of those they supervise. V. to breast feed an infant.

nutation (noo-tā′shən) N. act of nodding the head, esp. uncontrolled nodding.

nutrient (noo′trē-ənt) N. substance that must be supplied by the diet to provide for normal health of the body, and for energy supplies and materials for growth. Nutrients include proteins, fats, carbohydrates, vitamins, and minerals.

nutrition (noo-trĭsh′ən) N.
1. nourishment.
2. all of the chemical and physical processes involved in the ingestion, digestion, absorption, assimilation, and excretion of nutrients.
3. study of food and drink as related to the needs of the body.

nyctalopia (nĭk′tə-lō′pē-ə) *See* NIGHT BLINDNESS.

nyctophobia (nĭk′tə-fō′bē-ə) N. irrational fear of darkness.

nycturia *See* NOCTURIA.

Nydrazid N. trade name for the antibiotic isoniazid.

nymphomania (nĭm′fə-mā′nē-ə) N. psychosexual disorder of women, characterized by an insatiable desire for sexual gratification (*compare* SATYRIASIS). N. nymphomaniac, ADJ. nymphomaniacal

nystagmus (nĭ-stăg′məs) N. involuntary rhythmic eyeball movement; it may be congenital or result from brain disease or other disorders.

Nystan N. trade name for nystatin.

nystatin (nĭs′tə-tĭn) N. antifungal and antibiotic, available as a topical cream, as a suppository, in eyedrops, and for oral administration; it is used to treat gastrointestinal, skin, and vaginal infections.

O

O symbol for the element oxygen.

oat cell carcinoma (kär′sə-nō′mə) N. malignant neoplasm consisting of small epithelial cells that do not typically form masses but spread through the lymphatics; more than 25% of lung cancers are oat cell carcinomas. Surgery is usually not possible; chemotherapy and radiotherapy are often ineffective.

OB *See* obstetrics.

obesity (ō-bē′sĭ-tē) N. condition of being overweight; increase in the amount of fat in the subcutaneous tissues of the body. The most common cause is overeating, often dating to early childhood. Various disease conditions can also contribute to obesity (esp. such as thyroid, pituitary, and other endocrine gland problems). Treatment involves diet and sometimes counseling. Rarely, drug therapy or surgical treatment is recommended.

obligate ADJ. surviving only in a particular environment (e.g., an obligate parasite cannot survive without a particular host).

obligate aerobe (âr′ōb′) N. organism that cannot grow in the absence of oxygen (e.g., *Streptococcus pneumoniae*).

obligate anaerobe (ăn′ə-rōb′) N. organism that cannot grow in the presence of oxygen (e.g., *Clostridium botulinum*).

obsession N. abnormally persistent focus on a single idea (*compare* COMPULSION).

obsessive-compulsive ADJ. characterized by a tendency to repeat certain acts or rituals (e.g., washing the hands more than is necessary, usually to relieve anxiety).

obsessive-compulsive personality N. person who has an uncontrollable need to repeat certain acts or rituals; it may be mild or serious, involving irrational acts that interfere with normal social relationships and behavior.

obstetrician (ŏb′stĭ-trĭsh′ən) N. physician who specializes in obstetrics.

obstetrics (OB) (ŏb-stĕt′rĭks) N. that branch of medicine concerned with the care of women during pregnancy, childbirth, and the immediate postpartum period; it is often practiced in conjunction with gynecology. ADJ. obstetric; obstetrical

obstipation N. extreme constipation, caused by obstruction in the intestinal system.

obstruction N. blockage; something that blocks or prevents passage. *See also* INTESTINAL OBSTRUCTION.

obtund V. to blunt or deaden sensitivity, as to pain by use of an anesthetic agent.

obturator (ŏb′tə-rā′tər) N. device used to close or cover an opening (e.g., a device implanted to cover the opening in the roof of the mouth in cleft palate).

obtuse N. dull or blunt; of less than normal mental capacity.

occipital bone (ŏk-sĭp′ĭ-tl) N. one of the bones of the skull; the saucer-shaped skull bone that forms the back and part of the base of the cranium, articulating with the first vertebra of the backbone.

occipital lobe N. one of the five lobes of each cerebral hemisphere.

occipito- comb. form indicating an association with the back of the head (occiput) (e.g., occipitocervical, pert. to the back of the head and the neck).

occiput (ŏk′sə-pŭt′) N. back part of the head. ADJ. occipital

occlusion (ə-kloō′zhən) N.
1. blockage or closing off of a vessel or passageway in the body, as in a clot occluding a blood vessels.
2. manner in which the teeth in the opposing jaws meet in biting (*see also* MALOCCLUSION). V. occlude, ADJ. occlusive

occult (ə-kŭlt′) N., ADJ. hidden, difficult to observe (e.g., occult fracture, one that is at first not observable on an X ray).

occult blood N. a very small or hidden amount of blood, not observable and usually detected only by chemical tests or microscopic analysis (e.g., occult blood in the stool of someone with an intestinal disorder).

occupational disease N. illness or disability resulting from employment, usually from long-term exposure to a noxious substance (e.g., asbestos) or from continuous repetition of certain acts.

occupational hazard N. any condition of a job, such as exposure to radiation or chemicals, that can result in injury or illness.

occupational therapy N. therapeutic use of various activities in which handicapped or convalescing people learn and use, under the direction of a trained therapist, skills for daily life activities and for specific occupations, with the goal of providing recreation and exercise and maximizing the capabilities of the person.

ochronosis (ō′krə-nō′sĭs) N. condition marked by the accumulation of brown-black pigment in cartilage and other connective tissue, usually due to phenol poisoning.

ocular (ŏk′yə-lər) ADJ. pert. to the eye. N. eyepiece of an optical instrument.

oculist (ŏk′yə-lĭst) *See* OPHTHALMOLOGIST.

oculo- comb. form indicating an association with the eye (e.g., oculomycosis, any fungus-caused disease of the eye).

oculomotor nerve (ŏk′yə-lō-mō′tər) N. one of a pair of motor nerves, the third of cranial nerves, essential for eye movement.

oculus (ŏk′yə-ləs) N., *pl.* oculi, eye, usually designated oculus dexter (OD), the right eye; and oculus sinister (OS), the left eye. ADJ. ocular

odont-, odonto- comb. forms indicating an association with teeth (e.g., odontitis, inflammation of the pulp of a tooth).

odontalgia N. toothache; pain in a tooth or the region around a tooth.

odontiasis N. process of cutting teeth; teething.

odontology N. study of the anatomy and physiology of

teeth and the surrounding structures in the mouth.

odor N. scent or smell.

odoriferous ADJ. fragrant, possessing an easily perceived odor; depending on the context, the quality of the odor may be either pleasant or not.

odynophagia (ō-dĭn′ə-fā′jə) N. severe burning, squeezing pain on swallowing, due to disorder of the esophagus (e.g., gastroesophageal reflux, tumor, chemical irritation of the mucous membrane lining, or infection).

Oedipus complex (ĕd′ə-pəs) N. in psychoanalysis, repressed sexual feeling of a child toward the parent of the opposite sex and feelings of competition with the parent of the same sex, esp. a boy's sexual feeling toward his mother and sense of competition with his father. ADJ. Oedipal

-oid suffix meaning resembling (e.g., mastoid, like a breast or breast-shaped).

ointment N. semisolid preparation, usually containing a drug, applied externally (e.g., an anesthetic or antibacterial ointment applied to a skin irritation); also called unction.

Old World leishmaniasis (lēsh′mə-nī′ə-sĭs) *See* ORIENTAL SORE.

olecranon (ō-lĕk′rə-non′) N. projection of the ulna (one of the lower arm bones) that forms the outer bump of the elbow and fits into the fossa of the humerus (upper arm bone) when the arm is extended; also called olecranon process.

olfaction (ŏl-făk′shən) N. sense of smell. Special sensory cells in the mucous membrane lining of the nasal cavity respond to the presence of chemical particles (odors) dissolved in the mucus and transmit the impulses along the olfactory nerve to the brain for interpretation. ADJ. olfactory

olfactory center (ŏl-făk′tə-rē) N. group of neurons in the brain, located near the junction of the parietal and temporal lobes, concerned with the interpretation of odors.

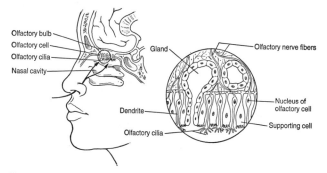

The sense of smell. Molecules strike the olfactory cilia of the olfactory cells in the upper portion of the nose. These cells are nerve cells whose impulses are sent to the brain.

olfactory nerve N. one of a pair of sensory nerves, the first cranial nerves, that transmit impulses from the mucous membranes of the nasal cavity to the olfactory center in the brain.

olig-, oligo- comb. forms meaning few, little, insufficient (e.g., oligodipsia, condition in which the sense of thirst is abnormally reduced or absent).

oligodactyly N. congenital condition characterized by the absence of one or more fingers or toes.

oligodendrocyte N. neuroglia cell of the nervous system.

oligodontia N. congenital condition in which some of the teeth are missing.

oligomenorrhea N. abnormally light or infrequent menstruation.

oligosaccharide N. carbohydrate compound made up of a small number of monosaccharide (single sugar molecule) units, typically two or three. Lactose (milk sugar) and sucrose (table sugar) consist of two monosaccharides. Polysaccharides contain larger numbers of monosaccharide units.

oligospermia (ŏl´ĭ-gō-spŭr´mē-ə) N. insufficient number of spermatozoa in the semen.

oliguria (ŏl´ĭ-gyŏor´ē-ə) N. production of an abnormally small amount of urine; it may be due to kidney disease, urinary tract obstruction, edema, imbalance in fluid and electrolytes in the body, or, occasionally, profuse sweating.

omentum (ō-měn´təm) N., *pl.* omenta, fold of peritoneal tissue attaching and supporting the stomach and adjacent organs. ADJ. omental

greater omentum N. tissue that covers the intestine; it is rich in fat, acts as a heat insulator, and prevents friction between abdominal organs.

lesser omentum N. tissue that links the stomach, the liver, and the first part of the small intestine.

omeprazole N. gastrointestinal agent (trade name Prilosec) that suppresses gastric acid secretion by inhibiting a specific enzyme system in the stomach lining; used in ulcer treatment and in severe esophagitis. *See* TABLE OF COMMONLY PRESCRIBED DRUGS—GENERIC NAMES.

omo- comb. form indicating an association with the shoulder (e.g., omoclavicular, pert. to the shoulder and clavicle collarbone).

omphal-, omphalo- comb. forms indicating an association with the umbilicus (navel) (e.g., omphalorrhagia, a flow of lymph from the umbilicus).

omphalocele (ŏm-făl´ə-sēl´) N. congenital defect in which abdominal organs protrude through the umbilical region—an umbilical hernia; it is usually treated surgically.

omphalus N. the umbilicus (navel). ADJ. omphalic

onchocerciasis (ŏng´kō-sər-kī´ə-sĭs) N. disease common in Central and South America and Africa in which the bite of black fleas transmits filariae (long, threadlike worms) under the skin, causing subcutaneous nodules, an itchy rash, and eye lesions. Treatment involves surgical incision of nodules to remove the worms and the use of anthelmintics (diethylcarbamazine). Also called river blindness.

onco- comb. form indicating an association with a tumor or mass (e.g., oncogenesis, process of neoplasm formation).

oncogene (ŏn'kə-jēn) N. gene in a virus that is able to produce a malignant change in an infected cell; several have been identified in human tissue as potential causes of cancer. Researchers are attempting to isolate anti-oncogenes that suppress tumors and may be used in the treatment of cancer. Certain oncogenes may play a role in normal growth and development; if they are damaged or mutated, cancer may result.

oncologist N. physician who specializes in oncology.

oncology (ŏng-kŏl'ə-jē) N. that branch of medicine concerned with the study and treatment of tumors.

oncotic pressure N. pressure within a blood vessel exerted by the presence of colloid molecules, such as proteins; this pressure tends to help retain fluid within the walls of the blood vessels, especially the capillaries. Loss of protein (colloid), such as in kidney failure, may allow the pressure to decrease. The vessels then leak, resulting in tissue fluid and swelling (edema).

Oncovin N. trade name for the antineoplastic drug vincristine.

oneirism (ō-nī'rĭz'əm) N. daydreaming. It is a normal phenomenon, but if engaged in to excess, is often a sign of autism or other obstacle to normal functioning.

oneiro- comb. form indicating an association with a dream or

dreaming (e.g., oneirology, study of dreams and dreaming).

onomatomania N. condition in which a person repeatedly uses or tries to recall a specific word or name; usually a form of obsession or other abnormal mental state.

ontogeny (ŏn-tŏj'ə-nē) N. development of an organism from fertilized egg through developmental and growth stages to maturity. ADJ. ontogenic

onych-, onycho- comb. forms indicating an association with nail or the nails (e.g., onychauxis, condition in which the nails are thickened).

onycholysis N. separation of the nail from its normal attachment to the nail bed; associated with trauma, certain infections, and other disorders of the skin.

onychosis N. any disease or disorder of the nails.

onyxis N. an ingrown nail.

oo- comb. form indicating an association with an ovum (egg) (e.g., oogonium, precursor cell from which an oocyte develops in the female fetus during embryonic development).

oocyte (ō'ə-sīt') N. cell from which a mature ovum develops.

oogenesis (ō'ə-jĕn'ĭ-sĭs) N. development of ova, female reproductive cells. During the reproductive years of a woman's life, at roughly monthly intervals, one or two oocytes present in the ovary since birth undergo a series of meiotic divisions that lead to the formation of a mature ovum (ova). The mature ovum has the haploid chromosome number and is released from the Graafian follicle at the time of ovulation, ready for fertilization. (*Compare* SPERMATOGENESIS.)

oophor-, oophoro- comb. forms indicating an association with the ovary (e.g., oophorocytosis, cyst formation in an ovary).

oophorectomy (ō'ə-fə-rĕk'tə-mē) N. surgical removal of one or both ovaries, usually performed to remove an ovarian tumor or cyst, to treat an ovarian abscess or endometriosis, or to remove the source of estrogen in some cases of cancer (e.g., breast cancer). If both ovaries are removed, sterility results and menopause occurs. Also called ovariectomy.

oophoritis (ō'ə-fə-rī'tĭs) N. inflammation of one or both ovaries often occurring with salpingitis (inflammation of the fallopian tubes).

oophorosalpingectomy N. surgical removal of one or both ovaries and the corresponding oviducts (fallopian tubes); performed to remove a cyst, tumor, or abscess or to treat endometriosis. *See also* OOPHORECTOMY.

ootid N. mature ovum after penetration by the spermatozoon but before fusion of the pronuclei (genetic material) to form a zygote.

opacification (ō-păs'ə-fĭ-kā'shən) N. clouding of a part or loss of transparency, esp. of the cornea or lens of the eye.

open fracture *See* COMPOUND FRACTURE under FRACTURE.

operant conditioning (ŏp'ər-ənt) N. in behavioral therapy, form of learning in which a person is rewarded for the desired response and punished for the undesired response; used to break harmful habits and reinforce desirable behavior.

operating microscope N. binocular microscope used in surgery to enable the surgeon to view clearly small and inaccessible parts of the body (e.g., parts of the eye or ear) (*see also* MICROSURGERY).

operating room (OR) N. room in a health care facility where surgical procedures are performed.

operation N. any surgical procedure. ADJ. operative

operator gene N. segment of deoxyribonucleic acid, DNA (the hereditary material) that regulates the transcription of structural genes in its operon and acts with a regulatory gene to control the activity of structural genes.

operculum (ō-pûr'kyə-ləm) N., *pl.* opercula, lid, covering, or plug, as the mucous plug that closes the uterus during pregnancy. ADJ. opercular

operon (ŏp'ə-rŏn') N. segment of deoxyribonucleic acid, DNA (the genetic material) containing several structural genes that determine related functions, an operator gene, and a regulatory gene that controls the function of the structural genes.

ophidism N. poisoning by snake venom. ADJ. ophidic

ophthalm-, ophthalmo- comb. forms indicating an association with the eye (e.g., ophthalmovascular, pert. to the blood vessels of the eye).

ophthalmectomy N. surgical removal of an eye.

ophthalmia neonatorum (ŏf-thăl'mē-ə nē'ō-nā-tôr'əm) N. type of conjunctivitis occurring in newborns, who contract the disease passing through the birth canal; the most serious form is due to gonorrhea. Routine administration of silver nitrate drops or topical antibiotics in the eyes of newborns largely prevents the disease; if it occurs, antibiotic therapy is indicated.

ophthalmic (ŏf-thăl′mĭk) ADJ. pert. to the eye.

ophthalmologist (ŏf-thəl-mŏl′ə-jĭst) N. physician who specializes in ophthalmology; formerly also called oculist (*compare* OPTOMETRIST; OPTICIAN).

ophthalmology (ŏf′thəl-mŏl′ə-jē) N. study of the eye, its development, structure, functions, defects, diseases, and treatment. ADJ. ophthalmologic

ophthalmoplegia (ŏf-thăl′mō-plē′jē-ə) N. condition characterized by paralysis of the motor nerves of the eyes, sometimes occurring in myasthenia gravis, botulism, thiamine deficiency, and disorders of the nerves of the cranial area.

ophthalmoscope (ŏf-thăl′mə-skōp′) N. device that allows clear visualization of the structures of the interior of the eye.

Ophthochlor N. trade name for an ophthalmic preparation containing chloramphenicol.

Ophthocort N. trade name for a fixed-combination ophthalmic preparation containing hydrocortisone and the antibacterials chloramphenicol and polymixin.

opiate (ō′pē-ĭt) N. drug that contains opium, is derived from opium, or is produced synthetically and has opiatelike characteristics. Opiates are central nervous system depressants: they relieve pain and suppress cough. Included among them are morphine, codeine, and heroin.

opisthorchiasis (ŏp′ĭs-thôr-kī′ə-sĭs) N. infestation of the liver and bile ducts with flukes of the genus Ophisthorchia, obtained from eating raw or inadequately cooked fish, common in eastern Asia. Symptoms include gastrointestinal disturbances and weight loss, often leading to damage to tissues of the liver and bile duct, and sometimes to cancer of the liver.

opisthotonos N. severe muscle spasm, sometimes occurring in the final stages of tetany, in which the back arches, the head bends back, and the heels are flexed toward the back.

OPISTHOTONOS

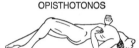

Opisthotonos may occur during tetanus.

opium (ō′pē-əm) N. substance derived from poppy plants (Papaver species) that contains morphine, codeine, papaverine, and other narcotic substances used to relieve pain.

opportunistic infection (ŏp′ər-tōō-nĭs′tĭk) N. infection caused by a microorganism that does not normally produce disease in humans; it occurs in persons with abnormally functioning immune systems, for example, those with acquired immune deficiency syndrome and those receiving immunosuppressive drugs (e.g., transplant patients).

opsonin (ŏp′sə-nĭn) N. component of serum that attaches to foreign particles (e.g., invading microorganism or other antigen) making them more vulnerable to phagocytosis by leukocytes.

opsonization (ŏp′sə-nĭ-zā′shən) N. process by which opsonins make an invading microorganism more susceptible to phagocytosis.

optic ADJ. pert. to the eye or to sight.

optic disk N. small spot on the retina, insensitive to light; blind spot.

optic nerve N. one of a pair of sensory nerves, the second cranial nerves, that arise in the retina and transmit visual impulses from the eye to the visual cortex of the brain.

optician (ŏp-tĭsh′ən) N. person who grinds and fits eyeglasses and contact lenses by prescription (*compare* OPHTHALMOLOGIST; OPTOMETRIST).

opto- comb. form indicating an association with sight (e.g., optoblast, a large nerve cell in the retina).

optometrist N. person who practices optometry.

optometry (ŏp-tŏm′ĭ-trē) N. practice of testing the eyes for visual acuity and prescribing corrective lenses or other visual aids (*compare* OPHTHALMOLOGY).

OR *See* OPERATING ROOM.

oral ADJ. pert. to the mouth.

oral cancer N. a malignant neoplasm of the lips or mouth most commonly occurring in men over the age of 60, often associated with tobacco use, esp. pipe smoking, and with alcoholism, syphilis, and poor oral hygiene. Premalignant leukoplakia or lip or mouth lesions may occur. Treatment depends on the size and location of the neoplasm and may include surgery, irradiation, and chemotherapy.

oral contraceptive (kŏn′trə-sĕp′tĭv) N. pill containing a combination of estrogen and progestin preparations that inhibits ovulation and thus prevents conception. It is a highly effective contraceptive if taken as directed, is generally acceptable to users, and has several beneficial side effects, including relief of dysmenorrhea and acne and regularization of menstrual cycles. However, oral contraceptives have been associated with side effects, some serious, that make them unadvised for some women. Serious adverse effects include increased tendency to develop thromboembolic disorders (e.g., stroke); less serious side effects experienced by many women include weight gain, breakthrough bleeding, breast tenderness, and depression. Oral contraceptives are generally not recommended for women with a history of breast or pelvic cancer, undiagnosed vaginal bleeding, cardiovascular disease, liver disease, renal disease, thyroid disorders, or diabetes. Also called birth control pill or, simply, the pill.

oral phase N. in psychoanalytic theory, first stage in a person's development, from birth through the first year, in which sucking and biting are prime sources of pleasure (*compare* ANAL PHASE; PHALLIC PHASE; LATENCY PHASE; GENITAL PHASE).

oral poliovirus vaccine (OPV) (pō′lē-ō-vī′rəs) *See* SABIN VACCINE.

Oramorph SR N. trade name for an oral form of the narcotic agent morphine; used in the control of severe pain; may be habit-forming.

orbit (ôr′bĭt) N. either of a pair of bony cavities in the skull that house the eyeball and associated structures; the eyeball socket. ADJ. orbital

orbito- comb. form indicating an association with the orbit or eye socket (e.g., orbitonasal, pert. to the eye socket and the nose).

orchi-, orchio- comb. forms indicating an association with testis or testes (e.g., orchidoptosis, abnormally low-slung testes).

orchialgia (ôr′kē-ăl′jē-ə) N. pain in the testes; it may be caused by a hernia in the groin; by a calculus in the lower ureter, or by disease of the testis itself.

orchiectomy (ôr′kē-ĕk′tə-mē) N. surgical removal of one or both testes, usually performed to treat cancer of the testes or serious injury to the testes or to control cancer of another organ (e.g., prostate) by removing the source of androgenic hormones. Removal of both testes results in sterility.

orchiopexy (ôr′kē-ə-pĕk′sē) N. surgical procedure to bring an undescended testis into the scrotum and attach it so that it will not retract.

orchis (ôr′kĭs) See TESTIS.

orchitis (ôr-kī′tĭs) N. inflammation of one or both testes, characterized by pain and swelling; it occurs in mumps, syphilis, and certain other diseases.

orchotomy N. surgical incision into the testis to obtain material for microscopic analysis, as, for example, in cases of abnormally low sperm count in semen.

Oreton N. trade name for a testosterone preparation.

orexigenic ADJ. pert. to a substance that increases appetite.

orf N. viral infection of sheep that can be transmitted to humans, causing a painless skin eruption that crusts and heals spontaneously.

organ N. part of the body that forms a structural unit concerned with a specific function; it often consists of more than one kind of tissue. An example is the lungs, organs that are responsible for the exchange of carbon dioxide and oxygen.

organ of Corti N. hearing organ of the inner ear; contains various cells and receptors that sense sound waves and transmit the sensations to the brain.

organelle (ôr′gə-nĕl′) N. specialized part of a cell (e.g., the MITOCHONDRION, RIBOSOME, OR GOLGI APPARATUS).

organic ADJ.
1. pert. to an organ or the organs of the body.
2. chemical compound containing carbon.

organic brain syndrome N. any mental abnormality resulting from transient or permanent disturbance of the structure or function of the brain; it may result from cerebral atherosclerosis; the effects of aging, drugs, or poisonous chemicals (e.g., lead); a tumor or other conditions.

organic disorder N. disorder caused by a structural or other detectable change in an organ (*compare* FUNCTIONAL DISORDER).

organism (ôr′gə-nĭz′-m) N. individual animal, plant, microorganism, or cell capable of carrying on life functions.

organo- comb. form indicating an association with an organ (e.g., organogenesis, formation of organs and organ systems during embryonic development).

orgasm N. sexual climax, usually involving strong involuntary contractions of the genital musculature, perceived as pleasurable.

Oriental sore N. cutaneous form of leishmaniasis; a skin disorder caused by the *Leishmania tropica* parasite, occurring in Africa, Asia, and areas around the Mediterranean Sea; it is characterized by ulcerative skin lesions. Treatment usually involves the use of antimony preparations. Also called Old World leismaniasis; tropical sore; Aleppo boil.

orientation N. person's awareness of self with regard to position, time, place, and personal relationships.

orifice (ôr′ə-fĭs) N. opening to a body cavity or chamber (e.g., aortic orifice, opening from the lower left heart chamber to the aorta).

Orinase N. trade name for the antidiabetic tolbutamide.

Ornade N. trade name for a fixed-combination drug containing a decongestant (phenylpropanolamine), an antihistamine (chlorpheniramine), and an anticholinergic (isopropamide); used to relieve symptoms of upper respiratory infection.

oro- comb. form indicating an association with the mouth (e.g., orolingual, pert. to the mouth and tongue).

oropharynx (ôr′ō-făr′ĭngks) N. that part of the pharnyx extending from the soft palate at the back of the mouth to the hyoid bone region and containing the palatine and lingual tonsils (*compare* NASOPHARYNX). ADJ. oropharyngeal

orphenadrine N. skeletal muscle relaxant (trade name Norflex) used in several forms to treat severe muscle strain and Parkinsonism. Adverse effects include rapid heartbeat and dry mouth.

ortho- comb. form indicating an association with straightening, normality, or appropriateness (e.g., orthostatic, pert. to an erect, correct stance).

orthodontics (ôr′thə-dŏn′tĭks) N. that branch of dentistry concerned with malocclusion and irregularities of the teeth and their correction. ADJ. orthodontic

orthomolecular medicine *See* TABLE OF ALTERNATIVE MEDICINE TERMS.

orthopedics (ôr′thə-pē′dĭks) N. that branch of medicine concerned with the musculoskeletal system (bones, joints, muscles, ligaments, tendons) and the treatment of disorders affecting it.

orthopedist (ôr′thə-pē′dĭst) N. specialist in orthopedics.

orthopnea N. condition in which the person can breathe normally or comfortably only when sitting erect or standing; it is associated with asthma, emphysema, angina pectoris, and many other respiratory and heart disorders. ADJ. orthopneic

orthoptic (ôr-thŏp′tĭk) ADJ. pert. to normal binocular vision.

orthoptics (ôr-thŏp′tĭks) N. practice of using nonsurgical measures, esp. eye exercises, to treat abnormalities of vision and coordinated eye movement, such as strabismus and amblyopia.

orthoptist N. specialist in orthoptics.

orthorexia nervosa (ôr′thə-rĕk-sē-ə) N. unhealthy fixation on eating healthy food. The patient may avoid certain types of food, such as those containing fats, preservatives, or animal products. It is characterized by the pathological obsession for biologically pure food, which leads to important dietary restrictions. Patients exclude from their diets foods that they consider to be impure because the food contains herbicides, pesticides, or artificial substances. Patients also worry in excess about the techniques and materials used in the food preparation. This obsession leads to loss of social relationships that further favors obsessive concerns about food. There is a higher prevalence in men and in those with a lower level of education. In orthorexia, patients initially want to improve their health, treat a disease, or lose weight. Finally, the diet becomes the most important part of their lives. As a result, the sufferers may become as hazardously thin as those suffering from anorexia. This condition is probably as common as anorexia nervosa and bulimia. ADJ. orthorexic (*compare* ANOREXIA NERVOSA; BULIMIA.)

orthostatic ADJ. pert. to an upright position (e.g., orthostatic hypotension, low blood pressure occurring in some people when they stand up).

Orudis N. trade name for the nonsteroidal anti-inflammatory agent ketoprofen.

os (ŏs) N.
1. bone, *pl.* ossa.
2. mouth or mouthlike part, *pl.* ora, (e.g., external os of the uterus) (*compare* ORO-).

osche- comb. form indicating an association with the scrotum (e.g., oscheocele, swelling of the scrotum).

oscilloscope (ə-sĭl′ə-skōp′) N. electronic instrument with a television-like screen that allows for the visual display of electronic signals.

osculum (ŏs′kyə-ləm) N. small opening.

-osis suffix indicating a condition, esp. a diseased condition (e.g., nephrosis), or an increase or excess (e.g., leukocylosis).

osmolality ADJ. concentration of dissolved substances per kilogram of solvent (often water). The term tonicity is used to describe the osmolality of a solution relative to plasma. Solutions with the same osmolality as plasma are considered isotonic; those with greater osmolality are hypertonic, and those with lower osmolality are hypotonic. Tonicity and osmolality are important considerations medically, particularly in determining the type of intravenous fluid to give a patient. Normal saline (0.9% sodium chloride solution) is isotonic to plasma while dextrose in water solutions (D5W) is hypotonic. When given in excess, hypotonic solutions, such as D5W, may abnormally dilute plasma concentrations of sodium and potassium, resulting in harm to the patient. Compare to osmolarity, which is the concentration of dissolved substance per liter of solution (such as plasma). Osmolarity is affected by the volume of the various solutes in the solution and the temperature, while osmolality is not.

OSMOTIC PRESSURE

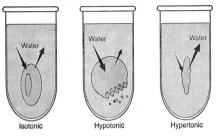

Isotonic   Hypotonic   Hypertonic

osmolarity ADJ. concentration of dissolved substance per liter of solution (such as plasma). Compare to osmolality, the concentration of dissolved substances per kilogram of solvent (often water). Osmolarity is affected by the volume of the various solutes in the solution and the temperature, while osmolality is not.

osmoreceptor (ŏz′mō-rĭ-sĕp′tər) N. group of cells in the hypothalamus that monitor blood concentration and influence the release of vasopressin from the posterior pituitary gland.

osmosis (ŏz-mō′sĭs) N. movement of a solvent through a membrane from a place of higher concentration to a place of lower concentration until the concentrations on both sides equalize. ADJ. osmotic

osmotic pressure (ŏz-mŏt′ĭk) N. pressure between two solutions of different concentrations separated by a semipermeable membrane.

osseo- comb. form indicating an association with bone (e.g., osseocartilaginous, pert. to bone and cartilage).

osseous (ŏs′ē-əs) ADJ. bony; of bone.

ossicle (ŏs′ĭ-kəl) N. small bone. The auditory ossicles are the three small bones (incus, stapes, and malleus) of the middle ear that transmit sound vibrations from the tympanic membrane to the inner ear.

ossification (ŏs′ə-fĭ-kā′shən) N. process of bone development.

osteitis (ŏs′tē-ī′tĭs) N. inflammation of a bone, caused by trauma, degeneration, or infection. *See also* OSTEOMYELITIS; PAGET'S DISEASE.

osteitis deformans (ŏs′tē-ī′tĭs dē-fôr′mănz′) *See* PAGET'S DISEASE.

osteo- comb. form indicating an association with bone (e.g., osteocampsia, bending of bone resulting from disease or nutritional deficiency).

osteoarthritis (ŏs′tē-ō-är-thrī′tĭs) N. most common form of arthritis, occurring mostly in the elderly, characterized by degenerative changes in the joints. Symptoms of pain after exercise or use, joint stiffness, and swelling develop, causing more disability when they affect the hip, spine, or knee. The cause is unknown but may involve many factors, sometimes aggravated by stress. Treatment includes rest, heat, anti-inflammatory and pain-relieving drugs, injection of corticosteroids into the joint areas and, if severe, surgery. (*Compare* RHEUMATOID ARTHRITIS.)

osteoblast (ŏs′tē-ə-blăst′) N. cell that functions in the formation of bone tissue.

osteoblastoma (ŏs′tē-ō-blă-stō′mə) N. benign tumor of bone and fibrous tissue, occurring in the vertebrae, femur, tibia, or arm bones, esp. in young adults. Symptoms include pain and resorption of normal bone tissue. Treatment is by surgical excision.

osteochondroma (ŏs′tē-ō-kŏn-drō′mə) N. benign tumor of bone and cartilage.

osteoclasis (ŏs′tē-ŏk′lə-sĭs) N. intentional fracture of a bone to correct a deformity.

osteoclast (ŏs′tē-ə-klăst′) N. cell that functions in the breakdown and resorption of bone tissue.

osteocyte (ŏs′tē-ə-sīt′) N. mature bone cell.

osteodystrophy (ŏs′tē-ō-dĭs′trə-fē) N. defect in bone development, usually due to renal disease or disturbances in phosphorus and calcium metabolism.

osteogenesis imperfecta (ŏs′tē-ə-jĕn′ĭ-sĭs ĭm′pər-fĕk′tə) N. genetic disorder (autosomal dominant disorder) of connective tissue characterized by abnormally brittle bones that are fractured by the slightest trauma. The disease varies from extreme, in which the child is born with multiple fractures, is deformed, and usually dies shortly after birth, through milder forms that typically manifest themselves after the child begins to walk and may ameliorate after puberty. In addition to bones that fracture easily, symptoms include translucent skin, blue sclerae, a tendency to bruise easily, and hyperextensibility of the ligaments. There is no cure; treatment involves measures to minimize the likelihood of fractures, esp. in young children.

osteolysis (ŏs′tē-ŏl′ĭ-sĭs) N. degeneration and dissolution of bone caused by disease, inadequate blood supply, or infection.

osteoma (ŏs′tē-ō′mə) N. tumor of bone tissue.

osteomalacia (ŏs′tē-ō-mə-lā′shə) N. abnormal softening of bone, due to loss of calcification resulting from a deficiency of phosphorus, calcium, or vitamin D, caused by a metabolic disorder resulting in malabsorption of these nutrients, or as a complication of another disease. Treatment involves administration of needed minerals and vitamins and correction of any underlying disorder.

osteomyelitis (ŏs′tē-ō-mī′ə-lī′tĭs) N. infection of bone and bone marrow, usually caused by bacteria (esp. staphylococci) introduced by trauma or surgery or by extension of another infection. Symptoms include bone pain, tenderness, fever, and muscle spasm in the affected region. Treatment is by rest of the affected area, pain-relieving drugs, antibiotics, and surgery to remove necrotic (dead) tissue, if necessary.

osteopathy (ŏs′tē-ŏp′ə-thē) N. treatment system that uses all the usual forms of medical therapy, including drugs and surgery, but places greater emphasis on the relationship of organs and the musculoskeletal system using manipulation to correct structural problems (*compare* CHIROPRACTIC; NAPRAPATHY).

osteopenia (ŏs'tē-ə-pē'nē-ə) N. generalized term for any decrease in the amount of bone tissue, regardless of cause.

osteopetrosis N. inherited disorder characterized by an increase in bone density, ranging from a mild form marked by short stature, fragile bones, and a tendency to develop osteomyelitis to a severe form in which the bone marrow cavity is obliterated and severe anemia, skull abnormalities, and cranial nerve pressure results, often leading to death; also called Albers-Schonberg disease; marble bones disease (*compare* OSTEOSCLEROSIS). ADJ. osteopetrotic

osteoporosis (ŏs'tē-ō-pə-rō'sĭs) N. abnormal loss of bony tissue, causing fragile bones that fracture easily; pain, esp. in the back; and loss of stature. The condition is common in postmenopausal women and also occurs in those immobilized or given steroid therapy for a long period and as a result of some endocrine disorders. Postmenopausal osteoporosis is sometimes treated with estrogen preparations.

osteosarcoma (ŏs'tē-ō-sär-kō'mə) N. malignant bone tumor, most common in children and young adults in whom it often affects the femur, but also occurring in older adults and affecting other body sites. Pain and swelling typically mark the tumor site. Treatment is by surgery, usually amputation of the limb, followed by chemotherapy.

osteosclerosis (ŏs'tē-ō-sklə-rō'sĭs) N. abnormal increase in bone density, resulting from a variety of diseases, including tumor formation, inadequate blood supply, or chronic infec-

tion (*compare* OSTEOPETROSIS). ADJ. osteosclerotic

ostium (ŏs'tē-əm) N., *pl.* ostia, opening (e.g., ostium appendicis vermiformis, opening between the appendix and the large intestine) (*See also* OS; STOMA). ADJ. ostial

ostomy (ŏs'tə-mē) N. surgical procedure in which an opening is made to allow the passage of urine from the bladder or feces from the intestines. *See also* COLOSTOMY; ILEOSTOMY.

ot-, oto- comb. forms indicating an association with the ear (e.g., otopharyngeal, pert. to the ear and pharynx).

otalgia (ō-tăl'jē-ə) *See* EARACHE.

otic (ō'tĭk) ADJ. pert. to the ear; also called auricular.

otitis (ō-tī'tĭs) N. inflammation of the ear, either otitis externa, otitis media, or otitis interna (labyrinthitis).

otitis externa (ĭk-stûr'nə) N. inflammation of the auricle of the external ear leading to the tympanic membrane (eardrum). It may be caused by infection (bacterial, viral, or fungal); allergic reaction to earrings, cosmetics, or drugs; and other factors. Treatment depends on the cause.

otitis interna *See* LABYRINTHITIS.

otitis media (mē'dē-ə) N. inflammation or infection of the middle ear, a common disorder of children, often occurring as an upper respiratory infection spreads through the eustachian tube. Pain, diminished hearing, and fever typically occur. Treatment is by antimicrobials, pain relievers, and decongestants.

otolaryngology (ō'tō-lăr'ən-gŏl'ə-jē) N. surgical specialty dealing with diseases of the ears, nose, throat, and upper respiratory tract. Sometimes called ENT (ears, nose, and throat).

otorrhea N. discharge from the external ear.

otosclerosis (ō′tō-sklə-rō′sĭs) N. hereditary condition in which ossification in the labyrinth of the inner ear causes tinnitus and eventually deafness. Surgery to remove the stapes (one of the middle ear bones) is usually successful.

otoscope (ō′tə-skōp′) N. instrument to examine the outer ear, tympanic membrane (eardrum), and middle ear.

ototoxic ADJ. harmful to the organs of hearing or balance or to the auditory nerve, as some drugs.

out-of-network provider N. provider who does not participate in the network of a managed care plan. *See* TABLE OF MANAGED CARE TERMS.

output N. amount produced, ejected, or expelled. Often used in reference to cardiac output, the amount of blood pumped by the heart each minute.

ovari-, ovario- comb. forms indicating an association with an ovary or the ovaries (e.g., ovariotubal, pert. to the ovaries and fallopian tubes).

ovarian cancer N. malignant neoplasm of the ovary, occurring in women most often between the ages of 40 and 60. Symptoms, which often do not appear until the disease is advanced, include abdominal discomfort, vaginal bleeding, irregular or excessive menstrual bleeding, constipation, and urinary problems. Treatment is by surgery, irradiation, and chemotherapy.

ovarian cyst N. sac, often filled with fluid or semisolid material, that develops in or on the ovary. It may be transient and functional or a sign of pathology; if it causes pain or is malignant, it is usually removed surgically.

ovariectomy (ō-vâr′ē-ĕk′tə-mē) *See* OOPHORECTOMY.

ovary N. one of a pair of female gonads, or sex organs, located in the lower abdomen. Under the influence of follicle-stimulating hormone (FSH) and luteinizing hormone (LH) from the pituitary gland, an ovum is released from a follicle on the surface of the ovary at roughly monthly intervals during a woman's reproductive life. The ovum then enters the fallopian tube (oviduct) for possible fertilization and for passage to the uterus. ADJ. ovarian

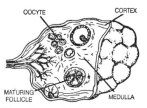

A typical ovary, showing internal maturation of ova.

Ovcon N. trade name for an oral contraceptive containing estradiol and norethindrone.

overbite N. condition in which the upper teeth extend abnormally over the lower teeth. *See also* MALOCCLUSION.

overcompensation (ō′vər-kŏm′pən-sā′shən) N. conscious or unconscious, exaggerated attempt to overcome or neutralize a real or imagined defect or unwanted characteristic. *See also* COMPENSATION.

Overeaters Anonymous N. fellowship, based on the Twelve Step Program, designed to help persons who are unable to control their desire to eat.

over-the-counter drug N. drug that is sold without a prescription (*compare* PRESCRIPTION DRUG).

ovi-, ovo- comb. forms indicating an association with an ovum or with ova (e.g., oviferous, capable of producing eggs).

oviduct (ō'vĭ-dŭkt') *See* FALLOPIAN TUBE.

ovotestis N. hermaphroditic gonad, containing both ovarian and testicular tissue.

Ovral N. trade name for an oral contraceptive containing estradiol and norgestrel.

ovulation (ō'vyə-lā'shən) N. expulsion of an ovum (egg) from the ovary after the rupture of a Graafian follicle in the ovary under the influence of pituitary and ovarian hormones. Ovulation typically occurs midway in the menstrual cycle, 14 days after the first day of the last menstrual period, and is sometimes marked by a sharp pain in the lower abdomen on the side of the ovulation ovary.

ovulation method of family planning N. method of family planning that uses observation of changes in the character and quantity of cervical mucus to determine the time of ovulation and thus the time during the woman's menstrual cycle when conception is most likely to occur. After several days of scanty mucus discharge, the time around ovulation is marked by an increase in mucus that becomes sticky, then clearer, slippery, and elastic, before again decreasing and becoming whitish and sticky before menstruation begins. This method is often combined with the basal body temperature method of family planning. *See also* CALENDAR METHOD OF FAMILY PLANNING; CONTRACEPTION.

Ovulen N. trade name for an oral contraceptive containing the estrogen compound mestranol and a progestin compound.

ovum (ō'vəm) N., *pl.* ova,
1. female germ cell produced in the ovary that, on uniting with a spermatozoon in fertilization,

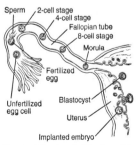

Events following fertilization. After the egg is fertilized in the fallopian tube, a number of cell divisions result in the morula and blastocyst, which implants in the uterine wall. The embryo eventually develops from the blastocyst.

OVUM

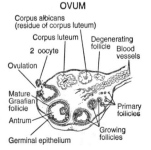

begins the formation of an embryo. During the menstrual cycle, the ovum matures, forming a Graafian follicle; during ovulation, this follicle (the developed ovum) ruptures through the ovarian surface; if fertilization occurs, the embryo proceeds through the fallopian tube and implants in the uterus. If fertilization does not occur, the follicle is sloughed, along with the uterine lining, during menstruation.
2. egg cell.

oxacillin (ŏk′sə-sĭl′ĭn) N. antibiotic of the penicillin family that is resistant to penicillinase, the penicillin-destroying enzyme released by some bacteria, esp. staphylococci. It is used to treat severe infections caused by penicillinase-producing staphylococci. Adverse effects include allergic reactions and gastrointestinal disturbances.

oxaprozin N. nonsteroidal anti-inflammatory agent (trade name Daypro) used in the once-a-day oral treatment of arthritis; side effects include stomach irritation and intestinal bleeding. *See* TABLE OF COMMONLY PRESCRIBED DRUGS—GENERIC NAMES.

oxazepam (ŏk-săz′ə-păm′) N. minor tranquilizer (trade name Serax) used to treat anxiety. Adverse effects include fatigue and dizziness.

oxidation (ŏk′sĭ-dā′shən) N. addition of oxygen, removal of hydrogen, or removal of electrons from an element or compound. Always accompanied by reduction (gain of electrons) of the oxidizing agent. The combination of simultaneous oxidation and reduction reactions is often termed an oxidation-reduction (redox) reaction. These occur commonly in blood when hemoglobin is oxygenated (oxidized), and then again when oxygen is delivered to the tissues (reduction). In the environment, organic matter is oxidized to more stable substances. (*Compare* REDUCTION.)

OXIDATION AND REDUCTION

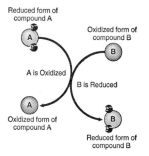

oxycephaly (ŏk′sē-sĕf′ə-lē) N. congenital malformation of the skull in which premature closure of the coronal and sagittal sutures results in accelerated upward growth of the head, giving it a long, narrow appearance.

oxycodone/acetaminophen (ə-sē′tə-mĭn′ə-fən) N. *See* TABLE OF COMMONLY PRESCRIBED DRUGS—GENERIC NAMES.

oxygen N. colorless, odorless gas essential for respiration and metabolism. *See also* TABLE OF IMPORTANT ELEMENTS.

oxygen deficit (dĕf′ĭ-sĭt) N. condition existing in cells during a period of temporary oxygen shortage, as, for example, during strenuous exercise, when energy is obtained through the breakdown of glucose in the absence of oxygen, and waste products, chiefly lactic acid, accumulate in the muscles and other tissues, creating a need for oxygen to rid the body of these waste products.

oxygen mask N. device used to administer oxygen. It is shaped to fit snugly over the mouth and nose, and may be secured in place with a strap or held with the hand. Oxygen flows at a prescribed rate through a catheter to the mask, often through a soft rubber bag that can be pumped by hand.

oxygen tent N. airtight enclosure for a patient's head and shoulders in which the oxygen content of the air can be raised above normal.

oxygen therapy N. the administration of oxygen for the treatment of conditions resulting from oxygen deficiency. It is used to combat acute arterial hypoxia that may result from pneumonia, pulmonary edema, or obstruction to breathing. It is also employed in congestive heart failure, coronary thrombosis, and after surgery.

oxygenation (ŏk′sĭ-jə-nā′shən) N. the process of treating or combining with oxygen.

oxyhemoglobin (ŏk′sē-hē′mə-glō′bĭn) N. complex of hemoglobin and oxygen that is the form in which oxygen is transported from the lungs to the cells of the body.

oxymetazoline hydrochloride (ŏk′sē-mĭ-tăz′ə-lēn′ hī′drə-klôr′īd′) N. over-the-counter decongestant nasal spray (trade name Afrin) used in the treatment of nasal congestion and allergy. This drug should not be used longer than three consecutive days without a physician's specific orders to do so. Otherwise, severe nasal irritation can result.

oxyopia N. unusually sharp vision.

oxytocic (ŏk′sĭ-tō′sĭk) N. drug that induces or accelerates labor by stimulating contractions of the muscles of the uterus.

oxytocin (ŏk′sĭ-tō′sĭn) N. hormone released by the posterior pituitary gland that causes contractions of the smooth muscles of the pregnant uterus and the release of milk from the breasts of lactating women. Preparations of oxytocin are sometimes used to induce or augment labor or to contract uterine musculature after childbirth to prevent hemorrhage.

ozena (ō-zē′nə) N. condition of the nose, sometimes following chronic inflammation of the nasal mucosa, characterized by a nasal discharge, an offensive odor, and crusting of nasal secretions.

ozone (ō′zōn′) N. toxic gas containing three atoms of oxygen per molecule (not the usual two) found in the upper atmosphere, where it shields out ultraviolet radiation from the sun. There is concern that the manufacture of various chemicals, as fluorocarbons used as propellants in aerosol sprays, and the effects of high-flying aircraft are destroying this protective layer and allowing excessive amounts of ultraviolet radiation to penetrate the earth's atmosphere, thus subjecting humans to increased dangers of skin cancer and other health problems.

ozone sickness N. abnormal condition, occurring among persons exposed to ozone in high-altitude aircraft, characterized by sleepiness, headache, chest pains and itchiness.

P

P symbol for the element phosphorus.

PABA *See* PARA-AMINOBENZOIC ACID.

pabulum N. any food or nutrient.

pacemaker N.
1. electrical (battery-operated) device used to maintain a normal heart rhythm by stimulating the heart muscle to contract. Some pacemakers stimulate the heart at a fixed rate; others stimulate the heart muscle on demand, sensing when heart contractions fall below a minimum rate.
2. *See* SINOATRIAL NODE.

pachy- comb. form meaning thick (e.g., pachycheilia, abnormal thickness of the lips).

pachyderma (păk′ĭ-dûr′mə) N. abnormal skin thickness.

Pacinian corpuscles N. small, bulblike sensory organs attached to the end of nerve fibers in subcutaneous and submucous areas, esp. in the palms, soles, joints, and genitals.

pack V. to treat the body or any part of it by wrapping it (e.g., with blankets or sheets), applying compresses to it, or stuffing it (e.g., gauze in a wound or tampon in a body opening) to provide cover, containment, or therapy (e.g., cold ointment), or to absorb blood.

packed cells N. preparation of red blood cells separated from the liquid plasma, used in the treatment of some cases of severe anemia to restore adequate levels of erythrocytes without overloading the circulatory system with too much fluid.

Paget's disease (păj′ĭts) N. disease of bone, common in the middle aged and elderly, in which there is excessive bone destruction and disorganized bone structure, sometimes leading to bone pain, frequent fractures, and skeletal deformities.

pain N. subjective unpleasant sensation resulting from stimulation of sensory nerve endings by injury, disease, or other harmful factors. Pain may be mild, severe, chronic, acute, burning, lancinating, sharp, or dull; it may be precisely located, diffuse, or referred. It is usually treated with analgesics. *See also* REFERRED PAIN.

pain threshold N. point at which a stimulus activates pain receptors to produce a feeling of pain. Individuals differ in pain threshold, some experiencing pain sooner than others with a higher pain threshold.

paint V. to apply a medicated solution (e.g., antiseptic or germicide) to the skin.

palate (păl′ĭt) N. structure that is the roof of the mouth and floor of the nasal cavity; it is divided into the hard palate and the soft palate. ADJ. palatal, palantine

palatine bone (păl′ə-tīn′) N. either of a pair of roughly L-shaped bones of the skull that form the posterior part of the hard palate, part of the floor of the orbit, and part of the nasal cavity.

palato- comb. form indicating an association with the palate (e.g., palatoglossal, pert. to the palate and tongue).

paleo- comb. form indicating an association with old, ancient, or primitive (e.g., paleocerebellum, anterior lobe of the cerebellum, which in evolutionary terms was one of the earliest parts of the hindbrain to develop in mammals).

palilalia (păl'ə-lā'lē-ə) N. abnormal condition in which a word is rapidly and involuntarily repeated; associated with Gilles de la Tourette syndrome and some brain disorders.

palindrome (pal-ən-drōm) N. words, phrases, or numbers that read the same forwards and backwards (e.g., "34543," "mom," "racecar"). In medicine, often refers to a nucleotide sequence on a DNA molecule in which the same sequence is found in each strand but in the opposite direction. *See also* DEOXYRIBONUCLEIC ACID; NUCLEOTIDE.

palliative (păl'ē-ā'tĭv) ADJ. bringing relief, but not curing (e.g., drugs that provide relief from pain and other symptoms of a disease but do not cure the disease).

pallium (păl'ē-əm) N. outer part of the cerebral hemispheres; the cerebral cortex.

pallor (păl'ər) N. abnormal paleness of the skin. ADJ. pallid.

palm (päm) N. lower side of the hand between the wrist and the fingers.

palmature N. condition in which the fingers are webbed.

palpable (păl'pə-bəl) ADJ. perceivable by touch.

palpation N. technique of examination in which the examiner feels the firmness, texture, size, shape, or location of body parts. V. palpate

palpebra (păl'pə-brə), *pl.* palpebrae. *See* EYELID.

palpebration N. winking, esp. if uncontrolled and persistent. V. palpebrate

palpitation (păl'pĭ-tā'shən) N. rapid, strong beating of the heart, associated with emotional arousal and certain heart abnormalities.

palsy (pôl'zē) N. condition associated with paralysis (e.g., Bell's palsy or cerebral palsy).

pan- comb. form meaning all (e.g., pansinusitis, inflammation of all the sinuses at the front of the head).

panacea (păn'ə-sē'ə) N. substance said to be a universal remedy.

Panadol N. trade name for the over-the-counter pain reliever acetaminophen.

pancarditis (păn'kär-dī'tĭs) N. inflammation of the entire heart, including the epicardium, the myocardium, and the endocardium.

pancreas (păn'krē-əs) N. compound gland, about 6 inches (15 centimeters) long, lying behind the stomach. It is both an exocrine gland, secreting pancreatic juice, which contains several digestive enzymes, into the pancreatic duct that unites with the common bile duct opening into the duodenum; and an endocrine gland, secreting the hormones insulin and glucagon from its islets of Langerhans directly into the bloodstream.

pancreatectomy (păng'krē-ə-tĕk'tə-mē) N. surgical removal of

OPPOSING ACTIONS OF INSULIN AND GLUCAGON

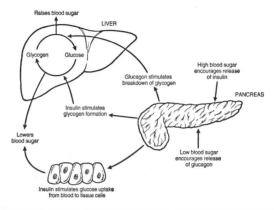

The antagonistic activities of insulin and glucagon, two hormones of the pancreas. When blood sugar is high, insulin affects the tissue cells and liver to remove glucose from the blood. Low blood sugar stimulates glucagon release, and glucagon affects the liver to increase the blood glucose level.

THE PANCREAS IN THE ABDOMEN

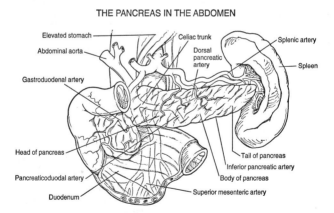

all or part of the pancreas, performed to remove a tumor, repair injury, or treat disease affecting the pancreas.

pancreatic duct (păng′krē-ăt′ĭk) N. pancreatic-juice-carrying duct leading from the pancreas and joining with the common bile duct to empty its secretions into the duodenal part of the small intestine.

pancreatic juice N. fluid secretion of the pancreas, containing water, salts, and enzymes, including trypsin and chymotrypsin; it is essential for the breakdown of starches, proteins, and fats.

pancreatico-, pancreato- comb. forms indicating an association with the pancreas (e.g., pancreaticoduodenal, pert. to the pancreas and duodenum).

pancreatin (păn′krē-ə-tĭn) N. extract from the pancreas, containing pancreatic enzymes, used to treat conditions (e.g., pancreatitis) characterized by insufficient pancreas secretion.

pancreatitis (păn′krē-ə-tī′tĭs) N. inflammation of the pancreas, usually marked by abdominal pain often radiating to the back, nausea, and vomiting. It may occur in an acute or chronic form, often associated with alcoholism, injury to the biliary tract, trauma, or infection. Treatment depends on the cause and severity; it may include surgical removal of all or part of the pancreas and administration of pain-relieving drugs and pancreatin.

pancytopenia (păn′sī-tə-pē′nē-ə) N. abnormal condition in which there is a marked decrease in all cells (red blood cells, white blood cells, and platelets) of the blood, usually associated with aplastic anemia or bone-marrow tumor.

pandemic (păn-dĕm′ĭk) N. widespread epidemic, occurring throughout a country, geographic area, or the world. ADJ. pandemic

pandiculation N. yawning and stretching actions, as when first awakening.

panencephalitis (păn′ĕn-sĕf′ə-lī′tĭs) N. inflammation of the entire brain, marked by progressive deterioration of mental and motor skills.

rubella panencephalitis N. rare, chronic deterioration of mental and physical skills, occurring in adolescents and associated with the rubella virus.

subacute sclerosing panencephalitis N. rare, often fatal, form of panencephalitis occurring as a complication of measles.

panhypopituitarism (păn′hī-pō-pĭ-too′ĭ-tə-rĭz′ əm) N. condition where all or most of the normal function of the pituitary gland is abnormally low or absent.

panhysterectomy N. surgical removal of the uterus, including the cervix, the Fallopian tubes, and the ovaries.

panic N. intense, overwhelming fear, producing terror, physiological changes, and often immobility or hysterical behavior.

panniculitis (pə-nĭk′yə-lī′tĭs) N. inflammation of fatty connective tissue; typically, it affects the fat of the abdomen or of the thigh, and results in pitting caused by loss of tissue in the affected areas.

panniculus (pə-nĭk′yə-ləs), *pl.* panniculi, N. tissue layer.

pannus (păn′əs) N. abnormal vascular membrane growing from the conjunctiva and covering the cornea of the eye; it is usually associated with inflammation of the cornea or conjunctiva.

pantothenic acid (păn′tə-thĕn′ĭk) N. member of the vitamin B complex. *See* TABLE OF VITAMINS.

Papanicolaou test (pä′pə-nē′kə-lou′) N. method of examining stained cells shed by mucous membranes, esp. of the cervix, used for early diagnosis of cancer and precancerous changes in cells. In its most common use, a smear of cervical cells is obtained during a routine pelvic examination. Also called Pap smear; Pap test.

papaverine (pə-păv′ə-rēn′) N. smooth muscle relaxant used to treat cardiovascular or visceral spasm. Adverse effects include jaundice.

papilla (pə-pĭl′ə) N., *pl.* papillae, small, nipplelike projection (e.g., the lacrimal papilla at the inner angle of the eye). ADJ. papillary

papillary muscle (păp′ə-lĕr′ē) N. any of several muscles associated with the atrioventricular valves of the heart. These muscles contract during systole to prevent regurgitation of blood into the atria.

papilledema (păp′ə-lĭ-dē′mə) N. swelling of the optic disc, the beginning of the optic nerve, usually associated with increased intracranial pressure.

papilliform ADJ. shaped like a papilla.

papilloma (păp′ə-lō′mə) N. benign growth on the skin or mucous membrane.

papule (păp′yōōl) N. small, firm, raised skin lesion, as in chicken pox (*compare* MACULE). ADJ. papular

para- prefix meaning near, beside (e.g., paranasal, near the nasal cavity) or indicating an abnormality (e.g., paracusis, abnormal hearing).

-para suffix meaning a woman who has given birth in a number of pregnancies (e.g., bipara, a woman who has given birth to a child after two separate pregnancies) (*compare* -GRAVIDA).

para-aminobenzoic acid (PABA) (păr′ə-ə-mē′nō-bĕn-zō′ĭk) N. part of folic acid, one of the members of the vitamin B complex (*see also* TABLE OF VITAMINS); a drug used as a sunscreen in many lotions and creams.

paracentesis (păr′ə-sĕn-tē′sĭs) N. procedure in which fluid is withdrawn from a body cavity, most often the abdomen, through a hollow needle; it is performed for therapeutic (e.g., to remove excess fluid from the abdomen) or diagnostic (e.g., to obtain a sample for analysis) purposes.

paracervical block N. type of regional anesthesia in which a local anesthetic agent is injected on each side of the cervix to achieve anesthesia during labor and childbirth.

paracrine ADJ. secretion of a chemical messenger or hormone from other than an endocrine gland; in paracrine communication, products of cells diffuse into the extracellular fluid to neighboring cells that may be some distance away. In a related fashion, cells may secrete chemical messengers that bind to receptors on the same cell that secreted it (autocrine communication). Chemical messengers may include amino acids, steroids, and protein peptides.

Parafon forte N. trade name for a fixed-combination drug containing the analgesic acetaminophen and the skeletal muscle relaxant chlorzoxazone, used to treat muscle-skeletal abnormalities associated with pain.

parainfluenza virus (păr′ə-ĭn′floo-ĕn′zə) N. virus causing upper respiratory infections, including the common cold, bronchiolitis, and croup, most commonly in children.

paraldehyde (pə-răl′də-hīd′) N. colorless, strong-smelling liquid, formerly used to induce sedation; no longer manufactured, but experts recommend using remaining supplies of the drug until gone because of its effectiveness.

paralysis (pə-răl′ĭ-sĭs) N., *pl.* paralyses, condition characterized by loss of sensation or of muscle function; it may be congenital or result from injury, disease, or poisoning (*See also* FLACCID PARALYSIS; PARAPLEGIA; QUADRIPLEGIA; SPASTIC PARALYSIS). ADJ. paralytic

paramedic (păr′ə-mĕd′ĭk) N. person specially trained in prehospital care of sick or injured patients; the paramedic is trained in the use of intravenous medications, placement of an endotracheal tube, defibrillation, and other advanced skills.

paramedical (păr′ə-mĕd′ĭ-kəl) ADJ. pert. to health-related activities or personnel supplemental to physicians and nurses and their activities; for example, ambulance attendants are paramedical personnel.

parameter (pə-răm′ĭ-tər) N. factor or quantity that can be clearly defined and usually, measured.

paramethadione N. anticonvulsant (trade name Paradione) used in the treatment of petit mal seizures. Adverse effects include dermatitis, sedation, blood disorders, disturbances of vision, and hepatitis.

parametritis N. inflammation of the tissues around the uterus.

paramyxovirus (păr′ə-mĭk′sə-vī′rəs) N. any of a family of viruses, including the parainfluenza viruses and the viruses responsible for measles and mumps.

paranasal sinus (păr′ə-nā′zəl) N. any of several air cavities in bones around the nose. More commonly referred to as nasal sinuses.

paranoia (păr′ə-noi′ə) N. rare mental disorder characterized by delusions of persecution, often organized into an elaborate and logical system of think-

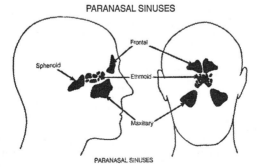

PARANASAL SINUSES

Frontal
Sphenoid
Ethmoid
Maxillary

PARANASAL SINUSES

ing and often centered on a specific theme, such as job persecution or a financial matter. Suspiciousness, hostility, and resistance to therapy are often characteristic of the paranoic person. ADJ. paranoid

paraparesis (păr′ə-pə-rē′sĭs) N. weakness of both legs.

paraphilia N. abnormal sexual activity. Kinds of paraphilia include exhibitionism, fetishism, pedophilia, voyeurism, and zoophilism.

paraplegia (păr′ə-plē′jē-ə) N. paralysis of the lower limbs, sometimes accompanied by loss of sensory and/or motor function in the back and abdominal region below the level of the injury; it most often occurs as a result of trauma (e.g., automobile or sports accident), but may also be congenital (e.g., spina bifida) or acquired as a result of alcoholism, syphilis, or disease affecting the spinal cord or associated nerves. Treatment depends on the cause and extent of damage; it may include surgery (e.g., laminectomy); use of special immobilization devices; and the administration of pain-relieving drugs and drugs to prevent infection, esp. of the bladder. (*See also* QUADRIPLEGIA.) ADJ. paraplegic

parapsychology (păr′ə-sī-kŏl′ə-jē) N. study of psychic phenomena, such as extrasensory perception, clairvoyance, and telepathy.

paraquat poisoning N. toxic condition resulting from ingestion of the pesticide paraquat and characterized by progressive damage to the esophagus, kidneys, and liver, often leading to death.

parasite (păr′ə-sīt′) N. organism that lives in or on another organism (the host), obtaining nourishment from it. ADJ. parasitic

parasitemia (păr′ə-sī-tē′mē-ə) N. presence of parasites in the blood.

parasympathetic nervous system (păr′ə-sĭm′pə-thĕt′ĭk) N. one of the two divisions of the autonomic nervous system (the other being the sympathetic nervous system), consisting of nerve fibers that leave the brain and sacral portion of the spinal cord, and extend to nerve cell clusters (ganglia) at specific sites, from which fibers are distributed to blood vessels, glands, and other internal organs. In general, parasympathetic nerves slow the heart rate; stimulate peristalsis; induce the secretion of bile, insulin, and digestive juices; dilate peripheral blood vessels; and contract the bronchioles, pupils, and esophagus. The system works in balance with the sympathetic nervous system, often opposing its actions.

parasympathomimetic ADJ. having an effect (as from a drug) similar to that caused by stimulation of the parasympathetic nervous system (e.g., slowing the heart rate).

parasystole (păr′ə-sĭs′tə-lē) N. independent and usually abnormal cardiac rhythm that originates and beats independently of, but contemporaneously with, the normal heart rhythm.

parathion poisoning (păr′ə-thī′ŏn) N. toxic condition caused by the inhalation or ingestion of the insecticide parathion. Symptoms include abdominal pain, nausea, vomiting, headache, convulsions, and difficulty

THE PARATHYROID GLAND AND ITS HORMONE

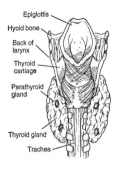

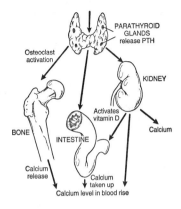

in breathing, sweating, and signs of stimulation of the parasympathetic nervous system.

parathyroid gland (păr′ə-thī′roid) N. one of four small endocrine glands, attached to the thyroid gland in the neck, that secretes parathyroid hormone, which acts to maintain normal levels of calcium in the blood and normal neuromuscular function. Decreased activity of the parathyroid glands can result in tetany.

parathyroid hormone (PTH) N. hormone synthesized and released into the bloodstream by the parathyroid glands. It regulates calcium and phosphorus distribution in the body and functions in muscle contraction and blood clotting. PTH increases the concentration of calcium in the blood in three ways. It enhances release of calcium from the bones, reabsorption of calcium from renal tubules, and absorption of calcium in the intestine. PTH also decreases the concentra-

tion of phosphate in the blood, primarily by reducing reabsorption in the proximal tubules of the kidney. Also called parathormone.

paregoric (păr′ə-gôr′ĭk) N. opium derivative used to treat diarrhea and to relieve pain. Adverse effects include constipation.

parenchyma (pə-rĕng′kə-mə) N. functional part of an organ, apart from supporting or connective tissue (*compare* STROMA).

parenteral (pă-rĕn′tər-əl) ADJ. pert. to administration of a substance (e.g., a drug), not through the digestive system, but, for example, by injection under or through the skin. Also includes intravenous administration of medications.

parenteral nutrition N. administration of nutrients by a route other than the digestive system, for example, by intravenous administration of fluids.

paresis (pə-rē′sĭs) N. slight or partial paralysis. ADJ. paretic

paresthesia (păr′ĭs-thē′zhə) N. sensation (e.g., tingling or pins and needles); usually associated with partial damage to a peripheral nerve.

paries (pâr′ē-ēz′) N., *pl.* parietes, wall of an organ or body cavity. ADJ. parietal

parietal (pə-rī′ĭ-təl) ADJ.
1. pert. to the inner walls of a body cavity, as opposed to the contents (viscera).
2. pert. to the parietal bone.

parietal bone N. either of two skull bones forming the top and sides of the cranium.

parietal lobe N. one of the main divisions of each hemisphere of the cerebral cortex, located beneath the crown of the head and concerned with sensory and associative nerve functions.

parieto- comb. form indicating an association with the parietal bone (e.g., parietofrontal, pert. to the parietal and frontal bones of the skull).

parity (păr′ĭ-tē) N. in obstetrics, designation based on the number of live-born children a woman has delivered; for example, a woman who is classified as para 3 has delivered three live children (*compare* GRAVIDA).

Parkinsonism (pär′kĭn-sə-nĭz′əm) N. slowly progressive neurological disorder characterized by resting tremor, shuffling gait, stooped posture, rolling motions of the fingers, drooling, and muscle weakness, sometimes with emotional instability. It most often occurs after the age of 60 and then its cause is unknown but it may occur in young people as a result of encephalitis, syphilis, or certain other diseases.

Treatment is by levodopa, and occasionally, in severe cases, by surgery. Also called Parkinson's disease.

paronychia (păr′ə-nĭk′ē-ə) N. infection of the skin fold at the margin of a nail. ADJ. paronychial

parosmia (pə-rŏz′mē-ə) N. disorder of the sense of smell.

parotexine HCl N. oral antidepressant (trade name Paxil) used to treat depression, associated anxiety, and lethargy; side effects may include nausea, sweating, tremor, decreased appetite, and ejaculatory disturbances in men.

parotid gland (pə-rŏt′ĭd) N. either of a pair of large salivary glands, located at the side of the face below and in front of the ear, that release saliva through the parotid ducts into the mouth.

parotitis (păr′ə-tī′tĭs) N. inflammation of one or both parotid glands, as in mumps.

parous (păr′əs) ADJ. having given birth to at least one viable child.

paroxetine N. *See* TABLE OF COMMONLY PRESCRIBED DRUGS—GENERIC NAMES.

paroxysm (păr′ək-sĭz′əm) N.
1. sudden, violent attack, esp. a seizure or convulsion.
2. marked increase in symptoms. ADJ. paroxysmal

parrot fever *See* PSITTACOSIS.

pars N., *pl.* partes, part of an organ (e.g., the pars nervosa of the pituitary gland).

particle physics N. the study of what things are made of. Particle physicists study the fundamental particles that make up all of matter, and how they interact with each other. Everything is made up of these building blocks—leptons, quarks, and force-carrying particles. Leptons and quarks are often called elementary particles. Four different force-carrying particles lead to the interactions between them. *See also* ATOM; FORCE-CARRYING PARTICLES; LEPTONS; QUARKS.

parthenogenesis N. type of reproduction in which an unfertilized ovum develops into a complete organism; it occurs in certain insects and other invertebrate animals. ADJ. parthenogenetic

partial abortion *See* ABORTION, INCOMPLETE.

participating provider N. provider who contracts with a health insurance plan to provide medical services. *See* TABLE OF MANAGED CARE TERMS.

parturition (pär'tyŏo-rĭsh'ən) N. *See* BIRTH.

passive ADJ. not active, not initiated by the self (e.g., passive movement, movement of body parts by a therapist or other agent, not by the efforts of the person).

passive immunity N. type of acquired immunity in which antibodies against a particular disease or against several diseases are transmitted naturally, through the placenta to an unborn child or through colostrum to a nursing infant; or artificially, through the administration (usually by injection) of antiserum. Passive immunity is not permanent. (*Compare* ACTIVE IMMUNITY.)

passive transport N. movement of small molecules across a cell membrane by diffusion; it does not require the expenditure of energy (*compare* ACTIVE TRANSPORT).

pasteurization (păs'chər-ĭ-zā'shən) N. process of applying heat (e.g., to temperatures of 140° Fahrenheit—60° Celsius) for a specified time (e.g., 60 minutes) to kill or retard the development of disease-causing microorganisms, esp. bacteria, in milk and other products.

patch test N. skin test for identifying an allergen. A paper or cloth patch containing suspected allergens (e.g., pollen, animal hair) is applied to the skin; the appearance of red, swollen skin or any rash when the patch is removed usually indicates allergy to a particular substance or substances.

patella (pə-tĕl'ə) N. flat, triangular bone at the front of the knee joint; also called sesamoid bone and, colloquially, kneecap. ADJ. patellar

patellar reflex N. deep tendon reflex in which tapping the tendon below the patella causes a contraction of the quadriceps muscle of the thigh and extension (kicking) of the lower leg; used diagnostically to test nerve function; also called knee-jerk reflex.

patent ADJ. open, as a tube or passageway. N. patency

patent ductus arteriosus *See* DUCTUS ARTERIOSUS.

patent medicine N. drug or other therapeutic substance that carries a specific trademark and is available without a prescription.

paternity test N. comparison of blood types among mother, child, and a man suspected of fathering the child in an effort to determine the father. If the child's blood group could not have resulted from the combination of the man's blood group with that of the woman, then the man is definitely not the father of the child. However, other results are not conclusive, since a finding that the man could be the father does not prove that he is the father.

pathogen (păth'ə-jən) N. microorganism capable of producing disease. ADJ. pathogenic

pathogenesis (păth'ə-jĕn'ĭ-sĭs) N. production of a disease, esp. the development of a disease from a specific cause or source.

pathognomonic ADJ. describing a sign or symptom that is specific to or characteristic of a particular disease (e.g., Koplik's spots on the mucous membranes of the mouth are pathognomonic for measles).

pathologic (păth'ə-lŏj'ĭk) ADJ. pert. to or arising from disease (e.g., pathologic fracture, fracture arising from bone disease, not from injury).

pathology (pă-thŏl'ə-jē) N. study of disease, its causes and effects, esp. the observable effects of disease on body tissues. ADJ. pathological

-pathy suffix indicating disease or abnormal state (e.g., craniopathy, skull disease).

Pavabid, Pavacap, Pavarine N. trade names for the smooth muscle relaxant papaverine.

pavor nocturnus (pā'vər nŏk-tûr'nəs) *See* SLEEP TERROR DISORDER.

Paxil N. trade name for the oral antidepressant, paroxetine. *See* TABLE OF COMMONLY PRESCRIBED DRUGS—TRADE NAMES.

Pb symbol for the element lead.

PCP *See* PHENCYCLIDINE HYDROCHLORIDE.

peak N. highest value of a measurement or recording, as the top temperature of a patient's fever period or the sharp elevation during an electrocardiographic tracing.

pectin (pĕk'tĭn) N. gelatinous substance found in fruits and used in jams and jellies.

pectinate ADJ. comb-shaped.

pectineal (pĕk-tĭn'ē-əl) ADJ. pert. to the pubis.

pectoral ADJ. pert. to the chest.

pectoralis major N. large, fan-shaped muscle of the upper chest wall that acts on the shoulder, flexing and rotating the arm. *See* MAJOR MUSCLES OF THE BODY, in Appendix.

pectoralis minor N. thin, triangular muscle of the upper chest, beneath the pectoralis major, that functions to draw the shoulder down and forward. *See* MAJOR MUSCLES OF THE BODY, in Appendix.

pectus (pĕk'təs) N. *See* CHEST. ADJ. pectoral

pederasty N. homosexual anal intercourse, esp. that between a man and a young boy who is the passive partner.

Pediamycin N. trade name for the antibacterial erythromycin.

pediatrician (pē'dē-ə-trĭsh'ən) N. a physician who specializes in pediatrics.

pediatrics (pē'dē-ăt'rĭks) N. that branch of medicine concerned with the development of children and the diagnosis and treatment of diseases and disorders affecting children.

pedicle (pĕd′ĭ-kəl) N. narrow, stemlike part of an organ.

pediculicide (pə-dĭk′yə-lĭ-sīd′) N. agent that kills lice.

pediculosis (pə-dĭk′yə-lō′sĭs) N. infestation with lice. Symptoms include intense itching, which often produces skin irritation that becomes secondarily infected. Treatment is by pediculicides.
  pediculosis capitis N. infestation of the scalp with lice; also called head lice.
  pediculosis corporis N. infestation of body skin with lice.
  pediculosis pubis N. infestation of pubic hair with crab lice.

pedophilia (pĕd′ə-fĭl′ē-ə) N. sexual activity, either homosexual or heterosexual, of an adult with a child.

peduncle (pĭ-dŭng′kəl) N. stalk-like connection. ADJ. peduncular

pelage N. all the body hair.

pellagra (pə-lăg′rə) N. disease caused by deficiency of niacin or tryptophan in the diet or by a defect in the metabolic conversion of tryptophan to niacin; it is characterized by dermatitis, inflammation of the tongue, diarrhea, and emotional and mental symptoms including depression, disorientation, and confusion. Treatment includes the administration of niacin and tryptophan and a well-balanced diet containing other vitamins.

pelvi-, pelvo- comb. forms indicating an association with the pelvis (e.g., pelvifemoral, pert. to the hip area where the pelvis and femur—upper leg bone—meet).

pelvic girdle N. bony structure, made up of the left and right hipbones, the sacrum, and the coccyx, to which the bones of the legs are attached.

pelvic inflammatory disease (PID) N. inflammatory condition of the female pelvic organs, often associated with bacterial infection. Symptoms include lower abdominal pain, fever, and foul-smelling vaginal discharge. Treatment is by antibiotics, pain-relieving drugs, if necessary; and, if an abscess develops, surgical drainage. Severe or recurrent attacks often lead to scarring of the fallopian tubes, sometimes causing infertility.

pelvimetry (pĕl-vĭm′ĭ-trē) N. measurement of the dimensions of the bony birth canal, done to determine whether vaginal birth is possible.

pelvis N. lower part of the trunk of the body, composed of the right and left hip bones (the innominate bone, made up of the ilium, ischium, and pubis), the sacrum and the coccyx; it protects the lower abdominal organs and provides for the attachment of the legs. The pelvis is usually lighter and wider in females than in males. ADJ. pelvic

pemphigoid N. any condition characterized by the appearance of bullae (blisters), often on reddish macules; treatment is by corticosteroids, but there may be spontaneous remission (*compare* PEMPHIGUS).

pemphigus (pĕm′fĭ-gəs) N. disease of the skin, characterized by thin-walled bullae (blisters) arising from normal skin or mucous membrane; the bullae frequently rupture, leaving raw patches that often become infected. Treatment is by corti-

costeroids (*compare* PEMPHI-
GOID).

-penia suffix indicating a deficiency or amount below
normal (e.g., erythropenia,
deficiency of red blood cells).

penicillamine N. drug (trade name
Cuprimine), used in the treatment of heavy metal poisoning,
Wilson's disease, and severe
arthritis. Adverse effects include
blood abnormalities, rash, and
fever.

penicillin (pĕn′ĭ-sĭl′ĭn) N. any of
a group of antibiotics including
ampicillin, oxacillin, penicillin
G, and penicillin V, known under many trade names (e.g., Pen-
Vee K, Pentids), and derived
from penicilium fungus or produced synthetically, which are
used to treat a wide variety of
bacterial infections. Some members of the penicillin family are
effective administered orally;
others must be given by injection. Some forms are inactivated by the enzyme pencil-
linase, produced by certain
bacteria; others, including cloxacillin and oxacillin, are peni-

THE PELVIS

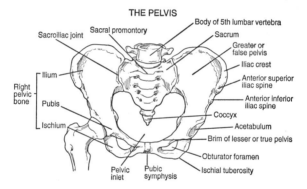

DIFFERENCES BETWEEN THE MALE PELVIS AND FEMALE PELVIS

Aspect	Comparison
Pelvis	Female pelvic bones are lighter, thinner, and have less obvious muscle attachments; the obturator foramina and the actetabula are smaller and farther apart than in the male.
Pelvic cavity	Female pelvic cavity has wider diameters and is shorter, roomier and less funnel-shaped than male; the distances between the ischial spines and between the ischial tuberosities are greater than in the male.
Sacrum	Female sacrum is relatively wider, and the sacral curvature is bent more sharply posteriorly than in the male.
Coccyx	Female coccyx is more movable than male.

cillinase-resistant. Hypersensitivity reactions, manifested by rash, fever, bronchospasm, and other symptoms, occur in some people given penicillin, and a small number develop a serious reaction leading to anaphylactic shock.

penicillin VK N. *See* TABLE OF COMMONLY PRESCRIBED DRUGS—GENERIC NAMES.

penicillinase (pĕn´ĭ-sĭl´ĭ-nās´) N. enzyme produced by certain bacteria, esp. staphylococci strains, that inactivates penicillin and causes resistance to the antibiotic.

penicillinase-resistant antibiotic N. antibiotic that is not rendered inactive by penicillinase; included are nafcillin, cloxacillin, oxacillin, and certain other semisynthetic penicillins.

penicilliosis N. infection with penicillium, usually a pulmonary infection.

penile implant (pē´nīl´) N. semirigid, cylindrical plastic device surgically placed within the penis to treat impotence. The penis is maintained in a semierect state at all times. There is usually no effect on the recipient's ability to urinate.

penis N. external reproductive organ of the male, which contains the urethra through which urine and semen pass. Most of the organ is composed of erectile tissue that becomes engorged under conditions of sexual excitement, causing the penis to become erect; it is then capable of entering the vagina during coitus and discharging semen in ejaculation. Urination occurs without erection. Also called phallus. ADJ. penile

pentazocine (pĕn-tăz´ə-sēn´) N. analgesic (trade name Talwin) used to treat moderate to severe pain. Adverse effects include nausea, dizziness, gastrointestinal upsets, and, in high doses, respiratory and circulatory depression; withdrawal symptoms after prolonged use may also occur.

Pentids N. trade name for the antibacterial penicillin G.

pentobarbital (pĕn´tə-bär´bĭ-tôl´) N. sedative (trade name Nembutal) used as a preoperative sedative, to control convulsions, and to treat insomnia and agitation. Adverse effects include respiratory and circulatory depression, withdrawal symptoms on discontinuance, and the potential for addiction.

Pentothal N. trade name for the barbiturate thiopental.

pentoxifylline (pĕn´tŏk-sĭf´ə-lēn´) N. drug (trade name Trental) for the treatment of claudication, thought to work by increasing the flexibility of the red blood cell, and thus its ability to flow through blood vessels.

Pen-Vee, Pen-Vee K N. trade names for the antibacterial penicillin V.

Pepcid N. trade name for the histamine blocker famotidine. *See* TABLE OF COMMONLY PRESCRIBED DRUGS—TRADE NAMES.

MALE GENITALIA

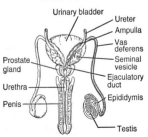

- Urinary bladder
- Ureter
- Ampulla
- Vas deferens
- Seminal vesicle
- Ejaculatory duct
- Epididymis
- Testis
- Prostate gland
- Urethra
- Penis

pepsin N. enzyme, secreted by the stomach, that catalyzes the breakdown of proteins.

pepsinogen (pĕp-sĭn′ə-jən) N. precursor of the digestive enzyme pepsin; it is stored in cells of the stomach walls and converted to its active form (pepsin) by hydrochloric acid in the stomach juices.

peptic ADJ. pert. to digestion or the enzymes of digestion.

peptic ulcer N. circumscribed erosion in, or loss of, the mucous membrane lining of the gastrointestinal tract. It may occur in the esophagus (esophageal ulcer), stomach (gastric ulcer), duodenum (duodenal ulcer), or jejunum (jejunal ulcer), the stomach and duodenum being the most common sites. Peptic ulcer may result from excess acid production or from a breakdown in the normal mechanisms protecting the mucous membranes and is often associated with stress and the intake of certain drugs (e.g., corticosteroids and certain nonsteroidal anti-inflammatory agents). *Helicobacter pylori*, a spiral-shaped bacterium found in the stomach, is generally acknowledged as the main cause for most peptic ulcers and many cases of chronic gastritis. Symptoms include gnawing pain, often worse when the stomach is empty, after certain foods have been eaten, or when the patient is under stress. Treatment includes avoidance of tobacco, alcohol, and irritating foods; drugs to decrease acidity (e.g., cimetidine); and a diet of small, frequent meals. If the ulcer perforates the wall of the gastrointestinal tract or hemorrhage occurs, surgery is usually required. *See also* HELI-COBACTER PYLORI; GASTRITIS. N. peptic ulcer disease

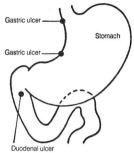

Gastric ulcer

Stomach

Gastric ulcer

Duodenal ulcer

Peptic ulcers may occur in the stomach (gastric ulcers) or in the first part of the small intestine (duodenal ulcer).

peptide (pĕp′tīd′) N. compound formed of two or more amino acids linked by peptide bonds. Proteins are made up of chains of polypeptides.

peptide bond N. a chemical bond linking two amino acids within a protein; during protein synthesis, the peptide bond forms between two amino acids that are held side by side on the ribosome. Chemically, a bond is formed between the carboxyl group (COOH) of one amino acid and the amino group (NH_2) of another, releasing water (H_2O) in the process. *See also* RIBOSOME.

perception (pər-sĕp′shən) N. process by which information received by the senses is recognized, interpreted, and analyzed to become meaningful. ADJ. perceptive

perceptual defect (pər-sĕp′chŏŏ-əl) N. any abnormality that interferes with the recognition and interpretation of sensory stimuli; it may occur in organic brain

PEPTIDE BOND

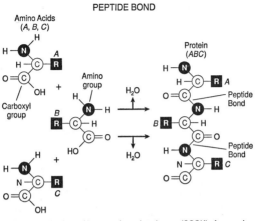

A peptide bond is formed between the carboxyl group (COOH) of one amino acid and the amino group (NH_2) of another, releasing water (H_2O) in the process. Here, three amino acids (A, B, C) have formed two peptide bonds, releasing two molecules of water in the process. The result is the protein ABC.

disorders and certain other disorders.

Percodan N. trade name for a fixed-combination narcotic analgesic containing oxycodone and aspirin; used to treat moderate to severe pain.

percussion (pər-kŭsh′ən) N. technique of physical examination in which the fingers or a small tool (percussor) are used to tap parts of the body in an attempt to determine the size and outline of internal organs and to detect the presence of fluid.

percutaneous (pûr′kyoo̅-tā′nē-əs) ADJ. through the skin.

perforate (pûr′fə-rāt′) V. to pierce or otherwise make a hole. N. perforation ADJ. perforated.

perforated eardrum N. puncture in the tympanic membrane (eardrum), resulting from trauma or other causes; it can interfere with normal hearing and cause other ear problems.

perforation (pûr′fə-rā′shən) N. rupture, either of a solid organ (e.g., spleen) or of a hollow viscus (e.g., duodenum).

perfusion (pər-fyoo̅′zhən) N. pumping a liquid (esp. blood) into an organ or tissue, usually by the way of blood vessels. Usually refers to delivery of oxygen and nutrients to cells, organs, and tissues via the circulatory system. Evaluation of a patient's level of organ perfusion is an important determination, especially to diagnose early shock. Decreased tissue perfusion results in subtle changes, such as aberrant mental status, far before a patient's vital signs (e.g., blood pressure, pulse, respiratory rate) appear abnormal.

Pergonal N. trade name for a preparation of gonadotropins extracted from the urine of menopausal women and used to induce ovulation in some cases of infertility.

peri- comb. form meaning around (e.g., periocular, around the eye).

Periactin N. trade name for the antihistamine and antipruritic cyproheptadine.

perianal ADJ. around the anus.

periapical (pĕr′ē-ā′pĭ-kəl) ADJ. pert. to tissues around the apex of a tooth (e.g., periapical abscess, infection around the root of a tooth).

periarteritis (pĕr′ē-är′tə-rī′tĭs) N. inflammation of the outer coats of one or more arteries.

periarteritis nodosa N. progressive disease of connective tissue characterized by nodules (often large) along arteries that may cause blockage of the artery and result in inadequate circulation to the affected area. Symptoms include pain, fever, and as the disease progresses, signs of lung, kidney, and intestinal damage. Treatment is by corticosteroids. Also called polyarteritis nodosa.

pericardial effusion (ĭ-fyoo′zhən) N. accumulation of fluid between the two layers of pericardium; may be due to inflammation (e.g., rheumatoid arthritis), tumor, or trauma (e.g., knife or gunshot wound); under certain circumstances, pressure from the fluid prevents adequate filling of the heart, resulting in life-threatening cardiac tamponade.

pericardiocentesis (pĕr′ĭ-kär′dē-ō-sĕn-tē′sĭs) N. placement of a needle, attached to a syringe, between the two layers of pericardium to remove either air (pneumopericardium) or fluid (pericardial effusion); used in the treatment of cardiac tamponade.

pericarditis (pĕr′ĭ-kär-dī′tĭs) N. inflammation of the pericardium, the double-layered sac that surrounds the heart, and the major blood vessels around it. It may be due to infection, trauma, neoplastic disease, or myocardial infarction, or it may result from unknown causes. Symptoms include fever, dry cough, difficulty in breathing, pain below the sternum (breastbone), often radiating upward, rapid pulse, and increasing anxiety and fatigue; untreated, it can lead to restricted heart action due to effusion. Treatment depends on the cause; it may include antibiotics, analgesics, removal of accumulated fluid, oxygen, and measures to lower fever.

pericardium (pĕr′ĭ-kär′dē-əm) N. double-layered sac surrounding the heart and large vessels entering and leaving the heart. The inner serous pericardium contains a layer that adheres to the surface of the heart and a layer that lines the inside of the outer, fibrous pericardium. The fibrous pericardium is tough and comparatively inelastic; it protects the heart and inner membranes. Between the two layers is the pericardial space, containing pericardial fluid that lubricates the membrane surfaces and allows easier heart movement. ADJ. pericardial

perilymph (pĕr′ə-lĭmf′) N. clear fluid in the inner ear, separating the osseous and membranous labyrinth.

perinatal (pĕr′ə-nāt′l) ADJ. pert. to the period a few months before and after birth.

perinatology (pĕr′ə-nā-tŏl′ə-jē) N. that branch of medicine concerned with the anatomy, physiology, and diagnosis and treat-

PERICARDIUM

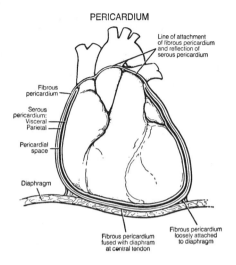

Line of attachment
of fibrous pericardium
and reflection of
serous pericardium

Fibrous
pericardium

Serous
pericardium:
Visceral
Parietal

Pericardial
space

Diaphragm

Fibrous pericardium
fused with diaphram
at central tendon

Fibrous pericardium
loosely attached
to diaphragm

ment of disorders of the mother and fetus or newborn child during late pregnancy, childbirth, and the puerperium.

perineotomy (pĕr′ə-nē-ŏt′ə-mē) N. surgical incision into the perineum.

perineum (pĕr′ə-nē′əm) N. region between the urethral opening and the anus, including the skin and underlying tissues. (In females it contains the vaginal opening.) ADJ. perineal

perineurium (pĕr′ə-no͞or′ē-əm) N. connective tissue covering around bundles of nerve fibers. ADJ. perineural

period N. colloquial term for the menses. Also refers to a cycle of time, to a phase or interval.

periodic ADJ. occurring at intervals.

periodic apnea of the newborn (ăp′nē-ə) N. condition of newborn infants characterized by an irregular breathing pattern, with periods of rapid breathing followed by brief periods of not breathing (apnea); it is normal in most infants, often associated with rapid eye movement (REM) sleep. Frequent episodes of apnea, not associated with REM sleep or periodic breathing patterns, may be a sign of neural, respiratory, circulatory, or other disorder and are thought to be associated with sudden infant death syndrome.

periodic breathing *See* CHEYNE-STOKES RESPIRATION.

periodicity (pĭr′ē-ə-dĭs′ĭ-tē) N. state of being recurrent at regular or irregular intervals; certain disease symptoms, such as wheezing, occur periodically without a pattern. Other events, such as a woman's menstrual cycle, are recurrent (periodic) and, normally, relatively regular.

periodontal (pĕr′ē-ə-dŏn′tl) ADJ. pert. to the area around a tooth.

periodontal disease N. disease of the tissues around a tooth, often leading to damage to the bony sockets of the teeth.

periodontics N. branch of dentistry concerned with the diagnosis and treatment of diseases of the tissues surrounding the teeth.

periosteum (pĕr′ē-ŏs′tē-əm) N. vascular membrane covering bones, except at the extremities, where bones articulate with other bones; it contains nerves and blood vessels that nourish and innervate the enclosed bone.

periostitis N. inflammation of the periosteum, the membrane of connective tissue that covers the bone except at the articular surfaces.

peripheral (pə-rĭf′ər-əl) ADJ. pert. to the outside, surface, or area away from the center of an organ or of the body.

peripheral nervous system N. one of the two main divisions of the human nervous system (the other being the central nervous system); the sensory and motor nerves outside the brain and spinal cord. It consists of 12 pairs of cranial nerves and 31 pairs of spinal nerves and the branches of these nerves that innervate the organs of the body. Sensory, or afferent, peripheral nerves transmit impulses to the central nervous system (the brain and spinal cord); motor, or efferent, peripheral nerves transmit impulses from the central nervous system to the muscles and organs of the body. Peripheral nerves that regulate respiratory, endocrine, cardiovascular, and other automatic functions comprise the autonomic nervous system.

peripheral vascular disease (pə-rĭf′ər-əl văs′kyə-lər) N. any abnormal condition, including atherosclerosis and Buerger's disease, affecting blood vessels outside the heart.

DEEP MUSCLES OF THE FEMALE PERINEUM

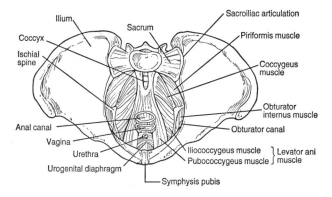

peristalsis (pĕr'ĭ-stôl'sĭs) N. rhythmic, wavelike contractions of the smooth muscle of the digestive tract that force food through the tube and wastes toward the anus. ADJ. peristaltic

perithelium (pĕr'ə-thē'lē-əm) N. tissue layer around small blood vessels. ADJ. perithelial

peritoneum (pĕr'ĭ-tn-ē'əm) N. serous membrane that covers the entire abdominal wall (parietal peritoneum) and envelops the organs contained in the abdomen (visceral peritoneum). ADJ. peritoneal.

peritonitis (pĕr'ĭ-tn-ī'tĭs) N. inflammation of the peritoneum, caused by bacteria or irritating substances (e.g., digestive enzymes) introduced into the abdominal cavity by a puncture wound, by surgery, by a ruptured abdominal organ, or through the bloodstream. A ruptured appendix is the most frequent cause, but peritonitis can also result from perforated peptic ulcer or rupture of the spleen or Fallopian tubes (as in ectopic pregnancy), or from other conditions. Symptoms include abdominal distension and pain, nausea, vomiting, rebound tenderness, chills, fever, rapid heart rhythm, and, if untreated, electrolyte imbalance, shock, and heart failure. Treatment involves control of the infection, usually with antibiotics; repair of any perforation; withdrawal of fluid from the abdominal cavity, if necessary; and maintenance of fluid and electrolyte balance.

peritonsillar abscess (pĕr'ĭ-tŏn'sə-lər) *See* QUINSY.

perleche (pər-lĕsh') *See* CHEILOSIS.

permanent tooth N. any of the set of 32 teeth that appear during and after childhood and, in the optimal case, last until old age. In each jaw there are 4 incisors, 2 canines, 4 premolars, and 6 molars. They replace the 20 deciduous (milk) teeth of early childhood, usually starting to erupt in the 6th year and continuing to erupt until the 18th to 25th year with the eruption of the third molars (wisdom teeth).

permeability N. ability of a substance, often a membrane or

THE PERITONEUM

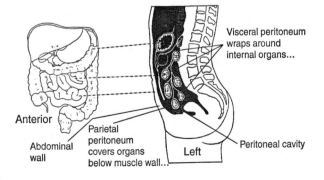

Visceral peritoneum wraps around internal organs...

Anterior

Abdominal wall

Parietal peritoneum covers organs below muscle wall...

Left

Peritoneal cavity

container, to allow the passage of liquids or substances in solution. ADJ. permeable.

pernicious (pər-nĭsh′əs) ADJ. dangerous or likely to lead to death, as a pernicious disease.

pernicious anemia N. type of anemia characterized by defective red blood cell production, the presence of megaloblasts in the bone marrow, and deterioration of nerve tissue in the spinal cord. It is caused by a lack of intrinsic factor, essential for the absorption of vitamin B_{12}, or to a deficiency of vitamin B_{12} in the diet. Symptoms include pallor, anorexia, weight loss, fever, weakness, and tingling of the extremities. Treatment includes the administration of vitamin B_{12}, folic acid, and iron.

pernio *See* CHILBLAIN.

peroneal (pĕr′ə-nē′əl) ADJ. pert. to the outer part of the leg.

peroneus N. either of two (peroneus brevis and peroneus longus) muscles of the lower leg, involved in movement of the foot.

perphenazine (pər-fĕn′ə-zēn′) N. tranquilizer and antidepressant (trade name Triavil) used to treat some types of depression, anxiety, and agitation; it is also an antiemetic, used to treat nausea and vomiting in adults. Adverse effects include ataxia, dyskinesia, blood abnormalities, and hypersensitivity reactions.

persistent vegetative state N. condition in which the patient is awake without being aware. In this state, the brainstem is functioning but the cerebral cortex is not, and the patient lies with the eyes open, looks around, but has no meaningful interaction with the environment.

persona (pər-sō′nə) N. in psychology, the personality role that a person assumes and presents to the world (*compare* ANIMA).

personality N. composite of a person's behavior and attitudes; a tendency to feel and behave in a certain way.

personality disorder N. any of a group of mental disorders (e.g., obsessive-compulsive) characterized by maladaptive and usually rigid patterns of behavior.

perspiration N.
1. sweat, the moisture passing through the sweat glands in the skin that functions to maintain body temperature (a cooling mechanism) and to rid the body of wastes.
2. action or process of sweating.

pertussis (pər-tŭs′ĭs) N. acute, contagious, respiratory disease, occurring most commonly in nonimmunized young children and characterized by attacks of coughing ending in inspiration with a loud whooping sound. It is caused by *Bordetella pertussis* bacteria; is transmitted directly (via contact with infectious particles spread by coughing or sneezing) or indirectly (through contaminated articles); has a 1- to 2-week incubation period; and typically lasts 6–8 weeks. The disease starts with sneezing, runny nose, dry cough, loss of appetite, and slight fever—the catarrhal stage. About 10 days later paroxysms of coughing with the characteristic whoop on inspiration begin, often accompanied by marked facial redness and signs of distress, the expulsion of large amounts of mucus, and frequently vomiting, after choking on mucus; this stage, the paroxysmal stage, lasts about 4–6 weeks. The convalescent stage, of about 2 weeks, is characterized by a persistent cough. Treatment includes rest, adequate fluid intake, oxygen, if necessary, and sometimes antibacterials to prevent secondary infection. One attack usually confers immunity. The disease can be prevented by pertussis vaccine, usually given along with diphtheria and tetanus toxoids (DPT) in a series of injections in early childhood. Cases are now appearing more frequently in recent years, after a period of time when vaccination had nearly completely eradicated the disease in the United States. Likely, this represents increasing numbers of children who have not been properly vaccinated, rather than the emergence of a new strain of bacteria causing the disease. Also called whooping cough.

perversion (pər-vŭr′zhən) N. action considered unnatural or abnormal, esp. a sexual activity deviating from what is considered normal.

pes (pās) N. foot or footlike part.

pes cavus See CLAWFOOT.

pes planus See FLATFOOT.

pessary (pĕs′ə-rē) N. plastic or metal device, usually ring-shaped, inserted into the vagina to correct the position of the uterus or to provide support in cases of uterine prolapse; it is usually used in cases where surgery to correct the problem is unwise (e.g., because of the advanced age or general poor health of the woman).

pesticide poisoning N. toxic condition brought on by ingestion or inhalation of a pesticide. See also MALATHION POISONING; PARATHION POISONING.

pestilence (pĕs′tə-ləns) N. general term for affliction, ailment; historically, refers to the fatal epidemic disease bubonic plague transmitted by the bite of an infected rat flea.

PET See POSITRON EMISSION TOMOGRAPHY.

petechia (pə-tē′kē-ə) N., pl. petechiae, tiny, reddish or purplish flat spot appearing on the skin as the result of tiny hemorrhages within the skin or subcutaneous layers. ADJ. petechial

petit mal N. form of epilepsy characterized by brief (usually momentary) episodes of unconsciousness, sometimes accompanied by muscular spasm, twitching, or loss of muscle tone. Treatment to prevent attacks includes anticonvulsants. (Compare GRAND MAL.)

petrissage (pā-trē-säzh′) N. massage technique in which the skin is gently lifted and squeezed, used to promote circulation and muscle relaxation.

Peyer's patches N. group of lymph nodes near the junction of the ileum and colon; in typhoid fever and certain other infectious diseases, they typically become enlarged and sometimes ulcerated.

peyote N. cactus from which the hallucinogen mescaline is derived.

pH N. measure of the acidity (amount of acid) or alkalinity (amount of base) of a solution. A pH of 7 is neutral; below 7, acid; above 7, alkaline. The pH scale is exponential, not linear; a drop in pH from 2 to 1 represents a tenfold ($10^1 = 10$) increase in acid content or decrease in base content, not simply a doubling or halving, respectively. Similarly, an increase in pH from 5 to 7 (2 pH units) represents a 100-fold ($10^2 = 100$) increase in the amount of base present or decrease in the amount of acid present. *See also* ACID-BASE BALANCE.

phaco- comb. form indicating an association with the lens of the eye (e.g., phacocele, protrusion of the lens).

phage (fāj) *See* BACTERIOPHAGE.

-phagia, -phagy suffixes indicating eating or an abnormality of appetite (e.g., coprophagia, eating of feces).

phago- comb. form indicating an association with eating or ingesting (e.g., phagomania, persistent concentration on food or an abnormal desire for food).

phagocyte (făg′ə-sīt′) N. cell that surrounds, engulfs, and digests microorganisms and cellular debris. Fixed phagocytes, including macrophages, do not circulate in the blood but are found in the liver, bone marrow, spleen, and other areas. Free phagocytes, such as leukocytes, circulate in the blood. ADJ. phagocytic

phagocytosis (făg′ə-sī-tō′sĭs) N. process by which certain cells (phagocytes) engulf and digest microorganisms and cellular debris (*compare* PINOCYTOSIS).

phalanges (fə-lăn′jēz) N., *sing.* phalanx, bones of the fingers and toes; the digits. The thumb and big toe each have two phalanges; the other fingers and toes each have three, for a total of 14 on each hand or foot. ADJ. phalangeal

phalangitis N. inflammation of a finger or toe.

phalanx (fā′lăngks′) N., *pl.* phalanges, any of the 14 bones of the fingers of one hand or a like number in the toes of one foot.

phallic phase (făl′ĭk) N. in psychoanalytic theory, the third stage in a person's development, usually between the ages of 3 and 6, when awareness and/or self-manipulation of the genitals is a prime source of pleasure (*compare* ORAL PHASE; ANAL PHASE; LATENCY PHASE; GENITAL PHASE).

phallo- comb. form indicating an association with the penis (e.g., phalloncus, tumor of the penis).

phalloplasty (făl′ə-plăs′tē) N. surgical repair or reconstruction of the penis done to treat congenital abnormality or injury.

phallus (făl′əs) N. *See* PENIS. ADJ. phallic

THE pH VALUES OF SOME BODY FLUIDS

Material	pH		Material	pH
Gastric juice	1.4		Tears	7.2
Urine	6.0		Blood	7.4
Saliva	6.8		Intestinal juice	7.8
Milk	7.1		Pancreatic juice	8.0

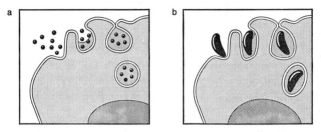

A comparison of pinocytosis and phagocytosis. (A) In pinocytosis, the cell takes liquids into the cell. (B) Phagocytosis involves the uptake of solid particles.

phantom limb syndrome (făn′təm) N. sense of pain, discomfort, or other sensation at the site where an arm or leg has been amputated.

pharmaceutical (fär′mə-soo͞o′tĭ-kəl) ADJ. pert. to drugs, esp. those used in medical treatment, or to a pharmacy.

pharmacist (fär′mə-sĭst) N. specialist in formulating and dispensing drugs.

pharmacokinetics N. study of the action of drugs in the body, including the method and rate of absorption and excretion, the duration of effect, and other factors.

pharmacology (fär′mə-kŏl′ə-jē) N. study of the preparation, properties, uses, and effects of drugs. A pharmacologist is a scientist with advanced training in pharmacology.

pharmacopoeia (fär′mə-kə-pē′ə) N. collection or stock of drugs. Often refers to a standardized treatise (e.g., United States Pharmacopoeia or USP) that contains formulas and information for the standard preparation and dispensing of drugs. The USP is issued every five years, with periodic supplements. A national committee of pharmacists, pharmacologists, physicians, chemists, biologists, and other scientific professionals write it. The initials USP after a drug name indicate that it is prepared in accordance with standards published in the pharmacopoeia (e.g., sterile saline, USP).

pharmacy (fär′mə-sē) N.
1. study of the preparation and dispensing of drugs.
2. location where medications and other medical supplies are dispensed and sold.

pharyngeal reflex (fə-rĭn′jē-əl) *See* GAG REFLEX.

pharyngeal tonsil *See* ADENOIDS.

pharyngitis (făr′ĭn-jī′tĭs) N. inflammation or infection of the pharynx, usually producing a sore throat; it may be caused by bacterial or viral infection. Treatment depends on the cause.

pharyngo- comb. form indicating an association with the pharynx (e.g., pharyngodynia, pharyngeal pain).

pharynx (făr′ĭngks) N. throat, muscular tube, extending from the base of the skull to the

PHARYNX

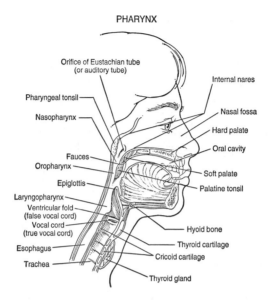

esophagus, that serves as a passageway for food from the mouth to the esophagus and for air from the nose and mouth to the larynx. It is divided into the nasopharynx, oropharynx, and laryngopharynx, and it connects with the eustachian tubes, the posterior nares, the mouth, the larynx, and the esophagus. ADJ. pharyngeal

Phenaphen N. trade name for the analgesic and antipyretic acetaminophen.

phenazopyridine N. analgesic (trade name Pyridium) used to relieve pain associated with urinary tract inflammation, including cystitis and urethritis. Adverse effects include gastrointestinal disturbances. The urine commonly turns an orange color during treatment with this agent.

phencyclidine hydrochloride (PCP) N. hallucinogenic drug no longer used in medicine; causes aggressive, sometimes paranoid, and often self-destructive behavior; persons who are agitated from PCP are very difficult to control and may require ten or more individuals to restrain them. Street name: angel dust.

phenelzine N. monoamine oxidase inhibitor (trade name Nardil) used to treat some forms of depression. Adverse effects include vertigo, constipation, dry mouth, and interaction with many foods and other drugs, sometimes producing serious effects.

Phenergan N. *See* TABLE OF COMMONLY PRESCRIBED DRUGS—TRADE NAMES.

pheniramine N. antihistamine, found in many preparations for allergies and respiratory infections, used to treat rhinitis, skin rashes, and pruritis. Adverse effects include sedation, dry mouth, and rapid heart rate.

phenobarbital (fē'nō-bär'bĭ-tôl') N. barbiturate used as a sedative to treat anxiety and as an anticonvulsant to treat some forms of epilepsy. Adverse effects include drowsiness, skin reactions, interaction with many other drugs, and possible development of dependence.

phenol (fē'nôl') N. disinfectant used to clean wounds and, in various lotions and ointments, to treat inflammations; it is poisonous if taken internally.

phenolphthalein (fē'nōl-thăl'ēn') N. laxative, found in many preparations under a variety of trade names. Adverse effects include abdominal cramps and possible allergic reactions.

phenomenon (fĭ-nŏm'ə-nŏn') N. observable event, which, in medicine, may be specific to a particular disease and therefore of diagnostic significance.

phenothiazine (fē'nō-thī'ə-zēn') N. any of a large group of drugs, many of which are used as tranquilizers, antiemetics, antihistamines, and adjuncts to anesthesia.

phenotype (fē'nə-tīp') N. observable characteristics of an organism that are the result of genetic makeup and environmental factors (*compare* GENOTYPE). ADJ. phenotypic

phensuximide N. anticonvulsant (trade name Milontin) used to treat petit mal. Adverse effects include gastrointestinal upset, drowsiness and other signs of central nervous system depression, and blood abnormalities.

phenylalanine (fĕn'əl-ăl'ə-nēn') N. amino acid essential for growth in children and for protein metabolism in children and adults; it is abundant in milk and eggs. *See also* PHENYLKETONURIA.

phenylephrine (fĕn'əl-ĕf'rēn) N. drug that constricts blood vessels, raising blood pressure; dilates the pupils of the eyes, and relieves nasal congestion. It is given by injection to raise blood pressure and is combined with other drugs in many nasal sprays and eyedrop preparations (under many trade names, including NeoSynephrine, Sinex, Dimetapp, and Histatapp) to relieve symptoms of allergy and the common cold (e.g., runny nose).

phenylketonuria (PKU) (fĕn'əl-kēt'n-oŏr'ē-ə) N. genetic disorder in which the absence of, or a deficiency in, the enzyme necessary for conversion of the amino acid phenylalanine into tyrosine causes the accumulation of phenylalanine and its metabolites in the body and the urine. Symptoms include eczema, an unusual odor to the urine, and progressive mental retardation. Treatment includes a diet low in, or free of, phenylalanine. Most states routinely test newborns for the defect; the test is referred to as the PKU test.

phenylpropanolamine (fĕn'əl-prō'pə-nōl'ə-mēn') N. drug used in many preparations to relieve the symptoms of allergic reactions, the common cold, and other respiratory infections. Adverse effects include nervousness, increased blood pressure, and loss of appetite.

phenytoin (fĕn′ĭ-tō′ĭn) N. anti-convulsant (trade name Dilantin) used to treat grand mal and other seizure disorders and to restore normal cardiac rhythm in cases of digitalis-induced arrhythmia. Adverse effects include ataxia, hypersensitivity reactions, and interaction with many other drugs. *See* TABLE OF COMMONLY PRESCRIBED DRUGS —GENERIC NAMES.

pheochromocytoma (fē′ō-krō′mō-sī-tō′mə) N. tumor of the adrenal gland that causes hyper-secretion of epinephrine and norepinephrine, resulting in intermittent hypertension and symptoms of headache, palpitations, sweating, and nervousness. Treatment is usually surgical removal of the tumor.

pheromone N. chemical substance secreted and released by an animal for detection and response by another, usually of the same species. Usually detected by smell and may affect behavior in various ways. Some animals secrete pheromones to warn of danger, others to attract mates. Pheromones probably play a minor role in human behavior, due to our relatively weak sense of smell.

phimosis (fī-mō′sĭs) N. condition in which the foreskin of the penis is abnormally tight, preventing retraction over the glans; it may be congenital or the result of infection. Treatment is usually by circumcision.

phleb-, phlebo- comb. forms indicating an association with a vein or veins (e.g., phlebangioma, saclike swelling of a vein).

phlebectomy (flī-bĕk′tə-mē) N. surgical removal of all or part of a vein, sometimes done to treat severe varicose veins.

phlebitis (flī-bī′tĭs) N. inflammation of the wall of a vein, most often occurring in the legs. Thrombosis may develop (*see also* THROMBOPHLEBITIS). Treatment includes rest and support of the area (e.g., by elastic stockings), nonsteroidal anti-inflammatory agents, and analgesics.

phlebothrombosis (flĕb′ō-thrŏm-bō′sĭs) N. abnormal condition marked by the formation of a clot within a vein without prior inflammation of the wall of the vein; it is associated with prolonged bed rest, surgery, pregnancy, and other conditions in which blood flow becomes sluggish or the blood coagulates more quickly than normal. The affected area, usually the leg, may become swollen and tender. The danger is that the clot may become dislodged and travels to the lungs (pulmonary embolism).

phlebotomy (flī-bŏt′ə-mē) N. incision of a vein for letting of blood, as in collecting blood from a donor or as treatment of polycythemia; also called venesection.

phlegm (flĕm) N. thick mucus of the respiratory passages.

phlegmon (flĕg′män) N. solid mass formed by inflamed connective tissue, such as forms around an appendix in appendicitis.

phobia (fō′bē-ə) N. anxiety disorder characterized by irrational and intense fear of an object (e.g., a dog), an activity (e.g., leaving the house), or physical conditions (e.g., height). The intense fear usually causes tremor, panic, palpitations, nausea, and other physical signs. Types of phobia include agoraphobia, claustrophobia, and zoophobia. Treatment includes desensitization therapy and other techniques of behavior therapy.

-phobia comb. form meaning abnormal fear (e.g., pyrophobia, abnormal fear of fire).

phocomelia (fō′kō-mē′lē-ə) N. developmental abnormality marked by the absence of the upper portion of the arm or leg so that the hands and/or feet are attached to the trunk of the body by short stumps; it is a rare anomaly, occurring as an effect of thalidomide taken during pregnancy; also called seal limbs (*compare* AMELIA).

phon-, phono- comb. forms indicating an association with sound, esp. the sound of the voice (e.g., phonasthenia, weakness or difficulty in speaking).

phosphatase N. enzyme that acts as a catalyst in reactions involving phosphorus.

phosphocreatine (fŏs′fō-krē′ə-tēn′) N. phosphate form of the muscle protein creatine, which is used as an energy source for muscle flexion. *See* CREATININE.

phospholipid (fŏs′fō-lĭp′ĭd) N. any of a class of compounds containing a nitrogenous base, phosphoric acid, and fatty acids. Phospholipids are found in many cells.

phosphorus (fŏs′fər-əs) N. nonmetallic element essential in the body for calcium, protein, and glucose metabolism and for the production of adenosine triphosphate (ATP). *See also* TABLE OF IMPORTANT ELEMENTS.

phosphorylation (fŏs′fər-ə-lā′shən) N. chemical process of adding a phosphorous-containing molecule (phosphate) to a substance. Phosphorylation reactions are essential to the normal production of energy in the body by forming ATP (adenosine triphosphate).

phot-, photo- comb. forms indicating an association with light (e.g., photolysis, breakdown of substances in light).

photalgia (fō-tăl′jē-ə) N. pain in the eye caused by bright light.

photocoagulation (fō′tō-kō-ăg′yə-lā′shən) N. destruction of tissue by an intense beam of light, used to destroy diseased retinal tissue or to create scar tissue to bind the retina in cases of detached retina.

photomicrograph N. photographic record of an object in a microscopic field taken by attaching a camera to a microscope.

photon (fō′tŏn′) N. unit of light energy.

photophobia (fō′tə-fō′bē-ə) N. abnormal intolerance to light, often associated with albinism, drug-induced pupil dilation, migraine, encephalitis, measles, and other diseases.

photopsia N. sensation of flashing lights, caused by irritation of the retina.

photoreceptor (fō′tō-rĭ-sĕp′tər) N. nerve endings capable of being stimulated by light, such as the rods and cones of the retina. Light strikes the photoreceptor (rods and cones), leading to a structural change in a chemical pigment that activates an enzyme. The net effect is that the movement of sodium is altered, leading to a nerve signal that is eventually perceived as sight and color.

photoretinitis (fō'tō-rĕt'n-ī'tĭs) N. damage to the retina caused by looking at the sun without adequate protection.

photosensitivity (fō'tō-sĕn'sĭ-tĭv'ĭ-tē) N. abnormal sensitivity of the skin to the sun; it is caused by a disorder (e.g., albinism) or is the result of certain drugs (e.g., tetracycline, phenothiazines). ADJ. photosensitive

phototherapy (fō'tō-thĕr'ə-pē) N. use of strong light to treat disorders such as acne and hyperbilirubinemia of the newborn.

phrenic (frĕn'ĭk) ADJ.
1. pert. to the diaphragm.
2. pert. to the mind.

phrenic nerve N. one of a pair of nerves, arising from cervical spinal roots and passing down the thorax to innervate the diaphragm and help control its movements during breathing.

phycomycosis N. any infection caused by fungi of the group Phycomycetes. These fungi inhabit soil and do not usually produce disease in humans.

physical ADJ. in medicine, pert. to the body, not the mind.

physical therapy N.
1. treatment by physical means.
2. health profession that is concerned with health promotion, prevention of physical disabilities, and rehabilitation of persons disabled by pain, disease, or injury. Physical therapy is involved with patient evaluation and treatment through the use of physical therapeutic measures as opposed to medicines, surgery, or radiation. Also called physiotherapy.

physiology (fĭz'ē-ŏl'ə-jē) N. branch of science dealing with the normal chemical and physical functioning of living organisms (*compare* ANATOMY).

physostigmine (fī'sō-stĭg'mēn') N. parasympathomimetic drug used in the treatment of tetanus and myasthenia gravis. Adverse effects include bronchospasm, digestive upsets, and excess salivation.

pia mater (pī'ə mă'tər) N. innermost of the three meninges covering the brain and spinal cord (the other two being the dura mater and arachnoid); it is highly vascular and closely applied to the brain and spinal cord, nourishing the nerve cells.

pian (pē-ăn') *See* YAWS.

pica (pī'kə) N. eating of nonfood substances, such as clay, chalk, hair, or glue; it occurs in some cases of nutritional deficiency, pregnancy, and some mental disorders.

Pick's disease (pĭks) N. form of presenile dementia occurring in middle-aged people, characterized by degeneration in the frontal and temporal lobes of the brain (not diffuse throughout the brain as in Alzheimer's disease) and manifested by changes in behavior and deterioration of intellectual abilities.

Pickwickian syndrome (pĭk-wĭk'ē-ən) N. extreme obesity, often with decreased lung function and sleepiness.

picornavirus (pē-kôr'nə-vī'rəs) N. any of a group of small ribonucleic acid (RNA) viruses, including the coxsackie virus and rhinoviruses.

piebald ADJ. having patches of nonpigmented hair or skin due to the absence of melanocytes in those areas (*compare* ALBIN-ISM; VITILIGO).

pigeon breast N. congenital condition in which there is abnormal forward projection of the sternum (breastbone); it is usually harmless and requires no treatment; also called pigeon chest.

pigeon toes N. abnormal posture in which the toes are turned inward, often associated with knock-knee.

pigment N. substance giving color, including blood pigments (e.g., hemoglobin), retinal pigments (e.g., rhodopsin), and melanin, found in the skin and iris of the eye.

pilar cyst (pī′lər) *See* WEN.

piles *See* HEMORRHOID.

Pill, the *See* ORAL CONTRACEPTIVE.

pilo- comb. form indicating an association with hair (e.g., pilosis, excessive development of hair).

pilocarpine (pī′lō-kär′pēn′) N. cholinergic agent used in eyedrops to treat glaucoma. Adverse effects include difficulty in breathing, excess salivation, and muscle tremors.

pilomotor reflex (pī′lə-mō′tər) N. erection of the hairs of skin in response to emotional stress, skin irritation, or cold; also called goose bumps; gooseflesh.

pilonidal fistula (fĭs′chə-lə) N. abnormal tract containing hairs extending from an opening in the skin, usually near the cleft at the top of the buttocks; also called pilonidae sinus.

pilosebaceous ADJ. pert. to a hair follicle and its sebaceous gland.

pilus (pī′ləs) N., *pl.* pili. *See* HAIR. ADJ. pilar

pimple N. small, inflamed, pus-containing swelling on the skin, usually due to infection of a pore obstructed with sebaceous secretions.

pin N. in orthopedics, rodlike metal device used to secure fragments of a bone.

pindolol (pĭn′də-lôl′) N. oral beta blocker (trade name Visken) used in the treatment of hypertension. It may also have stimulatory effects on the heart. Adverse effects include depression, cardiac arrhythmias, and aggravation of heart failure or asthma.

pineal gland (pĭn′ē-əl) N. small cone-shaped gland in the brain thought to secrete melatonin; also called pineal body; epiphysis.

pinealoma (pĭn′ē-ə-lō′mə) N. neoplasm of the pineal gland, usually causing headache, nausea, vomiting, and hydrocephalus.

pinguecula N. slightly elevated, irregular, yellow elastic-tissue deposit in the conjunctiva (mucous membrane lining of the eye) that may extend to, but does not cover, the cornea (*compare* PTERYGIUM).

pinkeye *See* CONJUNCTIVITIS.

pinna (pĭn′ə) N. *See* AURICLE.

pinocytosis (pĭn′ə-sī-tō′sĭs) N. process by which certain cells (e.g., some leukocytes) engulf and take in droplets of fluid (*compare* PHAGOCYTOSIS).

pinta (pĭn′tə) N. skin infection caused by the *Treponema carateum* spirochete and common in Central and South America; it is characterized by a slowly enlarging papule, followed by a generalized rash, and later by depigmentation (loss of normal pigment) of affected areas. Treatment is by penicillin.

piperacillin (pī-pĕr′ə-sĭl′ĭn) N. a synthetic penicillin-type antibiotic (trade name Pipracil) indicated in moderate to severe infections. Adverse effects include loose stools and liver abnormalities.

piperazine (pī-pĕr′ə-zēn′) N. anthelmintic used to treat infestations with pinworms and roundworms. Adverse effects include fever, vertigo, abdominal discomfort, and diarrhea.

piroxicam (pĭ-rŏk′sĭ-kăm′) N. nonsteroidal anti-inflammatory agent (trade name Feldene) used in the treatment of osteoarthritis, rheumatoid arthritis, and other inflammatory conditions. Adverse effects include gastrointestinal bleeding and nausea.

Pitocin N. trade name for oxytocin.

Pitressin N. trade name for the antidiuretic hormone vasopressin.

pitting (pĭt′ĭng) N.
1. small, depressed scars on the skin following severe acne or other disorder.
2. temporary indentation in the skin following pressure on edematous tissue.

pituitary dwarf (pĭ-tōō′ĭ-tĕr′ē) N. dwarf whose small size is due to lack of growth hormone from the anterior pituitary; the body is typically normally proportioned with no deformities; mental and, usually, sexual development is normal.

pituitary gland N. small endocrine gland attached to the hypothalamus that releases many hormones controlling many body activities and influencing the activity of many other endocrine glands. It is divided into anterior and posterior portions, each with separate functions. *See* ANTERIOR PITUITARY GLAND; POSTERIOR PITUITARY GLAND.

pityriasis (pĭt′ĭ-rī′ə-sĭs) N. any of several skin disorders, including dandruff.
   pityriasis alba N. common skin disorder, occurring most often in children and young adults, characterized by circumscribed round or oval patches of depigmentation (loss of normal pigment) or less than normal pigmentation.
   pityriasis rosea N. skin disease in which a mildly itchy rash develops over the trunk of the body several days after a single localized patch called herald patch.

pivot joint (pĭv′ət) N. synovial joint in which movement is limited to rotation (e.g., the articulation of the radius and ulna in the arm is a pivot joint).

PKD *See* POLYCYSTIC KIDNEY DISEASE.

PKU *See* PHENYLKETONURIA.

placebo (plə-sē′bō) N. inactive substance (e.g., distilled water or sugar) or less-than-effective dose of a harmless substance prescribed and administered as if it were an effective dose of a needed drug; used as a control in tests of drug efficacy and for treatment of certain patients who do not need or should not be given a drug they request.

placebo effect N. change, usually beneficial, occurring after a substance (a placebo) is taken that is not the result of any property of that substance but usually reflects the faith or expectations that the person has in the substance.

placenta (plə-sĕn′tə) N. highly vascular fetal organ through which the fetus absorbs oxygen, nutrients, and other substances from the mother and excretes carbon dioxide and other wastes. It forms around the eighth day of gestation as the blastocyst becomes implanted in the wall of the uterus. At the end of pregnancy the placenta weighs about one sixth of the weight of the infant. Its maternal side is rough, divided into lobules, and has fingerlike chorionic villi that project into the uterine wall. The fetal side is smooth, covered with the fetal membranes. The placenta is expelled after the birth of the child in the third stage of labor. Also called afterbirth. (*Compare* AMNION.) ADJ. placental

placenta previa (prē′vē-ə) N. condition of pregnancy in which the placenta is implanted abnormally in the lower, rather than the upper, part of the uterus so that it partially or completely covers the outlet from the uterus to vagina; it is a common cause of bleeding in late pregnancy. If severe hemorrhage occurs, immediate Cesarean section is required to save the mother's life. If the placenta is next to, but not blocking, the uterine outlet, vaginal delivery may be attempted.

Placidyl N. trade name for the sedative ethclorvynol.

plagiocephaly N. congenital malformation of the skull.

plague (plăg) N.
1. infectious disease caused by the bite of rat fleas infected with *Yersinia pestis*. *See also* BUBONIC PLAGUE.

2. any epidemic disease with a high death rate.

plano- comb. form meaning flat (e.g., planocellar, having flat cells).

plantar (plăn′tər) ADJ. pert. to the undersurface (sole) of the foot.

plantar reflex N. reflex in which drawing a blunt instrument over, or firmly stroking, the outer part of the sole from the heel toward the little toe causes the toes to bunch and curl downward. In those over the age of 1½–2 years an upward movement of the big toe after this stimulus is usually a sign of neurological damage, the Babinski reflex.

plantar wart N. wart occurring on the sole of the foot that, because of pressure, develops a callus (hardened) ring around its soft center and becomes painful. Treatment includes cryosurgery, electrodesiccation (cauterization), and application of topical acids.

plantigrade ADJ. pert. to walking on the entire sole of the foot, as in the human gait.

plaque (plăk) N.
1. flat, raised patch on the skin or mucous membrane.
2. deposit on the inner arterial walls in atherosclerosis.
3. deposit of saliva and bacteria on teeth that encourages the development of caries.

plasma (plăz′mə) N. acellular, straw-colored, fluid part of blood and lymph that contains water, electrolytes, glucose, fats, and proteins, and in which erythrocytes, leukocytes, and platelets are suspended. In addition to carrying the cellular elements, plasma helps maintain the fluid-electrolyte and the acid-base balances of the body and helps transport wastes (*compare* SERUM).

plasma cell N. lymphocyte-like cell found in bone marrow and sometimes in the blood that functions in immune responses; large numbers of plasma cells are found in multiple myeloma.

plasma protein N. any of various proteins in blood plasma, including fibrinogen and prothrombin, important for blood coagulation, and immunoglobulins, important in immune response.

plasmacytoma (plăz′mə-sī-tō′mə) N. neoplasm of plasma cells, occurring in bone marrow usually in association with multiple myeloma, or, less commonly, occurring in soft tissues, esp. those of the upper respiratory tract.

plasmapheresis (plăz′mə-fə-rē′sĭs) N. method of removing plasma from the blood. Blood is withdrawn from the body, and the cellular elements are separated and transfused back to the patient. The technique has been used to identify and analyze plasma proteins for diagnostic purposes and has been tried experimentally in the treatment of certain diseases.

plasmid (plăz′mĭd) N. small cellular inclusion consisting of deoxyribonucleic acid (DNA), capable of self-replicating, and involved in certain metabolic functions.

plasminogen (plăz-mĭn′ə-jən) N. inactive protein precursor to plasmin; found in many tissues and body fluids; prevents formation of abnormal blood clots as well as functions in the lysis (breakdown) of normally formed clots.

plasmo- comb. form indicating an association with plasma (e.g., plasmocyte, plasma cell).

plasmodium (plăz-mō′dē-əm) N. genus of parasites that includes the malaria-causing organisms.

plastic surgery N. that branch of surgery concerned with the alteration, reconstruction, and replacement of body parts to correct a structural or cosmetic defect. Common plastic surgery procedures include the repair of harelips and cleft palate, rhinoplasty, rhytidoplasty, the reconstruction of body parts destroyed by injury, and skin grafting.

plasticity N. literally, the ability to be molded, such as in a warmed plastic compound. In neurology, refers to changes in nerve synapse function that can occur as a result of the history of discharge at a synapse. Conduction can be strengthened or weakened on the basis of past experience. These changes are important in current studies of learning and memory. Plasticity has also been demonstrated in the brain. For example, if an arm is amputated, sensory nerve fibers serving other areas of the body grow into the area that contained nerve fibers serving the amputated arm. This explains why some individuals who have had an arm amputated may feel sensations as though the arm is still present when other areas of the body, such as the face, are stroked. Recent data indicate that similar, but less well defined, phenomena also occur in the motor nerve cells of the brain.

-plasty comb. form indicating plastic surgery on a specific body part (e.g., otoplasty, plastic surgery on the ear).

PLATE 462

FORMATION OF A PLATELET PLUG

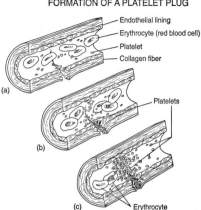

(a) A break occurs in the wall of a blood vessel. (b) Platelets adhere to each other and to the collagen fibers of the blood vessel wall. (c) The platelet plug helps control the loss of blood at the injury site.

plate N.
1. flat structure or part (e.g., the neural plate in the embryo, which develops into the neural tube).
2. *See* DENTURE.

plateau (plă-tō′) N. elevated, usually flat area esp. on a graph or flow chart; also refers to a period of little or no change or progress, such as in athletic training. Sometimes, the effects of a drug reach a plateau where no further beneficial effects are noted.

platelet (plāt′lĭt) N. disc-shaped, small cellular element in the blood, essential for blood clotting. Normally 200,000–300,000 platelets are found in 1 cubic centimeter of blood. Also called thrombocyte.

platy- comb. form indicating broadness or flatness (e.g., platyopia, broad face).

platysma (plə-tĭz′mə) N. broad muscle, on each side of the neck, extending from the lower jaw to the region of the clavicle and involved in mouth and jaw movement.

play therapy N. form of psychotherapy for children in which play with games and toys is used to gain insight into the child's feelings and thoughts and to help treat conflicts and psychological problems.

pleasure principle N. in psychoanalytic theory, tendency to pursue actions or objects that provide immediate gratification of instinctual drives and to avoid discomfort and pain (*compare* REALITY PRINCIPLE).

-plegia suffix indicating paralysis (e.g., hemiplegia, paralysis of one side of the body).

Plendil N. *See* TABLE OF COMMONLY PRESCRIBED DRUGS—TRADE NAMES.

plethora (plĕth'ər-ə) N. excess of blood or other body fluid. ADJ. plethoric

pleur-, pleuro- comb. forms indicating an association with the pleura (e.g., pleurobronchias, inflammation of the pleura and bronchi).

pleura (plŏŏr'ə) N., *pl.* pleurae, delicate membrane covering the lungs and the inner surface of the chest; it is divided into the visceral pleura, which covers the lungs, and the parietal pleura, which lines the chest wall and covers the diaphragm. Between the two layers of the pleura is a small space (pleural space) containing fluid that acts as a lubricant. ADJ. pleural

pleural cavity N. cavity in the thorax that contains the lungs.

pleural space N. small space between the visceral and parietal layers of the pleura.

pleurisy (plŏŏr'ĭ-sē) N. inflammation of the pleura, esp. the parietal layer, marked by difficulty in breathing and sharp pain that is worsened with inspiration. Causes include viral infections, pneumonia, tuberculosis, and cancer. Treatment depends on the cause.

pleurodynia (plŏŏr'ə-dĭn'ē-ə) N. acute inflammation of the muscles between the ribs, causing pain, tenderness, and often fever.

pleuropneumonia (plŏŏr'ō-nŏŏ-mōn'yə) N. pleurisy and pneumonia.

pleuropneumonialike organism (PPLO) *See* MYCOPLASMA.

plexus (plĕk'səs) N. network of intersecting nerves, blood vessels, or lymph vessels (e.g., brachial plexus).

pliable ADJ. capable of being bent or twisted easily; flexible.

plica (plī'kə) N., *pl.* plicae, fold of tissue (e.g., plica vocalis, vocal cord). ADJ. plical

plumbism *See* LEAD POISONING.

pluri- comb. form indicating more than one (e.g., pluriglandular, pert. to more than one gland).

plutonium (plōō-tō'nē-əm) highly poisonous radioactive element. (*See also* TABLE OF IMPORTANT ELEMENTS)

PMS N. abbrev. for premenstrual syndrome.

-pnea comb. form indicating an association with breathing (e.g., dyspnea).

pneuma-, pneumato- comb. forms indicating an association with air or gas (e.g., pneumarthrosis, gas in the joints).

pneumo-, pneumono- comb. forms indicating an association with the lungs (e.g., pneumogastric, pert. to the lungs and stomach).

pneumococcal (nŏŏ'mə-kŏk'əl) pert. to bacteria of the genus Pneumococcus.

pneumococcal vaccine N. active immunizing agent (trade name Pneumovax) effective against the 23 most common strains of Pneumococcus, associated with many, but not all, cases of pneumococcal pneumonia. Once vaccinated, a person has immunity for at least 5 years.

pneumoconiosis (nŏŏ'mō-kō'nē-ō'sĭs) N. any lung disease caused by chronic inhalation of dust, usually of occupational origin; types of pneumoconiosis includes abestosis, anthracosis, siderosis, and silicosis.

pneumocystosis (noo′mō-sĭ-stō′sĭs) N. infection with the organism *Pneumocystis carinii,* usually occurring only in infants or immunosuppressed persons (e.g., those with acquired immune deficiency syndrome); usually involves the lungs (pneumonia) and is characterized by fever, cough, rapid breathing, and cyanosis. This form of pneumonia may be fatal. Current treatment includes pentamidine and sulfa drugs (e.g., Bactrim); other agents are being tried experimentally. The responsible microbe has been thought to be a protozoan, though some studies suggest that it may be a fungus.

pneumoencephalography (noo′mō-ĕn-sĕf′ə-lŏg′rə-fē) N. technique for X-ray visualization of some brain tissues that involves the injection of oxygen or other gas into the ventricles of the brain to displace cerebrospinal fluid and provide a contrast medium.

pneumonectomy (noo′mə-nĕk′tə-mē) N. surgical removal of a lung, usually to treat cancer.

pneumonia (noo-mōn′yə) N. inflammation of the lungs, usually caused by infection with bacteria (esp. Pneumococcus), viruses, fungi, or rickettsiae. Symptoms include fever, chills, headache, cough, chest pain, and, as the disease progresses, difficult and painful breathing, the production of thick, purulent sputum, rapid pulse, and sometimes gastrointestinal complications. Treatment depends on the cause; it often includes antibiotics, analgesics, expectorants, rest, fluids, and oxygen. *See also* BRONCHO-PNEUMONIA.

pneumonitis (noo′mə-nī′tĭs) N. inflammation of the lung, caused by a virus or allergic reaction. Treatment includes removal of the offending agent, if possible, and corticosteroids.

pneumopericardium (noo′mō-pĕr′ĭ-kär′dē-əm) N. accumulation of air between the two layers of pericardium; it is most often caused by penetrating trauma (e.g., gunshot or knife wound) and may require pericardiocentesis to drain the air.

pneumothorax (noo′mō-thôr′ăks′) N. collection of air or gas in the pleural cavity, causing the lung to collapse. It may occur spontaneously but usually results from injury to the chest that allows the entrance of air. Symptoms include sudden, sharp chest pain, difficulty in breathing, rapid heart beat, weakness, and low blood pressure. Treatment involves aspiration of the air from the pleural cavity and the administration of oxygen and pain relievers.

pod-, podo- comb. forms indicating an association with the foot (e.g., podalgia, foot pain).

podiatry (pə-dī′ə-trē) N. medical specialty concerned with the foot and its structure and with the diagnosis and treatment of diseases and disorders of the feet; also called, less correctly, chiropody.

-poiesis comb. form meaning the production of (e.g., erythropoiesis, red blood cell production).

poison N. substance that when inhaled, ingested, or absorbed impairs health or causes death.

poison ivy, poison oak, poison sumac. *See* RHUS DERMATITIS.

polio- comb. form indicating an association with the gray matter of the brain and/or spinal cord (e.g., polioencephalitis, inflammation of the gray matter of the brain caused by a virus).

poliomyelitis (pō'lē-ō-mī'ə-lī'tĭs) N. infectious disease that affects the central nervous system. It is caused by the poliovirus and was once epidemic in many parts of the world, but now is largely prevented by vaccination with Salk or Sabin vaccines. Many infections are asymptomatic; some produce only mild symptoms of fever, malaise, headache, and gastrointestinal upsets; others cause paralysis, most often of the lower limbs. Treatment is largely symptomatic. Also called polio; infantile paralysis.

poliosis N. depigmentation (loss of normal pigment) of the hair.

poliovirus (pō'lē-ō-vī'rəs) N. organism that causes poliomyelitis.

poliovirus vaccine N. vaccine prepared from poliovirus to provide immunity to poliomyelitis. The live oral form of the vaccine, called the Sabin vaccine, is routinely given to children under the age of 18; inactivated polio vaccine, known as the Salk vaccine, usually is given subcutaneously to infants and unvaccinated adults.

pollex (pŏl'ĕks') N. thumb.

pollinosis (pŏl'ə-nō'sĭs) See HAY FEVER.

poly- comb. form indicating many or a large amount (e.g., polycystic, having many cysts).

polyarteritis (pŏl'ē-är'tə-rī'tĭs) N. inflammation of several arteries.

polyarteritis nodosa See PERIARTERITIS NODOSA.

Polycillin N. trade name for the antibacterial ampicillin.

polyclonal ADJ. arising from different cell types or lines. Often used regarding antibodies that arise from many different cellular sources in the body. Compare to monoclonal, arising from similar cell types or lines.

polycystic kidney disease (PKD) (pŏl'ē-sĭs'tĭk) N. abnormal condition in which the kidneys are enlarged and contain many cysts. It occurs in childhood and adult forms and often leads to kidney failure.

polycythemia (pŏl'ē-sī-thē'mē-ə) N. abnormal increase in the number of erythrocytes in the blood, often associated with pulmonary or heart disease, or exposure to high altitudes for a long period, but in many cases of unknown cause.

polydactyly (pŏl'ē-dăk'tə-lē) N. congenital abnormality characterized by the presence of more than the normal number of fingers or toes; it is usually corrected by surgery; also called hyperdactyly.

polydipsia (pŏl'ē-dĭp'sē-ə) N. excessive thirst, often associated with diabetes mellitus, diabetes insipidus, or kidney dysfunction.

polymerase (pä-lə-mə-rāz) N. enzyme that facilitates the synthesis of RNA or DNA from a template strand during replication. *See also* POLYMERASE CHAIN REACTION; REPLICATION.

polymerase chain reaction (PCR) N. laboratory method for enzymatically synthesizing in large quantities defined sequences of DNA or RNA. In medical diagnostics, PCR is a highly sensitive test that can detect small amounts of DNA or RNA (genetic material) in a blood or tissue sample using an amplification technique that multiplies the existing DNA/RNA so that it can more easily be detected. PCR assays are used to determine viral loads in persons infected with Human Immunodeficiency Virus (HIV). *See also* VIRAL LOAD.

polymorphism (pŏl′ē-môr′fĭz′əm) N. state of existing or occurring in several forms.

polymorphonuclear ADJ. having a nucleus with multiple lobules, as some leukocytes (white blood cells).

polymyositis (pŏl′ē-mī′ə-sī′tĭs) N. inflammation of many muscles.

polymyxin (pŏl′ē-mĭk′sĭn) N. antibiotic used to treat certain bacterial infections. Adverse effects include allergic skin reactions and kidney damage.

polyneuritic psychosis (pŏl′ē-nōō-rĭt′ĭk sī-kō′sĭs) *See* KORSAKOFF'S PSYCHOSIS.

polyneuritis (pŏl′ē-nōō-rī′tĭs) N. inflammation of all or most of the peripheral nerves.

polyostotic fibrous dysplasia (dĭs-plā′zhə) *See* ALBRIGHT'S DISEASE.

polyp (pŏl′ĭp) N. growth or nodule, usually benign, most commonly arising from a mucous membrane (e.g., in the nose, ear, or uterus).

polypeptide (pŏl′ē-pĕp′tīd′) N. molecule consisting of three or more amino acids; proteins are polypeptides.

polypharmacy N. act of prescribing or administering more than one drug to a patient. The possibility of drug interaction must be considered in these cases.

polysaccharide (pŏl′ē-săk′ə-rīd′) N. complex carbohydrate (e.g., starch) that can be broken down into simpler monosaccharides, such as sugar.

polysomy (pŏl′ē-sō′mē) N. presence of one or more extra chromosomes in somatic cells as a result of nondisjunction of chromosomes during gamete formation. It is usually associated with congenital defects.

Polysporin N. trade name for a fixed-combination, topical, ophthalmic drug, containing the antibacterials polymixin and bacitracin; used to treat eye infections.

polyuria (pŏl′ē-yōōr′ē-ə) N. production of large volumes of usually dilute, pale urine; it is often associated with diabetes mellitus, diabetes insipidus, renal disorder, or the intake of large amounts of fluid.

Poly-vi-flor N. trade name for an oral, pediatric, fixed combination of vitamins and minerals that includes sodium fluoride.

pons (pŏnz) N. any bridgelike part connecting two parts, esp. the pons varolii (varolius), between the medulla oblongata and the midbrain, which contains white matter and the nuclei of several cranial nerves.

Ponstel N. trade name for the anti-inflammatory and analgesic mefenamic acid used to treat mild to moderate pain; esp. effective against menstrual cramps (dysmenorrhea).

ponto- comb. form indicating an association with the pons of the brain (e.g., pontocerebellar, pert. to the pons and cerebellum).

popliteal (pŏp-lĭt′ē-əl) ADJ. pert. to the area behind the knee.

HEPATIC PORTAL SYSTEM

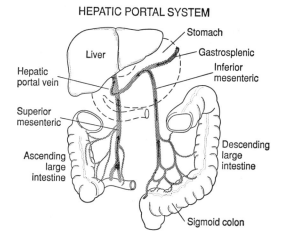

Stomach
Gastrosplenic
Inferior mesenteric
Hepatic portal vein
Liver
Superior mesenteric
Descending large intestine
Ascending large intestine
Sigmoid colon

popliteal artery N. artery extending from the femoral artery and branching to supply the legs and foot. *See* MAJOR ARTERIES AND VEINS OF THE BODY, in Appendix.

porcine ADJ. relating to or derived from swine (pigs); medically, used in reference to porcine heart valves that are used to replace diseased human heart valves; also pigskin is used as a temporary dressing in some burns.

pore N. small opening (e.g., openings of the sweat glands in the skin). ADJ. porous

porosity (pə-rŏs′ĭ-tē) ADJ. state of allowing liquids to flow through freely; degree of being porous.

porphyria (pôr-fēr′ē-ə) N. any of several inherited disorders characterized by disturbance of the metabolism of porphyrins, affecting primarily the liver or bone marrow. The affected person excretes large amounts of porphyrins in the urine and has photosensitivity, neuritis, and mental disturbances.

porphyrin (pôr′fə-rĭn) N. any of a number of pigments widely distributed in living tissue (in, e.g., hemoglobin, myoglobin, and cytochromes) and important in many oxidation reactions.

porta (pôr′tə) N. opening or entry, esp. one through which blood vessels pass into an organ (e.g., porta hepatis, the opening through which major blood vessels enter and leave the liver).

portacaval shunt (pôr′tə-kā′vəl) N. communication surgically created between the portal vein and the inferior vena cava so that blood drained from abdominal organs bypasses the liver and is channeled directly to the inferior vena cava for movement to the heart; it is used to decrease portal hypertension.

portal (pôr′tl) ADJ. pert. to the portal system.

portal hypertension (hī′pər-těn′shən) N. increase in pressure within the veins of the portal system caused by obstruction in the (hepatic) blood system, often associated with alcoholic cirrhosis of the liver. It causes enlargement of the spleen and collateral veins, and, if severe and untreated, systemic hypertension.

portal system N. system of veins that drains blood from abdominal organs (the digestive organs, pancreas, spleen, and gallbladder) and transports it to the liver. Also known as hepatic portal system.

portal vein (pôr′tl) N. short vein that receives branches from many veins leading from abdominal organs, including the splenic vein from the spleen and pancreas and the mesenteric vein from the intestine, and then enters the liver, ramifying there and ending in capillarylike sinusoids where the nutrients from the blood pass into liver cells. The blood then passes through the hepatic vein to the inferior vena cava.

port-wine stain N. flat birthmark, varying from pale pinkish red to deep purple; also called nevus flammeus.

positron emission tomography (PET) (tō-mŏg′rə-fē) N. computerized radiographic technique that allows examination of the metabolic activity of various tissues, esp. brain tissue. Radioactively tagged substances (usually glucose) taken by the patient give off positively charged particles (positrons) that interact with certain cells esp. neurons in the brain, giving off gamma rays. These rays are detected by special devices and converted through computer analysis into color-coded images that reveal the metabolic activity of the organ involved. PET is widely used in the diagnosis of brain disorders.

post- comb. form meaning after, behind (e.g., postadolescence, time in a person's life after adolescence).

post mortem ADJ. after death of the organism; also colloq. for autopsy.

posterior (pŏ-stēr′ē-ər) ADJ. pert. to, situated in, or toward the back or the back part of a structure (*compare* ANTERIOR).

posterior nares *See* NARES.

posterior pituitary gland (pĭ-tōō′ĭ-tĕr′ē) N. posterior lobe of the pituitary gland that secretes two hormones: antidiuretic hormone, or vasopressin, which acts on the kidney to reduce urine production; and oxytocin, which produces contractions of the pregnant uterus and causes milk to flow from the breasts of lactating women; also called neurohypophysis.

postero- comb. form indicating a posterior position (*compare* ANTERO-; RETRO-) (e.g., posteroanterior, from the back to the front).

postganglionic (pōst′găng-glē-ŏn′ĭk) ADJ. nerve fibers arising distal to (after) a ganglion; compare to preganglionic fibers that originate proximal to (before) a ganglion.

posthitis (pŏs-thī′tĭs) N. inflammation usually due to bacterial infection, of the foreskin of the penis, causing redness, swelling, and pain; often associated with inflammation of the glans. Treatment is by antibiotics. *See also* BALANITIS.

posthumous birth N.
1. birth of a child by Caesarean section after the death of the mother.
2. birth of a child after the father's death.

postictal ADJ. pert. to the period following a convulsion.

postmature infant N. infant born after 42 weeks gestation and usually showing signs of placental insufficiency. The child usually has dry, peeling skin, skin folds, and long nails, is prone to electrolyte imbalance and hypoglycemia, and may have lost weight the last few days in utero.

postmenopausal (pōst′měn-ə-pô′zəl) ADJ. pert. to the time after menopause.

postnasal drip (pōst-nā′zəl) N. discharge of nasal mucus into the pharynx, caused by rhinitis, sinusitis, or hypersecretion of mucus and usually associated with a feeling of nasal and throat obstruction and with unpleasant taste and odor. Treatment includes agents to constrict nasal vessels; irrigation of sinuses, if necessary; surgical correction of nasal polyps or deviated septum, if indicated; allergy treatment, and/or antibiotics.

postoperative (pōst-ŏp′ər-ə-tĭv) ADJ. pert. to the period after surgery, including the emergence from anesthesia and the abatement of the acute signs of anesthesia and surgery.

postpartum (pōst-pär′təm) ADJ. pert. to the first few days after childbirth.

postural hypotension (pŏs′chər-əl hī′pə-těn′shən) See ORTHOSTATIC HYPOTENSION under ORTHOSTATIC.

pot N. street term for marijuana.

potassium (pə-tăs′ē-əm) N. metallic element, essential to life. It is the major intracellular ion, functioning in nerve and muscle activity. See also TABLE OF IMPORTANT ELEMENTS.

potassium chloride N. salt of potassium used to treat potassium deficiency, which is usually the result of diuretic intake. See TABLE OF COMMONLY PRESCRIBED DRUGS—GENERIC NAMES.

potency (pōt′n-sē) N.
1. strength or power, as of a drug.
2. ability of a male to achieve and maintain an erection and thus engage in coitus. See also impotence.

potentiation N. synergistic effect, in which the effect of two drugs given simultaneously is greater than the effect of either drug given separately.

Pott's disease (pŏts) N. tuberculosis of the spine; it is rare and, if untreated, leads to bone destruction and skeletal deformity.

pouch N. saclike part.

poultice (pōl′tĭs) N. preparation of hot, moist material applied to any part of the body to increase local circulation, alleviate pain, or soften and lubricate the skin.

pox (pŏks) N. any of several diseases, usually viral, in which the skin breaks out in pustules or vesicles (small blisters). See CHICKEN POX; SMALLPOX.

PPLO See MYCOPLASMA.

PPO N. abbrev. for preferred provider organization.

prandial (prăn′dē-əl) ADJ. pert. to a meal.

Pravachol N. trade name for the oral lipid-reducing agent, pravastatin. *See* TABLE OF COMMONLY PRESCRIBED DRUGS—TRADE NAMES.

pravastatin (prăv'ə-stăt'ĭn) N. oral agent (trade name Pravachol) for the treatment of hyperlipoproteinemia; the most common side effect involves asymptomatic changes in the patient's liver tests. *See* TABLE OF COMMONLY PRESCRIBED DRUGS—GENERIC NAMES.

prazosin (prā'zō-sĭn) N. antihypertensive (trade name Minipress). Adverse effects include rapid heart beat, fainting, and a sudden drop in blood pressure.

pre- prefix meaning before (e.g., premenopausal, pert. to the time before menopause).

precancerous (prē-kăn'sər-əs) ADJ. pert. to a growth that is not malignant but probably will become so if left untreated.

precipitate (prĭ-sĭp'ĭ-tāt') V. to separate from solution; N. solid substance that has separated from solution.

precipitin (prĭ-sĭp'ĭ-tĭn) N. antibody that combines with its antigen to form a complex that settles out of solution as a precipitate. This reaction is used to identify an unknown antigen or to establish the presence of antibodies to a known antigen.

precocious (prĭ-kō'shəs) ADJ. pert. to earlier-than-expected development of physical or mental abilities (e.g., precocious dentition, eruption of deciduous or permanent teeth at an age earlier than expected).

precordial ADJ. pert. to the region of the chest over the heart (the precordium).

predisposition (prē'dĭs-pə-zĭsh'ən) N. tendency to be affected by a particular disease or to develop or react in a certain way; it may be genetic or result from environmental factors (e.g., nutritional factors).

prednisolone (prĕd-nĭs'ə-lōn') N. glucocorticoid used to treat inflammatory conditions. Adverse effects include those associated with most of the corticosteroids, including fluid and electrolyte imbalances and gastrointestinal and endocrine disturbances.

prednisone (prĕd'nĭ-sōn') N. glucocorticoid used to treat allergic reactions, rheumatoid arthritis, and other inflammatory conditions. *See* TABLE OF COMMONLY PRESCRIBED DRUGS—GENERIC NAMES.

preeclampsia (prē'ĭ-klămp'sē-ə) N. abnormal condition of pregnancy characterized by hypertension, edema, and the presence of protein in the urine. Abnormal metabolic functioning, ocular disorders, and other complications frequently occur in the pregnant woman, malnutrition and lowered birth weight, in the fetus. Untreated severe preeclampsia can lead to eclampsia and convulsions that threaten the lives of both the mother and the fetus.

preferred provider organization (PPO) N. form of health care insurance in which the patient is only able to see designated physicians who are members of the organization. Typically, a person is assigned a gatekeeper or attending physician who provides primary care and, if needed, refers the patient to another physician, such as a specialist. The gatekeeper physician must approve the referral, and the PPO needs to approve, often in advance, visits to the emergency department and hospital admissions; otherwise, the insurance plan will pay neither the physician's charges nor the hospital bills. *See also* HEALTH MAINTENANCE ORGANIZATION. *See* TABLE OF MANAGED CARE TERMS.

prefrontal lobe (prē-frŭn′tl) N. region of the brain at the front part of each cerebral hemisphere; it is concerned with learning, memory, emotions, and behavior.

preganglionic (prē-găng′glē-ŏn′ĭk) ADJ. nerve fibers arising proximal to (before) a ganglion; compare to postganglionic fibers that originate distal to (after) a ganglion.

pregnancy (prĕg′nən-sē) N. gestation; the period during which a woman carries a developing fetus in the uterus, from the time of conception to the birth of the child. Pregnancy lasts 266 days from the day of fertilization, but is usually calculated as 280 days from the first day of the last menstrual period. The fertilized ovum, or zygote, implants in the wall of the uterus and undergoes growth and development, nourished and protected by the placenta, which forms from embryonic and maternal tissue in the uterus. Pregnancy involves changes in virtually every system of a woman's body, including increase in total blood volume and cardiac output; increase in kidney filtration and increased urination; enlargement of the breasts and changes in the color of the nipple area as the breasts prepare to provide milk for an infant; skin changes, sometimes including chloasma; gastrointestinal changes, often manifested as heartburn, nausea, vomiting, and constipation; increased nutritional needs and weight gain (20–25 pounds or more); and numerous endocrine changes, including increased thyroid and adrenal function and the release of hormones from the placenta. ADJ. pregnant

pregnancy test N. one of several blood or urine tests to determine the presence of human chorionic gonadotropin (HCG), suggesting pregnancy. Serum (blood) tests are most reliable and have the lowest false-positive and false-negative rates, though some urine tests are very specific (low false-positive rate). The results of over-the-counter pregnancy tests should always be confirmed by a medical laboratory.

pregnanediol N. compound found in the urine of pregnant women and in the urine of women during certain phases of the menstrual cycle.

preinvasive cancer *See* CARCINOMA IN SITU.

Premarin N. trade name for an estrogen compound. *See* TABLE OF COMMONLY PRESCRIBED DRUGS—TRADE NAMES.

premature ADJ. occurring before the normal time; not fully developed, esp. a premature infant.

premature ejaculation N. emission of semen and loss of erection during early stages of sexual excitement before or immediately after insertion of the penis in the vagina. Numerous behavioral techniques are used to extend the time between erection and ejaculation.

premature infant N. infant born before 37 weeks of gestation regardless of birth weight. A premature infant is usually of low birth weight; has incompletely developed organ systems; appears thin, with little subcutaneous fat; has a large head; and pinkish, translucent skin. The cause of prematurity is unknown in many cases, but in some is associated with toxemia, multiple pregnancy, chronic disease, trauma, or poor nutrition. The prognosis depends on the maturity of the various organ systems of the infant's body and on the postnatal care given, the best care being provided in neonatal intensive care units. Treatment involves maintenance of stable body temperature and respiration, provision for adequate fluid and nutrient intake, and prevention of infection. Also called preterm infant.

premature labor N. labor beginning before the 37th or 38th week of gestation or before the fetus has reached a weight of 2,000 grams. Premature labor may occur spontaneously without apparent cause, or it may result from trauma, chronic disease, infection in the mother, placental problems, or other causes; predisposing factors are poor nutrition, low weight gain, smoking, and multiple pregnancies. In some cases labor can be inhibited and the pregnancy prolonged to allow further development of the fetus.

premature ventricular contraction (PVC) (věn-trĭk'yə-lər) N. irregularity of cardiac rhythm. Isolated PVCs may not be significant, but frequent, recurrent PVCs usually indicate heart abnormality and may be a precursor of ventricular fibrillation and inadequate cardiac output.

premenstrual syndrome (PMS) (prē-měn'strōō-əl) N. poorly understood syndrome of tension, irritability, edema, headache, mastalgia (breast pain), bloating, appetite changes, and changes in muscular coordination occurring in many women several days before the onset of the menstrual flow.

premolar (prē-mō'lər) N. any of eight teeth in adult dentition, two on each side of each jaw, situated behind the canines and in front of the molars; also called bicuspids.

Prempro N. *See* TABLE OF COMMONLY PRESCRIBED DRUGS—TRADE NAMES.

prenatal (prē-nāt'l) ADJ. occurring or existing before birth; used in reference to the pregnant woman or the growth and development of the fetus; also called antenatal.

prenatal development N. process of growth, differentiation, development, and maturation between fertilization and birth. The fertilized egg immediately begins dividing in the process of cleavage; passes through the stages of morula, blastocyst, gastrula; the three primary germ layers are laid down; and differentiation of the tissues, organs, and organ systems of the body occurs. By 14 weeks all the major organs and systems of the body have been formed; from then on there is further growth and maturation, so that at birth the average fetus is about 20 inches (50 centimeters) long and weighs between 7 and 8 pounds (approx. 3.2–3.6 kilograms).

prenatal diagnosis N. any of various diagnostic procedures to determine whether the fetus has a genetic or other abnormality. The procedures involve X rays and ultrasonography (sonograms), which can reveal structural abnormalities and allow growth to be followed; amniocentesis, in which amniotic fluid is withdrawn for analysis and identification of chromosome and metabolic defects; and fetoscopy, whereby fetal blood can be withdrawn and analyzed. *See also* GENETIC COUNSELING.

preoperative (prē-ŏp′ər-ə-tĭv) ADJ. pert. to the period before surgery, when the patient is prepared for surgery by limitations on food and fluids by mouth, by removal of body hair on the area to be incised, by premedication, and/or by other procedures.

preprandial ADJ. pert. to the time before a meal.

prepuberty (prē-pyoō′bər-tē) N. period of about 2 years immediately before puberty when growth and changes leading to sexual maturity occur. ADJ. prepubertal

prepuce (prē′pyoōs′) *See* FORESKIN.

presbyopia (prĕz′bē-ō′pē-ə) N. farsightedness developing with advancing age as the lens of the eye becomes less elastic. ADJ. presbyopic

prescription N. written order for medication, therapy, or a device given by a properly authorized medical practitioner, esp. a written order for a drug given by a physician to a pharmacist.

prescription drug N. drug that can be dispensed to the public only with a prescription (*compare* OVER-THE-COUNTER DRUG).

presenile dementia (prē-sē′nīl′ dĭ-mĕn′shə) *See* ALZHEIMER'S DISEASE.

presentation (prĕz′ən-tā′shən) N. position of the fetus in the uterus with reference to the part of the fetus directed toward the birth canal. Normally the head

appears first (cephalic presentation), but in some cases the buttocks, feet, shoulder, or side may present first. Abnormal presentations may cause difficulty in childbirth, and attempts to turn the fetus may be made; if normal delivery is deemed hazardous, a Cesarean section is performed.

pressor (prĕs′ôr′) ADJ. increasing or tending to increase blood pressure.

pressure (prĕsh′ər) N. force or stress applied to a surface.

pressure point N. point over an artery where the pulse can be felt and where pressure on the point may stop hemorrhage distal to (beyond) that point.

pressure sore *See* DECUBITUS ULCER.

preterm infant (prē′tûrm′) *See* PREMATURE INFANT.

Prevacid N. *See* TABLE OF COMMONLY PRESCRIBED DRUGS—TRADE NAMES.

prevalence (prĕv′ə-ləns) N. in epidemiology, number of occurrences of a disease or event during a particular period of time; it is usually expressed as a ratio, the number of events occurring per the number of units in the population at risk for the occurrence.

preventive medicine (prĭ-vĕn′tĭv) N. that branch of medicine concerned primarily with the prevention of disease; it concerns itself with immunization, eradication of disease carriers (e.g., malaria-carrying mosquitoes), screening programs, and other factors.

priapism (prī′ə-pĭz′əm) N. abnormal condition in which the penis is constantly erect, often with pain and seldom with sexual arousal; it may be caused by lesions in the central nervous system or the penis itself or be associated with certain systemic diseases.

prickly heat *See* MILIARIA.

Prilosec N. trade name for the gastrointestinal agent omeprazole. *See* TABLE OF COMMONLY PRESCRIBED DRUGS—TRADE NAMES.

Primacor N. trade name for the drug milrinone, used to treat severe congestive heart failure.

primaquine (prī′mə-kwĭn) N. drug used to treat malaria. High doses may cause gastrointestinal upsets and blood disorders.

primary ADJ.
1. first in occurrence, importance, or development.
2. not derived from any other source, as the original condition in a disease process.

primary amenorrhea (ā-měn′ə-rē′ə) *See* AMENORRHEA.

primary care provider (PCP) N. provider, often a general practitioner, family practitioner, or internist, responsible for the coordination and general medical care of a patient. *See* TABLE OF MANAGED CARE TERMS.

primary dysmenorrhea (dĭs-měn′ə-ə-rē′ə) *See* DYSMENORRHEA.

primary health care N. health care provided by a physician, nurse, or other health care professional in the first contact of the patient with the health care system. It may involve a private internist, a family physician, pediatrician, an ambulatory health care facility, or a hospital emergency department.

primary tooth *See* DECIDUOUS TOOTH.

Primaxin N. trade name for a fixed-combination parenteral antibiotic consisting of impenem and cilastatin. The spectrum of this agent is very broad, there is minimal resistance to it, and the side effects are few.

primidone N. anticonvulsant used to treat grand mal epilepsy and other seizure disorders. Adverse effects include drowsiness, dizziness, ataxia, and blood disorders.

primigravida (prī′mĭ-grăv′ĭ-də) N. woman pregnant for the first time.

primipara (prī-mĭp′ər-ə) N. woman who has delivered a child (or children, as in twins or triplets) for the first time. ADJ. primiparous

primitive (prĭm′ĭ-tĭv) ADJ. undeveloped, undifferentiated, rudimentary.

primordial (prī-môr′dē-əl) ADJ. pert. to an undeveloped or primitive state; first or original.

primordial dwarf N. dwarf whose small size is due to a genetic defect in the response to growth hormone; there are normal proportion of body parts and normal mental and sexual development; also called normal dwarf; true dwarf; hypoplastic dwarf.

primordium (prī-môr′dē-əm) N., *pl.* primordia, first recognizable stage in the differentiation and development of a particular organ or structure. ADJ. primordial

Prinivil N. trade name for the antihypertensive lisinopril. *See* TABLE OF COMMONLY PRESCRIBED DRUGS—TRADE NAMES.

prion (prē-än) N. short for proteinaceous infectious particle—infectious self-reproducing protein structures. Though their exact mechanisms of action and reproduction are unknown, it is now commonly accepted that prions are responsible for a number of previously known but little-understood diseases including kuru, Creutzfeldt-Jakob disease (CJD), and bovine spongiform encephalopathy (BSE or mad cow disease). These diseases affect the structure of brain tissue and all are fatal and untreatable. Not all prions are dangerous; in fact, prion-like proteins are found naturally in many (perhaps all) plants and animals. Disease occurs when the prion protein undergoes a change from its normal structure to an abnormal one. This change prevents the abnormal protein from being degraded properly. The change may occur spontaneously at an extremely low rate (resulting in sporadic cases) or at a higher rate if various mutations are present. *See also* BOVINE SPONGIFORM ENCEPHALOPATHY; CREUTZFELDT-JAKOB DISEASE; KURU.

prn in prescriptions, abbreviation for pro re nata, meaning as needed.

pro- prefix meaning before, in front of, preceding (e.g., proenzyme, precursor of an enzyme, as pepsinogen is the precursor of pepsin).

probenecid (prō-bĕn′ĭ-sĭd) N. drug that reduces the level of uric acid in the blood and is used in the treatment of gout. Adverse effects include urinary frequency, headache, skin rashes, and stomach upsets.

procainamide N. antiarrhythmic drug (trade name Pronestyl) to treat rhythm disturbances of the heart; it is most commonly used in patients who have frequent premature ventricular contractions, or cardiac arrest. Administration is either oral or intravenous, and side effects may include systemic lupus erythematosus or worsened cardiac arrhythmias.

procaine (prō′kān′) N. local anesthetic (trade name Novocaine) used for epidural, caudal, and other regional anesthesia; it is not used topically. Adverse effects include neurological and cardiovascular reactions.

procarbazine (prō-kär′bə-zēn) N. antineoplastic used to treat Hodgkin's disease and other neoplasms. Adverse effects include bone marrow depression, nausea, and vomiting.

Procardia N. trade name for the calcium blocker nifedipine. *See* TABLE OF COMMONLY PRESCRIBED DRUGS—TRADE NAMES.

process N. in anatomy, thin projection or prominence, as on the vertebrae.

prochlorperazine N. antipsychotic and antiemetic (trade name Compazine) used to treat schizophrenia and certain other mental disorders and to combat nausea and vomiting. Adverse effects include drowsiness, abnormal muscle movements, low blood pressure, liver toxicity, and blood abnormalities.

procidentia N. sinking of an organ. The uterus, for example, may descend into the vagina until most of the uterus lies outside of the vulva.

proct-, procto- comb. forms indicating an association with the rectum (e.g., proctalgia, pain in the rectum).

proctitis (prŏk-tī′tĭs) N. inflammation of the rectum, characterized by blood in the stool, frequent urge to defecate but inability to do so, and sometimes diarrhea. It may be associated with ulcerative colitis or Crohn's disease, or trauma, infection, or radiation may cause it.

proctocele (prŏk′tə-sēl′) *See* RECTOCELE.

proctologist N. physician who specializes in proctology.

proctology (prŏk-tŏl′ə-jē) N. that branch of medicine concerned with the diagnosis and treatment of disorders of the colon, rectum, and anus.

proctoscope (prŏk′tə-skōp′) N. instrument (a type of endoscope) used to examine the rectum and the end portion of the colon.

proctoscopy (prŏk′tŏs′kə-pē) N. medical procedure of using a lighted scope (proctoscope) to examine the rectum and anus by direct visualization.

procyclidine N. drug (trade name Kemadrin) used to reduce tremor in Parkinsonism and also to control the side effects of antipsychotic medications. Adverse effects include dry mouth, blurred vision, rapid heartbeat, and decreased sweating.

prodrome (prō′drōm′) N. earliest sign of a disease or a developing condition. ADJ. prodromal.

progenitor (prō-jĕn′ĭ-tər) N. parent or ancestor.

progeny (prŏj′ə-nē) N. offspring.

progeria (prō-jēr′ē-ə) N. rare, abnormal condition characterized by premature aging and the appearance of gray hair, wrinkled skin, and the posture of an aged person in a child or adolescent. The cause is unknown.

progesterone (prō-jĕs′tə-rōn′) N. hormone produced by the corpus luteum of the ovary, the placenta during pregnancy, and in small amounts by the adrenal cortex; it prepares the uterus for a fertilized egg. Natural and synthetic progesterones and progestational compounds (e.g., norethindrone) are used in oral contraceptives and in drugs to treat abnormal uterine bleeding. adj. progestational.

progestin (prō-jĕs′tĭn) N. any natural or synthetic progestational hormone.

prognosis (prŏg-nō′sĭs) N. prediction of the probable outcome of a disease, based on what is known about the usual course of the disease and on the age and general health of the patient.

progressive (prə-grĕs′ĭv) ADJ. increasing, worsening, as a progressive muscular disease.

projection (prə-jĕk′shən) N.
1. protruberance, something that juts out.
2. in psychology, unconscious defense mechanism in which a person attributes his/her own unacceptable ideas and attitudes to another person.

prokaryote (prō-kăr′ē-ōt′) N. organism containing cells without nuclei, the nuclear material being scattered throughout the cell. Bacteria, blue-green algae, and certain other microorganisms are prokaryotes. (*Compare* EUKARYOTE.)

prolactin (prō-lăk′tĭn) N. hormone produced in and secreted by the anterior pituitary gland that stimulates growth and development of mammary glands in females and the production of milk after delivery; also called lactogenic hormone; luteotropin.

prolapse (prō-lăps′) N. dropping or falling of an organ from its normal position, as in prolapse of the uterus into the vagina.

proliferation (prə-lĭf'ə-rā'shən) N. growth by rapid multiplication of parts, such as by cell division.

promethazine N. antihistamine (trade name Phenergan) used to treat allergies and to induce sedation; it is also an antiemetic, effective in treating nausea, esp. that of motion sickness. Adverse effects include drowsiness and dry mouth. *See* TABLE OF COMMONLY PRESCRIBED DRUGS—GENERIC NAMES.

promontory (prŏm'ən-tôr'ē) N. projecting part or process.

pronation (prō-nā'shən) N. action of lying face downward or turning the hand so that the palm is downward.

prone (prōn) ADJ. lying with the face and abdomen downward.

Pronestyl N. trade name for the antiarrhythmic drug, procainamide.

pronucleus (prō-noō'klē-əs) N., *pl.* pronuclei, nucleus of the ovum or the spermatozoon after fertilization but before fusion of the pronuclei to form the nucleus of the zygote. Each pronucleus contains the haploid chromosome number.

Propacet N. *See* TABLE OF COMMONLY PRESCRIBED DRUGS—TRADE NAMES.

propafenone N. antiarrhythmic (trade name Rhythmol) designed for treatment of severe, refractory, and life-threatening ventricular arrhythmias; side effects include gastrointestinal reactions or an increase in the frequency of dysrhythmias.

propagation (prŏp'ə-gā'shən) N. reproduction, the act of giving birth; regarding nerves, transmission of electrical impulses from one part to the other. In the heart, a wave of electrical stimulation propagates (passes) from top to bottom causing sequential contraction of the upper portions (atria) followed by the lower ones (ventricles).

propantheline N. drug (trade name Probanthine) that decreases smooth muscle activity and is used to treat peptic ulcer and certain other gastrointestinal disorders. Adverse effects include rapid heart rate, dry mouth, allergic reactions, and central nervous system disturbances.

prophase (prō'fāz') first of the four major phases of nuclear division (mitosis and meiosis) in which the nuclear membrane disappears and the chromosomes become recognizable individually and start to move toward the midplane of the developing spindle.

prophylactic (prō'fə-lăk'tĭk) ADJ. preventing the spread of disease, as a prophylactic agent. N. agent that prevents disease; often used colloq. for condom.

prophylaxis (prō'fə-lăk'sĭs) N. prevention of disease. ADJ. prophylactic

propoxyphene hydrochloride (prō-pŏk'sə-fēn' hī'drə-klôr'īd') N. mild narcotic analgesic (trade name Darvon) used to relieve mild to moderate pain. Adverse effects include liver disorders and oversedation.

propoxyphene acetaminophen N. *See* TABLE OF COMMONLY PRESCRIBED DRUGS—GENERIC NAMES.

propranolol (prō-prăn'ə-lôl') N. beta blocking agent (trade name Inderal) used in the treatment of hypertension and of angina pectoris and other heart ailments. Adverse effects include cardiac and gastrointestinal disturbances and hypersensitivity reactions. *See* TABLE OF COMMONLY PRESCRIBED DRUGS—GENERIC NAMES.

proprioceptor (prō′prē-ō-sĕp′tər) N. sensory nerve ending, located in muscles, tendons, and other organs, that responds to internal stimuli regarding body position and movement.

proptosis (präp-tō-səs) *See* EXOPHTHALMOS.

Propulsid N. *See* TABLE OF COMMONLY PRESCRIBED DRUGS—TRADE NAMES.

prosencephalon (prŏs′ĕn-sĕf′ə-lŏn′) *See* FOREBRAIN.

prostaglandin (prŏs′tə-glăn′dĭn) N. any of a group of hormone-like fatty acids produced in small amounts in many body tissues including the uterus, brain, kidneys, and semen. Prostaglandins act on target organs to produce wide-ranging effects. They affect capillary action, endocrine, nervous system, and smooth muscle activities, as well as many other body functions, including contractions of the uterus and regulation of blood pressure. Aspirin and certain other analgesics (nonsteroidal anti-inflammatory agents) are believed to act by interfering with the synthesis or reaction of certain prostaglandins.

prostate (prŏs′tāt′) N. firm, chestnut-sized gland in males at the neck of the urethra that produces a secretion that is the fluid part of semen. ADJ. prostatic

prostate cancer N. cancer of the male prostate gland. Except for skin cancer, cancer of the prostate is the most common malignancy in American men. The most common risk factor is age. More than 70 percent of men diagnosed with prostate cancer each year are over the age of 65. African American men have a higher risk of prostate cancer than white men. In most men the disease grows very slowly. The majority of men with low-grade, early prostate cancer (confined to the gland) live a long time after

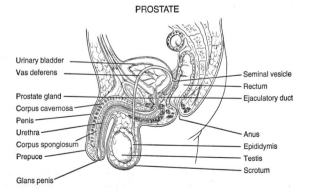

PROSTATE

Urinary bladder
Vas deferens
Prostate gland
Corpus cavernosa
Penis
Urethra
Corpus spongiosum
Prepuce
Glans penis

Seminal vesicle
Rectum
Ejaculatory duct
Anus
Epididymis
Testis
Scrotum

their diagnosis, dying of an unrelated cause. In some men, however, the disease is very aggressive, painful, and fatal. Prostate cancer often does not cause symptoms for many years. When symptoms do occur, they may include frequent urination, especially at night; inability or difficulty urinating; painful urination or ejaculation; blood in the urine or semen; and pain in the lower back, hips, or upper thighs. Two tests can be used to detect prostate cancer in the absence of any symptoms. One is the digital rectal exam (DRE), in which a physician feels the prostate through the rectum to find hard or lumpy areas. The other is a blood test used to detect a substance made by the prostate called prostate specific antigen (PSA). Together, these tests can detect many "silent" prostate cancers that have not caused symptoms. At present, however, it is not known whether routine screening saves lives. The diagnosis of prostate cancer can be confirmed only by a biopsy. Three treatment options are generally accepted for men with localized prostate cancer: radical prostatectomy, radiation therapy, and surveillance (also called watchful waiting). Radical prostatectomy is a surgical procedure to remove the entire prostate gland and nearby tissues. Sometimes lymph nodes in the pelvic area are also removed. Radical prostatectomy may be performed using a technique called nerve-sparing surgery that may prevent damage to the nerves needed for an erection. *See also* BIOPSY; PROSTATE; PROSTATE SPECIFIC ANTIGEN; PROSTATECTOMY.

prostate specific antigen N. protein produced only in the prostate gland; the level dramatically increases in patients with prostate cancer; used in diagnosis and in monitoring the response of the patient to treatment.

prostatectomy (prŏs′tə-tĕk′təmē) N. surgical removal of all or part of the prostate gland, performed to treat benign overgrowth or malignant neoplasm. ADJ. prostatic

prostatitis (prŏs′tə-tī′tĭs) N. inflammation of the prostate gland, usually the result of infection. Symptoms include pain in the perineal area, frequency or retention of urine, and, if severe, fever and chills. Treatment is by antibiotics.

prostatorrhea N. discharge from the prostate, usually the result of prostate infection.

prosthesis (prŏs-thē′sĭs) N. artificial device attached to the body to aid its function or replace a missing part; included among prostheses are artificial limbs, hearing aids, and implanted pacemakers.

prostration (prŏ-strā′shən) N. state of exhaustion. *See also* HEAT EXHAUSTION.

protease (prŏt-ē-āz) N. enzyme that breaks down proteins.

protease inhibitor N. class of anti-HIV (Human Immunodeficiency Virus) drugs designed to inhibit the enzyme protease and interfere with virus replication. Protease inhibitors prevent the cleavage of HIV precursor proteins into active proteins, a process that normally occurs when HIV replicates; used in therapy of AIDS and HIV infection. *See also* ACQUIRED IMMUNE DEFI-

CIENCY SYNDROME [AIDS]; HUMAN IMMUNODEFICIENCY VIRUS.

protein N. any of a large group of complex compounds, containing carbon, hydrogen, oxygen, nitrogen, and sometimes phosphorus and sulfur, and consisting of chains of amino acids joined by peptide bonds. Proteins form the structural part of most organs, and make up enzymes and hormones that regulate body functions. They are synthesized in the body from their constituent amino acids, obtained in the diet.

proteinuria (prōt'n-ōōr'ē-ə) N. presence of abnormally large amounts of protein, chiefly albumin, in the urine; it is usually associated with kidney disorder but can also result from fever or other causes.

proteolysis (prō'tē-ŏl'ĭ-sĭs) N. breakdown of complex proteins into their constituent amino acids through the action of proteolytic enzymes. ADJ. proteolytic

prothrombin (prō-thrŏm'bĭn) N. plasma protein that is a precursor of thrombin, a final step in blood coagulation; also called Factor II.

proton N. positively charged subatomic particle that forms the nucleus of all atoms.

protoplasm (prō'tə-plăz'əm) N. essential substance of all cells, including cytoplasm and nucleus. ADJ. protoplasmic

protozoal infection N. any disease, such as malaria, caused by a protozoan.

protozoan (prō'tə-zō'ən) N., pl. protozoa, single-celled, animal-like microorganism; some protozoa produce disease in humans.

protriptyline N. antidepressant used to treat depression. Adverse effects include dry mouth, gastrointestinal and cardiovascular disturbances, and the possibility of interaction with many other drugs.

Protropin N. trade name for a human growth hormone preparation that is available for administration to children who are deficient in this compound. Although intended primarily for children with documented deficiency, this drug has found its way into illicit use by weight lifters and other athletes. It is on the list of banned substances of the U.S. Olympic Committee.

protuberance (prō-tōō'bər-əns) N. projecting part, esp. a rounded projection (e.g., mental protuberance, projecting part of the chin).

Proventil (prō-věn'tl) N. trade name for the bronchodilator albuterol. *See* TABLE OF COMMONLY PRESCRIBED DRUGS—TRADE NAMES.

Provera N. trade name of a progestin. *See* TABLE OF COMMONLY PRESCRIBED DRUGS—TRADE NAMES.

provider N. hospital or health care facility, or a physician, nurse, physical therapist or other individual involved in providing medical care services to patients. *See* TABLE OF MANAGED CARE TERMS.

provitamin N. substance that in the body may be converted into a vitamin; a vitamin precursor.

proximal (prŏk'sə-məl) ADJ. nearer to or toward an axis or center, as the trunk of the body (*compare* DISTAL).

Prozac (prō′zăk′) N. trade name for fluoxetine hydrochloride. *See* TABLE OF COMMONLY PRESCRIBED DRUGS—TRADE NAMES.

prurigo (proo-rī′gō) N. any of a group of skin inflammations characterized by multiple blister-capped papules that are itchy and may become hardened and crusted as a result of repeated scratching. Causes include allergies, drug reactions, and endocrine imbalances. Treatment depends on the cause.

pruritus (proo-rī′təs) N. itching; causes include allergies, lymphoma, jaundice, infection, and other factors. Treatment depends on the cause, but antihistamines, corticosteroids, cool applications, or alcohol applications may obtain relief of the itching.

  pruritus ani N. common and chronic itchiness of the skin around the anus, often caused by contact dermatitis, pinworms, Candida infection, or hemorrhoids.

  pruritus vulvae N. persistent itching of the external female genitalia, often associated with Candida infection, trichomoniasis, or contact dermatitis.

PSA N. abbrev. for prostate specific antigen.

psammoma (să-mō′mə) N. small tumor containing sandlike particles and occurring in the meninges, ovaries, and certain other organs; also called sand tumor.

pseudo- comb. form meaning false (e.g., pseudojaundice, yellowing of the skin caused, not by excess bilirubin, but usually by excessive ingestion of carotene-containing foods).

pseudocyesis (soo′dō-sī-ē′sĭs) N. false pregnancy; a condition in which a woman experiences symptoms of pregnancy, including cessation of menstruation, enlargement of the breasts and abdomen, and weight gain, but is not pregnant; it is usually linked to hormonal changes brought about by emotional stress.

pseudogout (soo -dō-gout) N. form of arthritis characterized by a painful, sudden attack of a hot, very swollen, red joint, caused by calcium crystals in the joint. Severe attacks of pseudogout often occur in the knees and can incapacitate someone for days or weeks. The wrists, shoulders, ankles, elbows, or hands may also be affected. Clinically, the presentation may mimic gout, though the joint crystals found in gout are different (uric acid). Treatment involves nonsteroidal anti-inflammatory drugs (NSAIDs) or steroid injection into the affected joint. To prevent further attacks, low doses of colchicine (available only as a generic) or NSAIDs may be effective. Unfortunately, no treatment is available to dissolve the crystal deposits. If severe joint degeneration occurs over time, surgery to repair and replace damaged joints is an option. (*Compare* GOUT.)

pseudohermaphroditism (soo′dō-hər-măf′rə-dī-tĭz′əm) N. congenital condition in which either a male or a female has external genitalia resembling those of the opposite sex (e.g., a woman with an enlarged clitoris and labia resembling a penis and scrotum [*compare* ANDROGYNE]). ADJ. pseudohermaphroditic

pseudohypertrophic dystro′ (soo′dō-hī-pûr′trō′fĭk dĭ′

fē) *See* MUSCULAR DYSTROPHY, DUCHENNE'S.

pseudomembrane (soo'dō-měm'brān') N. false membrane, consisting of an exudate forming on skin or mucous membrane (e.g., the false membrane occurring in the throat in diphtheria).

psittacosis (sĭt'ə-kō'sĭs) N. infectious disease, caused by the bacterium *Chlamydia psittaci*, transmitted to humans by infected birds, esp. parrots; it is characterized by pneumonia-like symptoms, including fever, headache, and cough. Treatment is by tetracyclines. Also called parrot fever; ornithosis.

psoas N. either of two muscles of the abdomen and pelvis that flex the trunk and rotate the thigh. *See* MAJOR MUSCLES OF THE BODY, in Appendix.

psoas abscess (ăb'sĕs') N. accumulation of pus and other inflammatory material (e.g., white blood cells) within either of the two psoas muscles of the abdomen and pelvis that flex the trunk and rotate the thigh; may be caused by several bacteria, including those responsible for tuberculosis.

psoriasis (sə-rī'ə-sĭs) N. chronic skin disorder characterized by periods of remission and exacerbation of dry, scale-covered red patches esp. on the scalp, ears, genitalia, and skin over bony prominences; a type of arthritis may occur with the skin disorder. Treatment includes corticosteroids, ultraviolet light, and the use of medicated creams and shampoos.

psoriatic arthritis N. form of rheumatoid arthritis most often affecting small distal joints (esp. in the fingers and toes),

occurring in association with psoriasis.

psych-, psycho- comb. forms indicating an association with the mind (e.g., psychopharmacology, study of the effects of drugs on the mind and on the treatment of mental disorders).

psyche (sī'kē) N. mind, including conscious and unconscious processes; in psychoanalysis the total of the id, ego, superego, and all conscious and unconscious processes.

psychedelic ADJ.
1. describing a mental state with hallucinations, altered perceptions, and usually strong emotions.
2. pert. to a drug that produces these effects.

psychiatrist (sĭ-kī'ə-trĭst) N. physician who specializes in psychiatry.

psychiatry (sĭ-kī'ə-trē) N. that branch of medicine concerned with the study of the mind and the diagnosis, treatment, and prevention of mental, emotional, and behavioral disorders. ADJ. psychiatric

psychoactive (sī'kō-ăk'tĭv) ADJ. affecting the state of one's mind; usually refers to a drug (i.e., psychoactive drug).

psychoanalysis (sī'kō-ə-năl'ĭ-sĭs) N. branch of psychiatry, founded by Sigmund Freud, in which the processes of the mind are studied through techniques such as dream interpretation and free association to bring repressed conflicts into the consciousness, analyze them, and adjust behavioral patterns related to them. ADJ. psychoanalytic

psychogenic ADJ. originating in the mind, not in the body; referring esp. to symptoms or diseases of psychological, not physical, origin.

psychology (sī-kŏl′ə-jē) N. study of mental activity, esp. as it relates to behavior. ADJ. psychologic; psychological.

psychometrics (sī′kə-mĕt′rĭks) N. measurement of individual differences in psychological functions, such as intelligence, by means of standardized tests.

psychomotor (sī′kō-mō′tər) ADJ. pert. to mental and motor activities esp. in reference to disorders in which muscular activity is affected by brain disorder.

psychomotor development N. gradual and progressive acquisition and attainment of skills involving both mental and motor activity, as a child of 5 or 6 months learning to sit up, a child of 1–1½ years learning to walk, and a child of 3 years being able to feed him/herself.

psychopath (sī′kə-păth′) N. person with a personality disorder in which behavior is antisocial and, in the extreme, may be criminal; also called sociopath. ADJ. psychopathic

psychopathology N. study of the causes and manifestations of mental disorders.

psychopathy N. any disease of the mind; it may be congenital or acquired.

psychophysiology N. that branch of psychology that observes and records physiological changes and how they relate to mental activities.

psychosexual (sī′kō-sĕk′shoō-əl) ADJ. pert. to the psychological aspects of sex.

psychosexual development N. in psychoanalytic theory, the process during childhood and adolescence by which personality and mature sexual behavior emerge. The process is divided into stages, each characterized by sexual interest and gratification centered on a particular part of the body; the stages are the oral phase, anal phase, phallic phase, latency phase, and genital phase.

psychosis (sī-kō′sĭs) N. major mental disorder in which the person is usually detached from reality and has impaired perceptions, thinking, responses, and interpersonal relationships. Most people with psychoses require hospitalization; treatment involves the use of psychoactive drugs and psychotherapy (*compare* NEUROSIS). ADJ. psychotic

psychosomatic (sī′kō-sō-mătʹĭk) ADJ. pert. to the interaction of the mind and the body.

psychosomatic medicine N. that branch of medicine concerned with the relationship of mental and emotional reactions to body processes, esp. the way in which emotional conflicts affect physical symptoms.

psychosurgery (sī′kō-sûr′jə-rē) N. surgery of the brain, usually involving interruption of certain nerve pathways, to relieve severe abnormal psychological symptoms; the procedure is now employed only when other treatments (e.g., psychotherapy and drugs) have proved ineffective. Marked changes in personality and also often in cognitive and other mental processes occur.

psychotherapy (sī′kō-thĕr′ə-pē) N. treatment of mental disorders by psychological, not physical, techniques. There are many approaches to psychotherapy, including behavior modification, psychoanalysis, and group therapy.

psychotropic (sī'kə-trō'pĭk) ADJ. pert. to drugs that affect mood, such as tranquilizers and antidepressants.

pteroylglutamic acid (tĕr'ō-ĭl-glōō-tăm'ĭk) *See* FOLIC ACID.

pterygium (tə-rĭj'ē-əm) N. thickened flap of tissue extending from the nasal border of the cornea to the inner corner of the eye. The flaps usually arise when a preexisting pinguecula becomes irritated by wind or dust and begin to encroach upon the cornea. Treatment is surgical if the pterygium covers too much of the corneal surface.

ptomaine (tō'mān') N.
1. breakdown product resulting from the action of various bacteria on proteins (usually of foodstuffs).
2. colloquial term for food poisoning.

-ptosis (tō'sĭs) comb. form indicating a drop or prolapse of an organ from its normal position (e.g., metroptosis, dropping of the uterus).

ptosis N. drooping of one or both upper eyelids; it may be congenital or result from damage to the oculomotor nerve, myasthenia gravis, or other disorder.

ptyalin (tī'ə-lĭn) N. enzyme present in the mouth that starts the digestion of starches.

ptyalism (tī'ə-lĭz'əm) N. excessive salivation, sometimes occurring in pregnancy, certain poisonings, and neurological disorders.

ptyalith N. stone (calculus) in a salivary gland.

ptyalo- comb. form indicating an association with saliva (e.g.,

ptyalocele, saliva-containing tumor).

Pu symbol for the element plutonium.

puberty (pyōō'bər-tē) N. time at which sexual maturity occurs and the reproductive function becomes possible. It is characterized by the development of secondary sexual characteristics, such as breast development in girls and deepening voice in males, and by the start of menstruation in girls. The changes are brought about by pituitary gland-stimulated increases in sex hormones. ADJ. pubertal

pubes (pyōō'bēz) N. hair-covered surface covering the pubis at the front of the pelvis.

pubic bone (pyōō'bĭk) *See* PUBIS.

pubis (pyōō'bĭs) N., *pl.* pubes, one of the three bones that make up the innominate (hip) bone on each side of the body (the other two bones being the ilium and ischium); the two pubes meet at the front of the pelvis. ADJ. pubic

pubococcygeus exercises *See* KEGEL EXERCISES.

pudendal block N. form of regional anesthesia in which a local anesthetic agent is used to anesthetize the pudendal nerves in the region of the vulva, labia majora, and perirectal area to ease discomfort during childbirth.

pudendum (pyōō-dĕn'dəm) N., *pl.* pudenda, external genitalia, esp. those of a woman, including the mons veneris, labia majora, labia minora, and the opening of the vagina. (In males the pudendum includes the penis, scrotum, and testes.) ADJ. pudendal

puerile ADJ. pert. to children or childhood.

puerpera (pyoo-ûr′pər-ə) N. woman who has just delivered a baby.

puerperal (pyoo-ûr′pər-əl) ADJ. pert. to the period just after childbirth or to the woman who has just given birth.

puerperal fever N. bacterial infection and septicemia occurring in a woman after childbirth, usually due to unsanitary conditions. Symptoms include inflammation of the uterus, fever, rapid heartbeat, and foul lochia (vaginal discharge), followed, if untreated, by prostration, renal failure, shock, and death. The condition is now uncommon; when it occurs it is treated with antibiotics. Also called childbed fever.

puerperium (pyoo-oo′ər-pēr′ē-əm) N. time following childbirth during which the anatomic and functional changes of pregnancy resolve (e.g., the uterus shrinks).

pulmo-, pulmono- comb. forms indicating an association with the lungs (e.g., pulmogram, an X-ray film of the lungs).

pulmonary (pool′mə-nĕr′ē) ADJ. pert. to the lungs or respiratory system.

pulmonary artery N. artery that carries deoxygenated blood from the right ventricle of the heart to the lungs for oxygenation. The artery leaves the heart and passes upward before dividing, one branch going to each lung. *See also* PULMONARY CIRCULATION.

pulmonary circulation N. system of blood vessels transporting blood between the lungs and the lungs. Deoxygenated blood leaves the right ventricle by way of the pulmonary artery, which divides, sending branches to each lung. The deoxygenated blood gives off its carbon dioxide and takes in oxygen in the alveoli of the lungs. The freshly oxygenated blood is then transported by the pulmonary vein to the left atrium of the heart, where it enters the systemic circulation for transport throughout the body.

pulmonary edema (ĭ-dē′mə) N. accumulation of edema fluid in the lungs that results in an acute onset of severe shortness of breath and sometimes coughing of frothy sputum; it usually occurs rapidly as a consequence of coronary artery disease, but may also appear as a complication of an acute myocardial infarction; treatment consists of diuretics, nitroglycerin, morphine, and oxygen.

pulmonary embolism (ĕm′bə-lĭz′əm) N. blockage of a pulmonary artery by foreign matter or a thrombus (blood clot); it is characterized by difficult breathing, and sharp chest pain worsened by deep inspiration. If severe, shock and bluish discoloration of the skin (cyanosis) can develop, as can pleural effusion, heart rhythm abnormalities, and death. Predisposing factors include prolonged immobilization, esp. associated with surgery; blood-vessel-wall damage; and factors that increase the tendency of the blood to clot. Treatment is by anticoagulants and oxygen. In some cases, either surgery to remove the clot or administration of a thrombolytic drug may be used.

pulmonary function tests N. battery of breathing function tests using a spirogram or spirometer to determine the amount of and speed at which air moves in and out of the lungs.

pulmonary valve *See* SEMILUNAR VALVE.

pulmonary vein N. either of two blood vessels, one leaving each lung, that return oxygenated blood to the left atrium of the heart.

pulp N.
1. soft, spongy tissue, found in the spleen and certain other parts of the body.
2. connective tissue containing nerves and blood vessels that is at the center of a tooth under the dentin.

pulse (pŭls) N. regular, rhythmic beating of an artery resulting from the pumping action of the heart. The pulse is easily detected on superficial arteries (e.g., the radial artery at the wrist) and corresponds to each beat of the heart. The average adult pulse at rest is 60–80 beats per minute, but this may change with illness, emotional stress, exercise, or other factors.

pulseless disease (pŭls′lĭs) *See* TAKAYASU'S ARTERITIS.

punctum (pŭngk′təm) N. in anatomy, small area or point (e.g., punctum lacrimale, tiny opening of the tear ducts in the inner corners of the eyelids).

puncture (pŭngk′chər) V. to pierce with a sharp instrument. N. wound made by a sharp instrument; it may be made accidentally as a result of trauma or deliberately as in a diagnostic procedure to withdraw fluid for examination.

pupil (pyoo′pəl) N. circular opening in the center of the iris, lying behind the anterior chamber and cornea and in front of the lens,

through which light passes to the lens and retina. The diameter of the pupil changes with muscle action of the iris in response to changes in light and other stimulation. ADJ. pupillary.

pupillary reflex (pyoo′pə-lĕr′ē) N. reflex changes in the size of the pupil triggered by the amount of light entering the eye. Bright light stimulates the pupil to contract; dim light stimulates the pupil to widen.

pupillo- comb. form indicating an association with the pupil (e.g., pupillomotor, pert. to pupil movement).

purgative (pûr′gə-tĭv) N. *See* LAXATIVE.

purine (pyoor′ēn′) N. any of a group of nitrogen-containing compounds; some (adenine and guanine) are part of deoxyribonucleic acid (DNA) and ribonucleic acid (RNA) structure; some result from the digestion of proteins, and some are synthesized in the body.

Purkinje network (pər-kĭn′jē) N. network of specialized cardiac muscle fibers that carry the cardiac impulse from the atrioventricular node to the ventricles of the heart, causing them to contract. Sometimes called Purkinje fibers. *See* CARDIAC CONDUCTION SYSTEM.

purpura (pûr′pə-rə) N. any of several disorders in which the escape of blood into tissues below the skin causes reddish or purplish spots (petechiae); it may be due to a defect in capillaries caused by such agents as bacteria or drugs (nonthrombocytopenic purpura), or to a deficiency of platelets, due to such factors as drug reactions or infections or toxic disorders (thrombocytopenic purpura).

Typically, petechiae are smaller while purpuric lesions are larger and blotchier in nature.

purse-string operation *See* SHIRODKAR'S OPERATION.

purulent (pyoor'ə-lənt) ADJ. producing or containing pus.

pus (pŭs) N. thick, yellowish or greenish fluid, containing dead white blood cells, bacteria, and dead tissue, formed at an infection site.

pustule (pŭs'chool) N. small pus-containing elevation on the skin. ADJ. pustular

putrefaction (pyoo'trə-făk'shən) N. breakdown of proteins by bacteria, usually causing an unpleasant odor.

PVC *See* PREMATURE VENTRICULAR CONTRACTION.

pyelogram (pī'ə-lə-grăm') N. X ray of the kidney and ureters. In an intravenous pyelogram (IVP), a radiopaque dye that shows the outline of the kidney and associated structures is injected into the patient; the procedure is used to detect tumors, kidney stones, and other abnormalities of the urinary tract.

pyelonephritis (pī'ə-lō-nə-frī'tĭs) N. infection, usually bacterial, of the kidney. Acute pyelonephritis, usually resulting from the spread of a bladder infection, causes chills, fever, pain in the flank region, and urinary frequency. Chronic pyelonephritis, often associated with a stone or narrowing of the urinary passageways, develops more slowly and may, if untreated, lead to renal failure. Treatment involves antimicrobial drugs and removal of any obstruction.

pyemia (pī-ē'mē-ə) N. blood poisoning by pus-forming bacteria released from an abscess; abscesses may develop in various parts of the body. ADJ. pyemic

pyloric sphincter (sfĭngk'tər) N. muscular ring in the stomach separating the stomach from the duodenum; also called pyloric valve.

pyloric stenosis (stə-nō'sĭs) N. narrowing of the pyloric sphincter, blocking the passage of food into the duodenum from the stomach and often causing projectile (forceful) vomiting. It may be congenital or, in adults, result from an ulcer or neoplasm. Treatment is usually by surgery.

pylorus (pī-lôr'əs) N. tubular portion of the stomach, encircled by the pyloric sphincter, leading into the duodenum.

pyogenic ADJ. producing pus.

pyorrhea N.
1. discharge of pus.
2. purulent inflammation of tissues surrounding the teeth.

pyramidal tract (pĭ-răm'ĭ-dl) N. pathway in the medulla oblongata where nerve fibers pass from the brain to the spinal cord. In this area the fibers from one side of the brain cross to the opposite side of the spinal cord, giving the region a pyramid-shaped structure.

pyrectic ADJ. having fever. N. substance that produces fever.

pyrexia (pī-rĕk'sē-ə) *See* FEVER.

pyridoxine (pĭr'ĭ-dŏk'sēn) N. water-soluble vitamin, part of the B-complex group; it functions as a coenzyme in many metabolic processes; also called vitamin B$_6$. *See also* TABLE OF VITAMINS.

pyrilamine N. antihistamine used to treat many allergic reactions, including rhinitis and pruritus. Adverse effects include drowsiness, dry mouth, and skin rashes.

pyrimidine (pī-rĭm′ĭ-dēn′) N. any of several nitrogen-containing compounds, including cytosine, thymine, and uracil, important in the structures of deoxyribonucleic acid (DNA) and ribonucleic acid (RNA).

pyrogen N. substance (e.g., bacterial toxin) that raises body temperature.

pyromania (pī′rō-mā′nē-ə) N. uncontrollable urge to set fires.

pyrosis (pī-rō′sĭs) *See* HEARTBURN.

pyuria (pī-yŏŏr′ē-ə) N. presence of leukocytes (white blood cells) in the urine, usually a sign of urinary tract infection.

Q

Q fever N. acute illness, caused by the rickettsia *Coxiella burnetti,* transmitted to humans through contact with infected animals, esp. sheep, goats, and cattle; symptoms include high fever and signs of respiratory illness. Treatment is by tetracycline antibiotics.

qi *See* TABLE OF ALTERNATIVE MEDICINE TERMS.

qigong *See* TABLE OF ALTERNATIVE MEDICINE TERMS.

quadrant (kwŏd′rənt) N. one-fourth of a circle; anatomically, one of four regions divided equally for descriptive and diagnostic purposes. The four quadrants of the abdomen are formed by mentally drawing intersecting perpendicular lines through the navel (umbilicus). These lines form the right upper, left upper, right lower, left lower quadrants. The pain from appendicitis often localizes in the right lower quadrant while gall-bladder pain is typically in the right upper quadrant.

quadrantanopia N. condition characterized by loss of one fourth of a person's visual field.

quadri- comb. form indicating four (e.g., quadricuspid, tooth having four points on its surface).

quadriceps (kwŏd′rĭ-sĕps′) N. one of the extensor muscles of the legs. *See* MAJOR MUSCLES OF THE BODY, in Appendix.

quadripara N. woman who has given birth to a viable infant after each of four pregnancies.

quadriplegia (kwŏd′rə-plē′jē-ə) N. paralysis affecting all four limbs and the trunk of the body below the level of spinal cord injury. Trauma is the usual cause.

quadruplet (kwŏ-drŭp′lĭt) N. any of four offspring born at the same time from the same pregnancy.

quarantine (kwôr′ən-tēn′) N. isolation of people having communicable diseases or exposed to communicable diseases during the period of contagion in an effort to prevent the spread of the disease.

quarks N. one of two types of elementary particles (the other is leptons), incapable of independent existence, that combine to form particles such as protons and neutrons. Involved in strong interactions between particles. (*Compare* LEPTONS.)

QUADRANTS OF THE ABDOMEN

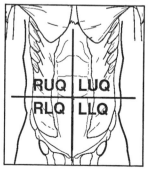

RUQ LUQ
RLQ LLQ

quartan (kwôrt′n) ADJ. occurring every 4th day, or about every 72 hours, as the fever and weakness of quartan malaria.

Queckenstedt's test (kwĕk′ən-stĕdz′) N. test to determine whether there is a blockage in the spinal canal or whether cerebrospinal fluid can flow freely.

quellung reaction N. swelling of the capsule surrounding a bacterium after it is exposed to specific antibodies or antisera; the reaction forms the basis of some tests to identify microorganisms.

quickening (kwĭk′ə-nĭng) N. pregnant woman's first awareness of the movement of the fetus, usually occurring about the 16th week of pregnancy but sometimes earlier.

quiescent (kwē-ĕs′ənt) ADJ. inactive.

quinacrine (kwĭn′ə-krēn′) N. anthelmintic and antimalarial used to treat certain worm infestations (e.g., cestodiasis) and malaria. Adverse effects include skin eruptions, nausea, vomiting, jaundice, liver dysfunction, and aplastic anemia.

quinapril N. *See* TABLE OF COMMONLY PRESCRIBED DRUGS—GENERIC NAMES

Quinidex N. trade name for the cardiac drug quinidine.

quinidine (kwĭn′ĭ-dēn′) N. drug (trade name Quinidex), used to treat certain heart arrhythmias. Adverse effects include gastrointestinal upsets, high blood pressure, and cardiac arrhythmia.

quinine (kwī′nīn′) N. antimalarial with antipyretic and analgesic properties. Adverse effects include tinnitus, deafness, visual disturbances, gastrointestinal upsets, blood disorders, and hypersensitivity reactions.

quinsy (kwĭn′zē) N. pus-filled inflammation of the tonsils and palate, usually a complication of tonsilitis. Incision of the abscess is usually necessary; also called peritonsillar abscess.

quintipara N. woman who has given birth to a viable infant after each of five pregnancies.

quintuplet (kwĭn-tŭp′lĭt) N. any of five offspring born at the same time from the same pregnancy.

R

Ra symbol for the element radium. *See also* TABLE OF IMPORTANT ELEMENTS.

rabbit fever *See* TULAREMIA.

rabbit test *See* FRIEDMAN TEST.

rabies (rā′bēz) N. acute, often fatal, viral disease affecting the brain and spinal cord, transmitted to humans by the bite of infected animals, esp. dogs, skunks, bats, foxes, and raccoons. After an incubation period that may range from a few days to 1 year, symptoms of fever, malaise, headache, and muscle pain are followed after a few days by severe and painful muscle spasms, esp. of the throat, delirium, difficulty in breathing, paralysis, coma, and death. The disease may be prevented in those bitten by an animal suspected of being rabid by a series of injections in combination with rabies immunoglobulin. The current vaccine is much less painful than older methods. Preexposure prophylaxis may be achieved in high-risk persons (e.g., veterinarians) by a series of vaccinations.

racemose (răs′ə-mōs′) ADJ. resembling a cluster of grapes (e.g., certain glands consisting of a number of small sacs).

rachi-, rachio- comb. forms indicating an association with the spine (e.g., rachialgia, spinal column pain).

rachis (rā′kĭs) *See* VERTEBRAL COLUMN.

rachischisis *See* SPINA BIFIDA.

rachitic (rə-kĭt′ĭk) ADJ. pert. to rickets.

rachitis (rə-kī′tĭs) N.
1. *See* RICKETS.
2. inflammation of the vertebral column.

racial immunity N. type of natural immunity shared by members of a race.

radial (rā′dē-əl) ADJ. pert. to the radius, one of the lower arm bones.

radial artery N. branch of the brachial artery that starts at the elbow, extends through the forearm, wraps around the wrist and extends into the hand, sending branches into the fingers. *See* MAJOR ARTERIES AND VEINS OF THE BODY, in Appendix.

radial keratotomy N. surgical procedure that corrects myopia; shallow incisions are made in the cornea, causing it to bulge.

radial nerve N. largest branch of the brachial plexus, the network of nerves supplying the arm.

radial pulse N. pulse of the radial artery, palpated at the wrist; it is the pulse commonly taken.

radiate (rā′dē-āt′) V. to spread from a focus or point of origin.

radiation (rā′dē-ā′shən) N. electromagnetic energy emitted in the form of rays or particles, including gamma rays, X rays, ultraviolet radiation, visible light, and infrared radiation. Some of these types of radiation are used in medicine for diagnosis (e.g., X rays) and treatment (e.g., radioactive elements such as radium, utilized in cancer treatment).

radiation sickness N. abnormal condition caused by exposure to ionizing radiation as, for example, from exposure to nuclear bomb explosions or exposure to radioactive chemicals in the workplace. Symptoms and prognosis depend on the amount of radiation, the exposure time, and the part of the body affected. Low to moderate doses cause nausea, vomiting, headache, and diarrhea, sometimes followed by hair loss and bleeding. Severe exposure causes sterility, damage to the fetus in pregnant women, and in many cases the development of cataracts, some forms of cancer, and other diseases. Severe exposure can cause death within hours. Also called radiation syndrome.

radiation therapy See RADIO-THERAPY.

radical (răd'ĭ-kəl) N. group of atoms acting as a single unit, but unable to exist independently for more than a short period of time; often called free radicals when the unit includes an oxygen atom that has a free electron. Free radicals may cause damage to a wide variety of tissues. As ADJ. refers to treatment that seeks a total cure, such as radical surgery. Compare to the opposite, conservative treatment.

radical mastectomy (mă-stěk'tə-mē) See MASTECTOMY.

radiculitis (rə-dĭk'yə-lī'tĭs) N. inflammation of the root (radicle) of a nerve.

radio- comb. form indicating an association with the emission of radiation (e.g., radiobiology, that branch of science dealing with the effects of radiation on living organisms).

radioactive (rā'dē-ō-ăk'tĭv) ADJ. emitting radiation, as some elements.

radioactive iodine excretion test N. evaluation of thyroid function in which the patient is given an oral tracer dose of radioactive iodine-131. The amount excreted in the urine and the amount accumulated in the thyroid gland are measured to indicate normal activity, underactivity, or overactivity of the gland. In the related radioactive iodine uptake (RAIU) test the amount of radioactive iodine taken up by the thyroid is measured.

radioactivity (rā'dē-ō-ăk-tĭv'ĭ-tē) N. emission of radiation (in the form of particles or waves) as a result of the disintegration (decay) of the nuclei of certain naturally occurring radioactive elements (e.g., uranium, radium) or of artificially produced radioactive isotopes (e.g., iodine-131).

radiodensity (rā'dē-ō-děn'sĭ-tē) N. in radiology, the ability of a substance to absorb X rays. The more radiodense (radiopaque) a material, the more X rays it absorbs. Put another way, the higher the radiodensity, the fewer X rays are able to penetrate a substance. See RADIOPAQUE, RADIOLUCENT.

radiography (rā'dē-ŏg'rə-fē) N. use of ionizing radiation, esp. X rays, to produce images on photographic plates or fluorescent screens (fluoroscopy); it is used to detect broken bones, the presence of ulcers, stones, or tumors in internal body organs, and many other disorders.

radioimmunoassay (rā′dē-ō-ĭm′ yə-nō-ăs′ā) N. method of determining the concentration of a protein in the serum by monitoring any reaction produced by the injection of a radioactively labeled substance known to react in a particular way with the protein being studied.

radioisotope (rā′dē-ō-ī′sə-tōp′) N. radioactive isotope of an element used in medicine for diagnostic and therapeutic purposes.

radiologist N. physician who specializes in radiology, administering, supervising, and interpreting X-ray, ultrasound, and other types of imaging studies.

radiology (rā-dē-ŏl′ə-jē) N. that branch of medicine concerned with X rays and other imaging techniques (e.g., ultrasound), radioactive substances, and their use in diagnosis and treatment.

radiolucent (rā′dē-ō-loo′sənt) ADJ. allows the passage of X rays to a variable degree, depending upon the radiodensity of the object x-rayed. *Compare* RADIOPAQUE.

radiopaque ADJ. (rā′dē-ō-pāk′) not allowing the passage of X rays or other forms of radiation (e.g., lead used as a shield around radioactive equipment, or radiopaque iodine isotopes used as contrast media in producing X-ray images). *Compare* RADIOLUCENT.

radiopaque dye N. chemical that does not permit the passage of X rays; used to outline the interior of certain organs during X-ray and fluoroscopic procedures.

radiosensitive ADJ. susceptible to radiation, as certain cancer cells that can be treated with radiotherapy.

radiotherapy (rā′dē-ō-thĕr′ə-pē) N. treatment of disease, esp. certain forms of cancer, by radiation given off by special machines or by radioactive isotopes. The radiation interferes with the division (mitosis) of cells and the synthesis of deoxyribonucleic acid (DNA) in the cells. Many cancer cells are destroyed by radiation; the major disadvantage is possible damage to cells and tissues in nearby areas. Also called radiation therapy.

radium (rā′dē-əm) N. radioactive metallic element used in radiotherapy. *See also* TABLE OF IMPORTANT ELEMENTS

radius (rā′dē-əs) N. outer and shorter of the two forearm bones, which partially revolves around the ulna (the other lower-arm bone); the radius articulates with the humerus (upper arm bone) at the elbow and with the ulna and carpal bones at the wrist.

radon (rā′dŏn) N. radioactive, gaseous, nonmetallic element, used in radiotherapy. Elevated levels of radon gas have been detected in homes in some areas. The need for its removal, although recommended by, for example, the Environmental Protection Agency, is the subject of much scientific controversy. *See also* TABLE OF IMPORTANT ELEMENTS.

rale (räl) N. abnormal chest sound, usually a bubbling or crackling noise on inspiration, heard through a stethoscope; it is associated with pneumonia, tuberculosis, congestive heart failure, and some other respiratory and cardiac disorders.

ramification (răm′ə-fī-kā′shən) N. branches or branching; nerve rami are smaller branches of larger nerves.

ramipril N. angiotensin converting enzyme inhibitor (trade name Altace); used once daily to treat hypertension. *See* TABLE OF COMMONLY PRESCRIBED DRUGS—GENERIC NAMES.

ramose ADJ. branched.

Ramsay Hunt syndrome N. abnormal condition caused by the varicella zoster virus (the virus that causes chicken pox and shingles), and characterized by ear pain, vertigo, facial nerve paralysis (sometimes permanent), and often hearing loss. Treatment is by corticosteroids.

ramus (rā′məs) N., *pl.* rami
1. small branch, esp. of a nerve or blood vessels.
2. thin process projecting from a bone. V. ramify

range of motion N. full measure that a limb or other body part can be moved.

ranitidine N. oral/parenteral H_2 histamine blocker (trade name Zantac) used in the treatment of peptic ulcer, gastritis, and gastroesophageal reflux. *See* TABLE OF COMMONLY PRESCRIBED DRUGS—GENERIC NAMES.

ranula (răn′yə-lə) N., *pl.* ranulae, cyst on the underside of the tongue, usually due to obstruction of a mucous or salivary gland.

raphe (rā′fē) N. line, ridge, or seam showing the union of two parts (e.g., palatine raphe, seam at the center of the hard palate).

rapid eye movement (REM) N. period of sleep characterized by rapid eye muscle contractions, detectable by electrodes placed over the skin near the eyes, during which dreaming occurs. REM sleep periods, lasting from a few minutes to about 30 minutes, alternate with nonrapid eye movement (NREM) periods during sleep.

raptus N.
1. intense excitement; ectasy.
2. sudden seizure or attack (e.g., raptus hemorrhagicus, sudden, profuse hemorrhage).

rash (răsh) N. skin eruption, usually characterized by red spots or generalized reddening. Rashes occur with chicken pox, measles, and rubella; in cases of local irritation and/or infection (e.g., diaper rash); and in

SLEEP CYCLES DURING A NIGHT'S SLEEP

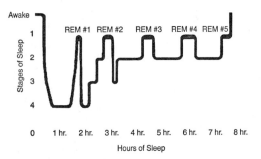

certain other diseases (e.g., butterfly rash or systemic lupus erythematosus).

rat typhus (tī′fəs) *See* MURINE TYPHUS.

ratbite fever N. either of two infectious diseases transmitted to humans by the bite of a rat or mouse; general symptoms include fever, headache, malaise, nausea, vomiting, and skin eruption. In the United States, the disease (also called Haverhill fever) is usually caused by *Streptobacillus moniliformis* and characterized by a rash on the palms and soles, painful joints, and a short (about 2 weeks) duration. In the Far East, the disease (also called sodoku) is usually caused by *Spirillum minus* and characterized by a rash on the extremities, lymph node enlargement, relapsing fever, and a longer duration. Treatment by penicillin is effective for both forms. Also called spirillum fever.

rate N. incidence or frequency of an event per unit of time (e.g., the heart rate is the number of beats per minute) or per number of possible occurrences (e.g., one illness per 100 people exposed to the illness). *See also* HEART RATE; SEDIMENTATION RATE; MORTALITY RATE.

rational (răsh′ə-nəl) ADJ. capable of, derived from, or using reason.

rationalization (răsh′ə-nə-lĭ-zā′shən) N. in psychiatry, defense mechanism in which a person justifies behavior or occurrences by giving reasonable, but not true, explanations.

rattle N. abnormal sound heard through a stethoscope in some types of respiratory disorders, it usually results from moisture in the air passages.

rauwolfia (ră-wŏlf′ē-ă) N. any of several alkaloids, including reserpine from the *Rauwolfia serpentina* shrub of Asia, used chiefly to treat hypertension.

Raynaud's disease (rā-nōz′) N. disease that typically affects women between the ages of 18 and 30 years, and is characterized by abnormal constriction of the arteries of the extremities, particularly the fingers; usually appears following exposure to cold.

Raynaud's sign *See* ACROCYANOSIS.

RBC *See* ERYTHROCYTE.

reaction N.
1. response to a stimulus, esp. in medicine.
2. response in opposition to a substance, drug, or treatment (e.g., hypersensitivity reaction).
3. in chemistry, change in a chemical acted on by another chemical.

reaction formation N. in psychiatry, defense mechanism in which a person unconsciously develops attitudes and behavior that are contrary to repressed unacceptable drives and impulses, and that serve to conceal them (e.g., a strong moral stance that hides an impulse to lust).

reaction time N. interval between the presentation of a stimulus and the subject's response to it.

Read method of childbirth N. system of natural childbirth, developed by Grantly Dick-Read, based on the idea that childbirth is a normal physiologic process and that pain during labor and childbirth is largely of psychological origin, the result of fear, ignorance, and tension. The method involves education of the woman on the physiologic process of childbirth, a series of breathing exercises to foster relaxation, and a series of other exercises to attain maximal physical conditioning for childbirth. (*Compare* BRADLEY METHOD OF CHILDBIRTH; LAMAZE METHOD OF CHILDBIRTH.) *See also* NATURAL CHILDBIRTH.

reagin (rē-ā′jĭn) N. antibody (an IgE immunoglobulin) formed against allergens (e.g., pollen) that attaches to cell membranes, causing the release of histamine and other substances responsible for the local inflammation characteristic of an allergy or for systemic anaphylaxis.

reality principle (rē-ăl′ĭ-tē) N. in psychoanalysis, modifying influences of environment and life circumstances on the pleasure principle, whereby behavior toward the immediate gratification of instinctual pleasures is changed in order to obtain long-term goals.

rebound (rē′bound′) V. to spring back (e.g., to recover from an illness). N. sudden contraction of a muscle following relaxation, occurring in cases where inhibitory reflexes are disturbed.

rebound tenderness N. pain elicited by the sudden release of a hand pressing on the abdomen; usually a sign of peritoneal inflammation.

receptor (rĭ-sĕp′tər) N.
1. ending of a sensory nerve, specialized to detect changes and trigger impulses in the sensory nerve (e.g., cells at the end of the olfactory nerve that detect odors in the nasal cavity).
2. structure or part of a structure or organ that receives, as the configuration on a cell surface for receiving an antigen.

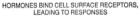

HORMONES BIND CELL SURFACE RECEPTORS, LEADING TO RESPONSES

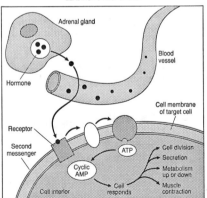

Hormones are released from the adrenal glands into the blood, where they move to their target cells; they bind cell surface receptors and interact with other proteins (curved arrows). A chemical signal is sent to the interior of the cell, causing a response. In this case the chemical signal causes the conversion of ATP to cyclic AMP, which acts as a second messenger, stimulating further events within the cell to occur.

Most drugs, neurotransmitters, and other chemical messengers in the body work by binding to one or more receptors. Pharmacologic research has identified many of these, leading to various drugs that block the receptor sites. Often, stimulation of a receptor leads to production of a second compound (second messenger) that actually transmits the "final information." Commonly used drugs, such as beta blockers, calcium channel blockers, and angiotensin converting enzyme blockers rely on inhibition at receptors.

recess (rē′sĕs′) N. small, hollow cavity (e.g., pharyngeal recess, a slitlike cavity in the wall of the pharynx).

recessive gene (rĭ-sĕs′ĭv) N. member of a pair of genes (an allele) that cannot express itself in the presence of its more dominant allele; it is expressed only in the homozygous state. For example, the gene for blue eyes is recessive and will not manifest itself if the gene for brown eyes (which is dominant) is also present; blue eyes will manifest themselves only if both genes are recessive. *See also* AUTOSOMAL RECESSIVE DISEASE.

reciprocal inhibition (rĭ-sĭp′rə-kəl) N. in behavior therapy, theory that the simultaneous presence of an anxiety-evoking stimulus and an anxiety-lessening situation will result in the stimulus producing less anxiety. The relaxing technique of deep breathing to decrease the pain and discomfort of childbirth is based on this idea.

recombinant DNA (rē-kŏm′bə-nənt) N. deoxyribonucleic acid (DNA) molecule in which genes have been artificially rearranged and genetic material from another organism, sometimes a member of another species, has been inserted. Replication of the new recombined DNA results in genetic changes in the organism. Recombinant DNA technology is being used to produce human insulin and growth hormone and is being investigated for many other medical applications.

recombinant human insulin (rē-kŏm′bə-nənt) *See* HUMULIN.

recovery (rĭ-kŭv′ə-rē) N. freedom from codependency; it often entails a long process of counseling and of reestablishing one's own identity and self-esteem.

recovery position N. position in which victims of cardiac arrest should be placed after cardiopulmonary resuscitation if they resume breathing and regain a pulse in order to avoid airway obstruction; the victim is rolled onto his or her side, so that the head, shoulders, and torso move together. If trauma is suspected, the victim must not be moved.

recrudescence (rē′krōō-dĕs′əns) N. return of symptoms of a disease soon after they disappeared and recovery appeared to be underway. ADJ. recrudescent

recruitment (rĭ-krōōt′mənt) N. condition in which the response to a stimulus increases to a maximum even though the strength of the original stimulus is unchanged. In neurology, this occurs because of activation of increasing numbers of nerve fibers. During generalized seizures, a few abnormal neurons fire at first. They rapidly recruit other neurons, causing them to fire and quickly, the entire brain is involved. A similar process occurs in the heart muscle when a single irritable cell recruits others, leading to a potentially life-threatening rhythm disturbance (arrhythmia).

rectal examination (rĕk′təl) N. process where a gloved finger probes the internal portion of the rectum, approximately one to three inches within the anus. Important in screening for bowel cancer, the presence of blood in stools, and, in males, prostate cancer.

rectal reflex N. normal response to the presence of feces in the rectum, allowing defecation; also called defecation reflex.

recto- comb. form indicating an association with the rectum (e.g., rectourethral, pert. to the rectum and the urethra).

rectocele (rĕk′tə-sēl′) N. protrusion of the rectum, and often part of the posterior wall of the vagina, into the vagina; it occurs when pelvic muscles have been weakened by childbirth, surgery, or other factors. Pain and difficulty in defecation and painful coitus may occur. Treatment is by surgery. Also called proctocele.

rectosigmoid (rĕk′tō-sĭg′moid′) ADJ. pert. to the sigmoid colon and the upper part of the rectum.

rectum (rĕk′təm) N. last portion of the large intestine, about 5 inches (12–13 centimeters) long, connecting the sigmoid colon and the anus. Feces are stored in the rectum before defecation. ADJ. rectal

rectus (rĕk′təs) N. any of several straight muscles (e.g., rectus abdominis, pair of muscles extending the length of the ventral part of the abdomen).

ADJ. indicating a straight or almost straight body part. See MAJOR MUSCLES OF THE BODY, in Appendix.

recumbent (rĭ-kŭm′bənt) ADJ. lying down or leaning backward.

recuperation N. recovery, or return to a normal state of health.

recurrent (rĭ-kûr′ənt) ADJ. incessant; recurring again and again.

red blood cell See ERYTHROCYTE.

red marrow See under BONE MARROW.

reduce V. in surgery, return of a dislocated part to its normal position by manipulation or operation, as in hernia correction when a displaced part is returned to its normal position in the body.

reduction N. process in which electrons are added to an atom or ion (as by removing oxygen or adding hydrogen); always accompanied by oxidation (loss of electrons) of the reducing agent. The combination of simultaneous oxidation and reduction reactions is often termed an oxidation-reduction (redox) reaction. (*Compare* OXIDATION.)

reduction division (rĭ-dŭk′shən) See MEIOSIS.

referred pain (rĭ-fûrd′) N. pain felt at a site in the body different from the diseased or injured part where the pain is expected. Angina pectoris, resulting from coronary artery insufficiency, often occurs in the left shoulder, and pain from gallbladder disease is frequently felt in the right shoulder area.

reflex (rē′flĕks′) N. involuntary function or movement of a part in response to a particular stimulus (e.g., the kneejerk or patellar reflex).

reflex arc N. nervous circuit involved in a reflex; at its simplest, it involves a sensory nerve linked with a motor nerve via an association nerve (also called an interneuron), supplying a muscle or gland, as in the patellar (kneejerk) reflex. Reflexes are very fast since the entire signal process takes place locally at the spinal cord level—information does not need to travel to the brain, be processed there, and return down the spinal cord to the effector. *See also* EFFECTOR.

reflex sympathetic dystrophy (sĭm-pə-thet-ik dis-trə-fē) *See* COMPLEX REGIONAL PAIN SYNDROME.

reflux (rē′flŭks′) N. abnormal backflow, as sometimes occurs with fluids in the esophagus (gastro-esophageal reflux) or other body parts.

refraction (rĭ-frăk′shən) N.
1. change in direction of light (or other energy) as it passes from one medium to another, as from air into glass.

2. means for determining the amount of refractive power of the eye and the need for corrective lenses. V. refract.

refractory (rĭ-frăc′tə-rē) ADJ. unresponsive, resistant to treatment.

refractory period N. in neurology, period of recovery needed by a neuron after excitation or by a muscle after contraction (depolarization), during which repolarization of the cell membrane occurs; a stimulus applied during the refractory period will not evoke a response.

refracture (rē-frăk′chər) V. to break a bone that, having been broken before, mended in an abnormal way.

regeneration (rĭ-jĕn′ə-rā′shən) N. replacement of lost tissue by an organism.

regional anesthesia (rē′jə-nəl ăn′ĭs-thē′zhə) N. anesthesia of an area of the body through administration of a local anesthetic that blocks a group of sensory nerve fibers. Kinds of regional anesthesia include epidural anesthesia, paracervi-

THE REFLEX ARC

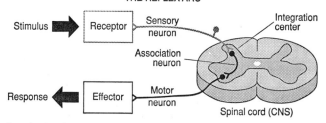

In a simple reflex arc, a receptor receives the stimulus and rapidly transfers it, via a sensory neuron, to the integration center in the spinal cord; the signal then continues through an association neuron (interneuron) to a motor neuron, which causes a response in the effector organ (usually a muscle). The signal remains localized in the spinal cord and does not travel to and from the brain.

THE COMPONENTS OF THE REFLEX ARC

Component	Description	Function
Receptor	The receptor end of a dendrite or a specialized receptor cell in a sensory organ	Sensitive to an internal or external change
Sensory neuron	Dendrite, cell body, and axon of a sensory (afferent) neuron	Transmits nerve impulse from the receptor to the brain or spinal cord
Interneuron	Dendrite, cell body, and axon of a neuron within the brain or spinal cord	Serves as a processing center; conducts nerve impulse from the sensory neuron to a motor neuron
Motor neuron	Dendrite, cell body, and axon of a motor (efferent) neuron	Transmits nerve impulse from the brain or spinal cord to an effector
Effector	A muscle or gland outside the nervous system	Responds to stimulation by the motor neuron and produces the reflex behavioral action

cal block, pudendal block, saddle block anesthesia, and spinal anesthesia.

regional enteritis (rē′jə-nəl ĕn′tə-rī′tĭs) *See* CROHN′S DISEASE.

regression (rĭ-grĕsh′ən) N. return to an earlier condition, esp. the retreat of an adult into childlike behavior. ADJ. regressive

regulatory gene (rĕg′yə-lə-tôr′ē) N. gene that regulates or suppresses the activity of one or more structural genes.

regurgitation N.
1. return of swallowed food into the mouth.
2. backflow of blood through a defective heart valve.

rehabilitation N. restoration of an individual or of a part of the body to normal function after injury, disease, or other abnormal state.

Reiki *See* TABLE OF ALTERNATIVE MEDICINE TERMS.

reinforcement (rē′ĭn-fôrs′mənt) N. in psychology, strengthening of a particular response or behavioral pattern by rewarding desirable behavior and punishing undesirable behavior.

Reiter′s syndrome (rī′tərz) N. inflammatory syndrome of unknown etiology, occurring predominantly in males. It usually begins several weeks after either a gastrointestinal or sexually-transmitted infection with the onset of conjunctivitis, urethritis, and arthritis, esp. of the ankles and sacroiliac joints. Treatment involves nonsteroidal anti-inflammatory agents, esp. phenylbutazone.

rejection (rĭ-jĕk′shən) N.
1. in medicine, immunological response whereby substances or organisms that the system recognizes as foreign are not

accepted, as in the body's attack against invading microorganisms (e.g., bacteria) or rejection of a transplanted organ. 2. in psychiatry, denying attention or affection to another person.

Relafen N. *See* TABLE OF COMMONLY PRESCRIBED DRUGS—TRADE NAMES.

relapse (rĭ-lăps′) V. to show again the signs of a disease from which the patient appeared to have recovered. N. recurrence of a disease after apparent recovery.

relapsing fever N. infectious disease caused by Borrelia microorganisms and transmitted by lice and ticks, most common in South America, Africa, and Asia. It is characterized by 2- or 3-day episodes of high fever, chills, headache, muscle pains, and nausea, sometimes with a rash and jaundice, recurring every week or 10 days for several months. Treatment is by antibiotics.

relaxant (rĭ-lăk′sənt) N. drug or device that reduces muscle tension or relieves anxiety.

relaxin (rĭ-lăk′sĭn) N. hormone, secreted by the corpus luteum during the last stages of pregnancy, that causes the cervix to dilate and prepares the uterus for labor.

releasing hormone (RH) N. any of several hormones released by the hypothalamus into a vein to the anterior pituitary gland, where they stimulate the release of anterior pituitary homones. Each releasing factor stimulates the pituitary to secrete a specific hormone (e.g., growth-hormone-releasing factor stimulates the release of growth hormone).

REM *See* RAPID EYE MOVEMENT.

remission (rĭ-mĭsh′ən) N. partial or complete disappearance of, or lessening of the severity of, the symptoms of a disease; it may be spontaneous or result from therapy, and be temporary or permanent.

remnant N. part or portion that is unused or left over; often used to refer to tissue from early development that is not completely absorbed during the growth process. Some feel that the appendix is a remnant of a structure that developmentally, may have served a useful function thousands of years ago.

renal (rē′nəl) ADJ. pert. to the kidney.

renal artery N. either of a pair of arteries arising from the abdominal aorta and supplying the kidneys, adrenal glands, and ureters. *See* MAJOR ARTERIES AND VEINS OF THE BODY, in Appendix.

renal calculus (rē′nəl kăl′kyə-ləs) *See* URINARY CALCULUS.

renal colic (rē′nəl kŏl′ĭk) N. sharp pain in the lower back radiating to the groin, usually associated with the passage of a calculus (stone) through the ureter.

renal failure N. inability of the kidneys to excrete wastes and function in the maintenance of electrolyte balance. Acute renal failure, characterized by inability to produce urine and an accumulation of wastes, is often associated with trauma, burns, acute infection, or obstruction of the urinary tract; its treatment depends on the cause and often includes antibiotics and reduced fluid intake. Chronic kidney failure, which may occur as a result of many systemic disorders,

DNA REPLICATION

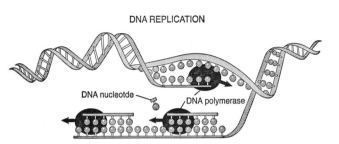

DNA nucleotde

DNA polymerase

causes fatigue and sluggishness, diminished urine output, anemia, and often complications of hypertension and congestive heart failure. Its treatment depends on the cause, often involving the use of diuretics, restricted protein intake, and, if the renal failure cannot be otherwise treated, hemodialysis. SYN. kidney failure.

renin (rē′nĭn) N. enzyme released by the kidney that affects blood pressure by catalyzing the formation of angiotensin I from angiotensinogen; angiotensin converting enzyme then converts angiotensin I to angiotensin II, a potent vasoconstrictor and stimulant of sodium and water retention. Angiotensin III is the final metabolically active product and is a strong stimulant of aldosterone secretion.

rennin (rĕn′ĭn) N. enzyme produced in the stomach that functions in the digestion of milk.

replacement (rĭ-plās′mənt) N. substitution of a missing part or substance, as the replacement of lost blood with a transfusion of donor blood.

replication (rĕp′lĭ-kā′shən) N. process of duplicating, copying, or reproducing, esp. in genetics, the process by which deoxyribonucleic acid (DNA) makes a copy of itself before cell division. In this process, the double-stranded molecule of DNA unwinds to become two separate strands, each of which acts as a template for the synthesis of a strand complementary to it. Though several enzymes are involved, the major one is DNA polymerase. The two new molecules, each with one parental strand and one new strand, then rewind to form the characteristic double-helix configuration. *See also* DOXYRIBONUCLEIC ACID; POLYMERASE.

repolarization (rē-pō′lər-ĭ-zā′shən) N. return to baseline electrochemical state of either a nerve or muscle tissue following depolarization. Involves a shift of sodium, potassium, and calcium ions.

repression (rĭ-prĕsh′ən) N.
1. inhibition of an action, as that of an enzyme or gene.
2. in psychoanalysis, unconscious defense mechanism whereby unacceptable thoughts, feelings, memories, and impulses are pushed from the conscious into the unconscious, where they are submerged but remain important in influencing behavior and are often the source of anxiety.

reproduction (rē′prə-dŭk′shən) N. process by which living organisms give rise to offspring; it may be asexual, involving only one parent that divides, buds, or otherwise produces an offspring of the same genetic makeup; or it may be sexual, involving the union of sex cells, or gametes, from two parents and recombination of the genetic material of the parents to produce an offspring with a new genetic makeup. Humans and higher animals reproduce sexually.

reproductive system (rē′prə-dŭk′tĭv) N. organs and tissues involved in the production and maturation of gametes and in their union and subsequent development to produce offspring. In the male the reproductive system includes the testes, vas deferens, prostate gland, seminal vesicles, urethra, and penis. In the female it includes the ovaries, Fallopian tubes, uterus, vagina, and vulva. The reproductive system is under the control of numerous hormones secreted by the pituitary gland, the sex organs (ovaries and testes), and the adrenal glands.

RES See RETICULOENDOTHELIAL SYSTEM.

rescue inhaler N. any of a number of inhaled bronchodilators, usually in an aerosol can form, taken for relief of acute respiratory symptoms, usually in either asthma or chronic obstructive pulmonary disease (COPD). These medications are not taken on a regular basis, but only as needed when symptoms occur that are not well controlled by the patient's usual ongoing medications. *See also* ASTHMA; BRONCHODILATOR; CHRONIC OBSTRUCTIVE PULMONARY DISEASE.

resection (rĭ-sĕk′shən) N. surgical removal of a portion of a structure or organ. v. resect.

reserpine (rĭ-sûr′pēn′) N. drug (trade name Rau-Sed) extracted from rauwolfia plants and used to treat hypertension. Adverse effects include depression, impotence, and gastrointestinal upset, including exacerbation of peptic ulcers.

reserve (rĭ-zûrv′) N. potential capacity to respond to maintain vital functions (e.g., pulmonary reserve, the extra volume of air that the lungs can inhale or exhale when breathing to the limits of capacity, as in times of stress).

resident (rĕz′ĭ-dənt) N. physician (graduate of a medical school) in one of the postgraduate years of clinical training, after the first internship year; the residency period is often concentrated on a particular medical specialty.

resilience N. ability to endure stress (physical or mental) and return to normal, even in situations that appear overwhelming; elasticity.

resistance (rĭ-zĭs′təns) N.
1. degree of immunity or resistance to a particular disease that the body possesses.
2. degree to which a disease-causing microorganism is unaffected by antibiotics or other drugs, as in penicillin-resistant bacteria.

resolution (rĕz′ə-loō′shən) N.
1. ability to distinguish fine details, as through a microscope.
2. period during which disease symptoms (e.g., swelling or other signs of inflammation) decrease or disappear.

resonance (rĕz′ə-nəns) N. echo-like sound produced by percussion of an organ or cavity during physical examination. ADJ. resonant.

resorcinol (rĭ-zôr′sə-nôl′) N. drug, used in ointments for acne and certain other disorders and in dandruff shampoos, that causes the skin to peel.

resorption (rē-sôrp′shən) N. process of being removed by absorption, such as pus in a wound.

respiration (rĕs′pə-rā′shən) N. processes involved in the exchange of gases—oxygen and carbon dioxide—between an organism and the environment, involving both external respiration, or breathing, in which oxygen is taken from the air by alveoli in the lungs and carbon dioxide is released from the blood to be exhaled; and internal respiration, whereby the oxygen in the blood is absorbed by cells throughout the body and waste product carbon dioxide is absorbed by the blood to be transported to the lungs.

respiratory (rĕs′pər-ə-tôr′ē) ADJ. pert. to respiration or the respiratory system.

respiratory acidosis (rĕs′pər-ə-tôr′ē ăs′ĭ-dō′sĭs) N. form of acidosis (excess hydrogen-ion concentration in the blood) in which reduced gas exchange in the lungs, caused by emphysema, pneumonia, asthma, chest trauma, drugs that depress respiration, or other condition, results in decreased carbon dioxide excretion. The excess carbon dioxide combines with water to form carbonic acid,

ORGANS OF THE HUMAN RESPIRATORY SYSTEM

Structure	Description	Function
Nasal cavity	Hollow space within nose	Conducts air to pharynx; mucous lining filters, warms, and moistens air
Sinuses	Hollow spaces in bones of the skull	Reduce weight of the skull; serve as resonant chambers; spaces for conditioning of air
Larynx	Enlargement at the top of the trachea	Passageway for air; houses vocal cords
Trachea	Rigid tube that connects larynx to bronchial tree	Passageway for air; mucous lining filters air
Bronchial tree	Branched tubes that lead from the trachea to the alveoli	Conducts air from the trachea to the alveoli; mucous lining filters air
Lungs	Soft, cone-shaped organs that occupy most of the thoracic cavity	Contain the air passages, alveoli, blood vessels, and other tissues of the lower respiratory tract

which increases the acidity of the blood, producing acidosis. Headache, hypertension, decreased mentation, cardiac arrhythmias, and possibly death may occur. Treatment involves correction of the underlying cause, if possible, and may involve oxygen, bronchodilators, and possibly a mechanical ventilator. (*Compare* RESPIRATORY ALKALOSIS.)

respiratory alkalosis (rĕs′pər-ə-tôr′ē ăl′kə-lō′sĭs) N. form of alkalosis (abnormally low hydrogen-ion concentration in the blood) in which there is greater than normal excretion of carbon dioxide, usually caused by hyperventilation associated with extreme anxiety, asthma or pneumonia, or by aspirin intoxication or metabolic acidosis. Deep, rapid breathing, dizziness, lightheadedness, and muscular spasm commonly occur. Abnormalities in the electrocardiogram that usually have no prognostic significance may be noted. Treatment involves correction and treatment of any underlying causes. Sometimes rebreathing of air that has been exhaled into a paper bag can be helpful, if potentially dangerous causes (e.g., diabetic ketoacidosis, pulmonary embolism, myocardial infarction) are excluded first. Sedatives to decrease the rate of breathing are used in cases of extreme anxiety. (*Compare* RESPIRATORY ACIDOSIS).

respiratory arrest N. complete cessation of breathing for any of a number of possible reasons. *Compare* CARDIAC ARREST.

respiratory center N. that part of the pons and medulla oblongata of the brain that controls the rate of breathing in response to changes in the levels of oxygen and carbon dioxide in the blood.

respiratory distress syndrome of the newborn N. acute lung disease of the newborn, esp. a premature newborn, in which the alveoli are airless and the lungs inelastic because of a deficiency of a surfactant substance necessary for normal alveolar function and lung expansion. Symptoms include rapid and shallow breathing, nasal flaring, and often edema of the extremities and the formation of a hyaline membrane in the collapsed alveoli. Treatment involves oxygen and fluid administration and use of a specially designed device to maintain positive airway pressure. Also called hyaline membrane disease.

respiratory failure N. inability of the heart and lungs to maintain an adequate level of gaseous exchange. This results in the accumulation of carbon dioxide in the blood which is converted to carbonic acid, leading to respiratory acidosis. Additionally, the blood may be poorly oxygenated, resulting in hypoxia. Treatment involves correction of any underlying cardiac or lung disorder, administration of oxygen, bronchodilators, and other measures (e.g., mechanical ventilation).

respiratory rate N. rate of breathing at rest, about 14 breaths per minute in an adult.

respiratory syncytial virus (RSV) (rĕs′pər-ə-tôr′ē sĭn-sĭsh′ē-əl) N. any of a group of myxoviruses responsible for many respiratory infections (including bronchiolitis, bronchopneumonia, and the common cold), esp. in children.

respiratory tract N. organs and structures associated with

RESTING POTENTIAL
Outside of Cell

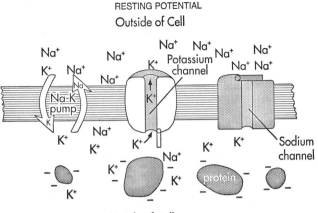

Inside of Cell

Ionic conditions leading to the establishment of a resting potential across the neuron membrane. Although both potassium and sodium channels exist, only the potassium channel is open, allowing for the passive loss of that ion to the outside.

breathing, gaseous exchange, and the entrance of air into the body. Included are the nasal cavity, pharynx, larynx (upper respiratory tract); the trachea, bronchi, bronchioles, and lungs (lower respiratory tract); and associated muscles.

respiratory tract infection (rĕs′ pər-ə-tôr′ē) N. any infection affecting the respiratory tract.

    lower respiratory infection N. infection of the trachea, bronchi, and/or lungs, as in bronchitis, bronchiolitis, or pneumonia.

    upper respiratory infection N. infection affecting the nasal cavity or pharynx, as in the common cold, pharyngitis (sore throat), sinusitis, rhinitis, or tonsillitis.

response (rĭ-spŏns′) N. reaction to a stimulus.

resting potential N. electrochem-ical difference between the two sides of a nerve or cardiac cell membrane when the cell is not conducting an impulse. In most nerve and cardiac cells, the resting potential is negative— the interior of the cell is negatively charged as compared to the extracellular space. The resting potential in cardiac cells is about –90 mV (millivolts), and in nerve cells, –60 mV. This potential is determined by the selective permeability of the cell membrane to potassium (K^+) and sodium (Na^+) ions. At rest, nerve and cardiac cell membranes are permeable to K^+, but they are relatively impermeable to other ions. The resting membrane potential is therefore determined by the K^+ gradient across the cell membrane. The gradient is maintained by various ion pumps and ion exchange mechanisms. (*Compare* ACTION POTENTIAL.)

restless legs syndrome N. condition characterized by restless movement, twitching, and unpleasant sensations of the legs, esp. the lower leg; it is sometimes associated with a sleep disturbance. Walking or moving the legs relieves it.

Restoril N. *See* TABLE OF COMMONLY PRESCRIBED DRUGS—TRADE NAMES.

resuscitation (rĭ-sŭs′ĭ-tā′shən) N. act of reviving a person or returning him/her to consciousness through the use of cardiopulmonary resuscitation and similar techniques.

retarded ADJ. abnormally slow, as in development or growth.

retch (rĕch) V. to attempt unsuccessfully to vomit.

rete (rē′tē) N. net or meshlike structure (e.g., rete testes, network of tubes carrying sperm from the seminiferous tubules in the testes to the vasa efferentia).

retention (rĭ-tĕn′shən) N.
 1. holding something inside a part, cavity, or organ, as in urinary retention.
 2. ability to remember information.

reticular (rĭ-tĭk′yə-lər) ADJ. having a netlike pattern.

reticular activating system N. system of nerve pathways in the brain concerned with the level of consciousness, from sleep and relaxation to full attention and concentration.

reticular formation N. cluster of nerve cells and nerve fibers in the brainstem connecting nerves to and from the spinal cord, cranial nerves, and areas of the brain; it constantly monitors the state of the body and functions in the control of breathing, heart rate, level of consciousness, and many other functions.

reticular protein N. connective tissue protein that forms a mesh or netlike structure.

STRUCTURE OF THE RETINA

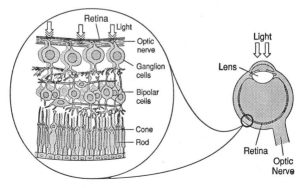

Light passes through the lens to the retina, striking rods and cones posteriorly. Nerve signals then past anterior through bipolar and ganglion cells to the optic nerve, then to the brain.

reticulocyte (rĭ-tĭk′yə-lō-sīt′) N. immature erythrocyte (red blood cell) with a network of threads and particles at the former site of the nucleus; normally making up about 1% of the total red blood cell count. (A mature erythrocyte lacks a nucleus.)

reticuloendothelial system (RES) (rĭ-tĭk′yə-lō-ĕn′dō-thē′lē-əl) N. unit of the body made up of phagocytic cells (e.g., Kupffer cells of the liver, macrophages, and cells of the spleen and bone marrow) and functioning in immune responses to infection and in ridding the body of cellular debris.

reticulum (rĭ-tĭk′yə-ləm) N. network, esp. of blood vessels or tubules.

Retin-A N. See TABLE OF COMMONLY PRESCRIBED DRUGS—TRADE NAMES.

retina (rĕt′n-ə) N. multilayered light-sensitive layer of the eye that receives images of objects and transmits visual impulses through the optic nerve to the brain for interpretation. The outer part of the retina, next to the choroid, contains the pigment rhodopsin; the inner layers, continuing to the vitreous humor, contain rods and cones (light-sensitive nerve cells) and their associated ganglia and fibers. ADJ. retinal

retinaculum (rĕt′n-ăk′yə-ləm) N. retaining structure or part that holds an organ or tissue in place (e.g., retinaculum unguis, the band of tissue holding the nail to the nail bed).

retinal detachment See DETACHED RETINA.

retinitis (rĕt′n-ī′tĭs) N. inflammation of the retina.

retino- comb. form indicating an association with the retina (e.g., retinomalacia, softening of the retina).

retinoblastoma (rĕt′n-ō-blă-stō′mə) N. congenital, hereditary neoplasm of retinal cells, the most common eye malignancy in childhood. Diminished vision, detached retina, and abnormal pupillary reflexes are common. Treatment includes removal of the eye.

retinol (rĕt′n-ôl′) N. form of vitamin A. See also TABLE OF VITAMINS.

retinopathy (rĕt′n-ŏp′ə-thē) N. disease of the retina of the eye; usually refers to damage from diabetes (diabetic retinopathy).

retraction (rĭ-trăk′shən) N. act of pulling, holding, or drawing a part back, as during surgery.

retractor (rĭ-trăk′tər) N. instrument used in surgery to hold back the edges of organs to maintain exposure of underlying structures.

retro- comb. form indicating a backward position or motion (*compare* ANTERO-, POSTERO-) (e.g., retroperitoneal—behind the peritoneum, as in the space between the peritoneum and the abdominal wall in which the kidneys are located).

retrobulbar neuritis (rĕt′rō-bŭl′bər noo-rī′tĭs) N. inflammation of the optic nerve behind the eye, usually causing blurred vision; it is a common sign of multiple sclerosis but may also result from other causes and heal completely.

retroflexion (rĕt′rō-flĕk′shən) N. bending backwards of an organ, esp. the upper part of the uterus.

retrograde (rĕt′rə-grād′) ADJ. moving or going backward; moving in a direction opposite to that considered normal. *Compare* ANTEROGRADE.

retrograde amnesia N. loss of memory for events immediately preceding an injury, illness, or emotional trauma (*compare* RETROGRADE MEMORY).

retrograde memory N. ability to recall recent events but not older knowledge previously familiar (*compare* RETROGRADE AMNESIA).

retrogression (rĕt′rə-grĕsh′ən) N. return to a less complex, less differentiated condition.

retroversion (rĕt′rō-vûr′zhən) N. backward displacement or inclination of an organ, esp. in reference to the uterus, the upper part of which may be tilted backward in relation to the lower part or cervix, which is pointed toward the pubic bone.

retrovirus N. type of virus that, when not infecting a cell, stores its genetic information on a single-stranded RNA molecule instead of the more usual double-stranded DNA (e.g., HIV). After a retrovirus penetrates a cell, it constructs a DNA version of its genes using a special enzyme called reverse transcriptase. This DNA then becomes part of the cell's genetic material. *See also* DEOXYRIBONUCLEIC ACID; HUMAN IMMUNODEFICIENCY VIRUS; RIBONUCLEIC ACID.

reverse transcriptase (tran-skrī′p-tāz) N. enzyme used by retroviruses to form a DNA sequence from their RNA. The resulting DNA is then inserted into the chromosome of the host cell. This enzyme is the target of many anti-AIDS (Acquired Immunodeficiency Syndrome) drugs, termed reverse transcriptase inhibitors. *See also* DEOXYRIBONUCLEIC ACID; HUMAN IMMUNODEFICIENCY VIRUS; RETROVIRUS; REVERSE TRANSCRIPTASE INHIBITORS; RIBONUCLEIC ACID.

reverse transcriptase inhibitor N. drug that blocks viral replication by interfering with the reverse transcriptase enzyme in retroviruses, preventing synthesis of DNA from RNA; used in therapy of AIDS and HIV infection. *See also* ACQUIRED IMMUNE DEFICIENCY SYNDROME; DEOXYRIBONUCLEIC ACID; HUMAN IMMUNODEFICIENCY VIRUS; RETROVIRUS; REVERSE TRANSCRIPTASE; RIBONUCLEIC ACID; HUMAN IMMUNODEFICIENCY VIRUS.

Reye's syndrome (rīz) N. poorly understood syndrome involving abnormal brain function and fatty infiltration of internal organs, esp. the liver. It occurs chiefly in children after an acute viral infection (esp. viruses associated with influenza and chicken pox); an association with aspirin intake has also been observed. Vomiting and confusion typically occur about a week after the viral infection, sometimes leading to disorientation, seizures, coma, and respiratory arrest. The cause is unknown, and there is no specific treatment. Intensive monitoring of all vital functions and correction of any imbalances may improve the prognosis.

Rezulin N. *See* TABLE OF COMMONLY PRESCRIBED DRUGS—TRADE NAMES.

RH *See* RELEASING HORMONE.

Rh factor N. antigen present in the erythrocytes (red blood cells) of about 85% of people; it is called Rh factor because it was first identified in the blood of rhesus monkeys. Persons having the factor are designated Rh-positive; those lacking the factor, Rh-negative. Blood for transfusions must be classified for Rh factor, as well as for ABO blood group, to prevent possible incompatibility reactions. If an Rh-negative person receives Rh-positive blood, hemolysis and anemia can result; a similar reaction can occur if an Rh-negative mother exposes an Rh-positive fetus (the fetus having inherited the Rh factor from the father) to antibodies to the factor. *See also* ERYTHROBLASTOSIS FETALIS; RHO-GAM.

Rh incompatibility (ĭn′kəm-păt′ə-bĭl′ĭ-tē) N. lack of compatibility between two blood samples because one contains Rh factor and the other does not.

rhabdomyosarcoma (răb′dō-mī′ō-sär-kō′mə) N. highly malignant tumor derived from striated muscle cells. There are three types. The embryonal form occurs mainly in infants and children, primarily affecting the head, neck, and genitourinary tract. The alveolar form occurs mainly in adolescents and young adults, affecting the muscles of the extremities, trunk, and orbital region. The pleomorphic form affects the limb muscles of older adults. Surgical excision is often impossible; treatment then involves chemotherapy and irradiation.

rhagades (răg′ə-dēz′) N. cracks in the skin, most common around the mouth.

rheology N. study of the flow characteristics, usu. of a liquid in a tube-like structure, such as the flow of blood in the vessels.

rheumatic aortitis (rōō-măt′ĭk ā′ôr-tī′tĭs) N. inflammation of the aorta, occurring in rheumatic fever.

rheumatic fever N. inflammatory disease, occurring primarily in children, as a result of a delayed reaction to an inadequately treated streptococcal infection of the upper respiratory tract (e.g., streptococcal throat). Symptoms, appearing several weeks after the acute infection, include fever, abdominal pain, vomiting, arthritis, and consequent pain affecting many joints, and palpitations and chest pain associated with inflammation of the heart; other signs include reddish patches on the skin and abnormal involuntary muscular movements. Treatment includes bed rest, restricted activity, and sometimes antibiotics, steroids, and pain relievers. Most cases resolve within 1 or 2 months, except for the residual effects of carditis. *See also* RHEUMATIC HEART DISEASE.

rheumatic heart disease N. damage to the heart muscle and heart valves caused by recurrent episodes of rheumatic fever. It is characterized by stenosis (narrowing) or regurgitation (leaking) of valves, changes in the size of the heart chambers, often with abnormal heart rhythm. Treatment depends on the nature and extent of heart damage and valve damage; it may include digitalis, diuretics, surgery to correct valve abnormalities, prevention of repeat attacks of rheumatic fever by prophylactic use of antibiotics, and other measures.

rheumatoid arthritis N. chronic, destructive disease characterized by joint inflammation. It usually begins in early middle age, most often in women, and is marked by periods of remission and exacerbation. Symptoms are varied, often including fatigue; low-grade fever; loss of appetite; morning stiffness; tender, painful swelling of two or more joints, most commonly in fingers, ankles, feet, hips, and shoulders; and small subcutaneous nodules near joints. There is no cure; treatment includes rest; exercises to maintain joint mobility; pain-relieving drugs; nonsteroidal anti-inflammatory agents (e.g., indomethacin, phenylbutazone); and, if other measures are not successful, corticosteroids. (*Compare* ANKYLOSING SPONDYLITIS; OSTEOARTHRITIS.) Gold preparations have been extremely successful in selected patients.

rheumatoid factor N. antibodies found in the serum of many people (about 70%) with rheumatoid arthritis, but also occurring in persons with certain other connective tissue disorders and other diseases.

rheumatology (roō'mə-tŏl'ə-jē) N. study of disorders characterized by degeneration or inflammation of connective tissues.

rhin-, rhino- comb. forms indicating an association with the nose (e.g., rhinopharyngeal, pert. to the nose and pharynx).

rhinencephalon (rī'nĕn-sĕf'ə-lŏn') N. that part of each cerebral hemisphere that contains the limbic system and the olfactory nerve.

rhinion N. point at the end of the suture between the two nasal bones.

rhinitis (rī-nī'tĭs) N. inflammation of the mucous membrane lining of the nose, usually associated with a nasal discharge; it may be caused by a viral infection, as in the common cold; or by allergic reaction, as in hay fever; also called coryza.

Rhinocort N. *See* TABLE OF COMMONLY PRESCRIBED DRUGS—TRADE NAMES.

rhinopathy (rī-nŏp'ə-thē) N. any disease or malformation of the nose.

rhinophyma (rī'nō-fī'mə) N. condition, usually associated with rosacea, in which there are marked swelling and redness and prominent vascularization of the skin on the nose. It may be associated with the intake of large amounts of alcohol. Treatment includes dermabrasion and plastic surgery.

rhinoplasty (rī'nō-plǎs'tē) N. plastic surgery technique in which the structure and shape of the nose are altered to correct a deformity, repair the effects of trauma, or (most often) improve the appearance.

rhinorrhea (rī'nə-rē'ə) N. persistent, usually watery, mucus discharge from the nose, as in the common cold.

rhinoscope (rī'nə-skōp') N. instrument for examining the nasal passages through the anterior nares or through the nasopharynx.

rhinosporidiosis (rī'nō-spə-rĭd'ē-ō'sĭs) N. fungus (*Rhinosporidium seeberi*) infection of the nose, often acquired by swimming in infected waters, characterized by reddish polyps on the mucous membranes of the nose, eyes, throat, and sometimes the genitals. Treatment is by cauterization.

rhinostenosis (rī'nō-stə-nō'sĭs) N. narrowing of the passage in the nasal cavity.

rhinotomy (rī-nŏt'ə-mē) N. surgical procedure in which an incision is made along one side of the nose to drain accumulated pus.

rhinovirus (rī'nō-vī'rəs) N. any of a group of small ribonucleic acid (RNA) viruses, responsible for almost one half of all respiratory infections, typically characterized by a scratchy throat, headache, runny nose, and other signs of nasal congestion.

rhizotomy (rī-zŏt'ə-mē) N. surgical procedure in which certain nerve roots are cut at the point where they emerge from the spinal cord; it is performed to relieve severe muscle spasm (posterior roots) or to relieve intractable pain (anterior roots).

rhodopsin (rō-dŏp'sĭn) N. purple pigment within the rods of the retina, essential for vision in dim light.

Rhogam N. trade name for Rh immunoglobulin, given to prevent Rh sensitization.

rhomboid N. any of several muscles of the upper back that function in the movement of the shoulder blade. *See* MAJOR MUSCLES OF THE BODY, in Appendix.

rhonchus (rŏn'kəs) N., *pl.* rhonchi, abnormal sound heard through a stethoscope, usually during expiration, as air passes through narrowed passageways obstructed by mucus, neoplasm, muscle spasm, or pressure. ADJ. rhonchal, rhonchial

rhus dermatitis (dûr'mə-tī'tĭs) N. type of contact dermatitis resulting from contact with plants of the genus Rhus, including poison ivy, poison oak, and poison sumac. Treatment is with calamine.

rhythm N. measured time or movement; one single event that is repeated; regular occurrence of an impulse, such as the cardiac rhythm.

rhythm method of family planning N. a natural family planning method based on determining the fertile time in a woman's menstrual cycle and either avoiding coitus at that time to try to prevent conception or engaging in coitus at that time to increase the chances of conception. Determination of the fertile time (around ovulation) may be based on the calendar method, on the basal body temperature method, or on changes in cervical mucus that typically occur around ovulation. *See also* CALENDAR METHOD OF FAMILY PLANNING; BASAL BODY TEMPERATURE METHOD OF FAMILY PLANNING; OVULATION METHOD OF FAMILY PLANNING; CONTRACEPTION.

Rhythmol N. trade name for the antiarrhythmic propafenone.

rhytidoplasty (rĭt'ĭ-dō-plăs'tē) N. procedure in plastic surgery in which an incision is made near the hairline and excess tissue excised, the face tightened, wrinkles removed, and the skin made to appear firm; also called, colloquially, face lift.

rib N. one of the 12 pairs of curved bones that form the skeletal framework of the chest and protect the heart and lungs. In the back, the head of each rib articulates with one of the 12 thoracic vertebrae. In the front, the first 7 ribs (the true ribs) attach to the sternum (breastbone). Each of the next 3 ribs

RIBS

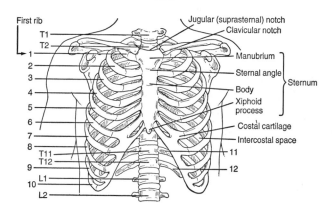

First rib
Jugular (suprasternal) notch
Clavicular notch
T1
T2
1
2
3
4
5
6
7
8
T11
T12
9
L1
10
L2
Manubrium
Sternal angle
Body
Xiphoid process
Costal cartilage
Intercostal space
11
12
Sternum

(the false ribs) attaches to the rib above it and thus indirectly to the sternum. The last 2 (the floating ribs) end freely in the musculature; also called costa. ADJ. costal

ribavirin N. inhaled antiviral agent (trade name Virazole), which may be used in the treatment of serious respiratory syncytial virus infection. Adverse reactions include exacerbation of pulmonary status and cardiac arrest.

riboflavin (rī′bō-flā′vĭn) N. water-soluble vitamin, one of the B-complex group, important as a coenzyme in metabolic processes; also called vitamin B_2. *See also* TABLE OF VITAMINS.

ribonucleic acid (RNA) (rī′bō-nōō-klē′ĭk) N. nucleic acid that in most cells transmits genetic information from the deoxyribonucleic acid (DNA) in the nucleus to the cytoplasm and functions in the synthesis of proteins. It is the genetic material of some viruses.

ribose (rī′bōs′) N. five-carbon sugar present in some vitamins and genetic material (RNA).

ribosome (rī′bə-sōm′) N. organelle composed of ribonucleic acid (RNA) and found in the cytoplasm of cells, where it serves as the site of protein synthesis.

rickets (rĭk′ĭts) N. condition caused by a deficiency of vitamin D, calcium, and/or phosphorus, occurring primarily in children and characterized by abnormal bone formation and resulting skeletal deformities, often accompanied by muscle pain and spleen and liver enlargement. Prevention and treatment include a diet adequate in calcium, phosphorus, and vitamin D and adequate exposure to sunlight. Also called rachitis. *See also* TABLE OF VITAMINS.

rickettsia (rĭ-kĕt′sē-ə) N. any of a group of bacteria-like microorganisms that live as parasites in ticks, fleas, lice, and mites and are transmitted to humans by these vectors. Rickettsia-caused diseases include Rocky Mountain spotted fever and typhus. ADJ. rickettsial

rickettsialpox (rĭ-kĕt′sē-əl-pŏks′) N. mild, infectious disease caused by *Rickettsia akari*, transmitted from mice to humans by mites. Symptoms include chills, fever, malaise, and chicken pox-like lesions that dry, form scabs, and fall off, leaving no scars. Chloramphenicol or tetracyclines are usually given.

ridge (rĭj) N. projecting edge, crest, or rim (e.g., pectoral ridge, crest of the largest tubercle in the bone of the upper part of the arm).

rifampin (rĭ-făm′pĭn) N. antibacterial used in the treatment of tuberculosis. Adverse effects include gastrointestinal upsets, discoloration of urine and sweat, and sometimes an influenza-like syndrome and liver toxicity.

Rift Valley fever N. self-limiting, usually short-lived viral infection in Africa, transmitted by mosquitoes or by handling infected animals, with symptoms of fever, malaise, headache, and photophobia.

right atrioventricular valve (ā′trē-ō-vĕn-trĭk′yə-lər) See TRICUSPID VALVE.

right-handedness N. tendency to use the right hand in writing and manipulating objects; also dextrality.

rigidity (rĭ-jĭd′ĭ-tē) N. condition of inflexibility, hardness, or stiffness. ADJ. rigid

rigor (rĭg′ər) N.
1. rigidity of the tissues of the body, as in rigor mortis.
2. sudden attack of shivering.

rigor mortis (môr′tĭs) N. rigid stiffening of the skeleton and some muscles shortly after death.

rima (rī′mə) N. crack, cleft, or opening (e.g., rima glottidis, space between the vocal cords).

ringworm (rĭng′wûrm′) N. any of several fungal infections of the skin, often characterized by ringlike skin lesions, including athlete's foot and jock itch. *See also* TINEA.

Risperdal N. *See* TABLE OF COMMONLY PRESCRIBED DRUGS—TRADE NAMES.

risperidone N. *See* TABLE OF COMMONLY PRESCRIBED DRUGS—GENERIC NAMES.

Ritalin (rĭt′l-ĭn) N. trade name for the central nervous stimulant methylphenidate.

river blindness *See* ONCHOCERCIASIS.

Rn symbol for the element radon.

RNA *See* RIBONUCLEIC ACID.

RNA polymerase (pä-lə-mə-rāz) *See* POLYMERASE.

Robaxin N. trade name for the skeletal muscle relaxant methocarbamol.

Rocephin N. trade name for the parenteral cephalosporin agent ceftriaxone.

Rocky Mountain spotted fever N. infectious disease caused by *Rickettsia rickettsii* and occurring throughout North and South America. It is characterized by fever, headache, muscle pains, mental confusion, and red macules that spread from the wrist and ankles over the trunk of the body; abdominal distension and hemorrhage sometimes occur. Treatment is by chloramphenicol and tetracycline. Also called mountain fever; spotted fever.

rod (rŏd) N.
1. rhodopsin-containing cylindrical element of the retina that functions in detecting low light.
2. straight, cylindrical structure, as the notochord of an embryo.

Rogaine N. trade name for a liquid form of the antihypertensive minoxidil, used to treat male-pattern (crown of the head) baldness. In tests on ideal candidates (men aged 20–40 with only recent and only partial hair loss), 15–20% showed noticeable improvement. The preparation must be used indefinitely, or hair loss will resume.

Rohipnol N. trade name for the benzodiazepine drug, flunitrazepam. Though no longer legally available in the United States, it is still used in other countries. Rohipnol gained notoriety as a commonly used agent for "date rape" by inducing unconsciousness and memory loss in victims.

Romazicon N. trade name for the benzodiazepine antagonist, flumazenil.

rooting reflex (rōō'tĭng) N. normal response of newborns whereby touching or stroking the side of the mouth and cheek causes the infant to turn toward the stimulated side and begin to suck.

Rorschach test N. personality assessment test consisting of 10 pictures of inkblots that the subject interprets, the interpretations being used by the examiner to assess personality and the integration of emotional and intellectual factors.

rosaceae (rō-zā'shē-ə) N. a skin disease of adults, more often women, in which the blood vessels, esp. of the nose, forehead, and cheeks, enlarge, giving the face a flushed appearance. The cause is unknown. Also called acne rosaceae.

roseola (rū-zē'ə-lə) N. any rose-colored rash, as in measles or roseola infantum.

roseola infantum N. benign illness of infants and young children. Characterized by abrupt, high fever; mild sore throat; and, a few days later, a faint, macular, pinkish rash that lasts for a few hours to a few days. Treatment involves fever-reducing agents (e.g., acetaminophen), and, if convulsions occur in association with high fever, anticonvulsants.

rostrum (rŏs'trəm) N. structure that looks like a beak (e.g., sphenoidal rostrum, ridge on the lower part of the sphenoid bone of the skull).

roughage (rŭf'ĭj) N. indigestible dietary fiber that stimulates intestinal function; derived from a variety of fruits, vegetables, and cereals.

roundworm N. worm of the phylum Nematoda, including several that produce disease in humans (*see also* TINEA).

Roxicet N. *See* TABLE OF COMMONLY PRESCRIBED DRUGS—TRADE NAMES.

-rrhea suffix indicating a flow or discharge from a body part (e.g., rhinorrhea, discharge from the nose).

RU 486 abortion-producing drug developed in France and marketed there and elsewhere abroad. Taken during the first 5 weeks of pregnancy, it blocks the action of the hormone progesterone, so that the uterine lining sloughs off the embryo.

rubefacient (roō′bə-fā′shənt) N. agent that causes reddening and warming of the skin, used as a counterirritant.

rubella (roō-bĕl′ə) N. contagious viral disease characterized by fever, mild symptoms of upper respiratory infection, and a diffuse, fine, red rash lasting for a short period, usually 3 or 4 days. The disease is usually mild and self-limiting; however, if contracted by a woman in early pregnancy, it may cause serious damage to the fetus. There is no treatment; prevention is by rubella vaccine, usually given to children as part of a normal immunization program; the vaccine should not be given to a pregnant woman or one who plans to become pregnant within 3 months. Also called three-day measles; German measles.

Rubin test (roō′bĭn) N. test that determines the patency of the fallopian tubes, used to help determine the cause of infertility. Carbon dioxide gas is introduced into the tubes through a cannula inserted in the cervix and attached to a manometer (device for measuring pressure in a gas). Increases in pressure shown on the manometer indicate that the tubes are blocked and the gas cannot escape into the abdominal cavity; a drop in pressure indicates open tubes.

rubor (roō′bôr′) N. redness, one of the signs of inflammation.

rudiment (roō′də-mənt) N. remains of a body part that was functional at an earlier stage of life; for example, Meckel's diverticulum is the rudiment of the embryonic yolk stalk.

ruga (roō′gə) N., *pl.* rugae, fold or ridge, as a ruga of the stomach.

rumination N. regurgitation of small amounts of food after feeding, seen in some infants.

rupture (rŭp′chər) N. tear or break. *See also* HERNIA.

ruptured intervertebral disc (ĭn′tər-vûr′tə-brəl) *See* HERNIATED DISC.

Russell's bodies (rŭs′əlz) N. inclusions found in plasma cells in cancer; also called cancer bodies.

S

S symbol for the element sulfur.

SA node *See* SINOATRIAL NODE.

Sabin vaccine (sā′bĭn) N. oral vaccine, consisting of live but attenuated (weakened) poliovirus, given to provide immunity to poliomyelitis, as part of the recommended immunization schedule for infants, usually in two or three doses before the age of 6 months and added doses at 18 months and at 4 or 5 years; also called oral poliovirus vaccine (OPV) and trivalent live oral poliomyelitis vaccine (TOPV) (*compare* SALK VACCINE).

sac (săk) N. pouch or baglike organ (e.g., pericardial sac, membrane surrounding the heart).

saccharide (săk′ə-rīd′) N. any of a large group of carbohydrates, including sugars and starches.

saccharin (săk′ər-ĭn) N. crystalline substance, much sweeter than sugar, used as a substitute for sugar in low calorie and no-sugar products.

saccule (săk′yōōl) N. small sac or pouch.

Sach's disease *See* TAY-SACHS DISEASE.

sacral (sā′krəl) ADJ. pert. to the sacrum.

sacral plexus (sā′krəl plĕk′səs) N. network of motor and sensory nerves branches of which innervate the pelvic region and lower limbs.

sacral vertebra (sā′krəl vûr′tə-brə) N. any of the five segments of the vertebral column that fuse in the adult to form the sacrum.

sacro- comb. form indicating an association with the sacrum (e.g., sacrococcygeal, pert. to the sacrum and coccyx).

sacroiliac (săk′rō-ĭl′ē-ăk′) ADJ. pert. to the joint in the pelvis where the sacrum and iliac bones join.

sacrum (sā′krəm) N. the large, triangular bone between the two hip bones at the back of the pelvis, formed by the fusion of five sacral vertebrae. Its base connects with the last lumbar vertebra, its apex with the coccyx.

saddle-block anesthesia (ăn′ĭs-thē′zhə) N. form of regional anesthesia in which the areas of the body that would touch a saddle if the patient were sitting astride one are anesthetized by injecting a local anesthetic agent into the spinal cavity; used sometimes for childbirth and gynecological procedures.

sadism (sā′dĭz′əm) N. pleasure obtained by inflicting physical or psychological harm and pain on another person, esp. the achievement of sexual gratification from inflicting pain or humiliation on another person, who may be a consenting or nonconsenting partner (*compare* MASOCHISM). N. sadist, ADJ. sadistic

sadomasochism (sā′dō-măs′ə-kĭz′əm) N. abnormal condition characterized by both sadism and masochism; in it pleasure is derived both from inflicting and from receiving physical or psychological pain.

safe period N. that time in a woman's menstrual cycle during which conception is least likely to occur, usually immediately before and after a period and not in midcycle, when ovulation is likely. *See also* CALENDAR METHOD OF FAMILY PLANNING.

safe sex N. use of sexual practices believed to decrease the chances of acquiring sexually transmitted diseases, esp. acquired immune deficiency syndrome (AIDS). Generally, this involves avoidance of promiscuity, abstinence from orogenital and rectal sex, and the use of condoms.

sagittal (săj′ĭ-tl) ADJ. pert. to a line from front to back in the midline of an organ or the body.

salicylate N. any of several commonly used drugs derived from salicylic acid, including aspirin, that have antipyretic, anti-inflammatory, and analgesic properties. Methyl salicyclate is a topical drug used as a counterirritant in ointments. *See also* SALICYLATE POISONING.

salicylate poisoning N. toxic condition caused by the ingestion of aspirin (acetylsalicylic acid) or other salicylates; it is characterized by vomiting, headache, rapid breathing, tinnitus, low blood sugar, electrolyte imbalance, and in severe cases by convulsions, respiratory arrest, and death. Treatment includes induced emesis and/or gastric lavage, saline cathartics, correction of electrolyte imbalance, and possibly dialysis. Some physicians advocate intravenous administration of sodium bicarbonate as part of the treatment.

saline (sā′lēn′) ADJ. containing a salt esp. sodium chloride. N. solution containing sodium chloride used as a plasma substitute and a means to correct electrolyte imbalances.

saliva (sə-lī′və) N. clear fluid, containing water, mucin, the enzyme ptyalin, and salts, secreted by the salivary glands and mucous glands of the mouth and serving to moisten food, aid in chewing and swallowing, and start the digestion of starches. ADJ. salivary

salivary duct N. duct through which saliva passes from a salivary gland to the mouth.

salivary gland (săl′ə-vĕr′ē) N. any of three pairs of glands that secrete saliva into the mouth. The parotid glands secrete a

SALIVARY GLANDS

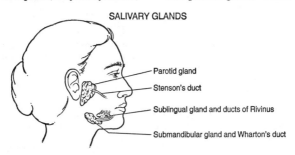

Parotid gland
Stenson's duct
Sublingual gland and ducts of Rivinus
Submandibular gland and Wharton's duct

serous fluid; the sublingual glands, a mucous fluid; and the submandibular glands, a fluid with both serous and mucous components.

Salk vaccine (sôlk) N. vaccine consisting of inactivated polio virus injected subcutaneously to provide immunity to poliomyelitis, used for infants, children with deficient immune systems, and unvaccinated adults; also called IPV (*compare* SABIN VACCINE).

salmeterol (săl-mē′tə-rôl′) N. *see* TABLE OF COMMONLY PRESCRIBED DRUGS—GENERIC NAMES.

salmonella (săl′mə-nĕl′ə) N. genus of Gram-negative, rod-shaped bacteria, some of which cause typhoid fever and some forms of gastroenteritis in humans.

salmonellosis (săl′mə-nĕ-lō′sĭs) N. form of food poisoning, caused by eating food contaminated with Salmonella bacteria; symptoms include sudden abdominal pain, nausea, vomiting, fever and diarrhea (sometimes bloody and watery). There is no specific treatment, but dehydration should be prevented.

salping-, salpingo- comb. forms indicating an association with a tube, esp. the Fallopian tubes (e.g., salpingectomy, surgical removal of one or both Fallopian tubes).

salpingitis (săl′pĭn-jī′tĭs) N. inflammation or infection of a Fallopian tube, usually the result of infection spreading from the vagina or uterus; if scar tissue forms, the tube may become blocked and disable fertilization in that tube. Treatment is by antibiotics or surgical removal of the tube.

salpingostomy (săl′pĭng-gŏs′tə-mē) N. surgically created opening in one or both fallopian tubes to restore patency that has been lost by chronic inflammation or to drain fluid.

salpinx (săl′pĭngks) N., *pl.* salpinges, tube

salt N. compound formed by the reaction of an acid and a base, esp. sodium chloride, table salt.

salt depletion N. loss of salt from the body by vomiting, diarrhea, profuse perspiration, or urination without replacement. *See also* ELECTROLYTE BALANCE.

salt-free diet *See* LOW-SODIUM DIET.

salubrious ADJ. healthful.

sand tumor *See* PSAMMOMA.

sangui-, sanguino- comb. forms indicating an association with blood (e.g., sanguifacient, blood-producing).

sanguineous ADJ. bloody; accompanied by bloodshed.

sanguis N. See BLOOD. ADJ. sanguineous

sanitarium (săn′ĭ-târ′ē-əm) N. institution for treatment of persons with long-term or chronic disorders. Prior to modern antibiotics, persons with tuberculosis were placed in a TB sanitarium. Also, colloq. for an institution that treats persons with mental disorders.

saphenous nerve (să-fē′nŭs) N. branch of the femoral nerve, supplying the inner aspect of the leg.

saphenous vein N. either of two veins of the leg that drain blood from the foot.

    long saphenous vein N. longest vein in the body; it runs from the foot up the medial side of the leg to the groin, where it joins the femoral vein. Also called great saphenous vein.

short saphenous vein N. vein running up the back of the lower leg from the foot to the knee.

sapr-, sapro- comb. forms indicating decay or putrefaction (e.g., saprophyte, organism that lives on dead tissue).

sarco- comb. form indicating an association with flesh (e.g., sarcolysis, breakdown of flesh).

sarcoid (sär'koid') ADJ. fleshy.

sarcoidosis (sär'koi-dō'sĭs) N. chronic disease of unknown cause characterized by the formation of nodules in the lungs, liver, lymph glands, and salivary glands. A relationship with tuberculosis is suspected, but has not been proven.

sarcolemma (sär'kə-lĕm'ə) N. membrane surrounding a muscle fiber. ADJ. sarcolemmic; sarcolemnous

sarcoma (sär-kō'mə) N. malignant neoplasm arising in bone, muscle, or other connective tissue (*compare* CARCINOMA).

sarcomere (sär'kə-mēr') N. contractile unit of which striated muscle is composed.

sarcoplasm (sär'kə-plăz'əm) N. cytoplasm of muscle.

sarcoplasmic reticulum (sär'kə-plăz'mĭk) N. network of tubules and sacs that function in muscle contraction and relaxation.

sartorius (sär-tôr'ē-əs) N. longest muscle in the body, extending from the pelvis to the calf of the leg; it functions in the movement of the thigh and lower leg. *See* MAJOR MUSCLES OF THE BODY, in Appendix.

satiety N. fullness; condition of being filled to satisfaction, especially with food.

saturated fatty acid N. fatty acid in which all the atoms are joined by single valence bonds; saturated fatty acids are found chiefly in animal fats (e.g., beef, pork, lamb, veal, milk products). A diet high in saturated fats has been associated with high serum cholesterol levels and in some studies with increased risk of coronary artery disease. (*compare* UNSATURATED FATTY ACID.)

satyriasis N. excessive and uncontrollable sexual desire in a male (*compare* NYMPHOMANIA).

scab (skăb) *See* ESCHAR.

scabicide N. a drug that destroys the itch mite (*Sarcoptes scabiei*).

scabies (skā'bēz) N. contagious disease caused by the itch mite (*Sarcoptes scabiei*) and characterized by itching and skin irritation, often leading to secondary infection. Treatment includes scabicides and antihistamines to relieve itching. All contacts, bedding, and clothing must be treated to prevent spread and reinfestation.

scale (skāl) N. flake of dead epidermis shed from the surface of the skin. V. to remove tartar or other encrusted material from the surface of a tooth.

scalenus N. any of four pairs of muscles extending from the cervical vertebrae to the second rib and involved in movement of the neck and in breathing movements.

scalenus syndrome N. symptoms caused by a scalenus muscle (esp. scalenus anterior) compressing the subclavian artery and part of the brachial plexus against the bones of upper thoracic or lower cervical vertebrae; loss of sensation, discomfort, and vascular symptoms in the affected shoulder and arm occur. *See also* THORACIC OUTLET SYNDROME.

scalp (skălp) N. skin covering the head, not including the ears and face.

scaphocephaly N. congenital malformation of the skull in which the skull is abnormally long and narrow; the condition is frequently accompanied by mental retardation.

scaphoid bone *See* NAVICULAR.

scapula (skăp′yə-lə) N., *pl.* scapulae, either of a pair of large, flat, triangular bones that form the back part of the shoulder girdle. The scapula articulates with the clavicle (collarbone) and overhangs the glenoid cavity into which the humerus (upper arm bone) fits, and provides for the attachment of many ligaments and muscles. Also called shoulder blade. ADJ. scapular.

scapulohumeral ADJ. pert. to the shoulder blade (scapula) and upper arm bone (humerus).

scar (skär) *See* CICATRIX.

scarlet fever (skär′lĭt) N. acute contagious disease, usually occurring in childhood, caused by a Streptococcus bacterium, and characterized by fever, sore throat, enlarged lymph nodes in the neck, and a bright red rash that typically spreads from the armpits and groin to the trunk of the body and limbs. Treatment is by antibiotics. Also called scarlatina.

scato- comb. form indicating an association with feces (e.g., scatophagy, eating of feces).

scavenger N. drug or cell that removes disintegrated tissues or abnormal compounds in the body. Anti-oxidant drugs function as free-radical scavengers, removing them from the body. Certain types of white blood cells remove foreign material or bacteria from the body, much as a scavenger bird would clean the carcass of a dead animal.

Schick test (shĭk) N. skin test to determine immunity to diphtheria. A small amount of diphtheria toxin is injected intradermally; the development of redness and swelling at the injection site constitutes a positive reaction and indicates suscepti-

SCAPULA

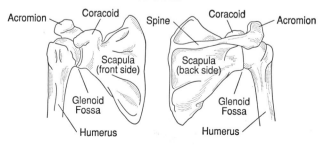

Acromion — Coracoid — Spine — Coracoid — Acromion

Scapula (front side) — Scapula (back side)

Glenoid Fossa — Glenoid Fossa

Humerus — Humerus

bility to diphtheria. A negative reaction indicates immunity.

schistosomiasis (shĭs′tə-sə-mī′ə-sĭs) N. infection with a parasite of the genus Schistosoma, transmitted to humans by contact with feces-contaminated fresh water or fresh-water organisms, esp. snails; it is common in the tropics and Far East, affecting a large percentage of the population in some areas. Symptoms depend on the part of the body infected, often the bladder, intestines, spleen, or blood vessels. Pain, disturbances of organ function, and anemia often result. Treatment is difficult and usually includes the use of antimony preparations. Also called bilharziasis.

schizo- comb. form indicating a split or division (e.g., schizonychia, condition in which the nails are split).

schizophrenia (skĭt′sə-frē′nē-ə) N. any of a group of mental disorders characterized by gross distortions of reality, withdrawal from social contacts, and disturbances of thought, language, perception, and emotional response. Symptoms are highly varied and may include apathy, catatonia or excessive activity, bizarre actions, hallucinations, delusions, and rambling speech. Some cases are mild; others severe, requiring prolonged or permanent hospitalization. There

is no known cause; a combination of hereditary or genetic predisposition factors is likely responsible in most cases.

schizophrenic (skĭt′sə-frĕn′ĭk) ADJ. pert. to schizophrenia. N. person with schizophrenia.

Schwann cells (shwän) N. cells that lay down the myelin sheath around the axon of certain nerve fibers.

sciatic nerve (sī-ăt′ĭk) N. nerve running from the lower spine down the thigh to the knee region, where it divides into two nerves that supply the lower leg.

sciatica (sī-ăt′ĭ-kə) N. pain felt in the back and down the back and outer part of the thigh and leg due to compression on sacral spinal nerve roots or the sciatic nerve, often associated with degeneration of an intervertebral disc. Treatment is by rest; intractable cases may require surgery.

scler-, sclero- comb. forms indicating hardness (e.g., scleradonitis, gland hardening) or the sclera of the eye (e.g., sclerocorneal, pert. to the sclera and cornea).

sclera (sklēr′ə) N. tough. opaque covering of the posterior part of the eye that maintains the size of the eyball and attaches to muscles involved in eye

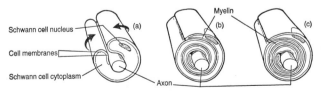

How the myelin sheath forms as the Schwann cell wraps itself around the axon in successive diagrams (a), (b), and (c). Myelin is the white, lipid-rich substance in the plasma membrane of the Schwann cell.

movement. It is pierced by the optic nerve. ADJ. scleral

scleroderma (sklēr'ə-dûr'mə) N. autoimmune disease affecting the blood vessels and connective tissue, occurring most often in middle-aged women. Skin changes in the face and fingers and rheumatoid-arthritis-like symptoms progress to areas where the skin becomes fixed to underlying tissue. In severe cases the skin of the face may become so taut as to interfere with chewing and swallowing, or there may be pulmonary and cardiac complications leading to death. Other cases remain benign and localized. Treatment includes corticosteroids and analgesics.

sclerosis (sklə-rō'sĭs) N. condition characterized by hardness of tissue resulting from inflammation, mineral deposits, or other causes.

scoliosis (skō'lē-ō'sĭs) N. abnormal lateral or sideward curve to the spine; common in childhood, it may be caused by congenital malformation, poliomyelitis, limbs of unequal length, or other factors. Early treatment involving surgery, casts, exercises, and braces may prevent progression of the curvature. (*compare* KYPHOSIS; LORDOSIS.)

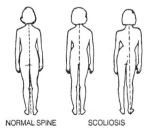

NORMAL SPINE   SCOLIOSIS

scopolamine (skə-pŏl'ə-mēn') N. anticholinergic drug used to treat nausea and vomiting, to sedate, and in ophthalmic procedures to dilate the pupils. Adverse effects are blurred vision, dry mouth, decreased sweating, and hypersensitivity reactions.

scopolamine patch N. small transdermal disc that contains the medication scopolamine and is placed behind the ear to prevent motion sickness; the disc delivers the medication over a period of three days; side effects include blurred vision, dryness of the mouth, and drowsiness. *See also* MOTION SICKNESS PATCH.

scratch test N. skin test for identifying an allergen. A small amount of a solution containing a suspected allergen is placed on a scratched skin area; if redness and wheal formation develop, allergy to that particular substance is demonstrated.

scrofula (skrŏf'yə-lə) N. form of tuberculosis characterized by abscess formation, usually in the lymph nodes of the neck. ADJ. scrofulous

scrotum (skrō'təm) N. pouch of skin containing the testes and parts of the spermatic cords below the abdomen. It is divided into two lateral portions by a ridge that continues ventrally to the undersurface of the penis and dorsally to the perineum. Because it holds the testes away from the abdomen, the scrotum allows the production of sperm at a temperature lower than that of the abdomen. ADJ. scrotal

scrub typhus (tī'fəs) N. disease of eastern Asia, surrounding islands, and Australia, caused by Rickesttsia organisms transmitted to humans by mites. Symptoms include a dark lesion at the site of the bite, lymph node enlargement, fever, muscle ache, rash, and in severe cases cardiovascular and nervous system involvement. Treatment is by antibiotics.

scurvy (skûr'vē) N. condition caused by a lack of ascorbic acid (vitamin C) in the diet and characterized by anemia, weakness, and spongy, bleeding gums. Treatment involves administration of vitamin C and a diet rich in ascorbic acid-containing fruits and vegetables.

seal limbs *See* PHOCOMELIA.

seasickness (sē'sĭk'nĭs) N. disorder consisting of nausea, vomiting, headache, and diaphoresis due to the motion of a boat or ship. Treatment is with medications such as dimenhydrinate (Dramamine) or motion sickness bands, which may also help to prevent symptom occurrence. Rest and a reduction in dietary and alcohol intake may also lessen the chances of developing seasickness. (*Compare* AIR SICKNESS; CAR SICKNESS; MOTION SICKNESS.)

sebaceous (sĭ-bā'shəs) ADJ. fatty, greasy, esp. pert. to the sebaceous glands.

sebaceous cyst (sĭ-bā'shəs sĭst) N. sac (cyst) filled with fatty matter (sebum) secreted by a sebaceous gland. The cyst occurs as a result of blockage in the gland, which then overdistends. Surgical removal of the gland is required for permanent relief.

sebaceous gland N. any of numerous sebum-secreting organs in the dermis throughout the body (except the palms and soles), esp. abundant on the scalp, face, nose, mouth, and ears. In most cases the sebum

is secreted into hair follicles but in some places (e.g., the labia minora, lips) it is secreted onto the surface. The sebum oils the hair and skin and helps to retain body heat and prevent sweat evaporation.

seborrhea (sĕb'ə-rē'ə) N. any of several conditions in which there is overactivity of the sebaceous glands and the skin becomes oily.

seborrheic dermatitis (sĕb'ə-rē'ĭk dûr'mə-tī'tĭs) N. a chronic skin disease associated with overactivity of the sebaceous glands and greasy scales on the scalp (cradle cap or dandruff), eyelids (blepharitis), or other parts of the skin. Treatment includes medicated shampoos, corticosteroids, antibiotics, and the treatment of any underlying disorder (e.g., diabetes mellitus or allergic reaction) causing the condition.

sebum (sē'bəm) N. secretion of the sebaceous glands, containing fat and cellular debris. With sweat, it moistens and protects the skin.

secobarbital (sĕk'ōbär'bĭ-tôl') N. sedative (trade name Seconal) used in the treatment of insomnia and convulsions. Adverse effects include respiratory depression, paradoxical excitement, and allergic reactions.

second messenger N. chemical signal that triggers a biochemical response; formation is usually stimulated by a drug, neurotransmitter, or hormone binding a cell surface receptor. One of the most common is cyclic AMP, whose function as a second messenger is vital in numerous biochemical processes in the body, as well as in the actions of many medications. *See also* CYCLIC AMP; SIGNAL TRANSDUCTION.

secondary amenorrhea (ā-měn′ə-rē′ə) *See* AMENORRHEA.

secondary dysmenorrhea (dǐs-měn′ə-rē′ə) *See* DYSMENORRHEA.

secondary sex characteristic N. any of the physical characteristics associated with sexual maturity but not directly involved in reproductive functioning. In males they include deep voice and facial and pubic hair; in females, breast development and pubic hair.

secretin (sǐ-krēt′n) N. hormone secreted by the small intestine when acidic, partially digested food enters it; it stimulates bile production and pancreatic secretion.

secretion (sǐ-krē′shən) N. process by which substances (e.g., enzymes and hormones) are released from specific organs or the blood for a particular purpose. V. secrete, ADJ. secretory

secretory phase (sǐ-krē′tə-rē) N. second half of the menstrual cycle, after ovulation during which progesterone secreted by the corpus luteum stimulates the development and thickening of the endometrium in preparation for the implantation of an embryo. If fertilization does not occur, the secretory phase ends as the corpus luteum involutes, progesterone levels decrease, and menstrual flow begins. Also called luteal phase.

section (sĕk′shən) N. act of cutting. V. to cut.

Sectral N. trade name for the beta blocker acebutolol.

secundi- comb. form meaning "second" (e.g., secundigravida,

woman pregnant for the second time).

sedation (sǐ-dā′shən) N. induced state of reduced activity and excitability; a state of calm and quiet, sometimes with sleep.

sedative (sĕd′ə-tǐv) N. agent that decreases activity and excitability, relieves anxiety, and calms the person. Some sedatives have a general effect; others affect the activities of certain organs (e.g., intestines or vasomotor system).

sedative-hypnotic (sĕd′ə-tǐv-hǐp-nŏt′ǐk) N. drug that depresses central nervous system activity, relieves anxiety, and induces sleep. Barbiturates, minor tranquilizers (e.g., diazepam and chlordiazepoxide), chloral hydrate, and many other drugs act as sedative-hypnotics.

sedimentation rate (sĕd′ə-mən-tā′shən) *See* ERYTHROCYTE SEDIMENTATION RATE.

seizure (sē′zhər) *See* CONVULSION.

Seldane N. trade name for the antihistamine drug, terfenadine.

self-breast examination *See* BREAST SELF-EXAMINATION.

self-limited ADJ. pert. to a disease that tends to end or resolve without treatment.

sella turcica N. concavity on the inside portion of the skull, in the sphenoid bone, that houses the pituitary gland.

semen (sē′mən) N. thick, whitish secretion discharged from the urethra during ejaculation. It contains spermatozoa and secretions of the prostate gland, seminal vesicles, and other glands. Also called seminal fluid. ADJ. seminal

SELLA TURCICA

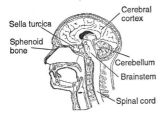

semi- prefix meaning "one-half" (e.g., semicoma, stuporous state from which arousal is possible; half a coma).

semicircular canal (sĕm'ĭ-sûr'kyə-lər) N. any of three bony, fluid-filled loops in the osseous labyrinth of the inner ear, concerned with the sense and maintenance of balance.

semilunar valve (sĕm'ē-lōo'nər) N. heart valve with half-moon-shaped cusps (semilunar), as the aortic valve or the pulmonary valve. *See also* TRICUSPID VALVE.

seminal duct (sĕm'ə-nəl) N. duct through which semen passes, as the ejaculatory duct.

seminal fluid *See* SEMEN.

seminal vesicle (vĕs'ĭ-kəl) N. either of a pair of accessory male sex glands that produce most of the fluid portion of semen, secreting it into the vas deferens before it joins the urethra.

seminiferous tubule (sĕm'ə-nĭf'ər-əs tōo'byōol) N. any of numerous long and convoluted tubes found in the testis; they are the sites of spermatozoa maturation.

seminoma (sĕm'ə-nō'mə) N. malignant tumor of the testis, usually occurring in older men.

Treatment is by surgery (orchidectomy).

semipermeable membrane (mĕm'brān') N. membrane (e.g., a cell membrane) that allows the passage of some molecules but not others.

senescence (sĭ-nĕs'əns) N. process of growing old; often refers to normal changes of aging, though these may occur prematurely due to a variety of conditions.

senile (sē'nīl') ADJ. pert. to or characteristic of old age or aging, esp. deterioration associated with aging. N. senility.

senile dementia (dĭ-mĕn'shə) N. mental disorder of the aged, resulting from atrophy and degeneration of the brain, with no signs of cerebrovascular disease. Symptoms, which are generally slowly progressive, include loss of memory, periods of confusion and irritability, confabulation (invention of fictitious details about a past event that may or may not have occurred), and poor judgment. Also called senile psychosis. (*Compare* ALZHEIMER'S DISEASE.)

senile memory *See* ANTEROGRADE MEMORY.

sensation (sĕn-sā'shən) N. one of the facilities by which information about the external environment is received and interpreted; there are five major senses: sight, hearing, smell, taste, and touch.

sense organ (sĕns) N. collection of specialized cells—receptor cells—capable of responding to a particular stimulus (e.g., an odor) and transmitting that message as an impulse along a sensory nerve to the central nervous system for interpretation.

sensibility (sĕn′sə-bĭl′ĭ-tē) N. ability to be affected by changes in the environment.

sensitivity (sĕn′sĭ-tĭv′ĭ-tē) N. capacity to feel or react to a stimulus. ADJ. sensitive; in statistics, proportion of people who actually had a given condition and are correctly identified by a test; a sensitive test has a low false-negative rate. An insensitive test has a high false-negative rate and should not be relied upon to exclude abnormality or disease. For example, an electrocardiogram for heart disease is relatively insensitive—many patients with coronary artery disease, including acute heart attacks, have a negative result. Other tests, such as nuclear medicine treadmill scans, are far more sensitive due to a much lower percentage of false-negative results.

sensitization (sĕn′sĭ-tĭ-zā′shən) N. acquired reaction in which antibodies develop in response to an antigen.

sensorineural hearing loss N. decreased hearing due to damage or disease of the auditory nerve (colloquially, "nerve deafness") (*compare* CONDUCTIVE HEARING LOSS).

sensory nerve (sĕn′sə-rē) N. nerve that conducts impulses from the periphery of the body (e.g., from sense organs) to the brain or spinal cord (*compare* MOTOR NERVE).

sepsis (sĕp′sĭs) N. destruction of tissue by bacterial toxins; contamination; infection (*compare* ASEPTIC).

septal defect N. congenital abnormality in the wall (septum) separating the left and right sides of the heart. It may occur between the two atria (atrial septal defect) or between the two ventricles (ventricular septal defect). The defect allows abnormal circulation of blood and causes numerous symptoms, depending on its location and size.

septicemia (sĕp′tĭ-sē′mē-ə) N. serious infection in which disease-causing organisms are present in the circulating blood usually resulting from spread of an infection from a specific site. Symptoms include fever, chills, nausea, diarrhea, headache, and prostration. Treatment is by antibiotics. Also called blood poisoning.

Septra N. *See* TABLE OF COMMONLY PRESCRIBED DRUGS—TRADE NAMES.

septum (sĕp′təm) N. partition or dividing wall in an organ (e.g., the septum dividing the left and right sides of the heart, and the septum dividing the nasal cavity). ADJ. septal, septate

sequela (sĭ-kwĕl′ə) N., *pl.* sequelae, abnormality following or resulting from a disease, injury, or treatment (e.g., paralysis following poliomyelitis).

sequestration (sē′kwĭ-strā′shən) N.
1. quarantine of a patient.
2. form of intervertebral disc herniation where a piece of the nucleus pulposus separates and floats freely in the spinal canal.
3. In the lung, a nonfunctioning area that receives its blood supply from the systemic circulation; pulmonary sequestration is often responsible for recurrent lung infections and may mimic a tumor on X ray.

Serax N. trade name for the tranquilizer oxazepam.

Serentil N. trade name for the phenothiazine tranquilizer mesoridazine.

Serevent N. *See* TABLE OF COMMONLY PRESCRIBED DRUGS—TRADE NAMES.

sero- comb. form indicating an association with serum (e.g., seroglobulin, globulin found in serum).

serology (sĭ-rŏl′ə-jē) N. that branch of science concerned with the study of blood serum, esp. the search for evidence of infection and the evaluation of immune reactions. ADJ. serologic; serological

serosa (sĭ-rō′sə) *See* SEROUS MEMBRANE.

serotonin (sĕr′ə-tō′nĭn) N. chemical widely distributed in the body, esp. in the brain, where it acts as a neurotransmitter; in the blood platelets, upon an injury, it acts as a vasoconstrictor; and in the small intestine it stimulates smooth muscle to contract.

serous membrane (sĕr′əs) N. smooth, transparent membrane, containing fibrous connective tissue, that lines many large cavities of the body (e.g., the pleural cavity, peritoneal cavity, and pericardial cavity). Serous membranes usually consist of two layers: a visceral layer covering the organs and a parietal layer lining the cavity walls. Between the two layers is a small space filled with serous fluid, derived from blood serum, that moistens the structures and allows frictionless movement. Also called serosa.

serratus N. any of several muscles with sawlike processes, esp. serratus anterior, muscle between the ribs and shoulder blade involved in shoulder and arm movement, particularly pushing-type motions. *See* MAJOR MUSCLES OF THE BODY, in Appendix.

Sertoli cells (sər-tō′lē) N. cells found in the seminiferous tubules of the testis, where they nourish developing spermatozoa.

sertraline HCl (sər′trə-lēn) N. antidepressant that works by inhibition of the uptake of the neurotransmitter serotonin; common side effects include nausea, diarrhea, tremor, insomnia, somnolence, and dry mouth. *See* TABLE OF COMMONLY PRESCRIBED DRUGS—GENERIC NAMES.

serum (sēr′əm) N. clear, thin, fluid of blood. Like plasma, it contains no cells or platelets; unlike plasma, it also contains no fibrinogen.

serum hepatitis (hĕp′ə-tī′tĭs) *See* HEPATITIS.

serum sickness N. reaction occurring 1 or 2 weeks after the injection of antiserum (donor serum containing desired antibodies) and caused by an antibody reaction to an antigen in the donor serum. Symptoms of fever, enlarged spleen, joint pain, and swollen lymph glands occur.

Serzone N. *See* TABLE OF COMMONLY PRESCRIBED DRUGS—TRADE NAMES.

sesamoid bone N. any of several small, round or oval bones lying within a tendon, such as the patella (kneecap). The patella is the largest sesamoid bone in the human body.

sex N. classification of male or female based on the physical, psychological, and behavioral characteristics of an animal that relate to reproduction, esp. in having specific chromosomes (Y in the human male) and producing special gametes (ova in females, sperm in males) and in having anatomical and physiological characteristics associated with femaleness or maleness. ADJ. sexual

sex chromatin (krō′mə-tĭn) N. chromatin found only in female cells; it usually occurs as a small object (Barr body) near the nucleus or as a drumstick-shaped appendage to the nucleus of some white cells. The presence or absence of sex chromatin is the basis of sex determination before birth through examination of cells obtained by amniocentesis.

sex chromosome (krō′mə-sōm′) N. chromosome that is responsible for sex determination and carries certain sex-linked genes. In mammals there are two sex chromosomes: X and Y. Human females have the XX combination; males, the XY combination.

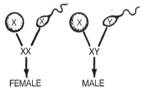

Pairing of sex chromosomes from the sperm and ovum determines the sex of the offspring at the time of fertilization.

sex hormone (hôr′mōn′) N. steroid hormone responsible for sexual development and reproductive function. The main female sex hormones are estrogens and progesterone; the male sex hormones are androgens (including testosterone).

sex-limited ADJ. pert. to a characteristic that is expressed differently in the two sexes.

sex-linked disorder N. disease or abnormality determined by the sex chromosomes. It may involve an abnormality in the number of sex chromosomes (e.g., Turner's syndrome or Kleinfelter's syndrome) or a gene defect on an X-chromosome (e.g., hemophilia).

sexual intercourse (sĕk′shoo-əl ĭn′tər-kôrs′) See COITUS.

sexually transmitted disease (STD) N. communicable disease transmitted by sexual intercourse or genital contact; sexually transmitted diseases include gonorrhea, some herpes infections, acquired immune deficiency syndrome (AIDS), syphilis, granuloma inguinale. Colloquial: venereal disease (VD).

sheath (shēth) N. tubular structure surrounding an organ or body part (e.g., synovial sheath of some tendons).

shell shock See COMBAT FATIGUE.

shiatsu (shē-ät′soo) N. Japanese method of massage that incorporates the technique of acupressure.

shigellosis (shĭg′ə-lō′sĭs) N. acute infection of the intestine with pathogenic Shigella bacteria; it is widespread in many lesser developed areas of the world and occurs sporadically in other areas. Symptoms include diarrhea, abdominal discomfort, and fever. Also called bacillary dysentery.

shin bone See TIBIA.

shingles (shĭng′gəlz) See HERPES ZOSTER.

Shirodkar's operation N. surgical procedure in which a purse-string suture is used to close the cervix in a pregnant woman whose incompetent cervix has failed to retain previous pregnancies; also called purse-string operation.

shock (shŏk) N. abnormal body state associated with inadequate oxygen delivery to the metabolic apparatus of the cell (the mitochondrion). This can occur for many reasons, including hypovolemia (*see also* HYPOVOLE-MIC SHOCK), cardiac failure (cardiogenic shock), obstruction to blood flow (obstructive shock), and maldistribution of the blood flow (distributive shock). Shock is characterized by reduced cardiac output, circulatory insufficiency, rapid heartbeat, and pallor. Low blood pressure, though classically associated with shock, is a late sign, especially in children. Treatment is primarily that of the underlying condition. Intravenous fluid therapy helps most patients, at least initially.

shock therapy (shŏk thĕr'ə-pē) *See* ELECTROCONVULSIVE THERAPY.

short-acting ADJ. pert. to a drug or other agent that has a short period of effectiveness, usually beginning shortly after administration (*compare* LONG-ACTING).

shoulder blade (shōl'dər) *See* SCAPULA.

shoulder joint N. ball-and-socket joint in which the humerus articulates with the scapula.

shunt (shŭnt) V. to redirect the flow of a body fluid from one vessel to another. N. device implanted to redirect the flow of a body fluid.

Si symbol for the element silicon.

sial-, sialo- comb. forms indicating an association with saliva or the salivary glands (e.g., sialadenitis, inflammation of the salivary glands).

sialolith (sī'ə-lō-lĭth') N. stone formed in a salivary gland.

Siamese twins (sī'ə-mēz') N. twins born joined together at one or more body parts and often sharing a body part. Most Siamese twins can be separated surgically, the prognosis depending on the site of connection and the extent of shared organs. Also called conjoined twins.

sibling (sĭb'lĭng) N. one of two or more children who have both parents in common.

sickle cell (sĭk'əl) N. abnormal red blood cell (erythrocyte) with a crescent shape and abnormal form of hemoglobin.

sickle-cell anemia (sĭk'əl sĕl ə-nē'mē-ə) N. hereditary blood disease, occurring mostly in blacks, in which abnormal hemoglobin (hemoglobin HbS) causes red blood cells (erythrocytes) to become sickle-shaped, fragile, and nonfunctional, leading to anemia. Persons inheriting the trait from only one parent may show few symptoms; those homozygous

SHOULDER

Articular Surface: Head of Humerus
Acromion
Coracoid Process
A/C Joint
Greater Tuberosity
Bicipital Groove
Glenohumeral Joint
Lesser Tuberosity

for the trait (inheriting it from both parents) have chronic anemia, an enlarged spleen, lethargy, weakness, blood clot formation, and joint pain.

sickle-cell trait N. heterozygous sickle-cell anemia with both normal and abnormal hemoglobin present. There are usually few or no symptoms, the main concern being possible transmission to offspring. *See also* SICKLE-CELL ANEMIA.

sideropenia N. iron deficiency, caused by inadequate iron intake in the diet or increased loss from the body, as occurs in hemorrhage or chronic bleeding. The major manifestation is anemia, corrected by iron administration.

siderosis (sĭd′ə-rō′sĭs) N. form of pneumoconiosis in which iron dust or particles affect the lungs, causing fibrosis; it occurs among welders and other metal workers.

SIDS *See* SUDDEN INFANT DEATH SYNDROME.

sigmoid colon (sĭg′moid′) N. that part of the colon extending from the end of the descending colon to the rectum.

sigmoidectomy (sĭg′moi-dĕk′tə-mē) N. surgical removal of all or part of the sigmoid colon, usually to remove a malignant tumor.

sigmoidoscope (sĭg-moi′də-skōp′) N. instrument, consisting of a tube and light, inserted through the anus to allow visualization of the sigmoid colon.

sigmoidoscopy (sĭg′moi-dŏs′kə-pē) N. procedure of examining the sigmoid colon utilizing a sigmoidoscope.

sign (sīn) N. observable indication of a disease (e.g., Babinski reflex) (*compare* SYMPTOM).

signal transduction N. biochemical events that conduct the signal of a ligand (e.g., hormone or drug) from the cell exterior, through the cell membrane, and into the cytoplasm. This involves a number of molecules, including receptors and second messengers. *See also* CYCLIC AMP; LIGAND; SECOND MESSENGER.

sildenafil N. *See* TABLE OF COMMONLY PRESCRIBED DRUGS—GENERIC NAMES.

silicon (sĭl′ĭ-kən) N. nonmetallic element; occurs in traces in bones and teeth. *See also* TABLE OF IMPORTANT ELEMENTS.

silicosis (sĭl′ĭ-kō′sĭs) N. form of pneumoconiosis produced by inhaling silica dust; common among sandblasters, some miners, and others who work with sand.

silver nitrate N. topical anti-infective agent used on wound dressings and placed in the eyes of newborns to prevent gonorrheal infection.

simple fracture *See* FRACTURE.

simple mastectomy (mă-stĕk′tə-mē) *See* MASTECTOMY.

simvastatin N. oral agent (trade name Zocor) used in the treatment of hypercholesterolemia; the most common side effects are gastrointestinal in nature (e.g., constipation). *See* TABLE OF COMMONLY PRESCRIBED DRUGS—GENERIC NAMES.

Sinequal N. trade name for the antidepressant doxepin.

sinew (sĭn′yōō) *See* TENDON.

singultus *See* HICCUP.

532

sinistrality (sĭn'ĭ-străl'ĭ-tē) *See* LEFT-HANDEDNESS.

sinoatrial node (SA node) (sī'nō-ā'trē-əl) N. area of modified cardiac muscle in the right atrium near the entry of the superior vena cava that generates impulses that travel through the muscles of both atria, causing them to contract. Cells in the node have an intrinsic rhythm independent of nerve impulse stimulation. Normally the node fires about 60–80 beats per minute, with certain hormones and other factors (e.g., exercise) causing faster rate. An artificial pacemaker can be used in cases of defective sinoatrial node. Also called pacemaker. (*Compare* ANTRIOVENTRICULAR NODE.)

sinus (sī'nəs) N.
1. air cavity within a bone, esp. the nasal sinuses in the bones of the face and skull.
2. wide channel containing blood (e.g., venous sinuses in the dura mater, draining blood from the brain). *See* PARANASAL SINUSES.

sinus headache N. pain in the head resulting from congestion and/or infection in the paranasal sinuses. Typically the discomfort is localized over the forehead or behind the eyes and is increased by bending over. Treatment involves decongestants, analgesics, and sometimes antibiotics.

sinusitis (sī'nə-sī'tĭs) N. inflammation of one of the paranasal sinuses occurring as a result of an upper respiratory tract infection, an allergic response, a change in atmospheric pressure, or a defect of the nose. As sinus secretions accumulate, pain, fever, tenderness, and headache develop; serious complications include spread of the infection to the bone or brain. Treatment is by antibiotics (if infection is present), decongestants, steam inhalation, and in some chronic cases, surgical drainage.

skeletal muscle (skĕl'ĭ-tl) *See* STRIATED MUSCLE.

skeleton (skĕl'ĭ-tn) N. framework of the body, made up of 206 bones that provide structure and form for the body, protect delicate internal organs, provide for the attachment of muscles, produce red blood cells, and serve as blood reservoirs. The skeleton is divided into two major parts: the axial skeleton, which includes the skull, vertebral column, sternum, and ribs; and the appendicular skeleton, which includes the pectoral (shoulder) girdle (clavicle and scapula), the pelvic (hip) girdle, and the arms and legs. ADJ. skeletal.

skin N. outer covering of the body, the largest organ of the body. It protects the body from injury and invasion by microorganisms, helps (through hair follicles and sweat glands) to maintain body temperature, serves as a sensory network, lubricates and waterproofs the exterior, and serves as an organ of excretion. The skin consists of an outer layer: the epidermis and an inner layer: the dermis (corium).

skin cancer (skĭn) N. neoplasm of the skin. Skin cancer is the most common and most curable malignancy. Sun or other source of ultraviolet-ray exposure (e.g., tanning salons) is a strong causative factor. Treatment depends on the location and extent of the neoplasm; it may involve surgery, radiotherapy, and/or chemotherapy.

skin graft (skĭn grăft) N. portion of skin cut and removed from

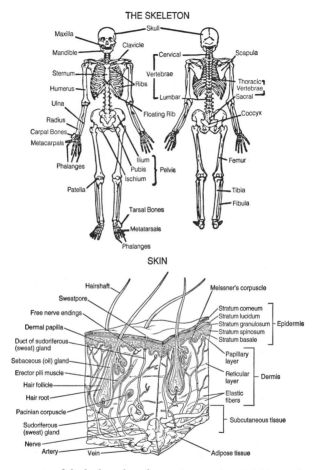

THE SKELETON

SKIN

one area of the body and used to cover a part that has lost skin because of burns, injury, or other factors. A skin graft is usually taken from another part of the body of the same person (autograft), but sometimes from another person (homograft) as a temporary measure.

skull (skŭl) N. bony skeleton of the head, consisting of the cra-nium, made up of 8 bones that contain and protect the brain; and the facial skeleton, consist-ing of 14 bones.

SLE *See* SYSTEMIC LUPUS ERY-THEMATOSUS.

sleep (slēp) N. state of reduced consciousness and depressed metabolism occurring normally at regular intervals, ranging

SKULL

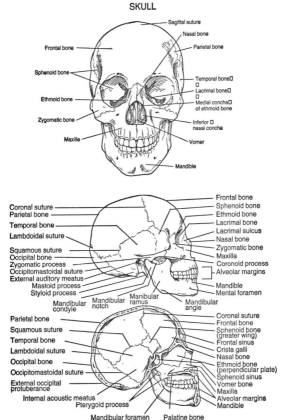

Sagittal suture
Nasal bone
Frontal bone
Parietal bone
Sphenoid bone
Temporal bone
Lacrimal bone
Medial concha
of ethmoid bone
Ethmoid bone
Inferior
nasal concha
Zygomatic bone
Maxilla
Vomer
Mandible

Coronal suture
Parietal bone
Temporal bone
Lambdoidal suture
Squamous suture
Occipital bone
Zygomatic process
Occipitomastoidal suture
External auditory meatus
Mastoid process
Styloid process
Mandibular condyle
Mandibular notch
Manibular ramus
Frontal bone
Sphenoid bone
Ethmoid bone
Lacrimal bone
Lacrimal sulcus
Nasal bone
Zygomatic bone
Maxilla
Coronoid process
Alveolar margins
Mandible
Mental foramen
Mandibular angle

Parietal bone
Squamous suture
Temporal bone
Lambdoidal suture
Occipital bone
Occipitomastoidal suture
External occipital protuberance
Internal acoustic meatus
Pterygoid process
Mandibular foramen
Coronal suture
Frontal bone
Sphenoid bone (greater wing)
Frontal sinus
Crista galli
Nasal bone
Ethmoid bone (perpendicular plate)
Sphenoid sinus
Vomer bone
Maxilla
Alveolar margins
Mandible
Palatine bone

from as much as 20 hours a day in some infants to as little as 5 or 6 hours a day in some adults, esp. the aged. Sleep can be divided into two parts: non-rapid eye movement sleep, representing about 75% of total sleep, during which dreaming does not occur; and rapid eye movement sleep, during which dreaming does occur.

sleep apnea (ăp′nē-ə) N. condition in which the patient has transient periods of apnea during sleep; typically, these last less than 30 seconds. Obstructive sleep apnea is caused by obstruction (e.g., large tonsils, adenoids, or thyroid gland), whereas central sleep apnea is an alteration of the central nervous system stimulus to breathe during sleep. Symptoms include excessive daytime sleepiness, snoring, and congestive heart failure. Patients may actually die in their sleep

SKULL

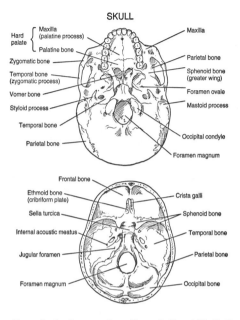

Hard palate { Maxilla (palatine process) / Palatine bone }
Zygomatic bone
Temporal bone (zygomatic process)
Vomer bone
Styloid process
Temporal bone
Parietal bone

Maxilla
Parietal bone
Sphenoid bone (greater wing)
Foramen ovale
Mastoid process
Occipital condyle
Foramen magnum

Frontal bone
Ethmoid bone (cribriform plate)
Sella turcica
Internal acoustic meatus
Jugular foramen
Foramen magnum

Crista galli
Sphenoid bone
Temporal bone
Parietal bone
Occipital bone

from cardiac arrhythmias caused by hypoxia. Treatment may include removal of an offending blockage, tracheostomy, or medication.

sleep terror disorder N. disorder of sleep, occurring mostly in children, in which episodes of abrupt awakening, with feelings of terror, panic, and anxiety, often with screaming and marked movements, occur without awareness of a frightening dream and with total amnesia of the event afterward; also called pavor nocturnus.

sleeping pill N. colloquial term for a sedative taken for insomnia or as an aid to sleep.

sleepwalking (slēp′wô′kĭng) *See* SOMNAMBULISM.

slipped disc (slĭpd) *See* HERNIATED DISC.

Slo-Bid N. trade name for a bronchodilator containing aminophylline and used to treat some respiratory disorders, esp. those marked by spasm of the airways.

slough N. separation of dead matter or tissue from normal or living tissue. Often used in reference to the skin, where dead tissue sloughs off a wound during treatment and healing. v. to shed or fall away from, as tissue (e.g., skin) that has died and been replaced by new tissue.

slow virus N. virus that remains dormant in the body for a long time, with years elapsing before symptoms may occur. Several human diseases (e.g., kuru) are thought to be caused by slow viruses.

slurry N. thin, watery mixture of a solid substance, often a drug, and a liquid.

small intestine (ĭn-tĕs'tĭn) N. longest part of the digestive tract, about 24 feet (7 meters), extending from the pylorus of the stomach to the ileocecal junction. It is divided into the duodenum, jejunum, and ileum and is a major site for food digestion and absorption of nutrients.

small-for-gestation-age (SGA) infant (jĕ-stā'shən) N. infant whose size and weight are significantly less than expected for the age of the baby, whether term or premature. Factors associated with smallness include chronic disease, infection, malnutrition, and smoking in the mother.

smallpox (smôl'pŏks') N. highly contagious viral disease characterized by fever, weakness, and a pustular rash that may result in permanent scarring. The disease was once widespread, but since 1979 has been eradicated throughout the world as a result of vaccination programs. The virus is now believed to exist only in deepfreeze lockers in two laboratories in Atlanta (Centers for Disease Control) and Moscow. Also called variola.

smear (smēr) N. thin film of tissue spread on a slide for microscopic examination.

smegma (smĕg'mə) N. white, cheesy secretion of glands of the foreskin.

smooth muscle N. one of three major types of muscle in the body (the other two are striated muscle and cardiac muscle), made up of spindle-shaped cells. It is under autonomic nervous system control, and contracts involuntarily with slow, long-term contractions. Smooth muscle occurs in many organs, including the blood vessels, intestines, and bladder.

snare (snâr) N. instrument with a wire hoop used to remove polyps, small tumors, or other growths, esp. in body cavities.

sneeze (snēz) N. involuntary sudden expulsion of air through the nose and mouth, resulting from irritation of the mucous membrane of the upper respiratory tract, as from a cold or allergic reaction.

Snellen chart (snĕl'ən) N. chart commonly used to test visual acuity.

snow blindness N. temporary and painful disorder of the cornea of the eye, caused by excessive exposure to ultraviolet light reflected from snow.

socialization (sō'shə-lĭ-zā'shən) N. process by which a person learns to adapt to, and be productive within, the expectations and standards of a group or society.

sociopath (sō'sē-ə-păth') *See* PSYCHOPATH.

socket (sŏk'ĭt) N. bony hollow into which a structure fits; the orbits are informally referred to as "eye sockets."

sodium (sō'dē-əm) N. metallic element that is one of the most important elements in the body, essential for acid-base balance, water balance, nerve transmission, and muscle contraction. *See also* TABLE OF IMPORTANT ELEMENTS.

sodium bicarbonate N. antacid used in the treatment of indigestion and gastric acidity. Adverse effects include electrolyte imbalance.

sodium chloride N. common table salt, used in the replenishment of fluids and electrolytes and in irrigating mediums and enemas.

sodium fluoride (sō'dē-əm floͦor'īd') N. salt of sodium used to prevent tooth decay.

sodoku *See* RATBITE FEVER.

sodomy (sŏd'ə-mē) N. in medical usage, anal intercourse; which is usually homosexual, but may involve an animal or be heterosexual.

soft diet N. diet containing low-residue, easily digested soft foods, such as milk, cheese, custards, strained vegetables, potatoes, rice, breads, and ground meats; advised for those with acute infections or intestinal disorders.

soft palate (păl'ĭt) N. structure containing muscles and mucous membranes and extending from the back of the hard palate in the posterior of the mouth, part of it hanging between the mouth and the pharynx.

solar plexus (sō'lər plĕk'səs) N. network of nerve fibers and ganglia where sympathetic and parasympathetic nerve fibers combine at the upper part of the back of the abdomen.

soleus (sō'lē-əs) N. any of several superficial muscles of the lower leg. *See* MAJOR MUSCLES OF THE BODY, in Appendix.

solubility (sŏl'yə-bĭl'ĭ-tē) N. the ability of a particular substance to dissolve in a particular solvent.

solution (sə-loͦo'shən) N. homogenous mixture, usually liquid, of two or more substances.

solvent (sŏl'vənt) N. liquid capable of dissolving other substances; liquid in which another substance (solute) is dissolved.

Soma (sō'mə) N. *See* TABLE OF COMMONLY PRESCRIBED DRUGS —TRADE NAMES.

somatic cell (sō-măt'ĭk) N. nonreproductive cell of the body (*compare* GERM CELL).

somatic chromosome (sō-măt'ĭk krō'mə-sōm') *See* AUTOSOME.

somatomedins N. proteins produced by the liver and other tissues that, in conjunction with growth hormone, stimulate growth. These compounds are closely related to insulin; their secretion is reduced in untreated diabetes and restored to normal by insulin treatment.

somatotropin (sə-măt'ə-trō'pĭn) *See* GROWTH HORMONE.

somn-, somni-, somno- comb. forms indicating an association with sleep (e.g., somniloquism, sleep talking).

somnambulism (sŏm-năm'byə-lĭz'əm) N. condition, occurring primarily in children and often associated with anxiety, fatigue, or stress, in which the person performs motor activity, usually leaving bed and walking around, while sleeping and has no memory of it on awakening. *See also* SLEEPWALKING.

somnolent (sŏm'nə-lənt) ADJ. sleepy or drowsy. N. somnolence

sonogram (sŏn'ə-grăm') *See* ULTRASONOGRAPHY.

soporific (sŏp'ə-rĭf'ĭk) ADJ. pert. to a substance or process that causes sleep.

sore (sôr) N. wound or lesion, ADJ. tender, painful

sotalol N. antiarrhythmic drug (trade name Betapace) that works as a beta blocker and also increases the length of the action potential; indicated in the treatment of life-threatening ventricular arrhythmias (e.g., ventricular tachycardia, ventricular fibrillation); side effects include aggravation of congestive heart failure and increased incidence of arrhythmias.

space N. area, region, segment, or cavity of the body; small structural area between tissues or parts of an organ, such as the interstitial space.

spasm (spăz'əm) N.
1. sudden, involuntary muscle contraction.
2. sudden constriction of a blood vessels or other hollow organ. *See also* BRONCHOSPASM. ADJ. spasmodic

spasmo- comb. form indicating an association with spasm (e.g., spasmolytic, drug that relieves smooth muscle spasm).

spastic (spăs'tĭk) ADJ. pert. to spasm or uncontrolled skeletal muscle contraction. N. spasticity.

spastic bladder N. type of neurogenic bladder caused by spinal cord lesion, multiple sclerosis, or trauma, and characterized by loss of bladder sensation, incontinence, and interrupted voiding (*compare* FLACCID BLADDER).

spastic colon *See* IRRITABLE BOWEL SYNDROME.

spastic paralysis (spăs'tĭk pə-răl'ĭ-sĭs) N. loss of muscle function with involuntary spasm or contraction of one or more muscles (*compare* FLACCID PARALYSIS).

specificity N. proportion of people who do not have a given condition and are correctly identified by a test; a specific test has a low false-positive rate. A nonspecific test has a high false-positive rate and should not be relied upon to suspect or diagnose an abnormality or disease. Some types of urine pregnancy tests are very nonspecific—any type of contaminant (such as dirt, blood, or vaginal secretions) may give a false-positive result when, in reality, the patient is not pregnant. A serum pregnancy test is both sensitive and specific.

specimen (spĕs'ə-mən) N. small sample of something; part of a whole, intended upon analysis to reveal the characteristics of the whole (e.g., a urine specimen used for urinalysis).

SPECT N. acronym for Single Photon Emission Computed Tomography. A nuclear medicine procedure in which the gamma camera rotates around the patient and takes pictures from many angles, which a computer then uses to form a tomographic (cross-sectional) image. The calculation process is similar to that in X-ray Computed Tomography (CT) and in Positron Emission Computed Tomography (PET).

spectinomycin (spĕk'tə-nō-mī'sĭn) N. antibiotic used to treat gonorrhea and certain other infections. Adverse effects include nausea, fever, dizziness, and rashes.

speculum (spĕk'yə-ləm) N. instrument inserted into and used to hold open a body cavity (e.g., vagina) for examination.

sperm (spûrm) *See* SPERMATOZOON.

sperm count N. estimate of the number of spermatozoa in an ejaculate, used as an indication of male fertility. An ejaculate normally contains between 300,000,000 and 500,000,000 spermatozoa; significantly lower numbers usually indicate sterility.

spermatic cord (spər-măt′ĭk) N. cord containing arteries, veins, nerves, and lymphatics and extending from the lower abdomen to the testis.

spermatid (spər′mə-tĭd) N. male germ cell that becomes a mature spermatozoon in the last stage of sperm formation.

spermatocele (spər-măt′ə-sēl′) N. sperm containing swelling on the epididymis or testis.

spermatocide N. chemical that kills sperm; found in many contraceptive creams, jellies, and foams; also called spermicide.

spermatogenesis (spər-măt′ə-jĕn′ĭ-sĭs) N. process of spermatozoa development from early stages of spermatogonia through other stages leading to spermatids and finally mature spermatozoa (*compare* OOGENESIS).

spermatozoon (spər-măt′ə-zō′ŏn′) N., *pl.* spermatozoa, male sex cell that fertilizes an ovum. It develops in the seminiferous tubules of the testis. Tadpolelike, it is tiny (about 1/500 inch) with a head, neck, and tail.

spermicidal (spûr′mĭ-sīd′l) ADJ. destructive to spermatozoa.

spheno- comb. form indicating an association with the sphenoid bone (e.g., sphenofrontal, pert. to the frontal and sphenoid bones of the skull).

sphenoid bone (sfē′noid′) N. bone at the base of the skull.

spherocyte (sfēr′ə-sīt′) N. abnormal spherical-shaped red blood cell (erythrocyte).

sphincter (sfĭngk′tər) N. circular band of muscle that constricts or closes an opening in the body (e.g., pyloric sphincter).

sphygmo- comb. form indicating an association with the pulse (e.g., sphygmogram, recording of the strength and rate of the pulse).

sphygmomanometer (sfĭg′mō-mă-nŏm′ĭ-tər) N. medical instrument used to measure blood pressure; it consists of an inflatable cuff connected by a rubber tube to a column of mercury with a graduated scale for both systolic and diastolic pressure.

spicule (spĭk′yōōl) N. sharp, needlelike part.

spider angioma (ăn′jē-ō′mə) N. dilatation of superficial capillaries with an elevated red dot from which blood vessels radiate.

spina bifida (spī′nə bĭf′ĭ-də) N. relatively common congenital defect in which there is a malformation of a posterior vertebral arch; unless the defect affects a large area or spinal cord material protrudes (myelomeningocele), there are few or no symptoms. The condition can be diagnosed by amniocentesis at about the 16th week of pregnancy.

spinal canal (spī′nəl) N. canal within the vertebral column through which the spinal cord passes.

spinal column *See* VERTEBRAL COLUMN.

spinal cord N. major part of the central nervous system, which conducts sensory and motor impulses to and from the brain and is a site of reflex activity. It is a cylindrical tube, extending from the base of the brain through the vertebral canal to the upper part of the lumbar region. It has an inner core of gray matter, containing mostly nerve cells, surrounded by white matter with nerve fibers. The entire cord is surrounded by meninges (protective membranes). From it arise 31 spinal nerves.

spinal curvature (spī′nəl kûr′və-chŏŏr′) N. abnormality in curvature of the vertebral column. *See also* KYPHOSIS; LORDOSIS; SCOLIOSIS.

spinal fluid *See* CEREBROSPINAL FLUID.

spinal fusion (spī′nəl fyōō′zhən) N. fixation of an unstable part of the spinal column, usually done surgically by a bone graft, sometimes through traction or immobilization.

spinal immobilization (spī′nəl ĭ-mō′bə-lĭ-zā′shən) N. set of techniques used by emergency care providers to prevent movement of the cervical vertebrae following an injury; usu-ally involves placing a semi-rigid collar around the patient's neck and strapping him or her to a backboard.

spinal nerve N. any of 31 pairs of nerves connected to the spinal cord. Each spinal nerve divides into branches, some serving the voluntary nervous system, others the autonomic nervous system.

spinal puncture, spinal tap (spī′nəl pŭnk′chər) *See* LUMBAR PUNCTURE.

spinal tract N. any ascending or descending pathway for sensory or motor nerve impulses found in the white matter of the spinal cord.

spindle (spĭn′dl) N. collection of fibers seen in a dividing cell that function in chromosome movement in mitosis and meiosis. The fibers radiate from two poles and meet in the middle at the equator.

spine (spīn) N.
1. *See* VERTEBRAL COLUMN.
2. process (thin projection or prominence) of a bone. ADJ. spinal

SPINAL CORD

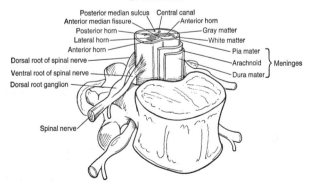

Posterior median sulcus — Central canal
Anterior median fissure — Anterior horn
Posterior horn — Gray matter
Lateral horn — White matter
Anterior horn
Dorsal root of spinal nerve — Pia mater
Ventral root of spinal nerve — Arachnoid } Meninges
Dorsal root ganglion — Dura mater
Spinal nerve

spinocerebellar disorder N. any of several inherited disorders characterized by progressive degeneration of the spinal cord and cerebellum and usually marked by increasing spasticity, ataxia, and incoordination.

spirochete (spī′rə-kēt′) N. motile, spiral-shaped microorganism, including the causative agents of syphilis and leptospirosis.

spirograph (spī′rə-grăf′) N. instrument for recording breathing movements; the recording is a spirogram. Also spirometry; *see* PULMONARY FUNCTION TESTS.

spironolactone N. antihypertensive (trade name Aldactone) that blocks the action of aldos-

terone on the renal tubules. Adverse effects include headache, gastrointestinal upset, and hyperkalemia.

splanchnic (splăngk′nĭk) ADJ. pert. to the internal organs.

splanchnic nerve N. any of a series of nerves of the sympathetic part of the autonomic nervous system, innervating viscera and blood vessels.

spleen (splēn) N. large, dark-red, oval organ situated on the left side of the body between the diaphragm and stomach. It is part of the lymphatic and reticuloendothelial systems, functioning to destroy wornout red blood cells; it also stores blood

SPINAL NERVES

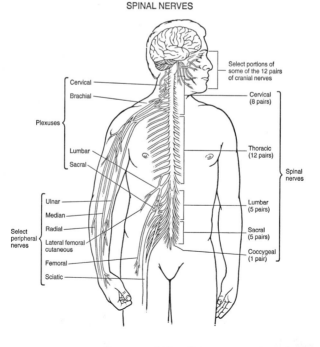

Select portions of some of the 12 pairs of cranial nerves

Cervical

Brachial

Plexuses

Lumbar

Sacral

Ulnar

Median

Radial

Lateral femoral cutaneous

Femoral

Sciatic

Select peripheral nerves

Cervical (8 pairs)

Thoracic (12 pairs)

Lumbar (5 pairs)

Sacral (5 pairs)

Coccygeal (1 pair)

Spinal nerves

and produces red blood cells before birth. Also called lien. ADJ. splenic; lienal.

splen-, spleno- comb. forms indicating an association with the spleen (e.g., splenitis, inflammation of the spleen).

splenectomy (splĭ-nĕk'tə-mē) N. surgical removal of the spleen.

splenitis (splĭ-nī'tĭs) N. inflammation or infection of the spleen.

splenomegaly (splĕ'nō-mĕg'ə-lē) N. enlargement of the spleen, caused by malaria, certain types of anemia, certain infectious diseases (e.g., infectious mononucleosis), and other disorders.

splint (splĭnt) N. orthopedic device to immobilize, support, or restrain an injured part; it may be rigid (plaster, metal) or flexible (leather).

spondyl-, spondylo- comb. forms indicating an association with the spinal column or a vertebra (e.g., spondylarthritis, arthritis affecting the spinal column).

spondylitis (spŏn'dl-ī'tĭs) N. inflammation of a joint of the spinal column, usually characterized by pain and stiffness; it may occur after injury, as the result of rheumatoid arthritis or

infection. *See also* ANKYLOSING SPONDYLITIS.

spondylolisthesis N. forward dislocation of one vertebra over the one below it, causing pressure on spinal nerves.

spondylosis (spŏn'dl-ō'sĭs) N. condition in which vertebral joints become fixed or stiff, causing pain and restricted mobility.

spontaneous (spŏn-tā'nē-əs) ADJ. occurring without apparent cause, as in spontaneous recovery from a disease.

spontaneous abortion *See* ABORTION.

sporadic (spə-răd'ĭk) ADJ. occurring occasionally or in a few isolated situations, as in the sporadic appearance of a disease.

sporotrichosis (spôr'ō-trĭ-kō'sĭs) N. chronic fungal infection of the skin and lymph nodes caused by the fungus *Sporothrix schenckii*, found in soil and decaying vegetation; it causes skin lesions and subcutaneous lymph nodules in lymph channels. Treatment is by antifungal agents.

spotted fever *See* ROCKY MOUNTAIN SPOTTED FEVER.

sprain (sprān) N. injury to ligaments around a joint, causing

SPLEEN

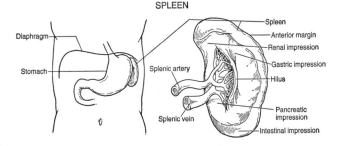

Diaphragm

Stomach

Splenic artery

Splenic vein

Spleen
Anterior margin
Renal impression
Gastric impression
Hilus
Pancreatic impression
Intestinal impression

pain, swelling, and skin discoloration. The severity of symptoms and degree of immobility depend on the site of injury and extent of damage of tissues. Treatment includes support, rest, and cold compresses at the time of injury.

sprue (sproō) N. chronic disorder, occurring in tropical and nontropical forms and affecting both children and adults, characterized by malabsorption of nutrients and symptoms of diarrhea, poor appetite, weight loss, and atrophy of the membrane lining (villi) of the digestive tract; also called tropical sprue. *See also* CELIAC DISEASE.

sputum (spyoō′təm) N. material usually containing mucus and cellular debris, sometimes pus or blood, coughed up from the lungs and expectorated through the mouth. Differences in the amount, color, and contents of sputum are important in the diagnosis of some respiratory ailments.

squama (skwā′mə) N.
1. platelike part; a thin plate of bone.
2. part resembling a fish scale (e.g., squamocellular, having scale-shaped cells). ADJ. squamous

squint (skwĭnt) *See* STRABISMUS.

St. Vitus Dance *See* SYDENHAM'S CHOREA.

stain (stān) N. pigment or dye, esp. one used to impart color to microorganisms or cell parts for microscopic study.

stapedectomy (stā′pĭ-dĕk′tə-mē) N. surgical removal of the stapes of the middle ear, performed to restore hearing in cases where the stapes has become ossified, fixed, and unable to vibrate in response to sound waves.

stapes (stā′pēz) N. one of the three ossicles (small bones) of the middle ear; it resembles a tiny stirrup and transmits vibrations from the incus (another of the three ossicles) to the inner ear.

staphylococcal infection (stăf′ə-lō-kŏk′əl) N. infection with pathogenic species of Staphylococcus bacteria; usually characterized by abscess formation. Common staphylococcal infections include carbuncles, furuncles, and some forms of food poisoning.

staphylococcus (stăf′ə-lō-kŏk′əs) N. genus of spherical bacteria typically occurring in grapelike clusters; several species are pathogenic to humans, producing boils, some form of food poisoning, and other types of infection.

startle reflex (stär′tl) *See* MORO REFLEX.

starvation (stär-vā′shən) N. condition resulting from lack of essential nutrients over a prolonged period and characterized by weight loss, widespread physiologic and metabolic disturbances, and increased susceptibility to infection.

stasis (stā′sĭs) N. abnormal condition in which the customary flow of a fluid (e.g., blood) is slowed or stopped.

static (stăt′ĭk) ADJ. at rest, in equilibrium; not changing.

status asthmaticus (stā′təs) N. prolonged, severe asthma attack in which spasm of the bronchi does not respond to standard treatments. Cyanosis (bluish discoloration of the skin) and other signs of lack of oxygen may occur, along with respiratory failure. Treatment involves aggressive bronchodilator therapy, corticosteroids, and possibly artificial respiration.

status epilepticus (ĕp′ə-lĕp′tĭ-kəs) N. condition in which there are continual seizures without intervals of consciousness; it can lead to severe brain damage and death. Therapy includes maintenance of adequate oxygen supply and anticonvulsants.

steatorrhea (stē′ə-tə-rē′ə) N. greater than normal amounts of fat in the feces, with the feces frothy, foul-smelling, and floating; it is associated with malabsorption syndromes and disorders of fat metabolism.

Steinert's disease See MUSCULAR DYSTROPHY, MYOTONIC.

stenosis (stə-nō′sĭs) N. abnormal narrowing or constriction of a passageway or opening, as in aortic stenosis.

stent (stĕnt) N. a woven piece of wire, inserted percutaneously through a catheter and used to maintain the lumen of a coronary artery that has been narrowed by atherosclerosis.

sterility (stə-rĭl′ĭ-tē) N.
1. pert. to a living organism: state of being unable to reproduce.
2. pert. to a nonliving object: state of being free from disease-causing microorganisms. ADJ. sterile

sterilization (stĕr′ə-lĭ-zā′shən) N.
1. surgical procedure in which a man or woman is rendered incapable of reproducing; in males the procedure is vasectomy; in females, a form of tubal ligation.
2. means of rendering objects free of microorganisms that may produce disease by boiling, subjecting to steam in an autoclave, or using disinfectants and antiseptics.

stern-, sterno- comb. forms indicating an association with the sternum (e.g., sternoclavicular, pert. to the sternum—breastbone, and clavicle—collarbone).

sternum (stûr′nəm) N. breastbone; an elongated, flattened bone forming the middle of the thorax, which articulates with the clavicles and first 7 ribs and serves for the attachment of numerous muscles. It is composed of three parts: upper manubrium; middle body, or gladiolus; and lower xiphoid process.

steroid (stĕr′oid′) N. one of a large group of substances produced by or related to those produced by the adrenal gland. These include corticosteroids and mineralocorticoids, as well as sex hormones. See ADRENAL GLAND.

stethoscope (stĕth′ə-skōp′) N. instrument used for listening to body sounds, such as those of the heart and lungs. A simple stethoscope consists of a bell-shaped structure that is placed

CORONARY ARTERY STENT

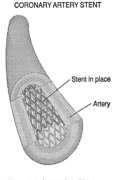

Stent in place

Artery

Woven metal stent placed into a coronary artery helps maintain patency of the lumen.

on the patient's skin and is connected by plastic or rubber tubes to earpieces for the examiner.

stilbestrol (stĭl-bĕs′trôl′) *See* DIETHYLSTILBESTROL.

stillbirth N. birth of a fetus that shows no signs of life (e.g., respiration, heartbeat, or movement).

Still's disease (stĭlz) N. form of rheumatoid arthritis, primarily affecting children, in which large joints become inflamed and bone growth may be affected, causing skeletal deformities. Treatment includes nonsteroidal anti-inflammatory agents, analgesics, and rest; also called juvenile rheumatoid arthritis.

stimulant (stĭm′yə-lənt) N. agent, such as a drug, that activates or increases the activity of a body part or system. Amphetamines and caffeine are central nervous system stimulants.

stimulus (stĭm′yə-ləs) N., *pl.* stimuli, anything that causes a reaction or response (e.g., an odor activating olfactory receptor in the nasal cavity). V. stimulate, N. stimulation

stirrup (stûr′əp) *See* STAPES.

stitch (stĭch) N.
1. suture.
2. sharply localized pain, a form of cramp, commonly occurring in the abdomen after strenuous exercise, esp. after eating.

Stokes-Adams syndrome (stōks′) *See* ADAMS-STOKES SYNDROME.

stoma (stō′mə) N. opening or pore on the surface, esp. a surgically created opening of an internal organ on the surface of the body, as in colostomy or tracheostomy.

stomach (stŭm′ək) N. expandable, saclike organ, located below the diaphragm in the upper left part of the abdomen, which forms part of the digestive tract between the esophagus and the duodenum. The stomach receives partly digested food from the esophagus through the cardiac sphincter. In the stomach the food is churned by muscular layers of the stomach and mixed with the secretions of the gastric glands, chiefly hydrochloric acid and the enzyme pepsin. The semiliquid mass (chyme) then passes through the pyloric sphincter to the duodenum.

stomatitis (stō′mə-tī′tĭs) N. inflammation of the mouth; it may result from vitamin deficiency, infection, exposure to irritating substances, or systemic diseases.

stomato- comb. form indicating an association with the mouth (e.g., stomatogastric, pert. to the mouth and stomach).

stone N. hard mass. *See also* GALLSTONE; RENAL CALCULUS.

stool (stōōl) *See* FECES.

strabismus (strə-bĭz′məs) N. condition in which the eyes are not properly aligned; it may be inherited or result from trauma or injury to the eye or brain. Strabismus may be convergent, in which the eyes are directed inward toward each other; or divergent, in which one or both eyes are directed outward. Some forms of strabismus can be corrected in early childhood by the child wearing a patch over the normal eye, so that the deviating eye must be used; other types can be corrected surgically but some amblyopia will often remain. Also called squint.

STOMACH

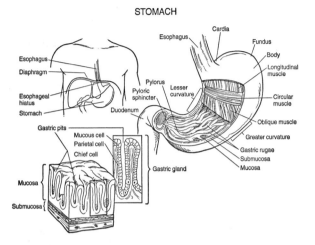

strain N.
1. injury to a muscle or tendon, resulting in swelling and pain usually caused by overuse.
2. group or line of microorganisms having characteristics that separate them from others of their species.

strangulation (străng′gyə-lā′shən) N. constriction of a tubular structure that prevents passage of material; for example, strangulation of the bowel prevents the passage of feces. Also refers to constriction of the blood supply to an organ, resulting in lack of oxygen, such as a strangulated hernia. ADJ. strangulated.

stratum (strā′təm) N., *pl.* strata, layer of tissues or cells (e.g., the layers of the skin).

stratum corneum (strā′təm kôr′ nē-əm) N. horny, outermost layer of the epidermis, containing dead cells that slough off; it is thick over the palms and soles, thinner in more protected areas. Also called horny layer.

stratum germinativum N. innermost layer of the epidermis, containing dividing cells and melanocytes (pigment cells) that resupply the outer skin layers. The outer part of this layer forms a prickle-cell portion with cells connected by spines or intercellular bridges; the inner part of this layer is the basal layer with dividing cells; also called stratum basale.

stratum granulosum N. layer of epidermis just under the stratum corneum or, in the area of the palms and soles just under the stratum lucidum; it contains cells with visible granules that die and move to the surface.

stratum lucidum N. layer of epidermis just under the stratum corneum, most noticeable in the skin of the palms and soles.

strawberry hemangioma (hǐ-măn′jē-ō′mə) N. congenital, bright red, superficial vascular tumor, resembling a strawberry; it tends to decrease in size and eventually to disappear during childhood.

streak N. in anatomy, a line or furrow.

streptococcal sore throat N. infection of the oral pharynx and tonsils with streptococcus, producing fever, sore throat, chills, lymph node enlargement, and occasionally gastrointestinal disturbances. Treatment is by antibiotics, usually penicillin or erythromycin, and analgesics. Complications include sinusitis, ear infection, or if inadequately treated, rheumatic fever. Also called strep throat.

streptococcus (strĕp′tə-kŏk′əs) N. genus of bacteria, many species of which produce disease in humans, including tonsillitis, pneumonia, and urinary tract infections. Some strains of streptococcus have become resistant to penicillin.

streptokinase N. enzyme produced by some strains of streptococcus that liquefies blood clots by converting plasminogen to plasmin; it is used in some cases of myocardial infarction and pulmonary embolism to dissolve the clot blocking the blood vessels and restore normal blood flow. Adverse effects include hemorrhage, fever, and gastrointestinal upsets.

streptomycin (strĕp′tə-mī′sĭn) N. antibiotic used to treat tuberculosis and many other bacterial infections. Adverse effects include ear and kidney damage.

stress N. any factor—physical (e.g., infection), emotional (e.g., anxiety), or other—that requires a change in response or affects health in any way, esp. having an adverse effect on the functioning of the body or any of its parts. Continual stress brings about widespread neurological and endocrine responses that, over a period of time, cause changes in the functioning of many body organs, often leading to disease (e.g., hypertension and allergic responses).

stress fracture See FATIGUE FRACTURE.

stress test N. test that measures the function of a system when it is subjected to controlled amounts of stress. For example, the treadmill test measures the effect of stress on cardiovascular and respiratory function; the fetal stress test measures the adequacy of fetal-placental function and the condition of the fetus.

stretch mark See STRIA.

stria (strī′ə) N. streak or narrow line, often resulting from tension in the skin, as on the skin of abdomen after pregnancy. Also called stretch mark. ADJ. striated.

striated muscle (strī′ā′tĭd) N. one of three major types of muscle (the other two are smooth muscle and cardiac muscle); it makes up the major part of the body's musculature and is called skeletal muscle because it is attached to the skeleton and voluntary muscle because it is under voluntary control. Striated muscle is composed of parallel, multinuclear fibers, each made of numerous myofibrils that have striations due to the position of actin and myosin protein filaments. When a muscle contracts, the two sets of filaments slide past each other, reducing the length of the fibril.

stricture (strĭk′chər) N. narrowing of any tubular structure

SKELETAL MUSCLE CELL

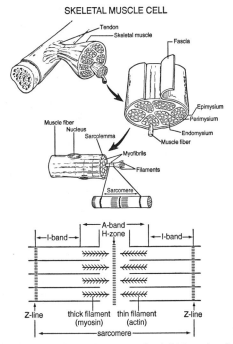

The microscopic and submicroscopic structure of a skeletal muscle cell.

(e.g., esophagus, ureter) caused by inflammation, a tumor, pressure from an adjacent organ, or muscle spasm.

stridor (strī'dər) N. abnormal breathing sound, usually heard on inspiration, occurring when the trachea or larynx is obstructed (e.g., by neoplasm or by inflammation).

stroke (strōk) *See* CEREBROVASCULAR ACCIDENT.

stroma (strō'mə) N., *pl.* stromata, supporting tissue of an organ, as opposed to its functional tissue (*compare* PARENCHYMA). ADJ. stromal

stronglyoidiasis (strŏn'jə-loi-dī'ə-sĭs) N. infection of the intestine with *Strongyloides stercoralis* roundworm, usually acquired when larvae in the soil penetrate the skin and migrate to the intestines, producing diarrhea and malabsorption. Treatment is by anthelmintics.

stump (stŭmp) N. that part of a limb remaining on the body after amputation of part of the limb.

stupor (stoo'pər) N. a state of unresponsiveness and near unconsciousness, occurring in some neurologic and psychotic disorders. ADJ. stuporous

stutter (stŭt′ər) v. to speak with frequent repetition of words or parts of words. The most common cause of stuttering is emotional, though brain injury or disease may play a role. Treatment involves specialized speech therapy.

stye (stī) *See* HORDEOLUM.

styptic (stĭp′tĭk) N. substance used as an astringent, often to control bleeding.

sub- comb. form meaning "under" (e.g., sublingual, under the tongue), "almost," "just before" (e.g., subclinical, not yet showing symptoms).

subacute (sŭb′ə-kyōōt′) ADJ. less than acute; pert. to a disease present in a person with no symptoms of it.

subacute bacterial endocarditis (sŭb′ə-kyōōt′ băk-tîr′ē-əl ĕn′dō-kär-dī′tĭs) N. chronic bacterial infection of the valves of the heart, often associated with surgical or dental procedures or drug abuse. Symptoms of fever, heart murmur, enlarged spleen, and abnormal tissue in the heart develop slowly. Treatment involves prolonged administration of an antibiotic; acute episodes are also treated with fever reducers and pain relievers, rest, and adequate fluid intake.

subarachnoid space (sŭb′ə-răk′noid′) N. space located under the arachnoid membrane and above the pia mater of the meninges and containing cerebrospinal fluid. A type of spinal anesthesia, often used for obstetrical and gynecological procedures, is achieved by injecting an anesthetic agent into the subarachnoid space.

subclavian artery (sŭb-klā′vē-ən är′tə-rē) N. either of two arteries that supply blood to the neck and arms. The right subclavian artery branches from the innominate artery; the left subclavian artery directly from the aortic arch. *See* MAJOR ARTERIES AND VEINS OF THE BODY, in Appendix.

subconscious (sŭb-kŏn′shəs) ADJ. partially conscious; partially aware and responsive. N. in psychoanalytic theory, the portion of the mind where mental processes occur without an individual being aware.

subcutaneous (sŭb′kyōō-tā′nē-əs) ADJ. beneath the skin, as a subcutaneous injection.

subcutaneous test *See* INTRADERMAL TEST.

subdural (səb-dōōr′əl) ADJ. beneath the dura mater and above the arachnoid membrane of the meninges.

sublimation (sŭb′lə-mā′shən) N. replacement of a socially unacceptable means of satisfying desires by means that are socially acceptable, esp. the diversion of components of the sex drive to nonsexual goals.

subliminal (sŭb-lĭm′ə-nəl) AJD. Below or outside the range of conscious awareness or sensory perception.

sublingual (sŭb-lĭng′gwəl) ADJ. below the tongue.

sublingual gland N. either of a pair of salivary glands located on the floor of the mouth below the tongue.

subluxation (sŭb′lŭk-sā′shən) N. partial dislocation of a joint. *See also* LUXATION.

submandibular gland (sŭb′măn-dĭb′yə-lər) N. either of a pair of salivary glands located near the lower jaw and secreting serous fluid components of saliva.

subnormal ADJ. below the normal range; often refers to subnormal body temperatures.

substrate (sŭb′strāt′) N. material acted upon by an enzyme.

succinylcholine N. striated muscle relaxant used as an adjunct to anesthesia during certain surgical procedures. Adverse effects include respiratory depression and cardiac arrhythmias.

succus *See* JUICE.

succussion N. sound heard when a person with a large amount of fluid in a body cavity moves or is shaken.

sucking blisters (sŭk′ĭng) N. blisterlike pads on the lips of newborns that form as the baby begins to suck and seem to help to seal the lips around the nipple.

suckle V. to provide nourishment, esp. by breastfeeding.

suckling reflex N. involuntary sucking movement of newborns.

sucralfate (sōō-krăl′fāt′) N. oral tablet (trade name Carafate) used in the treatment of peptic ulcer which is thought to work by actually binding to the ulcer site and coating it. The most common adverse effect is constipation.

sucrose (sōō′krōs′) N. table sugar.

suction curettage (sŭk′shən kyōōr′ĭ-täzh′) *See* VACUUM ASPIRATION.

sudden infant death syndrome (SIDS) N. unexpected and sudden death of an apparently healthy infant during sleep with no autopsy evidence of disease.

It is the leading cause of death in infants between 2 weeks and 1 year of age. The cause is unknown, but certain risk factors have been identified: lying face downward; prematurity; low birth weight; male sex; winter months; mothers who are very young, smoke, or are addicted to a drug; and recent mild upper respiratory tract infection. Also called cot death; crib death.

sudo- comb. form indicating an association with sweat (perspiration) (e.g., sudorific, producing sweat).

sudoriferous gland (sōō′də-rĭf′ər-əs) N. any of several million structures in the skin that produce sweat (perspiration). Most of the glands are eccrine, producing sweat that contains salt and the waste product urea; a few, associated with the hair of the armpits and pubic region, are apocrine, secreting a thicker fluid. *See also* ECCRINE GLAND; APOCRINE GLAND.

suicide (sōō′ĭ-sīd′) N. deliberate taking of one's own life; the leading cause of death in college-age Americans. Risk factors include repeated failure or humiliation, the breakup of a love affair or marriage, mental illness (e.g., schizophrenia or depression), incurable disease, and substance abuse. Among the warning signs are changes in appetite or sleep patterns, impaired concentration, agitation, giving away possessions, and such statements as, "I'd be better off dead." Preventive measures include psychotherapy, referral services, and telephone "help lines."

Sulamyd N. trade name for the sulfonamide antibacterial sulfacetamide.

sulcus (sŭl′kəs) N. small groove or furrow on the surface of an organ (e.g., sulcus that separates convolutions on the surface of the cerebral hemispheres).

sulfacetamide N. topical sulfonamide most commonly used to prevent infection from injury to the cornea and to treat eye infections. Adverse effects include local irritation.

sulfadiazone, sulfameter, sulfamethazine, sulfamethizole, sulfamethoxazole, sulfamethoxypyridazine, sulfapyridine See SULFONAMIDE.

sulfonamide N. any of a large group of antibacterial drugs that act by halting the growth and reproduction of bacteria but do not kill the bacteria. Sulfonamides are used to treat bacterial urinary tract infections and certain other infections. Adverse effects include jaundice and blood abnormalities. Sulfonamides are not given in pregnancy, to young children, or to persons with impaired liver or kidney functions.

sulfonylurea N. any of a group of drugs, including tolazamide and tolbutamide, that reduce the level of glucose in the blood and are used in the treatment of diabetes mellitus.

sulfur (sŭl′fər) N. nonmetallic element active against parasites and fungi. See also TABLE OF IMPORTANT ELEMENTS.

sulindac (sə-lĭn′dăk) N. nonsteroidal anti-inflammatory agent used in the treatment of osteoarthritis, rheumatoid arthritis, and ankylosing spondylitis. Adverse effects include tinnitus, dizziness, skin rash, gastrointestinal upsets, and the possibility of drug interactions.

sumatriptan N. injectable medication (trade name Imitrex) used in the treatment of migraine headache; generally, relief occurs within ten minutes after its injection; side effects include atypical sensations (tingling, warmth, burning, tightness), flushing, injection-site reactions, and dizziness. Rarely, this agent can result in myocardial infarction when administered to persons with known ischemic heart disease. See TABLE OF COMMONLY PRESCRIBED DRUGS—GENERIC NAMES.

Sumycin N. See TABLE OF COMMONLY PRESCRIBED DRUGS—TRADE NAMES.

sunscreen (sŭn′skrēn′) N. ointment or cream placed on the skin to protect against ultraviolet rays from the sun or other source.

sunstroke (sŭn′strōk′) See HEATSTROKE.

superego (soo′pər-ē′gō) N. in psychoanalysis, part of the psyche that functions as a conscience and for the formation of ideals; it forms as parental and societal standards are incorporated into a child's mind (compare EGO; ID).

superfecundation N. fertilization of two or more ova released during the same menstrual cycle by spermatozoa from separate acts of coitus.

superfetation N. fertilization of a second ovum after a pregnancy has commenced; this results in two fetuses of different degrees of maturity developing in the uterus at the same time; also called superimpregnation.

superficial (soo′pər-fĭsh′əl) ADJ. pert. to the skin or other surface.

superinfection (soo'pər-ĭn-fĕk'shən) N. infection occurring during treatment with antimicrobials for another infection; it usually is caused by a change in the normal microscopic inhabitants of tissue (e.g., a vaginal yeast infection occurring during antibiotic treatment for a bacterial infection); secondary infection caused by an opportunistic pathogen (e.g., fungus-caused pneumonia occurring in a person debilitated or immunosuppressed because of another illness or treatment).

superior vena cava (soo-pēr'ē-ər vē'nə) N. vein that returns deoxygenated blood from the upper half of the body to the right atrium of the heart; it is the second longest vein in the body (*compare* INFERIOR VENA CAVA).

supine (soo-pīn') ADJ. lying on the back.

suppository (sə-pŏz'ĭ-tôr'ē) N. semisolid substance that melts when placed in the vagina, urethra, or rectum; it can be used to deliver drugs, esp. in babies or those with vomiting.

suppurate (sŭp'yə-rāt') V. to produce pus. ADJ. suppurative.

supra- comb. form indicating a position above or over (e.g., suprapubic, above the pubis).

sura N. calf of the leg.

surfactant (sər-făk'tənt) N. substance that acts on a surface, esp. certain lipoproteins that facilitate gaseous exchange in the alveoli by preventing alveolar collapse. Premature infants frequently experience respiratory distress because of a lack of surfactant. *See also* RESPIRATORY DISTRESS SYNDROME OF THE NEWBORN. Patients who inhale fresh water in near-drowning episodes have surfactant washed away with subsequent alveolar collapse and various levels of respiratory failure.

surgery (sûr'jə-rē) N. that branch of medicine concerned with the treatment of injuries and diseases by operations and manipulation. ADJ. surgical

Surmontil N. trade name for the antidepressant drug, trimipramine.

surrogate (sûr'ə-gĭt) N. substitute; person or object replacing another.

surrogate mother N. woman who, usually (but not always) by formal contract and for a stipulated sum of money, bears a child for a couple characterized by a wife who either is infertile or has an illness that would be exacerbated by pregnancy. The surrogate is artificially inseminated with the husband's semen, carries the fetus to term, and is expected to turn the baby over at birth to the natural father and his wife. In some cases, however, the natural mother has refused to surrender the baby or has sought visitation rights; as a result of ensuing litigation some states are considering legislation that would declare surrogate motherhood contracts to be void and unenforceable.

surveillance (sər-vā'lēns) N. monitoring, close observation; in epidemiology, refers to ongoing determination of the presence and severity of various diseases, usually done by the Centers for Disease Control in Atlanta. In immunology, the concept that the immune system routinely monitors the body for foreign materials and abnormal cells; when recognized, they are destroyed. Some theories hold that cancer develops due to a failure in the immune surveillance system.

susceptibility (sə-sĕp′tə-bĭl′ĭ-tē) N. condition of being easily affected by a disease-causing organism; condition of being more than normally vulnerable. ADJ. susceptible.

suspension (sə-spĕn′shən) N. mixture in which fine particles are suspended in a fluid where they are supported by buoyancy. Often refers to a form of liquid medication, such as an oral antibiotic; water is added to powdered drug, forming a suspension. During its preparation, the suspension must be thoroughly agitated to assure equal distribution of the medicine particles. This is also why many medications must be thoroughly shaken prior to taking them.

suture (soo′chər) N.
1. natural seam border in the skull formed by the close joining of bony surfaces.
2. material (e.g., silk catgut, wire) used for surgical stitches.
v. to stitch torn or cut edges together with suture material.

swallowing N. act of moving food from the mouth through the pharynx and esophagus to the stomach.

sweat (swĕt) *See* PERSPIRATION.

sweat duct N. any tiny tubule conveying sweat from a sudoriferous gland to the skin surface.

sweat gland *See* SUDORIFEROUS GLAND.

swelling (swĕl′ĭng) N. abnormal protuberance or localized enlargement.

Sydenham's chorea (sĭd′n-əmz kô-rē′ə) N. condition, usually affecting children and associated with rheumatic fever, characterized by involuntary, purposeless movements (chorea) that occur for several weeks and then usually subside; a streptococcal infection of vascular tissue of the brain area is thought to be responsible; also called St. Vitus dance.

symbiosis (sĭm′bē-ō′sĭs) N. in biology, close association of organisms of two different species, usually to their mutual benefit.

symbolism (sĭm′bə-lĭz′əm) N. in psychiatry, process of representing an object or idea by something else.

sympathectomy (sĭm′pə-thĕk′tə-mē) N. surgical interruption of a nerve pathway in the sympathetic nervous system; performed to minimize the effects of sympathetic nervous system function (e.g., to inhibit excess sweating or to improve blood circulation to a particular area, as in Buerger's disease).

sympathetic nervous system (sĭm′pə-thĕt′ĭk) N. one of the two divisions of the autonomic nervous system (the other being the parasympathetic nervous system), consisting of fibers that leave the central nervous system, pass through a chain of ganglia near the spinal cord, and are distributed to heart, lungs, intestine, blood vessels, and sweat glands. In general, sympathetic nerves dilate the pupils, constrict peripheral blood vessels, and increase heart rate. The system works in balance with the parasympathetic nervous system.

sympathomimetic (sĭm′pə-thō-mĭ-mĕt′ĭk) ADJ. having an effect (as from a drug) similar to that caused by stimulation of the sympathetic nervous system (e.g., dilating the bronchi).

symphysis (sĭm′fĭ-sĭs) N. joint in which fibrocartilage unites adjacent bony surfaces. For example, the pubic symphysis is where the two pelvic (innominate) bones unite anteriorly.

symptom (sĭm′təm) N. subjective indication of a disease; it may or may not be accompanied by an objective sign (*compare* SIGN).

synapse (sĭn′ăps) N. tiny gap between two neurons or between a neuron and a muscle across which nerve impulses are transmitted through the action of neurotransmitters (e.g., acetylcholine). When an impulse reaches the end of one neuron, it causes the release of a neurotransmitter that diffuses across the gap to trigger an impulse in the other neuron or muscle. ADJ. synaptic.

synapsis (sĭ-năp′sĭs) N. pairing of homologous chromosomes during an early stage of meiosis.

syncope (sĭng′kə-pē) N. brief loss of consciousness due to temporarily insufficient flow of blood to the brain; it may be caused by injury, emotional shock, prolonged standing, or other events. In many cases the feeling is preceded by lightheadedness and can be prevented by sitting with the head between the knees. Also called fainting.

syncytium (sĭn-sĭsh′ē-əm) N. mass of protoplasm containing several nuclei, as in muscle fibers.

syndactyly (sĭn-dăk′tə-lē) N. congenital defect characterized by partial or total webbing of some or all of the fingers and toes.

syndrome (sĭn′drōm′) N. complex of signs and symptoms presenting a clinical picture of a disease or disorder.

synechia N. adhesion between the iris and the cornea (anterior synechia) or between the iris and the lens (posterior synechia), developing as a result of trauma or surgery to the eye or

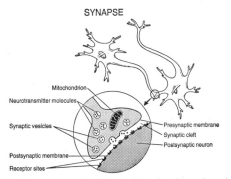

SYNAPSE

Mitochondrion
Neurotransmitter molecules
Synaptic vesicles
Presynaptic membrane
Synaptic cleft
Postsynaptic neuron
Postsynaptic membrane
Receptor sites

A typical synapse. The neuron portion at the top is equipped to make and release neurotransmitter; the receiving neuron's membrane has receptors to match the shape of arriving molecules of the neurotransmitter at ion channels.

as a complication of cataract or glaucoma. Treatment depends on the cause; untreated it can lead to blindness.

synergist N. substance that augments the activity of another substance, agent, or organ, as one drug augmenting the effect of another. N. synergism, ADJ. synergistic.

synovial fluid N. transparent, viscous fluid secreted by synovial membranes and acting as a lubricant for many joints and connective tissues; also called synovia.

synovial joint N. freely movable joint; types of synovial joints are ball-and-socket joint, gliding joint, hinge joint, and pivot joint.

synovial membrane N. membrane, secreting synovial fluid, that covers freely movable joints; also called synovium.

synovitis (sĭn′ə-vī′tĭs) N. inflammation of the synovial membrane lining a joint, resulting in pain and swelling; it may be caused by injury, infection, or rheumatic disease (e.g., rheu-matoid arthritis). Treatment depends on the cause.

Synthroid N. *See* TABLE OF COMMONLY PRESCRIBED DRUGS—TRADE NAMES.

syphilis (sĭf′ə-lĭs) N. sexually-transmitted disease caused by the *Treponema pallidum* spirochete; it is transmitted by sexual contact or through the placenta (congenital syphilis). Symptoms occur in stages—primary stage: chancre filled with spirochetes most often in anal or genital region, but can occur elsewhere; secondary stage: malaise, nausea, vomiting, fever, bone and joint pain, rash, and mouth sores; third stage: soft tumors (gummas) that ulcerate and then heal, leaving scars; they may form anywhere in the body and may or may not be painful. Various parts of the body, including the heart, nervous system, and lungs may be damaged, leading to death. These three stages occur over a prolonged period, often 15 or more years, before the tertiary stage takes hold. Congenital syphilis may result in the child's being born blind or deformed. Treatment is by penicillin, often in very large doses for a prolonged period.

syringe (sə-rĭnj′) N. device for withdrawing, injecting, or instilling a fluid. It usually includes a glass or plastic barrel with a close fitting plunger at one end and a needle at the other end.

syringomyelia (sə-rĭng′gō-mī-ē′lē-ə) N. progressive disease of the spinal cord in which the tissue develops cavities surrounded by scar tissue; more common in males, it results in sensory loss, weakness, and muscle atrophy.

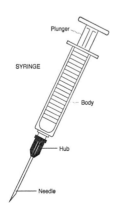

Plunger

SYRINGE

Body

Hub

Needle

systemic (sĭ-stĕm′ĭk) ADJ. affecting the body as a whole, rather than individual parts.

systemic circulation (sĭ-stĕm′ĭk sûr′kyə-lā′shən) N. system of blood vessels (arteries, veins, and capillaries) that supplies all of the body except the lungs. *See also* PULMONARY CIRCULATION.

systemic lupus erythematosis (sĭ-stĕm′ĭk lōō′pəs) N. chronic inflammatory disease of unknown cause, affecting women more frequently than men. Symptoms include arthritis, a red rash over the nose and cheeks (butterfly rash), fatigue, and weakness, followed by fever, photosensitivity, and skin lesions starting in the neck region and spreading to mucous membranes and other tissues, damaging the tissues involved. Glomerulonephritis, pericarditis, anemia, and neuritis may develop. Renal failure and neurological abnormalities often occur as the disease progresses. The disease may be controlled by corticosteroids; salicylates and antimalarial drugs are also sometimes used; the patient is warned to avoid fatigue and exposure to the sun. Also called disseminated lupus erythematosus, lupus erythematosus. (*Compare* DISCOID LUPUS ERYTHEMATOSUS.)

systole (sĭs′tə-lē) N. contraction of the heart, esp. of the ventricles, driving blood into the aorta and pulmonary artery. ADJ. systolic

systolic murmur (sĭ-stŏl′ĭk) N. murmur heard during systole.

systolic pressure *See* BLOOD PRESSURE.

-stomy suffix meaning surgical opening (e.g., tracheostomy).

T

T cell N. small circulating lymphocyte that matures in the thymus and is the chief agent of cell-mediated immunity, involved particularly in transplant rejection and delayed hypersensitivity reactions. Special T cells, called helper T cells and suppressor T cells, affect the production of B cells, the chief agents of the humoral (antibody-mediated) immune response.

tabes dorsalis (tā′bēz dôr-sā′lĭs) N. abnormal condition, usually associated with syphilis, characterized by progressive degeneration of sensory neurons, usually with symptoms of severe stabbing pains in the trunk and legs, unsteady gait, defective reflexes, incontinence, and impotence.

tablet (tăb′lĭt) N. small, solid dosage form of a drug.

tachi-, tacho-, tachy- comb. forms indicating an association with speed (e.g., tachypnea, rapid breathing).

tachycardia (tăk′ĭ-kär′dē-ə) N. abnormally rapid heart rate (over 100 beats per minute in an adult). Heart rate normally increases in response to fear and excitement and also in conditions characterized by lack of oxygen, as in congestive heart failure, hemorrhage, or shock.

tactile (tăk′təl) ADJ. pert. to the sense of touch.

taenia N. genus of large parasitic tapeworms, many of which are among the most common parasites affecting humans. Included are the beef tapeworm (*T. saginata*) and the pork tapeworm (*T. solium*).

Tagamet (tăg′ə-mĕt′) N. trade name for cimetidine. *See* TABLE OF COMMONLY PRESCRIBED DRUGS—TRADE NAMES.

Takayasu's arteritis (är′tə-rī′tĭs) N. disorder characterized by an absence of pulse in both arms and in the carotid arteries, transient paraplegia, and facial muscle weakness and atrophy caused by progressive occlusion of the left subclavian and left common carotid arteries above the aortic arch; also called pulseless disease.

talipes (tăl′ə-pēz′) N. any of several deformities of the foot, including talipes equinus, in which the toes are pointed downward, and talipes calcaneus, in which the toes are pointed upward so that the person walks on the heel of the affected foot.

talo- comb. form indicating an association with the ankle (talus) (e.g., talofibular, pert. to the talus and fibula).

talus (tā′ləs) N. bone of the ankle; it articulates with the tibia and fibula of the lower leg and with the calcaneus (heelbone) below; also called astragalus; ankle bone.

Talwin N. trade name for the analgesic pentazocine.

Tambocor N. trade name for the antiarrhythmic flecainide.

tamoxifen (tə-mŏk′sə-fĭn) N. *See* TABLE OF COMMONLY PRESCRIBED DRUGS—GENERIC NAMES.

tampon N. plug of cotton or sponge inserted into a body passage or cavity (e.g., the vagina or nose) to absorb exuded fluids, esp. blood.

tamponade (tăm′pə-nād′) N. cessation of the flow of blood to an organ or other part of the body by pressure, as in cardiac tamponade, when accumulated fluid compresses the heart.

tanning N. process by which pigmentation of the skin darkens because of exposure to ultraviolet light.

tapeworm infection (tāp′wûrm′) N. intestinal infection caused by a species of parasitic tapeworm, usually the result of eating raw or undercooked meat or fish that is an intermediate host to the tapeworm or its larva. Symptoms include diarrhea and weight loss; diagnosis is made when worms and eggs are found in the stool.

tapotement (tə-pōt′mənt) N. type of massage, sometimes used on the chest wall of patients with bronchitis to loosen mucus, in which the body is tapped rhythmically with the fingers or sides of the hand with short rapid movements.

tardive (tär′dĭv) ADJ. late-occurring, esp. in reference to symptoms of a disease.

tardive dyskinesia (tär′dĭv dĭs′ kə-nē′zhə) N. abnormal condition characterized by involuntary and repetitious movements of muscles of the face, trunk, and limbs; most often occurring as a side effect in people treated with phenothiazine drugs for Parkinsonism, or in patients taking antipsychotic medications.

target cell N.
1. abnormal red blood cell (erythrocyte) with a ringed appearance; associated with several types of anemia.
2. any cell with a specific receptor for antigen, antibody, hormone, or other substance.

target organ N.
1. in radiology, organ intended to receive the greatest therapeutic or diagnostic dose of a radioactive substance.
2. in endocrinology, organ most affected by a particular hormone; for example, the thyroid gland is the target organ of thyroid-stimulating hormone from the pituitary.

tarsal bone (tär′səl) N. any of seven bones making up the ankle.

tarsal gland N. any of numerous tiny sebaceous glands lining the inner surfaces of the eyelids. Bacterial infection of a tarsal gland produces a stye; also called Meibomian gland.

tarsitis (tär-sī′tĭs) N. inflammation of the eyelid.

tarsus (tär′səs) N.
1. seven bones of the ankle and proximal part of the foot; they articulate proximally with the tibia and fibula (lower leg bones) and with the metatarsals distally. ADJ. tarsal.
2. connective tissue that is the basis of each eyelid.

tartar (tär′tər) N. hard deposit that forms on the teeth and gums.

taste N. sense that occurs in response to the contact of dissolved material with specialized nerve receptors (taste buds) on the tongue; the impulses are then transmitted to taste centers in the brain for interpretation. There are four basic tastes: bitter (detected mostly in the back of the tongue); sour (sides of the tongue); sweet, and salty (front of the tongue). All other tastes are a combination of these.

taste bud N. any of numerous special sensory nerve endings located on the tongue and roof of the mouth that respond to different materials, triggering

impulses conducted to the taste centers in the brain; also called gustatory organ. *See also* TASTE.

tattoo (tă-tōō′) N. design made on skin by puncturing the skin and adding pigment; typically, cannot be removed, washed away or erased without special techniques, sometimes including plastic surgery. Unless sterile surgical technique is used, transmission of diseases such as hepatitis or AIDS may occur. Traumatic tattooing refers to embedding of fine dirt particles in the skin following an abrasion or close-range exposure to gunfire (powder burns). If promptly removed, little or no permanent scarring occurs. Otherwise, the particles are absorbed by scavenger cells (macrophages) in the skin, and may be permanent.

taxis (tăk′sĭs) N. in surgery, restoration by manipulation only of a dislocated organ or part to its normal position.

TASTE AREAS OF THE TONGUE

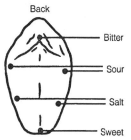

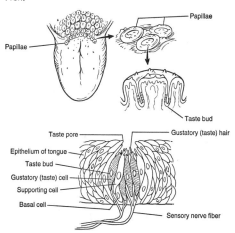

taxonomy (tăk-sŏn'ə-mē) N. science of classifying and naming organisms on the basis of natural relationships. ADJ. taxonomic

Tay-Sachs disease (tā'săks') N. inherited disease (autosomal recessive disease) characterized by progressive mental and physical degeneration and early death. It is caused by lack of the enzyme hexosaminidase, which results in an accumulation of sphingolipids in the brain. The disease occurs almost exclusively among Ashkenazic and Sephardic Jews. Symptoms appear by age 6 months; progressive degeneration follows, with blindness, development of a cherry red spot on the retina, spasticity, dementia, and death before the age of 4. There is no treatment. The disease can be diagnosed prenatally through amniocentesis. Also called amaurotic familial idiocy.

tear duct (tēr) N. duct, such as the lacrimal duct or the nasolacrimal duct, that transports tears.

tearing (tēr'ĭng) N. watering of the eye resulting from excessive tear production caused by irritation (as from a foreign object), infection, or strong emotion.

technician (tĕk-nĭsh'ən) N. skilled worker; may refer to one's degree of expertise, such as a surgeon being a superb technician.

teething (tē'thĭng) N. eruption of deciduous teeth (baby teeth, milk teeth) through the gums, usually extending from 4–6 months to about 30 months, when all 20 milk teeth have appeared. Discomfort in the gum area may occur, and symptoms of drooling, biting of hard objects, and irritability are common.

telangiectasia (tĕl-ăn'jē-ĕk-tā'zhə) N. localized collection of widened and distended capillaries and other small blood vessels, visible as a red spot that typically blanches on pressure. The spots may be found on the skin or mucous membranes.

telencephalon (tĕl'ĕn-sĕf'ə-lŏn') N. that part of the brain that includes the cerebral hemispheres, basal ganglia, olfactory bulb, and olfactory tracts.

telepathy (tə-lĕp'ə-thē) N. supposed ability of one person to know the thoughts of another; communication of thought from one person to another by nonphysical means. ADJ. telepathic

telophase (tĕl'ə-fāz') N. last of the four main stages of division within a cell nucleus, in which the new daughter chromosomes are at the poles of the division spindle, the nuclear membrane forms around them, the nucleolus reappears, and cytoplasmic division begins. *See also* MITOSIS; MEIOSIS.

temazepam (tə-măz'ə-păm') N. oral benzodiazepine (trade name Restoril) used in the treatment of insomnia; side effects include oversedation, dizziness, and confusion. *See* TABLE OF COMMONLY PRESCRIBED DRUGS —GENERIC NAMES.

temperature (tĕm'pər-ə-choor') N. in humans and other animals, measure of the heat associated with the metabolism of the body. Normal human temperature taken orally is considered to be 98.6° Fahrenheit (37° Celsius), but it may vary from person to person, and even in the same person depending on the time of day and level of activity.

template N. molecule that serves as the pattern for synthesizing another molecule; DNA provides a template for RNA synthesis. *See also* TRANSCRIPTION.

temple (tĕm′pəl) N. region of the head in front and above each ear.

temporal (tĕm′pər-əl) ADJ. pert. to the temple of the head or the corresponding lobe of the brain.

temporal arteritis (tăm′pər-əl är′tə-rī′tĭs) N. inflammation of the cranial arteries, esp. a temporal artery on the side of the head; it occurs most often in elderly women and produces symptoms of headache, chewing difficulty, and sometimes impaired vision.

temporal artery (tĕm′pər-əl är′tə-rē) N. any of three arteries on each side of the head. *See* MAJOR ARTERIES AND VEINS OF THE BODY, in Appendix.

temporal bone N. one of a pair of skull bones, forming the lower part of the cranium (skull) and containing cavities associated with the ear.

temporal lobe N. division of the cerebral cortex, lying at each side within the temple of the skull; it includes parts of the brain associated with speech, sound, and smell.

temporalis N. any of several muscles associated with chewing.

temporo- comb. form indicating an association with the temple (temporal) region of the head (e.g., temporomandibular, pert. to the mandible [lower jaw] and the temporal bone of the skull).

temporomandibular joint (TMJ) (tĕm′pə-rō-măn-dĭb′yə-lər) N. joint where the jawbone (mandible) joins or articulates with the temporal bone of the skull.

TEMPOROMANDICULAR JOINT (TMJ)

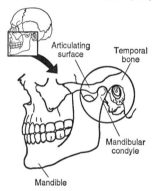

tenderness (tĕn′dər-nĭs) N. soreness sensed on being touched; touch sensitivity. ADJ. tender

tendinitis (tĕn′də-nī′tĭs) N. inflammation of a tendon, usually resulting from strain or injury. Treatment includes rest and corticosteroid injections. *See also* TENNIS ELBOW.

tendon (tĕn′dən) N. one of many whitish, glistening, fibrous bands of tissue that connect muscles to bone; tendons are inelastic and strong and occur in various thicknesses and lengths; also called sinew (*compare* LIGAMENT).

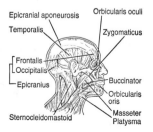

tenesmus (tə-nĕz′məs) N. spasm of the rectum and desire to defecate without the production of significant amounts of feces. It is associated with irritable bowel syndrome and other conditions.

tennis elbow (tĕn′ĭs) N. painful inflammation of the tendon at the outer border of the elbow caused by overuse of lower arm muscles. Treatment is by rest, nonsteroidal anti-inflammatory agents, and, if necessary, corticosteroid injections.

teno- comb. form indicating an association with a tendon (e.g., tenodynia, tendon pain).

Tenoretic N. trade name for the fixed-combination antihypertensive consisting of the beta blocker atenolol and the diuretic chlorthalidone.

Tenormin N. trade name for the beta blocker atenolol. *See* TABLE OF COMMONLY PRESCRIBED DRUGS—TRADE NAMES.

tenosynovitis (tĕn′ō-sĭn′ə-vī′tĭs) N. inflammation of the sheath surrounding a tendon, caused by repeated strain, trauma, or certain systemic conditions (e.g., gout, rheumatoid arthritis, or gonorrhea). Treatment includes rest of the affected area, corticosteroid injections, treatment of any underlying cause, and, if severe, surgical intervention.

tension (tĕn′shən) N.
1. condition of being taut or tense, as in muscle tension.
2. psychophysiological state, usually a response to stress, characterized by an increase in heart rate, muscle tone, and alertness, and usually accompanied by irritability, anxiety, and uneasiness.

tension headache N. pain, chiefly located at the back of the head and often spreading forward, occurring as a result of tensing the body as a response to overwork, strong emotion, or psychological stress.

tensor (tĕn′sər) N. any of several muscles of the body that tense an attached structure (e.g., tensor tympani, the muscle that tenses the tympanic membrane eardrum).

tentorium (tĕn-tôr′ē-əm) N. tent-like body part, esp. the tentorium that covers the cerebellum and supports the occipital lobes of the cerebrum above.

tepid ADJ. moderately warm.

teras (tĕr′əs) N., *pl.* terata, grossly deformed fetus (monster) that usually does not survive. ADJ. teratic

terato- comb. form indicating an association with a monster (e.g., teratology, study of developmental abnormalities).

teratogen (tə-răt′ə-jən) N. substance or agent that interferes with normal embryonic development and causes one or more abnormalities in the fetus. The specific agent and its action, on the stage of embryonic development during which exposure occurs, on genetic predisposition, and on other modifying factors determine the type and extent of the defect. Among the agents known to be teratogens are X rays and other forms of ionizing radiation; drugs such as thalidomide and alcohol; infectious agents, such as those that cause rubella and toxoplasmosis; and various chemicals that may be in the environment. The time of greatest vulnerability for the fetus is between the 3rd and 12th week of gestation, when most of the major organ systems are formed. ADJ. teratogenic

teratogenesis (tĕr′ə-tə-jĕn′ĭ-sĭs) N. development of defects in the embryo.

teratoma (tĕr′ə-tō′mə) N. tumor made up of tissue not normally found at that site, occurring most often in the testes and ovaries; some can become malignant.

terazosin (tə-rā′zə-sĭn) N. oral antihypertensive (trade name Hytrin). Adverse effects include syncope, postural hypotension, depression, sleep disturbance, and, rarely, impotence. *See* TABLE OF COMMONLY PRESCRIBED DRUGS—GENERIC NAMES.

teres (tēr′ēz) N. either of two muscles (teres major and teres minor) in the shoulder region, responsible for some shoulder and arm movements.

MAJOR SUPERFICIAL BACK MUSCLES

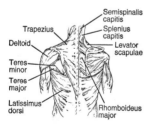

terfenadine (tər-fĕn′ə-dēn′) N. antihistamine (trade name Seldane) used in the treatment of allergy and rhinitis. Side effects include dry mouth, dizziness, and rarely, cardiac arrhythmias. This drug should not be given concomitantly with the antibiotic erythromycin because of an increased risk of heart rhythm problems.

term infant (tûrm) N. infant born after the normally expected duration of pregnancy after the 37th and before the 43rd week of gestation regardless of weight (*compare* POSTMATURE INFANT; PREMATURE INFANT).

testicle (tĕs′tĭ-kəl) *See* TESTIS.

testicular cancer (tĕ-stĭk′yə-lər) N. malignant neoplasm of the testis, occurring most often in men between the ages of 20 and 35, often affecting an undescended testis and more frequently the right testis. In its early stages testicular cancer is often asymptomatic, and it may metastasize, later causing urinary and pulmonary symptoms and an abdominal mass. Treatment depends on the nature of the tumor and includes surgery (orchidectomy), radiation, and/or chemotherapy.

testis (tĕs′tĭs) N., *pl.* testes, either of a pair of male gonads, or sex glands, that produces sperm and secretes androgens. The adult testes, each about 1½

MALE REPRODUCTIVE DUCTS

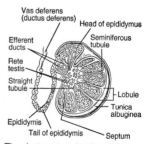

The duct system leading from the testis. Sperm cells form in the seminiferous tubules and pass through the rete testis and efferent ducts to emerge in the epididymis. The tail of the epididymis leads to the vas deferens, which carries sperm cells away from the testis.

inches (4 centimeters) long and oval-shaped, are suspended in the scrotum below the abdomen. Each testis consists of many hundred seminiferous tubules where sperm develop. The sperm pass from there through efferent ducts to the epididymis, after which they pass into the vas deferens for movement toward the penis. Also: testicle. ADJ. testicular.

testosterone (tĕs-tŏs′tə-rōn′) N. male sex hormone, produced chiefly in the testes, but also in small amounts in the adrenal glands and in the ovaries of women. It is responsible for the development of male secondary sex characteristics (e.g., deep voice and facial hair). Preparations of testosterone are used in the treatment of deficiency conditions, breast cancer in women, and certain other conditions. Adverse effects of the use of these preparations include fluid retention, masculinization in women, and acne.

tests N. generic term for numerous possible types of medical studies, ranging from blood tests to X rays, to sophisticated surgical procedures (e.g., open lung biopsy).

test-tube baby N. baby born as a result of fertilization occurring outside the mother's body. Ova are removed from a woman's body (usually using a laparoscope) and mixed with sperm in a culture medium. If fertilization occurs and cleavage results, the blastocyst is then implanted in the woman's uterus and pregnancy continues.

tetanus (tĕt′n-əs) N. acute and serious infection of the central nervous system caused by an exotoxin produced by the *Clos-tridium tetani* bacterium. The bacterium, common in the soil, esp. in farm areas, infects wounds with dead tissue, as in a puncture wound, laceration, or burn. Symptoms include fever, headache, irritability, and painful spasms of the muscles, causing lockjaw and laryngeal spasm, and, if untreated, leading to muscle spasm of virtually every organ. Prompt and thorough cleaning of wounds is important to prevent tetanus. Treatment of the disease includes use of tetanus toxoid and antibiotics, maintenance of an airway if laryngeal spasm occurs, control of muscle spasms, and sedation. Also called lockjaw.

tetanus antitoxin (ăn′tē-tŏk′sĭn) N. a tetanus immune serum given for short-term immunization against tetanus in cases of possible exposure to the tetanus organism. Adverse effects include pain at the site of injection and possible allergic reactions.

tetanus immune globulin (ĭ-myoon′ glŏb′yə-lĭn) N. preparation prepared from the globulin of a person immune to tetanus and given to provide short-term protection from the disease in cases of possible exposure to the tetanus organisms; it is considered safer than tetanus antitoxin, the chief disadvantage being pain at the site of injection.

tetany (tĕt′n-ē) N. disorder, usually caused by a disorder of calcium metabolism, associated with hypoparathyroidism, vitamin D deficiency, or alkalosis and characterized by muscular twitching, cramps, and convulsions.

tetrachloroethylene N. drug used to treat hookworm infestation. Adverse effects include nausea, abdominal cramps, and sometimes liver toxicity.

tetracycline (tĕt′rə-sī′klēn′) N. any of a family of antibiotics derived from Streptomyces bacteria, including chlortetracycline, oxytetracycline, and doxycycline. They are known under many trade names, and are used to treat a variety of bacterial and rickettsial infections. Tetracyclines are not used during pregnancy or in young children because they cause discoloration of children's teeth. Other adverse effects include gastrointestinal disturbances, suprainfections, and allergic reactions. *See* TABLE OF COMMONLY PRESCRIBED DRUGS—GENERIC NAMES.

tetrahydrocannabinol (THC) N. active principle in hemp-plant derivatives such as marihuana, hashish, and ganja. Considered a mild hallucinogen, it causes sensory and perceptual disturbances, euphoria and other mood changes, decreased motor coordination, and various physiological changes, including alterations in pulse rate, respiration rate, and pupil size. THC is a drug of abuse but has also been used to relieve the nausea and vomiting associated with chemotherapy for cancer.

tetralogy of Fallot (tĕ-trăl′ə-jē fă-lōz′) N. congenital heart defect characterized by four anomalies: pulmonary stenosis, ventricular septal defect, malposition of the aorta, and hypertrophy of the right ventricle. The infant exhibits cyanosis and other signs of lack of oxygen, failure to thrive, poor development, and later clubbing of the fingers and toes. Treatment is by surgical repair, usually done when the child is 4–5 years old. *See also* BLUE BABY.

thalamus (thăl′ə-məs) N. one or two large, oval masses of gray matter deep in the cerebral hemispheres concerned with relaying sensory impulses to the cerebral cortex; the thalamus is also the site where crude sensations of pain, pressure, and temperature originate. ADJ. thalamic

thalassemia (thăl′ə-sē′mē-ə) N. hereditary (autosomal recessive) form of anemia, occurring most often in people of Mediterranean origin, characterized by abnormal hemoglobin synthesis. Persons homozygous for the trait, inheriting it from both parents—"thalassemia major"—are severely affected in childhood with anemia, enlarged spleen, failure to thrive, iron accumulation in the tissues, respiratory difficulty, and retarded growth and development. There is no cure; treatment involves repeated transfusions. Persons heterozygous for the trait, inheriting it from only one parent—"thalassemia minor"—may have few or no symptoms. The disease can be detected prenatally through amniocentesis. Also called Cooley's anemia.

thalidomide (thə-lĭd′ə-mīd′) N. sedative drug, no longer used because of its teratogenic properties when taken during pregnancy.

thanatology (thăn′ə-tŏl′ə-jē) N. study of death and dying.

THC *See* TETRAHYDROCANNABINOL.

theca (thē′kə) N. sheath or capsule covering.

thelarche (thē-lär′kē) N. beginning of female breast development, usually occurring between the ages of 9 and 13, before puberty.

thenar (thē′när′) N. palm, esp. the raised, fleshy part of the palm at the base of the thumb. ADJ. thenal

Theobid N. trade name for a bronchodilator containing aminophylline, and used to treat some respiratory disorders, esp. those marked by spasm of the airways.

Theodur N. trade name for a popular aminophylline derivative; used in the treatment of asthma and chronic obstructive pulmonary disease.

theophylline (thē-ŏf′ə-lĭn) N. See AMINOPHYLLINE.

therapeutic abortion (thĕr′ə-pyŏŏ′tĭk) See ABORTION.

therapeutic touch See TABLE OF ALTERNATIVE MEDICINE TERMS.

therapeutics (thĕr′ə-pyŏŏ′tĭks) N. that branch of medical science specifically concerned with treatment. ADJ. therapeutic

therm-, thermo- comb. forms indicating an association with heat (e.g., thermalgesia—heat-caused pain).

thermal (thûr′məl) ADJ. pert to heat or the production of heat.

thermocautery (thûr′mō-kô′tə-rē) N. destruction of tissue by heat, as by direct flame or electric current.

thermocoagulation (thûr′mō-kō-ăg′yə-lā′shən) N. congealing tissue by heat (electric current).

thermography N. technique for sensing (by means of an infrared detector) and recording the heat produced by different parts of the body; it is used to study blood flow and detect tumors (which may show as hot spots), esp. those of the breast (mammothermography). Its validity as a medical test has been seriously questioned in medical literature over recent years.

thermolabile (thûr′mō-lā′bĭl) ADJ. easily changed or destroyed by heat.

thermometer (thər-mŏm′ĭ-tər) N. device for measuring temperature, usually consisting of a glass tube marked with degrees Fahrenheit or Celsius and containing mercury or alcohol, which rises or falls as it expands or contracts with changes in temperature.

thermotherapy (thûr′mō-thĕr′ə-pē) N. use of heat, as with heating pads, hot compresses, and hot water bottles, to treat a disease or disorder (e.g., to promote circulation in peripheral vascular disease or to relax tense muscles).

theta rhythm (rĭth′əm) N. brainwave frequency of relatively low frequency and low amplitude; the drowsy waves characteristic of a person who is awake but relaxed and sleepy; also called theta wave. It is one of four brain-wave patterns (*compare* ALPHA RHYTHM; BETA RHYTHM; DELTA RHYTHM).

thiamine (thī′ə-mĭn) N. member of the B-complex group of vitamins essential for functioning of the cardiovascular and nervous systems and for metabolism; also called thiamin; vitamin B_1; antiberiberi factor. See *also* TABLE OF VITAMINS.

thiazide (thī′ə-zīd′) N. any of a group of compounds, many of which are widely used diuretics.

thigh (thī) N. section of the leg between the hip and the knee.

thigh bone See FEMUR.

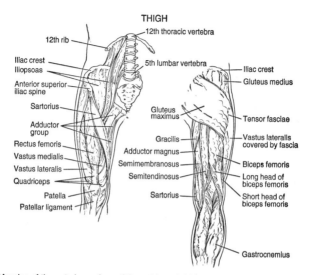

THIGH

12th thoracic vertebra
12th rib
Iliac crest
Iliopsoas
Anterior superior iliac spine
5th lumbar vertebra
Iliac crest
Gluteus medius
Sartorius
Gluteus maximus
Tensor fasciae
Adductor group
Gracilis
Vastus lateralis covered by fascia
Rectus femoris
Adductor magnus
Vastus medialis
Semimembranosus
Biceps femoris
Vastus lateralis
Semitendinosus
Long head of biceps femoris
Quadriceps
Sartorius
Short head of biceps femoris
Patella
Patellar ligament
Gastrocnemius

Muscles of the anterior surface of the pelvis and thigh.
Muscles on the posterior surface of the right thigh.

thioguanine N. antineoplastic drug used to treat acute leukemias and other malignant neoplastic diseases. Adverse effects include bone marrow depression and gastrointestinal disturbances.

thiopental (thī′ō-pĕn′tăl′) N. strong, short-acting barbiturate used as anesthesia for very short surgical procedures and as an induction to another anesthetic agent. It depresses respiration and heart activity and may be habit-forming.

thioridazine (thī′ə-rĭd′ə-zēn′) N. major tranquilizer (trade name Mellaril) used to treat schizophrenia and many other psychotic disorders. Adverse effects include low blood pressure, liver toxicity, and blood disorders.

thiotepa (thī′ō-tē′pə) N. antineoplastic drug used to treat certain malignancies. Adverse effects include nausea, vomiting, and bone marrow depression.

Thomsen's disease *See* MYOTONIA CONGENITA.

thoracic aorta (thə-răs′ĭk ā-ôr′tə) N. large upper part of the descending aorta supplying the heart, chest muscles, ribs, and stomach.

thoracic duct N. one of the two major trunks of the lymphatic system; it drains lymph from the abdomen and lower limbs and from the left side of the thorax and head and empties it into the junction of the left subclavian and left internal jugular vein.

thoracic medicine N. that branch of medicine concerned with diagnosis and treatment of diseases of the chest.

thoracic nerves N. 12 spinal nerves on each side of the thorax distributed to the walls of the thorax and abdomen.

thoracic outlet syndrome N. condition characterized by tingling sensation in the fingers and caused by compression on a nerve of the arm.

thoraco- comb. form indicating an association with the chest (e.g., thoracocentesis, draining of fluid through a needle from the chest for diagnostic or therapeutic purposes).

thorax (thôr′ăks′) N. bone and cartilage cage, formed in the front by the sternum and rib cartilage and in the back by the thoracic vertebrae and dorsal parts of the ribs, that encloses the lungs, heart, esophagus, and other structures; also called chest. ADJ. thoracic.

Thorazine (thôr′ə-zēn′) N. trade name for chlorpromazine.

threatened abortion *See* ABORTION.

three-day measles (mē′zəlz) *See* RUBELLA.

threshold (thrĕsh′ōld′) N. minimal point at which a stimulus evokes a response.

thrill (thrĭl) N. fine vibration that can be felt on placing the hand on the body.

throb (thrŏb) N. deep, pulsating type of pain or discomfort.

thromb-, thrombo- comb. forms indicating an association with a blood clot (thrombus) (e.g., thromboclasis, breaking up of a clot).

thrombasthenia (thrŏm′băs-thē′nē-ə) N. rare, inherited (autosomal recessive) disease in which platelets do not function normally to produce a blood clot, and hemorrhage ensues. Treatment is by platelet transfusion.

thrombectomy (thrŏm-bĕk′tə-mē) N. surgical removal of a thrombus (blood clot) from a blood vessel to restore circulation to the affected part.

thrombin (thrŏm′bĭn) N. coagulation factor, formed in plasma from prothrombin, calcium, and thromboplastin, that acts to change fibrinogen to fibrin, necessary for a blood clot.

THORAX

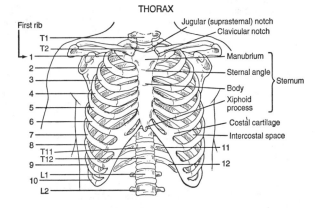

First rib — T1, T2
1, 2, 3, 4, 5, 6, 7, 8 — T11, T12, 9, L1, 10, L2

Jugular (suprasternal) notch
Clavicular notch
Manubrium
Sternal angle — Sternum
Body
Xiphoid process
Costal cartilage
Intercostal space
11
12

thromboangiitis obliterans (thrŏm'bō-ăn'jē-ī'tĭs) *See* BUERGER'S DISEASE.

thrombocyte (thrŏm'bə-sīt') *See* PLATELET.

thrombocytopenia (thrŏm'bō-sī'tə-pē'nē-ə) N. condition characterized by a lower than normal number of platelets and resulting in bleeding and easy bruising. Causes of the reduced platelet level include drug reactions and neoplastic disease of blood-forming tissue. Treatment depends on the cause.

thrombocytopenic purpura (thrŏm'bō-sī'tə-pē'nĭk pûr'pə-rə) *See* PURPURA.

thrombocytosis (thrŏm'bō-sī-tō'sĭs) N. increase in the number of platelets in the blood, causing greater tendency for clots to form; it is associated with many chronic infections, neoplasms, and other diseases.

thromboembolism (thrŏm'bō-ĕm'bə-lĭz'əm) N. condition in which a blood vessel is blocked by an embolus carried in the bloodstream from its site of formation. The area affected by the diminished blood supply may become cyanotic (bluish) and numb. Often the first symptom is excruciating pain. Treatment includes anticoagulants, rest, moist heat, and surgery, especially if a major vessel (aorta, pulmonary artery, femoral or iliac arteries) is involved. ADJ. thromboembolic.

thrombolysis N. process of breaking up and removing blood clots, during which fibrin is dissolved. This is a normal and ongoing process in the body. The principles of thrombolysis have been utilized therapeutically via administration of drugs that dissolve blood clots

associated with disease (e.g., such as in a coronary artery during an acute myocardial infarction). *See also* FIBRINOLYSIS; THROMBOLYTIC THERAPY.

thrombolytic therapy N. administration of a pharmacological agent with the intention of causing thrombolysis of an abnormal blood clot, such as in the coronary (myocardial infarction) or pulmonary (pulmonary embolism) arteries. Available agents include streptokinase, urokinase, tissue plasminogen activator, and APSAC. These preparations may be given either intravenously or directly into the blocked artery (intra-arterial).

thrombophlebitis (thrŏm'bō-flĭ-bī'tĭs) N. inflammation of a vein (*see also* PHLEBITIS), in conjunction with the formation of a blood clot (thrombus). It occurs as a result of trauma to the blood vessels; prolonged immobilization and consequent venous stasis; hypercoagulability of the blood; infection; or irritation. Treatment includes rest of the affected area (most often the legs), moist heat, and the use of anticoagulants and agents (e.g., streptokinase) to dissolve clots. Close monitoring to detect signs of pulmonary embolism, myocardial infarction, or other serious complication is essential.

thromboplastin (thrŏm'bō-plăs'tĭn) N. substance found in most tissues and some blood cells that starts the blood coagulation process, converting prothrombin to thrombin.

thrombosis (thrŏm-bō'sĭs) N. condition in which a blood clot (thrombus) forms within a blood vessel. Thrombosis in an artery supplying the brain results in a stroke (cerebrovascular accident); in an artery supplying the heart, in a myocardial infarction; in a vein, thrombophlebitis. A thrombus may also move from its site of origin. *See also* EMBOLISM.

thrombus N., *pl.* thrombi, blood clot attached to the interior wall of a vein or artery (*compare* EMBOLUS).

thrush *See* CANDIDIASIS.

thymine N. base found in DNA (deoxyribonucleic acid).

thymo- comb. form indicating an association with the thymus (e.g., thymoma, tumor, usually benign, of the thymus).

thymosin N. hormone secreted by the thymus, present in greatest amounts in childhood and decreasing in amount throughout life.

thymus N. bilobed gland situated below the thyroid gland and behind the sternum and involved in the function of the lymphatic

system and the immune system. The gland increases in size until puberty; thereafter it becomes smaller and decreases in functional activity during adulthood. ADJ. thymic.

thyro- comb. form indicating an association with the thyroid gland (e.g., thyromegaly, thyroid gland enlargement).

thyrocalcitonin *See* CALCITONIN.

thyroid cartilage (thī'roid') N. large cartilage of the larynx, forming the Adam's apple.

thyroid gland N. large endocrine gland situated at the base of the neck. It consists of two lobes, one on each side of the trachea, connected by an isthmus. Under the influence of thyroid-stimulating hormone (TSH) released from the anterior pituitary gland, the thyroid secretes the hormone thyroxine into the bloodstream; it is essential for normal growth and development in children and normal

POSITION OF THE THYMUS IN THE UPPER THORAX

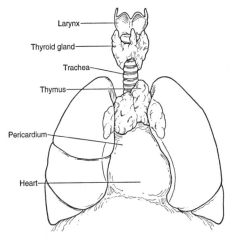

Larynx —
Thyroid gland —
Trachea —
Thymus —
Pericardium —
Heart —

THYROID GLAND

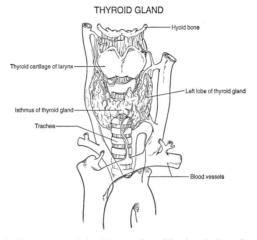

metabolic rates in adults. Disorders of the thyroid include goiter, myxedema, and cretinism.

thyroid storm N. crisis in uncontrolled hyperthyroidism in which the release of thyroid hormone into the bloodstream causes rapid pulse, fever, respiratory distress, and restlessness, leading to delirium, heart failure, and death. Treatment is by antithyroid drugs.

thyroidectomy N. surgical removal of the thyroid gland, usually done to remove tumors or to treat hyperthyroidism that does not respond to other therapies.

thyroiditis N. inflammation of the thyroid gland. Acute thyroiditis is usually due to bacterial or other infection and is marked by abscess formation and signs of infection; chronic forms include several hereditary conditions (e.g. Hashimoto disease) and responses to irradiation of the thyroid.

thyroid-stimulating hormone (TSH) N. hormone secreted by the anterior pituitary gland that controls the release of thyroid hormone (thyroxine) from the thyroid. It is influenced by thyrotropin-releasing factor from the hypothalamus.

thyrotoxicosis (thī′rō-tŏk′sĭ-kō′ sĭs) *See* EXOPHTHALMIC GOITER.

thyrotropin-releasing factor (TRF) (thī′rə-trō′pĭn) N. substance released by the hypothalamus that controls the release of thyroid-stimulating hormone from the anterior pituitary gland.

thyroxine (T$_4$) (thī-rŏk′sēn′) N. one of two principal hormones secreted by the thyroid gland to regulate metabolism; the other is triiodothyronine, also known as T$_3$. Sometimes called thyroid hormone.

tibia (tĭb′ē-ə) N. inner and larger bone of the lower leg (the second longest bone in the body); it articulates proximally with the femur (thigh bone), form-

TIBIA AND FIBULA

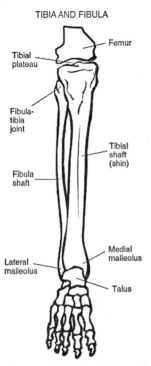

ing part of the knee joint, and with the fibula (the other lower leg bone) and talus (ankle bone) distally; also called shin bone.

tibio- comb. form indicating an association with the tibia (e.g., tibiofemoral, pert. to the tibia and the femur).

tic (tĭk) N. a repeated, largely involuntary, spasm or twitch, esp. of part of the face (*compare* BLEPHARISM).

tic douloureux (tĭk) *See* TRIGEMINAL NEURALGIA.

tick (tĭk) N. blood-sucking parasite, some species of which cause diseases in humans, including Lyme disease, Rocky Mountain spotted fever, and tularemia.

Tietze's syndrome (tē'tsēz) N. disorder characterized by swelling of rib cartilage, causing pain; it may accompany a chronic respiratory disorder, but in many cases the cause is unknown and it resolves without treatment.

timolol N. *See* TABLE OF COMMONLY PRESCRIBED DRUGS— GENERIC NAMES.

Timoptic N. *See* TABLE OF COMMONLY PRESCRIBED DRUGS— TRADE NAMES.

tine test (tīn) N. tuberculin skin test in which a disc with several tines bearing tuberculin antigen is used to puncture the skin. The development of hardened skin around the area indicates active disease or previous exposure and the need for further testing.

tinea (tĭn'ē-ə) N. any of a group of fungus-caused skin diseases, usually characterized by skin lesions, scaling and itchiness; also called roundworm.

   tinea capitis N. contagious fungal infection of the scalp characterized by bald patches, reddening, and crust formation. Treatment is by the antifungal griseofulvin.

   tinea corporis N. fungal infection of nonhairy parts of the skin, most common in warm areas. Treatment is by antifungal agents.

   tinea cruris N. fungal infection of the groin, most common in males, and often associated with warmth and local irritation; also called jock itch.

   tinea pedis *See* ATHLETE'S FOOT.

   tinea unguium N. fungal infection of the nails that can cause complete crumbling of the nails, esp. the toenails. Treatment is by griseofulvin.

tinnitus (tĭ-nī′təs) N. ringing in the ears; it may be a sign of trauma to the ear area, Meniere's disease, or an accumulation of earwax.

tissue (tĭsh′o͞o) N. collection of cells specialized to perform a particular function. The cells may be all of the same type (e.g., in nervous tissue) or of different types (e.g., in connective tissue). An aggregate of tissues with a specific function is an organ.

tissue plasminogen activator (TPA) (tĭsh′o͞o plăz-mĭn′ə-jən ăk′tə-vā′tər) N. thrombolytic agent (trade name Activase) that causes fibrinolysis at the site of blood clot formation; used currently in the treatment of acute myocardial infarction.

tissue typing (tĭsh′o͞o tī′pĭng) N. series of tests to determine the compatibility of tissues from a donor and a recipient before transplantation.

titer (tī′tər) N. concentration of a solution; in bacteriology, meas-urement of the number of organisms (bacterial titer) or viruses (viral titer) present, or the level of an antibody in the blood (antibody titer).

titrate v. to adjust the concentration of a solution (such as an injectable drug) so that the smallest possible amount (or lowest concentration) of the active ingredient is used that will achieve the desired effect. N. titration

Tobradex N. *See* TABLE OF COMMONLY PRESCRIBED DRUGS—TRADE NAMES.

tobramycin/dexamethasone N. *See* TABLE OF COMMONLY PRESCRIBED DRUGS—GENERIC NAMES.

tocainide (tō-kā′nĭd′) N. oral anti-arrhythmic (trade name Tonocard) useful as second-line therapy against ventricular arrhythmias, such as frequent premature ventricular contractions. Serious adverse effects have been reported, including blood disorders and changes in the patient's level of consciousness; therefore this agent is recom-

HUMAN TISSUES AND THEIR FUNCTIONS

Tissue	Function
Epithelial	Provides protection and support; lines organs
Connective	Holds together specialized areas of human body
Bone	Provides support
Cartilage	Provides flexibility; absorbs shock
Fibrous connective tissue	Connects muscles to bone; bone to bone
Blood	Transports oxygen, nutrients, wastes, antibodies, hormones
Muscle	Contracts to provide body movement
Nerve	Conducts electrical impulses between all parts of the body and between the external environment and body

mended only when less dangerous drugs have failed.

tocopherol N. any of a group of fat-soluble compounds with vitamin E activity, occurring in many fish, seed, and vegetable oils and functioning as important antioxidants. *See also* TABLE OF VITAMINS.

toe N. digit of the foot.

Tofranil N. trade name for the tricyclic antidepressant imipramine.

tolazamide N. antidiabetic used in the treatment of adult-onset, stable diabetes mellitus. Adverse effects include nausea, diarrhea, and weakness.

tolazoline N. vasodilator used to treat spasms of peripheral blood vessels (e.g., Raynaud's sign—acrocyanocis).

tolbutamide N. oral antidiabetic used in the treatment of adult-onset diabetes mellitus. Adverse effects include low blood sugar and skin reaction.

tolerance N. ability to endure large exposures to a substance without an adverse effect; typically, the patient demonstrates decreased sensitivity to subsequent doses of the same substance. Clinically, patients may develop tolerance to a medication, so that it no longer has the desired effect at the usual dose. Similarly, microorganisms may develop tolerance to antibiotics, rendering particular agents useless in treatment.

Tolinase N. trade name for the antidiabetic tolazamide.

tomography *See* COMPUTED TOMOGRAPHY.

-tomy suffix meaning a surgical incision into an organ (e.g.,

gastrotomy, incision into the stomach).

tone N. normal state of balanced tension and responsiveness of the body, esp. the muscles; also called tonus. ADJ. tonic

tongue N. mucous-membrane-covered, muscular organ attached to the floor of the mouth by the frenulum linguae. The surface is covered with papillae and taste buds. The tongue manipulates food during chewing and swallowing; functions in the production of speech and different sounds; and is the main organ of taste; also called glossa; lingua. ADJ. lingual

tonic
1. ADJ. pert. to normal muscle tone.
2. marked by tension, as in tonic muscle spasm. N. substance taken to increase one's sense of vigor.

tonicity N. state of normal muscle tone, ready to contract. Also osmolality of a solution relative to plasma. Solutions with the same osmolality as plasma are considered isotonic; those with greater osmolality are hypertonic, and those with lower osmolality are hypotonic.

Tonocard N. trade name for the antiarrhythmic tocainide.

tonometer N. instrument used to measure tension or pressure, esp. intraocular pressure in testing for glaucoma.

tonsil N. mass of lymphoid tissue, esp. one of the paired masses at the back of the mouth (palatine tonsils or lingual tonsils) concerned with response to infection. The adenoids or pharyngeal tonsils are posterior and superior, within the nasopharynx.

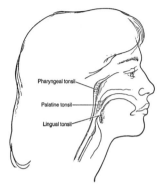

Pharyngeal tonsil

Palatine tonsil

Lingual tonsil

tonsillectomy N. surgical removal of the palatine tonsils, usually performed to prevent recurrent streptococcal infections; often performed together with adenoidectomy.

tonsillitis N. inflammation or infection of a tonsil, esp. the palatine tonsils. Acute tonsillitis, often caused by bacterial, esp. streptococcal, infection, produces sore throat, fever, headache, enlarged lymph glands in the neck region, and difficulty in swallowing. Treatment is by rest, fluids, and antibiotics. Surgery (tonsillectomy) is sometimes performed to prevent recurrent streptococcal attacks. *See also* STREPTOCOCCAL THROAT.

tooth N. any of the hard structures in the mouth used to cut, grind, and process food. Each tooth contains an enamel-covered crown above the gum and a neck with a dentin-covered pulp-filled cavity that stretches to the cementum-covered root embedded in the socket of the jaw. Normally two sets of teeth appear during life: a deciduous (milk) set of 20 teeth that appears during infancy and a permanent set of 32 teeth that appears gradually during childhood and early adulthood. The 32 adult teeth differ somewhat

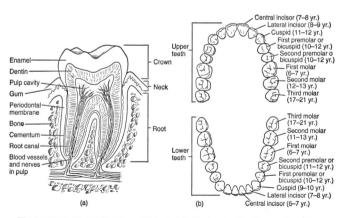

The human teeth: (a) Structure of a typical tooth showing the three major regions of the tooth and the structures associated with each region. (b) The permanent teeth of an adult, with the date of eruption of each tooth.

in shape and function. *See also* CANINE; INCISOR; MOLAR; PREMOLAR; DECIDUOUS TOOTH; PERMANENT TOOTH.

topical ADJ. pert. to the surface of a part, as a drug applied to the skin surface.

topical anesthesia N. surface anesthesia obtained by applying a topical agent, such as benzocaine or lidocaine, to the skin or mucous membrane.

Toprol-XL N. trade name for an extended-release preparation of the antihypertensive drug, metoprolol. *See* TABLE OF COMMONLY PRESCRIBED DRUGS—TRADE NAMES.

Toradol N. trade name for the nonsteroidal, anti-inflammatory pain medication, ketorolac tromethamine.

torpor (tôr′pər) N. state of decreased responsiveness and sluggishness; occurring in some mental disorders, some types of poisoning, and some metabolic disorders; also called torbidity. ADJ. torpid.

torsion (tôr′shən) N. twisting.

torticollis (tôr′tĭ-kŏl′ĭs) N. abnormal condition in which the head leans to one side because of contraction of the neck muscles on that side; it may be congenital or result from injury. Treatment depends on the cause and severity of the condition; it may include immobilization, pain relievers (if the muscle spasm produces severe pain), and surgical intervention. Also called wryneck.

tortuous ADJ. twisting; having many twists or turns.

total parenteral nutrition (TPN) (pă-rĕn′tər-əl) N. administration of a nutritionally adequate solution (containing, e.g., proteins, electrolytes, and vitamins) through a catheter into the vena cava; used to provide nutrients in cases of long-term coma, severe burns, and severe gastrointestinal or malabsorption syndromes; also called hyperalimentation.

Tourette's syndrome (too-rĕts′) N. *See* GILLES DE LA TOURETTE SYNDROME.

tourniquet (toor′nĭ-kĭt) N. device, such as a tight bandage or rubber tube, pressed on an artery to stop the flow of blood in a hemorrhage; used only when other measures cannot be used or have not succeeded.

tox-, toxi-, toxico-, toxo- comb. forms indicating an association with a poison or poisoning (e.g., toxicogenic, producing poisons).

toxemia (tŏk-sē′mē-ə) N. blood poisoning (septicemia) caused by bacterial toxins and characterized by systemic symptoms such as fever and vomiting.

toxemia of pregnancy N. abnormal condition of pregnancy characterized by high blood pressure, fluid retention and edema, and protein in the urine. The cause is unknown. Severe cases may lead to preeclampsia and eclampsia.

toxic (tŏk′sĭk) ADJ.
1. pert. to a poison.
2. pert. to a disease that is progressive.

toxic shock syndrome (TSS) N. serious acute infection caused by toxin elaborated by certain strains of *Staphylococcus aureus;* it occurs most often in menstruating women using high-absorbency tampons but also occasionally occurs in non-tampon-using women, men, and children. Onset is sudden with fever, achy joints and muscles, headache, reddish skin (a sunburnlike flushing that starts on the face and spreads to the torso), sore throat, and gastrointestinal disturbances, including watery diarrhea; dehydration, circulatory collapse, and renal and liver abnormalities may follow, leading to death.

toxicity n. extent or degree to which something is poisonous.

toxicology (tŏk′sĭ-kŏl′ə-jē) N. study of poisons and their effects on living organisms.

toxin (tŏk′sĭn) N. poison, esp. one produced or occurring in a plant or microorganism.

toxoid (tŏk′soid′) N. weakened toxin that, when introduced into the body, causes antibody formation and the development of immunity to the specific disease caused by the toxin.

toxoplasmosis (tŏk′sō-plăz-mō′sĭs) N. common infection with the parasite *Toxoplasma gondii,* transmitted to humans by contact with infected cats or their feces or litter boxes or by eating poorly cooked meat containing cysts of the parasites. The infection often produces only mild illness with few or minimal symptoms, such as malaise, low-grade fever, and swollen lymph glands. However, it is dangerous if contracted by a pregnant woman because it can cause serious damage to the fetus.

TPA abbrev. of tissue plasminogen activator.

TPN *See* TOTAL PARENTERAL NUTRITION.

trabecula (trə-bĕk′yə-lə) N., *pl.* trabeculae, mass of connective tissue that divides an organ into

parts (e.g., in the penis) or stabilizes and secures an organ, as with the spleen. ADJ. trabecular

trace element N. element necessary in minute quantities for nutrition and normal functioning (e.g., copper and molybdenum).

tracer (trā′sər) N. in radiology, radioactive isotope (e.g., iodine-131) introduced into the body to allow biological structures to be seen as part of diagnostic X-ray techniques.

trachea (trā′kē-ə) N. tube extending from the larynx to the bronchi that conveys air to the lungs. It is about 4 inches (11 centimeters) long, covered in the front by the isthmus of the thyroid gland, and in contact in the back with the esophagus. Also called windpipe. ADJ. tracheal

tracheitis (trā′kē-ī′tĭs) N. inflammation of the trachea, resulting from infection, irritation, or allergic reaction.

tracheo- comb. form indicating an association with the trachea (e.g., tracheobronchial, pert. to the trachea and the bronchi).

tracheobronchitis (trā′kē-ō-brŏn-kī′tĭs) N. common respiratory infection characterized by inflammation of both the trachea and the bronchi.

tracheostomy (trā′kē-ŏs′tə-mē) N. surgically created opening into the trachea, with a tube inserted to establish an airway when the pharynx is obstructed by tumor, edema, or other cause. Also called tracheotomy.

trachoma (trə-kō′mə) N. chronic infection of the eye, caused by *Chlamydia trachomatis,* common in many tropical areas, esp. where sanitation is limited;

in the United States it occurs primarily in the Southwest, esp. on American Indian reservations. Early inflammation, pus, and tearing may lead to scar formation, causing blindness. Treatment is by antibiotics.

tract (trăkt) N.
1. group of organs and tissues concerned with a common function or arranged serially (e.g., the digestive tract or the respiratory tract).
2. group of nerve fibers passing from one part of the central nervous system to another part.

traction (trăk′shən) N. in orthopedics, to place a bone or limb under tension to immobilize the part, align parts in a particular way, or relieve pressure.

traditional Chinese medicine *See* TABLE OF ALTERNATIVE MEDICINE TERMS.

tragus N., *pl.* tragi, projection of cartilage of the auricle.

trait (trāt) N. characteristic, esp. one that is inherited.

tramadol N. *See* TABLE OF COMMONLY PRESCRIBED DRUGS— GENERIC NAMES

trance (trăns) N. sleeplike state characterized by detachment from one's surroundings, as in deep concentration, or diminished motor activity, as in hypnosis or catalepsy.

Trandate N. trade name for the antihypertensive labetalol.

tranquilizer (trăng′kwə-līz′ər) N. drug that produces a calming effect, lessening anxiety and tension. Most tranquilizers induce drowsiness and can cause dependence.

major tranquilizer N. drug, usually a derivative of phenothiazine or butyrophenone, used to treat psychotic conditions in which a calming effect is desired.

minor tranquilizer N. any of several drugs, including diazepam (Valium) and chlordiazepoxide (Librium), used to relieve anxiety, tension, and irritability; many also reduce skeletal muscle spasm.

trans- comb. form meaning across, through (e.g., transabdominal, through the wall of the abdomen).

TRANSCRIPTION

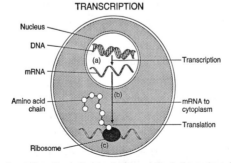

An overview of protein synthesis showing (a) transcription in the nucleus, (b) movement of mRNA to the cytoplasm, and (c) translation at the cellular ribosome.

transcendental meditation *See* TABLE OF ALTERNATIVE MEDICINE TERMS.

transcription (trăn-skrĭp′shən) N. in genetics, process by which the genetic information contained in DNA (deoxyribonucleic acid) in the nucleus is transferred to messenger RNA (ribonucleic acid), which then leaves the nucleus to direct protein synthesis in the ribosomes.

Transderm Scop N. trade name for the scopolamine patch.

transdermal (trăns-dûr′məl) ADJ. through the skin, referring to absorption of drugs that are either placed directly on the skin (such as creams and ointments) or applied in time-release forms, such as skin patches that gradually release small amounts of medication. Popular drugs available for transdermal administration include nitroglycerin, clonidine, estrogen, and scopolamine.

Transderm-Nitro N. trade name for a transdermal-patch form of nitroglycerin used in angina and congestive heart failure.

transducer (trăns-doo′sər) N. instrument that converts electrical energy into mechanical energy. Also acts as a transmitter and receiver of ultrasound information.

transduction *See* SIGNAL TRANSDUCTION.

transfer RNA (tRNA) (trăns′fər) N. that form of ribonucleic acid that attaches the correct amino acid to the protein chain being synthesized at the ribosome of a cell according to the coded directions of messenger RNA (transcribed from the genetic message of DNA in the nucleus).

transference (trăns-fûr′əns) N. in psychoanalysis, patient's assignment of qualities, emotions, and attitudes of a person significant in his/her early life, usually a parent, to the therapist; used as a means of understanding and dealing with emotional conflicts.

transferrin (trăns-fĕr′ĭn) N. blood protein that binds and transports iron.

transfusion (trăns-fyoo′zhən) N. introduction of whole blood or components of blood (e.g., plasma, platelets, or packed erythrocytes) from one person (the donor) or from pooled material into the bloodstream of another (the recipient). Donor and recipient blood must be typed to determine whether they are compatible. *See also* BLOOD TYPING.

transfusion reaction N. response by the body to the introduction of blood that is not compatible with its own. Signs of an adverse reaction range from fever, hive formation, and headache to severe asthmatic attacks, deep chest and back pain, difficulty in breathing, vascular collapse, renal failure, shock, and death.

transient global amnesia (trăn′shənt) N. temporary loss of memory that occurs in otherwise healthy persons. Memory for recent events is absent, but remote memory is retained. The spells are abrupt in onset and typically last several hours. The cause is unknown. Generally, no treatment is necessary.

transient ischemic attack (TIA) N. usually very brief episode in which there is insufficient blood supply to the brain, usually caused by atherosclerotic

TRANSLATION IN PROTEIN SYNTHESIS

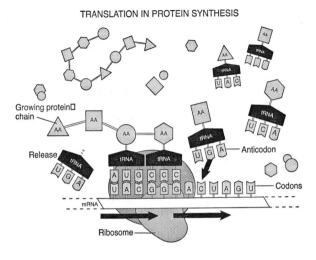

plaque or embolus. Symptoms depend on the site affected and the size of the blockage and may include dizziness, disturbance of vision, and numbness.

translation (trăns-lā′shən) N. process by which the genetic information carried in coded form by messenger RNA (after its transcription from deoxyribonucleic DNA in the nucleus) directs the formation of a specific protein at a ribosome in the cytoplasm.

translocation (trăns′lō-kā′shən) N. in genetics, the rearrangement of genetic material on a chromosome or the transfer of part of one chromosome to another chromosome. Translocations can result in serious congenital disorders.

transmission (trăns-mĭsh′ən) N. passing of information from one cell, tissue, or region of the body to another. Also may refer to passing of a disease from one person to another, such as the common cold.

transmural ADJ. involving the entire wall or thickness of a structure; a transmural myocardial infarction (heart attack) involves the entire wall of the affected portion of heart muscle (myocardium).

transplacental (trăns′plə-sĕn′tl) ADJ. passing across or through the placenta, as nutrients and wastes.

transplant (trăns-plănt′) V. to transfer an organ or tissue from one person (the donor) to another (the recipient) or from one body part to another to replace a diseased organ or to restore normal function. The organs most commonly transplanted are the skin and kidneys; corneal, bone, cartilage, and vessel transplants also occur, and, less commonly, heart and liver transplants. The major problem with donor-recipient transplants is the tendency of the recipient's body to reject the transplanted tissue as foreign; donor and recipient are carefully matched by blood-typing and tissue-typing procedures (the best donors are identical twins) to minimize the chances of rejection. N. any organ or tissue transferred from one person to another or from one part of the body to another part. N. transplantation

transport (trăns′pôrt′) N. movement of materials within the body, esp. across cell membranes. *See* ACTIVE TRANSPORT; PASSIVE TRANSPORT.

transposition (trăns′pə-zĭsh′ən) N.
1. abnormal placement of an organ or part so that it is on the side opposite its normal position.
2. in genetics, shifting of genetic material from one chromosome to another, often resulting in congenital defects.

transsexualism (trăns-sĕk′shoo-ə-lĭz′əm) N. condition in which a person assumes the psychological identity of the sex opposite to his or her biological gender. N., ADJ. transsexual

transudation (trăn′soo-dā′shən) N. passage of a liquid through a membrane, as into the intercellular space of a tissue or through a capillary wall.

transverse (trăns-vûrs′) ADJ. situated at right angle to the long axis of the body or organ.

transverse colon N. that part of the colon that extends across the midabdomen from the ascending colon on the right side to the beginning of the descending colon on the left side.

trapezium N. bone of the wrist.

trapezius (trə-pē′zē-əs) N. large, flat triangular muscle of the shoulder and upper back region involved in movement of the shoulder and arm.

trapezoid bone N. smallest of the wrist bones.

trauma (trô′mə) N.
1. physical injury caused by accident, violence, or disruptive action (e.g., a fracture).
2. severe emotional shock. ADJ. traumatic

traumatology (trou′mə-tŏl′ə-jē) N. that branch of medicine concerned with the surgical repair of wounds and injuries arising from accidents; accident surgery.

trazodone N. oral antidepressant (trade name Desyrel). Adverse effects include priapism, sleepiness, and double vision (diplopia). *See* TABLE OF COMMONLY PRESCRIBED DRUGS—GENERIC NAMES.

treadmill test N. an exercise device consisting of a moving platform, on which a patient walks while having his/her heart and breathing rates monitored; it is used to determine the effect of exertion on heart function.

treatment N. act of caring for a patient such as by medication or other therapy.

trefoil peptides N. proteins in the shape of a three-leafed clover that are acid-resistant; help prevent damage to the stomach lining by gastric acid (hydrochloric acid) secreted during digestion.

trematode (trĕm′ə-tōd′) N. parasitic flatworm, some of which cause disease in humans (e.g., schistosomiasis).

tremor (trĕm′ər) N. rhythmic, quivering movements from involuntary alternating contraction and relaxation of skeletal muscles; tremor may occur as a result of age (senile tremor) or disease (e.g., Parkinsonism, multiple sclerosis, and many degenerative diseases of the nervous system); some forms are hereditary.

trench mouth (trĕnch) N. infection of the mouth and gums marked by ulcers on the mucous membranes; it often occurs as a secondary infection in malnourished or debilitated people. Treatment depends on the cause, the primary illness, and the health of the person.

Trental N. trade name for pentoxifylline.

treponema (trĕp′ə-nē′mə) N. genus of spirochetes, some of which produce disease in humans (e.g., *Treponema pallidum,* the cause of syphillis).

tretinoin (trĕt′ĭ-noin′) N. *See* TABLE OF COMMONLY PRESCRIBED DRUGS—GENERIC NAMES.

TRF *See* THYROTROPIN-RELEASING FACTOR.

tri- prefix meaning three (e.g., trilaminar, having three layers).

triad N. set of three similar things considered as a unit.

triage N. classification process, used in military medicine, in disasters, and in hospital emergency departments, whereby the wounded, injured, or sick are sorted according to the severity of their injuries or illnesses and their need for immediate treatment, so that those most likely to survive with treatment will be given medical care first. In many systems, those awaiting treatment are grouped as follows:

those with life-threatening conditions who can be saved with immediate treatment; those with serious conditions that should be treated within 1 or 2 hours; and those with noncritical conditions for whom treatment can be delayed until more urgent cases are treated.

triamcinolone (trī′ăm-sĭn′ə-lōn′) N. synthetic corticosteroid used as an anti-inflammatory agent. Adverse effects include gastrointestinal and endocrine disturbances and, if used topically, skin rashes. *See* TABLE OF COMMONLY PRESCRIBED DRUGS—GENERIC NAMES.

triazolam (trī-ā′zə-lăm) N. sleeping pill (trade name Halcion), widely prescribed for insomnia. Side effects include lightheadedness, dizziness, and drowsiness.

tricarboxylic acid cycle (trī′kär-bŏk-sĭl′ĭk) *See* KREBS CYCLE.

triceps (trī′sĕps′) N. muscle having three heads, esp. the triceps brachii muscle of the back surface of the upper arm, which functions to extend the forearm and adduct the upper arm (*compare* BICEPS). *See* MAJOR MUSCLES OF THE BODY, in Appendix.

trichiasis (trī-kī′ə-sĭs) N. abnormal turning in of the eyelashes that causes irritation of the eye; it may result from inflammation of the eyelids.

trichinosis (trĭk′ə-nō′sĭs) N. infestation with the parasitic roundworm *Trichinella spiralis,* transmitted by eating undercooked meat, esp. pork. Symptoms vary greatly in severity and include nausea, diarrhea, abdominal pain, and fever, sometimes progressing to muscle pain, tenderness, and stiffness as the roundworm larvae migrate from the intestinal tract to the muscles, where they become encysted. There is no specific cure; treatment is aimed at alleviating symptoms. Once all the larvae become encysted completely, symptoms usually disappear. Also called myositis trichinosa.

tricho- comb. form indicating an association with hair (e.g. trichology, study of hair).

trichobezoar N. hair ball, sometimes formed in the alimentary canal.

trichomoniasis (trĭk′ə-mə-nī′ə-sĭs) N. infection of the vagina (occasionally the urethra in males) caused by the *Trichomonas vaginalis* protozoan and characterized by a foul-smelling, pale yellowish vaginal discharge, burning, and itching. Treatment is by the antimicrobial metronidazole, usually given orally.

trichuriasis (trĭk′yə-rī′ə-sĭs) N. infestation with the roundworm *Trichuris trichiura,* common in tropical areas, esp. those with poor sanitation. Symptoms include diarrhea, nausea, and abdominal pain.

tricuspid (trī-kŭs′pĭd) ADJ. having three cusps or points.

tricuspid valve N. heart valve with three cusps, situated between the right atrium and the right ventricle of the heart, where it allows the passage of blood from the atrium to the ventricle and closes to prevent backflow when the ventricle contracts; also called right atrioventricular valve.

trifocal glasses (trī-fō′kəl) N. eyeglasses containing three different types of lenses, each used for a separate purpose (e.g., near vision, far vision, and reading).

trigeminal nerve (trī-jĕm′ə-nəl) N. one of a pair of motor and sensory nerves, the fifth and largest cranial nerves; involved in facial sensibility, chewing, and other muscular actions of the face.

trigeminal neuralgia (trī-jĕm′ə-nəl noo-răl′jə) N. condition resulting from pressure on or degeneration of the trigeminal nerve, causing paroxysms of severe, stabbing pain radiating along a branch of the nerve, usually from the angle of the jaw; also called tic douloureux.

triglyceride (trī-glĭs′ə-rīd′) N. compound consisting of a fatty acid and glycerol that is the principal lipid in the blood, usually bound to a protein, forming a lipoprotein. The amount and the proportion of different types of triglycerides in the blood are important in the diagnosis of many diseases, including heart disease and diabetes mellitus.

trigone N. triangle-shaped space; often referring to the base of the urinary bladder between the openings of the ureters and the urethra.

triiodothyronine (T$_3$) (trī-ī′ə-dō-thī′rə-nēn′) N. one of two principal hormones secreted by the thyroid gland to regulate metabolism; the other is thyroxine, also known as T$_4$.

trimester (trī-měs′tər) N. one of the three periods, each of approximately 3 months, into which pregnancy is divided.
first trimester N. that part of pregnancy extending from the first day of the last menstrual period through 12 weeks of gestation.
second trimester N. that part of pregnancy extending from

the 13th through the 27th week of gestation.

third trimester N. that part of pregnancy extending from the 28th week until delivery.

trimethoprim/sulfamethoxasole N. *See* TABLE OF COMMONLY PRESCRIBED DRUGS—GENERIC NAMES.

trimipramine N. antidepressant (trade name Surmontil) used to treat depression, anxiety, and occasionally insomnia. Adverse effects include symptoms of Parkinsonism, rapid heartbeat, hypotension, and increased occular pressure.

Trimox N. *See* TABLE OF COMMONLY PRESCRIBED DRUGS—TRADE NAMES.

triplet (trĭp′lĭt) N. any of three offspring born at the same time from the same pregnancy.

triploid (trĭp′loid′) ADJ. pert. to an organism or cell that has three complete sets of chromosomes, not the normal two. In humans, triploid fetuses are usually spontaneously aborted or stillborn; in the few cases of live birth, they are grossly deformed and die quickly.

trismus (trĭz′məs) N. prolonged spasm of jaw muscles.

trisomy (trī-sō′mē) N. condition in which one more than the normal number of two chromosomes exists in a cell. This chromosomal aberration is associated with many congenital defects, the type and severity of the abnormal condition depending on which chromosome is affected. Trisomy 21, for example, is Down's syndrome.

Tri-Vi-Flor N. trade name for an oral, pediatric, fixed-combination drug, containing fluorine and vitamins A, C, and D.

tRNA *See* TRANSFER RNA.

trochanter (trō-kăn′tər) N. one of two bony projections (the greater trochanter and the lesser trochanter) on the proximal end of the femur that serve for the attachment of muscles.

troche (trō′kē) N. lozenge containing a drug.

trochlear nerve (trŏk′lē-ər) N. one of a pair of motor nerves, the fourth and smallest cranial nerve, essential for eye movement.

troglitazone N. *See* TABLE OF COMMONLY PRESCRIBED DRUGS—GENERIC NAMES.

trophoblast (trō′fə-blăst′) N. layer of tissue that forms the wall of the blastocyst in early development; aids in implantation in the uterine wall; and after implantation divides into two layers, one becoming the chorion, the other the outer layer of the placenta. ADJ. trophoblastic

trophoblastic cancer N. malignant neoplasm of the uterus derived from the epithelium of the chorion, often associated with hydatid mole, sometimes with normal or tubal pregnancy or abortion. Treatment is by hysterectomy and chemotherapy. *See* CHORIOCARCINOMA.

tropical medicine N. that branch of medicine concerned with the diagnosis and treatment of diseases, such as schistosomiasis, malaria, and yellow fever, found most commonly in tropical regions.

tropical sore *See* ORIENTAL SORE.

tropical sprue *See* SPRUE.

troponin (trōp′pə-nĭn) N. muscle fiber protein that normally inhibits muscle contraction. Following nerve stimulation, calcium binds to troponin, blocking its inhibitory effect; normal contraction then occurs. Troponin is often released following myocardial infarction (heart attack). Its presence in the blood may be helpful in early diagnosis and treatment. *See* SARCOMERE.

true dwarf (dwôrf) *See* PRIMORDIAL DWARF.

trunk N. body excluding the head and limbs; main stem of any lymphatic vessel, blood vessels, or nerve.

truss (trŭs) N. device to prevent protrusion of abdominal organs through a weakness in the abdominal wall.

truth serum *See* AMOBARBITAL.

trypanosomiasis (trĭ-păn′ə-sō-mī′ə-sĭs) N. infection with a parasite of the Trypanosoma genus. *See also* CHAGAS' DISEASE.

trypsin (trĭp′sĭn) N. enzyme involved in the digestion of proteins. The inactive form, trypsinogen, is secreted by the pancreas and converted to active trypsin in the duodenum.

tryptophan (trĭp′tə-făn′) N. amino acid essential for growth and normal metabolism. It is a precursor of niacin.

tsetse fly (tsĕ′tsē) N. insect that carries the parasites that cause trypanosomiasis.

TSH *See* THYROID-STIMULATING HORMONE.

TSS *See* TOXIC SHOCK SYNDROME.

tubal ligation (tōō′bəl lī-gā′shən) N. sterilization procedure in which both fallopian tubes are ligated (tied) in two places and the intervening space is removed or crushed so that the tube is effectively blocked and conception cannot occur. It is a common method of contraception.

tubal pregnancy N. type of ectopic pregnancy in which the conceptus implants in the fallopian tube; it is the most common type of ectopic pregnancy (about 90%), with prior injury to the tube and pelvic infection being predisposing factors. Symptoms, which occur as the embryo grows and ruptures the tube, include sudden, sharp pain on one side of the abdomen and bleeding, but diagnosis is often difficult. Treatment is removal of the products of conception and removal or repair of the ruptured tube.

tubercle (tōō′bər-kəl) N.
1. nodule (e.g., on a bone).
2. nodule caused by *Mycobacterium tuberculosis*.

tuberculin test (tōō-bûr′kyə-lĭn) N. test to determine past or present infection or exposure to tuberculosis, based on a skin reaction to injection, scratching, or puncturing of the skin with tuberculin, a purified protein derivative of the tuberculosis bacterium. Types of tuberculin tests include the Mantoux test and the tine test.

tuberculosis (tōō-bûr′kyə-lō′sĭs) N. chronic infection with bacterium *Mycobacterium tuberculosis,* transmitted by inhalation or ingestion of droplets; it usually affects the lungs but may also affect other organs. Early symptoms include fever, loss of appetite, fatigue, and vague chest pain; later, night sweats, difficulty in breathing, production of purulent sputum, and signs of severe lung involvement occur. Treatment is by antituberculosis drugs (e.g., isoniazid), rest, and proper nutrition. *See also* POTTS'S DISEASE.

tubule (tōo′byōol) N. small tube (e.g., the seminiferous tubules of the testis).

tularemia (tōo′lə-rē′mē-ə) N. infectious disease of animals, caused by *Pasturella tularensis,* transmitted to humans by insects or direct contact. Symptoms include headache, fever, ulcers on the skin, lymph node enlargement, gastrointestinal symptoms, or other manifestations. Treatment is by antibiotics; also called rabbit fever; yatobyo.

tumefaction (tōo′mə-făk′shən) N. process by which a tissue becomes swollen by accumulation of fluid within it.

tumescence (tōo-mĕs′əns) N. swelling, usually because of the presence of blood or other fluid in the tissue.

tumor (tōo′mər) N. growth of tissue characterized by uncontrolled cell proliferation. A tumor may be benign or malignant; localized or invasive. Also called neoplasm.

tunica (tōo′nĭ-kə) N. covering or layer of an organ.

tunica albuginea testes *See* ALBUGINEA.

tunnel vision N. condition in which peripheral sight is diminished and vision is limited to the area in front of the eyes.

turbidity N. state of being cloudy, as a solution. ADJ. turbid

turgid ADJ. swollen, hard, or full, usually as the result of fluid accumulation. N. turgor

Turner's syndrome (tûr′nərz) N. chromosomal abnormality in females in which there is only one X chromosome (instead of the normal two); it is characterized by dwarfism, cardiac abnormalities, underdeveloped reproductive organs, and often varying degrees of mental retardation or learning problems. Treatment is by hormone therapy and surgical correction of cardiovascular or skeletal abnormalities.

Twelve Step Program N. general term for program used by any of a number of fellowships (e.g., Alcoholics Anonymous, Overeaters Anonymous, Gamblers Anonymous) for self-development and mutual assistance; the program consists of twelve suggested steps, twelve traditions, a few slogans, nonsectarian prayers, books and pamphlets, and many meetings that members attend as often as they choose; typically, members are very supportive of each other and share compassion, understanding, care, and brotherly love; the various programs have helped close to one million people throughout the world.

twin N. either of two offspring born at the same time from the same pregnancy. Twins may result from a single fertilized ovum that divides early in development to form two separate embryos (monozygotic—identical twins) or from two ova fertilized at the same time (dizygotic—fraternal twins).

Tylenol #3 N. *See* TABLE OF COMMONLY PRESCRIBED DRUGS—TRADE NAMES.

tympanic membrane (tĭm-păn′ĭk) N. thin, semitransparent membrane that separates the outer ear from the middle ear. When sound waves enter the outer ear, they cause the membrane to vibrate; these vibrations are transmitted through the three ossicles (small bones) of the middle ear to the inner

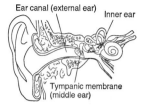

Ear canal (external ear)

Inner ear

Tympanic membrane
(middle ear)

ear and the main organ of hearing (the organ of Corti). Also called eardrum; myringa.

tympanoplasty (tĭm′pə-nə-plăs′tē) N. surgical correction or repair of injuries or defects in the tympanic membrane or bones of the middle ear to improve hearing.

typhoid fever (tī′foid′) N. serious, sometimes fatal infection with the bacterium *Salmonella typhi,* characterized by high fever, watery diarrhea, delirium, cough, rosy spots on the abdomen, and an enlarged spleen. Treatment is by antibacterials; typhoid vaccine provides short-term prevention.

typhus (tī′fəs) N. infection caused by Rickettsia organisms and characterized by headache, chills, fever, rash, and malaise.

tyramine N. amino acid. Persons taking monoamine oxidase inhibitors should avoid foods containing tyramine (e.g., chocolate, cola drinks, beer, some wines, some cheeses).

tyrosine (tī′rə-sēn′) N. amino acid found in most proteins, and a precursor of several hormones.

tyrosinemia (tī′rə-sĭ-nē′mē-ə) N. hereditary (autosomal recessive) defect in tyrosine metabolism caused by an enzyme lack and resulting in liver and kidney disturbances and mental retardation. Treatment is by a diet low in tyrosine and phenylalanine.

U

ulalgia N. pain in the gums.

ulcer (ŭl′sər) N. circumscribed lesion of the skin or mucous membrane of an organ formed by necrosis of tissue resulting from an infectious, malignant, or inflammatory process. Two types of ulcers are decubitus ulcers (bedsores) and peptic ulcers. Also known as ulceration. ADJ. ulcerative, ulcerous

ulcerative colitis (ŭl′sə-rā′tĭv kə-lī′tĭs) N. serious and chronic inflammatory disease of the large intestine and rectum characterized by recurrent episodes of abdominal pain, fever, chills, and profuse diarrhea, with stools containing pus, blood, and mucus. It affects children, often interfering with their normal growth, and young adults, often preventing many normal life activities. Treatment consists of anti-inflammatory agents, including corticosteroids; severe cases may require surgery with removal of parts of the intestinal tract. Complications include arthritis, kidney and liver disease, inflammation of other mucous membranes, and increased risk of developing cancer of the colon. (*Compare* CROHN'S DISEASE.)

ulcero- comb. form indicating an association with ulcers (e.g., ulcerogenic, causing ulcers to form).

ulemorrhagia N. bleeding of the gums.

ulitis N. inflammation of the gums.

ulna (ŭl′nə) N. larger of the two lower arm bones (the other being the radius) extending from the elbow, where it articulates with the humerus, to the wrist on the little finger side of the arm; also called elbow bone. ADJ. ulnar.

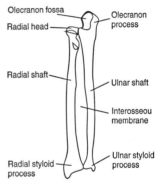

Olecranon fossa
Olecranon process
Radial head
Radial shaft
Ulnar shaft
Interosseou membrane
Ulnar styloid process
Radial styloid process

RADIUS AND ULNA

ulnar artery N. large artery that branches from the brachial artery and supplies muscles of the forearm, wrist, and hand. *See* MAJOR ARTERIES AND VEINS OF THE BODY, in Appendix.

ulnar nerve N. nerve, a branch of the brachial plexus, that supplies the skin and muscles of the little-finger side of the forearm and hand; it is the funny bone of the elbow.

ultracentrifuge N. high-speed centrifuge (machine to separate particles or media) with rotation fast enough to cause viruses to settle out, even in plasma; used in many forms of biochemical analysis to separate and measure proteins and viruses.

ultralente insulin N. generic name for long-acting (up to 36 hours) insulin preparation.

Ultram N. *See* TABLE OF COMMONLY PRESCRIBED DRUGS—TRADE NAMES.

ultrasonography (ŭl'trə-sə-nŏg'rə-fē) N. process by which the reflection of high-frequency sound waves is used to develop an image (sonogram) of a structure; used in medicine to study fetal growth and detect abnormalities, and to study the heart and many other organs.

ultrasound (ŭl'trə-sound') N. sound waves at very high frequencies used in the technique of ultrasonography to aid diagnosis.

ultraviolet radiation (ŭl'trə-vī'ə-lĭt rā'dē-ā'shən) N. invisible short-wavelength radiation; it is contained in sunlight, but much of it is absorbed by the atmosphere before reaching the earth, where it causes tanning and burning of the skin. Artificial sources of ultraviolet radiation (e.g., iron or mercury vapor arc in ultraviolet lamps) are sometimes used in medicine to treat rickets and certain skin disorders. Also called ultraviolet light.

umbilical cord (ŭm-bĭl'ĭ-kəl) N. flexible cordlike structure that connects the fetus to the placenta during pregnancy. It contains arteries that carry blood to the placenta and a vein that returns blood to the fetus and the remains of the yolk sac and allantois. In the newborn it is usually about 24 inches (60 centimeters) long. ADJ. umbilical

umbilical hernia N. protrusion of the intestine and omentum through a weakness in the abdominal wall near the umbilicus;

it often closes spontaneously after birth, but large hernias may require surgical closure.

umbilicus (ŭm-bĭl'ĭ-kəs) N. navel: the point on the abdomen where the umbilical cord is connected to the fetus; in adults it is marked by a depression or occasionally a small protrusion; also called, colloquially, belly button.

umbo (ŭm'bō) N. rounded projection; a knoblike center. ADJ. umbonate

unasyn N. parenteral antibiotic that is a fixed combination of ampicillin and sulbactam; used in moderate to severe infections. Adverse effects include diarrhea and rash.

unconditioned reflex (ŭn'kən-dĭsh'ənd) N. instinctive, unlearned response to a stimulus; also called instinctual response; instinctive reflex; inborn reflex (*compare* CONDITIONED REFLEX).

unconscious (ŭn-kŏn'shəs)
1. ADJ. unaware of one's surroundings; unable to respond to sensory stimuli.
2. N. in psychiatry, part of the mind where thoughts, ideas, and emotions are not subject to ready recall and are outside of awareness.

unconsciousness (ŭn-kŏn'shəs-nĭs) N. state of complete or partial unawareness of the surroundings and lack of response to sensory stimuli. It may be caused by many conditions, including shock; lack of respiratory efficiency; drugs or poisons; many metabolic disorders, including severe electrolyte imbalance; severe hypoglycemia; and kidney failure; as well as trauma, seizures, tumors, and other causes.

unction (ŭngk′shən) N. See OINT-MENT.

uncus N. hook-shaped structure, esp. that projecting from the lower surface of the cerebral hemispheres.

undescended testis (ŭn′dĭ-sĕn′ dĭd tĕs′tĭs) See CRYPTORCHID ISM.

undulant fever (ŭn′jə-lənt) See BRUCELLOSIS.

ungual (ŭng′gwəl) ADJ. pert. to the fingernails or toenails.

unguis (ŭng′gwĭs) N. fingernail or toenail. See also NAIL.

uni- prefix meaning one, single (e.g., unicellular, composed of a single cell).

unilateral (yoo′nə-lăt′ər-əl) ADJ. affecting only one side (e.g., unilateral paralysis, paralysis of only one side of the body).

union N. healing process; the growing together of the edges of a wound or broken bone.

unit N. defined quantity; division of quantity accepted as a standard; single undivided whole.

universal donor (yoo′nə-vûr′səl) N. person with type O, Rh-negative blood; this blood can be used with minimal risk for transfusion to people with types O, A, AB, and B blood.

universal precautions N. routine use of certain barrier devices (e.g., gloves, gowns, mask, eyeshields) to prevent the transmission of infectious disease.

unsaturated fatty acid (ŭn-săch′ ə-rā′tĭd) N. fatty acid in which some of the atoms are joined by double or triple valence bonds that are easily split, enabling other substances to join to them. Monounsaturated fatty acids, found in olive oil, chick-en, almonds, and some other nuts, have one double or triple bond per molecule. Polyunsaturated fatty acids, found in fish, corn, and soybean and safflower oil, have more than one double or triple bond per molecule. A diet high in polyunsaturated fatty acids and low in saturated fatty acids has been linked in some studies to low serum cholesterol levels (*compare* SATURATED FATTY ACIDS).

upper respiratory infection (rĕs′pər-ə-tôr′ē) See RESPIRATORY TRACT INFECTION.

upper respiratory tract See RESPIRATORY TRACT.

urachus N. in the fetus, canal connecting the bladder and the allantois; it remains in the adult as an umbilical ligament. ADJ. urachal

uracil (yoor′ə-sĭl) N. nitrogencontaining base found in ribonucleic acid (RNA).

uragogue N. agent that increases urinary flow.

urano- comb. form indicating an association with the roof of the mouth or the palate (e.g., uranoplasty, surgical correction of a defect in the palate).

urarthritis (yoor′är-thrī′tĭs) N. arthritis associated with gout.

uratemia (yoor′ə-tē′mē-ə) N. presence of uric acid salts in the blood, occurring in gout.

uraturia (yoor′ə-toor′ē-ə) N. presence of uric acid salts in the urine, esp. their presence in abnormally large amounts, as in gout.

urban typhus (tī′fəs) See MURINE TYPHUS.

urea (yoo-rē′ə) N.
1. main breakdown product of proteins and the form in which

nitrogen is excreted from the body in the urine.

2. diuretic preparation used to reduce cerebrospinal and intraocular fluid pressure.

uremia (yoŏ-rē′mē-ə) N. presence of excessive amounts of urea and other nitrogen-containing wastes in the blood; it occurs in kidney failure, producing symptoms of nausea, vomiting, and lethargy, and leading if uncorrected to death.

ureter (yoŏ-rē′tər) N. either of a pair of thick-walled tubes, about 12 inches (30 centimeters) long, that transport urine from the kidney to the urinary bladder. ADJ. uretal, ureteral, ureteric

ureter-, uretero- comb. forms indicating an association with the ureter (e.g., ureterectasis, bulging of the ureter).

ureteritis (yoŏ-rē′tə-rī′tĭs) N. inflammation of the ureter, caused by infection or the passage of a stone.

ureterocele (yoŏ-rē′tə-rō-sēl′) N. prolapse of the end portion of the ureter into the bladder; it may lead to obstructed urine flow and is usually treated by surgery.

ureterostenosis N. abnormal narrowing of the ureter.

urethra (yoŏ-rē′thrə) N. small tubular structure that drains urine from the bladder, passing it to the outside. In women it is very short, located behind the pubis between the clitoris and the vaginal opening; in men it is much longer, passing from the bladder through the prostate gland into the penis, and serving as the passageway for semen during ejaculation. ADJ. urethral

urethritis (yoŏr′ĭ-thrī′tĭs) N. inflammation of the urethra, usually with symptoms of painful urination. It is most commonly caused by bladder or kidney infection and is treated by antibacterials and pain relievers.

urethro- comb. form indicating an association with the urethra (e.g., urethrophraxis, obstruction of the urethra).

urethrocele (yoŏ-rē′thrə-sēl′) N. herniation or protrusion of the urethra into the vagina; it may be congenital or acquired, the result of pressure during pregnancy or childbirth, obesity, or poor muscle tone. Treatment depends on the size and location of the hernia and on whether or not it produces symptoms of incontinence and painful urination and coitus. Treatment is usually by surgery.

-uria suffix indicating a characteristic or constituent of urine (e.g., ammoniuria, presence of ammonia in the urine).

uric acid (yoŏr′ĭk) N. product of protein metabolism present in the blood and excreted in urine. Deposits of uric acid and its salts occur in gout.

uricaciduria N. greater than normal levels of uric acid in the urine, associated with gout or urinary system malfunction.

urinalysis (yoŏr′ə-năl′ĭ-sĭs) N. analysis of urine by physical, chemical, or microscopic means to reveal color, turbidity, pH, and the possible presence of microorganisms, blood, pus, or crystals, or abnormal levels of ketones, proteins, sugar, and other compounds. Urinalysis is an important aid in diagnosing urinary system disorders, metabolic disorders, and other conditions.

urinary bladder (yōͦor'ə-nĕr'ē) N. muscular sac in the pelvis that stores urine for discharge through the urethra. The urine is carried to the bladder through the ureters from the kidneys; also called bladder.

urinary calculus (kăl'kyə-ləs) N. stone formed in any part of the urinary system (kidney, ureter, bladder); some are small enough to pass in the urine, with or without pain; others must be removed surgically; also called kidney stone; renal calculus.

urinary frequency N. greater than normal frequency of the urge to void without an increase in the total daily volume of urine; it is associated with inflammation of the bladder or urethra or dysfunction in the bladder, and is often accompanied by burning and discomfort. Treatment depends on the cause.

urinary hesitancy (hĕz'ĭ-tən-sē) N. difficulty in beginning the flow of urine and decrease in the force of the urine stream. In men it is associated with prostate gland enlargement; in women with narrowing of the opening of the urethra or obstruction between the bladder and urethra; it may also be caused in either sex by emotional stress and other factors.

urinary incontinence (ĭn-kŏn'tə-nəns) N. inability to control the flow of urine and involuntary passage of urine from the body; it may be caused by central nervous system lesions, multiple sclerosis, neoplasm, trauma, aging, or other factors. Treatment depends on the cause.

urinary tract N. organs and tubes involved in the production and excretion of urine; it includes the kidneys, ureters, urinary bladder, and urethra.

urinary tract infection N. any infection of any of the organs of the urinary system; more common in women than in men and most often caused by bacteria. Symptoms include frequency, burning pain on urination, and sometimes blood or pus in the urine. Treatment is by antibacterials and pain-relievers. Types of urinary tract infections are cystitis, urethritis, and pyelonephritis.

urinary urgency N. sudden, compelling urge to urinate, accompanied by discomfort in the bladder. Sometimes called hyperactive bladder. If ignored, may produce urinary incontinence. Treatment depends upon the cause. *See also* URINARY INCONTINENCE.

urination (yōͦor'ə-nā'shən) N. act of passing urine through the urethral opening to outside the body.

urine (yōͦor'ĭn) N. fluid secreted by the kidneys, transported through the ureters to the bladder, where it is stored until excreted from the body through the urethra. Normal urine is straw-colored and slightly acid. Changes in the color, acidity, and other characteristics of urine are important clues to many diseases. ADJ. urinary

uro-, urono- comb. forms indicating an association with urine or the urinary tract (e.g., urolith, a urinary stone).

urobilin (yōͦor'ō-bī'lĭn) N. brown pigment found in feces and sometimes in small amounts in urine.

urobilinogen (yŏor′ō-bī-lĭn′ə-jən) N. compound formed in the intestine from the breakdown of bilirubin; some is excreted in the feces, some resorbed and excreted in bile or urine.

urocele (yŏor′ə-sēl′) N. swelling of the scrotum from the urine that has entered the tissues.

urochesia (yŏor′ə-kē′zē-ə) N. discharge of urine from the rectum.

urodynia (yŏor′ə-dĭn′ē-ə) N. pain during urination.

urogenital (yŏor′ō-jĕn′ĭ-tl) ADJ. pert. to the urinary and reproductive systems.

urokinase (yŏor′ō-kī′nās) N. enzyme produced in the kidney that activates fibrinolysis. A urokinase preparation is used in the treatment of pulmonary embolism and some myocardial infarctions to dissolve blood clots.

urologist N. physician who specializes in urology.

urology (yŏo-rŏl′ə-jē) N. that branch of medicine concerned with the anatomy, physiology, disorders, and treatment of the urinary tract in both men and women and of the reproductive tract in men.

uropathy (yŏo-rŏp′ə-thē) N. any disease of the urinary tract.

urticaria (ûr′tĭ-kâr′ē-ə) N. itchy skin eruption characterized by well-defined, red-margined, pale-centered transient wheals; it is usually the result of an allergic reaction to drugs, food, or insect bites, but in some cases, esp. chronic ones, the cause cannot be identified. Treatment is by avoidance of the offending agent, and, when an eruption occurs, antihistamines; also called hives. ADJ. urticarial

utero- comb. form indicating association with the uterus (e.g., uteroabdominal, pert. to the uterus and the abdomen).

uterus (yŏo′tər-əs) N. that part of the female reproductive system specialized to allow the implantation, growth, and nourishment of a fetus during pregnancy. The nonpregnant uterus is a hollow, pear-shaped organ, about 3 inches (7.5 centimeters) long, suspended in the pelvic

FEMALE REPRODUCTIVE SYSTEM

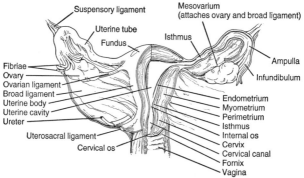

cavity by ligaments. Its upper end is connected to the fallopian tubes, its lower end narrows into a neck, or cervix, that opens into the vagina. The uterus has an inner mucus layer, the endometrium, which undergoes cyclic changes during the menstrual cycle and helps form the placenta in pregnancy; a muscular layer, the myometrium, contractions of which expel the fetus during labor and childbirth; and an outer connective tissue, the parametrium, that extends into the broad ligament. Also called womb. ADJ. uterine.

utricle (yoo′trĭ-kəl) N. larger of two pouches in the membranous labyrinth of the ear; it functions in the maintenance of balance. ADJ. utricular

uvea (yoo′vē-ə) N. layer of the eye containing the iris, ciliary body, and choroid. ADJ. uveal

uveitis (yoo′vē-ī′tĭs) N. inflammation of the uvea, characterized by irregularly shaped pupil, tearing, pain, pus discharge, and opaqueness. Infection, allergic response, or trauma may cause it, or it may occur as a complication of certain diseases (e.g., diabetes mellitus). Treatment depends on the cause.

uvula (yoo′vyə-lə) N. small, fleshy mass hanging from the soft palate in the mouth.

uvulitis (yoo′vyə-lī′tĭs) N. inflammation of the uvula usually caused by allergic reaction or infection.

V

vaccination (văk′sə-nā′shən) N. introduction of attenuated (weakened) or killed viruses or microorganisms (or occasionally of substances extracted from these agents) into the body to induce immunity by causing the production of specific antibodies. Vaccination has eradicated smallpox throughout the world; has decreased the incidence of poliomyelitis and diphtheria to very low levels in North America and Europe, and is also available against other diseases, including measles and mumps. V. vaccinate

vaccine (văk-sēn′) N. preparation of attenuated (weakened) or killed disease-producing viruses or microorganisms (or of substances extracted from them) administered by mouth or by injection to induce active immunity to the specific disease (*compare* ANTISERUM).

vaccinia (văk-sĭn′ē-ə) *See* COWPOX.

vacuole (văk′yōō-ōl′) N. small space in a cell, esp. one containing material taken in by the cell. ADJ. vacuolar

vacuum aspiration (văk′yōō-əm ăs′pə-rā′shən) N. method of induced abortion in which the embryo and placenta are removed by suction applied to the dilated cervix. It is performed only in early pregnancy, up to about the 14th week of gestation. Also called suction curettage.

vagal (vā′gəl) ADJ. pert. to the vagus nerve.

vagina (və-jī′nə) N. muscular tube lined with mucous membrane that forms the lower part of the female reproductive tract, situated behind the bladder and in front of the rectum and extending from the vaginal opening to the cervix of the uterus. It receives the penis during coitus, ejaculation of semen usually occurring in the upper vagina, from where the sperm move upward to fertilize an ovum. The vagina is normally sufficiently elastic to allow the passage of a fetus. ADJ. vaginal

vaginal birth after Cesarean (VBAC) N. delivery of an infant through the birth canal (vagina) for women who had previously given birth by Cesarean section. Once viewed as a sometimes safer option than a planned Cesarean section, the benefits of VBAC are being questioned by some experts in the field of maternal and child health. VBACs were dealt a serious blow when research showed that some women (fewer than 1%) who attempted to have a VBAC suffered uterine ruptures. In 1999 the American College of Obstetricians and Gynecologists (ACOG) altered its recommended guidelines regarding the procedure, recommending that only hospitals with an immediately available surgical team allow VBACs. *See also* CESAREAN SECTION.

vaginal cancer (văj′ə-nəl) N. malignancy of the vagina; it most often results from the spread of cancer from another organ, esp. the uterus or ovaries, but may occur as a primary neoplasm, esp. in women exposed while in the uterus to diethylstilbestrol (given to their mothers to prevent spontaneous abortion). Treatment depends on the size and location of the lesion and the age and health of the woman; it may include removal of the vagina, hysterectomy, and/or irradiation.

vaginal discharge N. discharge made up mostly of secretions from cervical glands from the vagina. A clear or whitish discharge is normal, varying in amount and consistency from woman to woman and in each woman during different phases of the menstrual cycle or pregnancy. Inflammation of the vagina and cervix often causes the discharge to change in amount, color, and odor.

vaginismus (văj′ə-nĭz′məs) N. contraction of the muscles around the vagina, causing its opening to close; it usually occurs as a fear or anxiety reaction before coitus or pelvic examination; but may also be caused by injury or dryness of the vagina or inflammation of the vagina or bladder.

vaginitis (văj′ə-nī′tĭs) N. inflammation of the vagina, often producing pain, itchiness, burning on urination, and increased, sometimes foul-smelling, discharge. It may be caused by infection (e.g., candidiasis), poor hygiene, dietary deficiency, or local irritation (e.g., from a contraceptive). Treatment depends on the cause.

vagino- comb. form indicating an association with the vagina (e.g., vaginoperineal, pert. to the vagina and perineum).

vago- comb. form indicating an association with the vagus nerve (e.g., vagoglossopharyngeal, pert. to both the vagus and glossopharyngeal nerves).

vagotomy (vā-gŏt′ə-mē) N. cutting of branches of the vagus nerve, usually performed with stomach surgery, to reduce the secretion of gastric juice and thus lessen the chances of ulcer recurrence.

vagus nerve (vā′gəs) N., *pl.* vagi, one of a pair of motor and sensory nerves, the tenth and longest cranial nerves, functioning in swallowing, speech, breathing, heart rate, and many other body functions. ADJ. vagal

valence (vā′ləns) N. relative capacity of atoms to combine electrically with others; in immunology, refers to the capacity to unite with or react to various antigens or biological substrates.

valgus ADJ. pert. to a deformity in which part of a limb is turned outward or twisted away from the center of the body (e.g., talipes valgus, a deformity in which the foot is twisted outward).

valine (văl′ēn′) N. amino acid needed for growth in children and nitrogen balance in adults.

Valium (văl′ē-əm) N. trade name for the tranquilizer diazepam. *See* TABLE OF COMMONLY PRESCRIBED DRUGS—TRADE NAMES.

vallecula N. groove or depression on the surface of an organ.

valley fever *See* coccidioidomycosis.

varix (văr′ĭks) N., *pl.* varices, enlarged and twisted (tortuous) blood vessels or lymph vessel.

vas deferens (văs′ dĕf′ər-ənz) N. either of a pair of ducts that is the extension of the epididymis of the testis, ascending into the abdominal cavity, where it passes over the bladder and joins the seminal vesicle.

vascular (văs′kyə-lər) ADJ.
1. pert. to a blood vessel.
2. consisting of or supplied with, blood vessels.

vascularization (văs′kyə-lər-ĭ-zā′shən) N. process by which body tissue becomes vascular and develops capillaries.

vasculitis (văs′kyə-lī′tĭs) N. inflammation of a blood vessel, caused by allergic reaction or certain systemic disease.

vasectomy (və-sĕk′tə-mē) N. a surgical procedure to render a male sterile by severing the vas deferens so that sperm cannot pass from the epididymis to the ejaculatory duct. Potency is not affected. The operation is sometimes reversible. *See also* VASO-VASOSTOMY.

vaso- comb. form indicating an association with a vessel or duct (e.g., vasoconstriction, narrowing of the opening of a blood vessels).

vasoconstriction (vā′zō-kən-strĭk′shən) N. decrease in the diameter of the blood vessels which may occur for many reasons, both normal and abnormal.

vasoconstrictor (vā′zō-kən-strĭk′tər) N. agent that causes a narrowing of the opening of a blood vessel. Cold, stress, nicotine, epinephrine, norephinephrine, angiotensin, vasopressin, and certain drugs are vasoconstrictors, maintaining or increasing blood pressure.

vasodilation (vā′zō-dī-lā′shən) N. widening of blood vessels, esp. arteries, usually due to certain nerve impulses or drugs that relax the musculature of the arteries.

vasodilator N. agent that dilates or widens blood vessels. Some vasodilators, including nitroglycerine and hydralazine, are used in the treatment of certain heart ailments.

vasomotor (vā′zō-mō′tər) ADJ. pert. to the nerves and muscles that control the diameter of blood vessels.

vasopressin (vā′zō-prĕs′ĭn) *See* ANTIDIURETIC HORMONE.

vasopressor N. agent that causes vasoconstriction and therefore an increase in blood pressure.

Vasotec N. trade name for the antihypertensive enalapril. *See* TABLE OF COMMONLY PRESCRIBED DRUGS—TRADE NAMES.

vasovasostomy (vā′zō-vā-zŏs′tə-mē) N. surgical procedure that attempts to restore the function of the vas deferens on either or both sides after the vas has been severed in a vasectomy. In many cases the function of the vas deferens is restored but fertility does not result, usually because antibodies that interfere with sperm production developed after the earlier vasectomy.

vasovesiculitis N. inflammation of the vas deferens and seminal vesicles, usually occurring with prostatitis and causing pain in the scrotum and groin and fever. Treatment is by antibiotics.

vastus (văs′təs) N. any of three muscles that form part of the quadriceps muscle of the thigh. *See* MAJOR MUSCLES OF THE BODY, Appendix.

VD *See* VENEREAL DISEASE.

vector (věk′tər) N. person, animal, or microorganism that carries and transmits disease. Mosquitoes, for example, are vectors of malaria and yellow fever, carrying disease-producing parasites. (*Compare* CARRIER.)

Veetids N. *See* TABLE OF COMMONLY PRESCRIBED DRUGS—TRADE NAMES.

vegetarian (věj′ĭ-târ′ē-ən) N. person who restricts his/her diet to foods of vegetable origin, including fruits, grains, and nuts.

vegetative (věj′ĭ-tā′tĭv) ADJ. pert. to growth and nutrition, as opposed to reproduction (propagative).

vehicle (vē′ĭ-kəl) N. inert agent that carries the active ingredients of a medication.

vein (vān) N. any of many vessels that carry blood to the heart; it may be part of the pulmonary venous system, portal system, or (most veins) the systemic venous system. All veins except the pulmonary vein carry deoxygenated blood from the tissues of the body to the vena cava and heart. The walls of veins are thinner and less elastic than the walls of arteries and contain valves that maintain the flow of blood toward the heart. (*Compare* ARTERY.) ADJ. venous

vena cava (vē′nə kā′və) N. either of two large veins returning deoxygenated blood from the peripheral circulation to the right atrium of the heart.

VENOUS VALVES

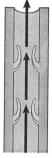 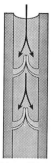

Valves Open   Valves Closed

inferior vena cava N. the large vein, formed by the union of the two iliac veins, that receives blood from parts of the body below the diaphragm and transports it to the heart.

superior vena cava N. the large vein that draws blood from the head, neck, chest, and arms and transports it to the heart.

venereal (və-nēr′ē-əl) ADJ. pert. to or caused by sexual intercourse or genital contact, as a venereal disease. *See* SEXUALLY TRANSMITTED DISEASE.

venereal disease (VD) N. colloq. for sexually transmitted disease.

venesection (věn′ĭ-sěk′shən) *See* PHLEBOTOMY.

venipuncture (vē′nĭ-pŭngk′chər) N. procedure in which a vein is punctured through the skin to withdraw blood for analysis, to start an intravenous drip, to instill medication, or to inject a radiopaque dye for a radiographic examination of a part of the body.

venlafaxine N. *See* TABLE OF COMMONLY PRESCRIBED DRUGS—GENERIC NAMES.

veno- comb. form indicating an association with a vein (e.g., venopressor, substance that causes veins to narrow).

venogram (vē′nə-grăm′) N. X-ray film of veins injected with a radiopaque contrast medium.

venography (vĭ-nŏg′rə-fē) N. technique of preparing X-ray images of a vein injected with a radiopaque contrast medium.

venom (vĕn′əm) N. toxic fluid secreted by some snakes and other animals and transmitted in their bites or stings. Some venoms produce local irritation and swelling at the site of the bite or sting; other venoms produce systemic, sometimes fatal, effects usually focused on the circulatory or nervous system.

venous blood (vē′nəs) N. blood found in the veins. Except in the pulmonary vein, venous blood is poor in oxygen and rich in carbon dioxide, which is carried to the right side of the heart for transport to the lungs, where it is given off. (The pulmonary vein carries freshly oxygenated blood from the lungs to the left atrium of the heart.)

venous blood gases N. oxygen and carbon dioxide levels in venous blood.

venous pressure N. stress exerted by the circulating blood on the walls of the veins. *See also* BLOOD PRESSURE.

venous sinus (vē′nəs sī′nəs) N. any of several sinuses that collect blood from the dura mater covering the brain and drain it into the internal jugular veins.

venous thrombosis (vē′nəs thrŏm-bō′sĭs) N. presence of a blood clot in a vein in which the wall of the vein is not inflamed. Pain and swelling may occur.

venter (vĕn′tər) N., *pl.* ventres, bellylike part, as the bulging part of a muscle.

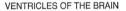

VENTRICLES OF THE BRAIN

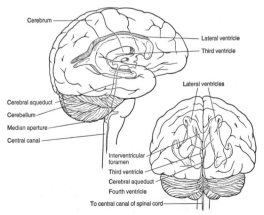

Cerebrum
Lateral ventricle
Third ventricle
Cerebral aqueduct
Cerebellum
Median aperture
Central canal
Lateral ventricles
Interventricular foramen
Third ventricle
Cerebral aqueduct
Fourth ventricle
To central canal of spinal cord

ventilation (vĕn′tl-ā′shən) N. breathing; the process by which gases are moved into and out of the lungs. v. ventilate

ventilator N. mechanical device, used in respiratory failure from many causes, that provides artificial respiration for the patient, usually via an endotracheal tube; also called, colloquially, breathing machine.

Ventolin (vĕn′tl-ĭn) N. trade name for the bronchodilator albuterol. *See* TABLE OF COMMONLY PRESCRIBED DRUGS—TRADE NAMES.

ventral (vĕn′trəl) ADJ. pert. to or toward the front side of the body (*compare* DORSAL).

ventricle (vĕn′trĭ-kəl) N.
1. either of the two lower chambers of the heart. The left ventricle receives oxygenated blood from the pulmonary vein through the left atrium and pumps it to the aorta, from which it is sent throughout the body. The thinner-walled right ventricle receives deoxygenated blood from the venae cavae through the right atrium and pumps it through the pulmonary artery to the lung for the exchange of gases.
2. any of four fluid-filled cavities in the brain containing cerebrospinal fluid. ADJ. ventricular.

ventricular aneurysm (vĕn-trĭk′yə-lər ăn′yə-rĭz′əm) N. localized dilation or saccular protrusion on the wall of the left ventricle of the heart occurring after a myocardial infarction.

ventricular fibrillation (vĕn-trĭk′yə-lər fĭb′rə-lā′shən) N. serious disturbance in cardiac rhythm, characterized by disorganized impulse conduction and ventricular contraction. Unconsciousness occurs and death may follow within minutes if defibrillation and other life-saving measures are not immediately provided.

ventricular septal defect (vĕn-trĭk′yə-lər) N. common congenital heart defect, characterized by an abnormal opening in the septum dividing the ventricles, which allows blood to pass from the left to the right ventricle. Small openings may cause no symptoms and may heal spontaneously during childhood. Larger openings may cause symptoms of congestive heart failure and usually require surgical repair of the defect. An acute ventricular septal defect can occur as a complication of myocardial infarction.

ventricular tachycardia (vĕn-trĭk′yə-lər tăk′ĭ-kär′dē-ə) N. cardiac arrhythmia resulting in a heart rate greater than 150 beats per minute; often, the heart is unable to pump blood effectively, and the patient may develop cardiac arrest; the treatment of life-threatening ventricular tachycardia is defibrillation.

ventriculo- comb. form indicating an association with a ventricle of the heart or brain (e.g., ventriculoatrial shunt, surgically created passageway with plastic tubing leading from the ventricle of the brain to the right atrium of the heart to drain excess fluid from the brain in cases of hydrocephalus).

venule (vĕn′yo̅o̅l) N. small vein, esp. one that extends from a capillary network and merges to form a vein.

verapamil N. oral/parenteral calcium channel blocker (trade names Isoptin and Calan) used in the treatment of hypertension, congestive heart failure, angina,

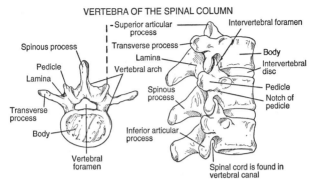

VERTEBRA OF THE SPINAL COLUMN

Superior articular process

Intervertebral foramen

Spinous process

Transverse process

Lamina

Body

Pedicle

Vertebral arch

Intervertebral disc

Lamina

Spinous process

Pedicle

Transverse process

Notch of pedicle

Body

Inferior articular process

Vertebral foramen

Spinal cord is found in vertebral canal

arrythmia, and migraine. Adverse effects include nausea, bradycardia, and hypotension with the intravenous form. *See* TABLE OF COMMONLY PRESCRIBED DRUGS—GENERIC NAMES.

Verelan N. trade name for a once-a-day, long-acting preparation of verapamil; used to treat hypertension.

vermicide N. agent that kills worms, esp. those in the intestines.

vermiform appendix (vûr′mə-fôrm′) *See* APPENDIX.

vermifuge N. agent that causes the evacuation of worms.

vernix caseosa (vûr′nĭks kā′sē-ō′sə) N. cheese-like substance that covers the skin of a fetus and newborn, serving as a protective cover.

verruca (və-roo′kə) *See* WART.

Versed N. trade name for midazolam.

version (vûr′zhən) N. changing the position of a fetus in the uterus, usually done to aid delivery.

vertebra (vûr′tə-brə) N., *pl.* vertebrae, any of the 33 bones of the spinal column (vertebral

column, or backbone), including 7 cervical (neck region), 12 thoracic (chest region), 5 lumbar, 5 sacral (fused), and 4 coccygeal (fused). Except for the first two—the atlas and axis—each vertebra consists of a centrum, or body, a neural arch enclosing a cavity through which the spinal cord passes, and processes for the attachment of muscles. The vertebrae are connected by ligaments and separated by intervertebral discs, which cushion adjacent vertebrae. ADJ. vertebral.

vertebral column (vûr′tə-brəl) N. firm, flexible, bony column that is the longitudinal axis and chief supporting structure of the human body, extending from the base of the skull to the coccyx. It consists of 26 separate bony parts: 7 cervical vertebrae, 12 thoracic vertebrae, 5 lumbar vertebrae, a sacrum (composed of 5 fused sacral vertebrae), and a coccyx (composed of 4 fused coccygeal vertebrae). Intervertebral discs separate the vertebrae, which serve for the attachment of muscles. The vertebral column normally has several curves, most visible from a lateral view: a cervical curve, convex ven-

VERTEBRAL COLUMN

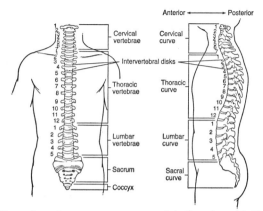

trally; a thoracic curves, concave ventrally; a lumbar curve, convex ventrally; and a pelvic curve, concave ventrally. Also called rachis; spinal column; spine.

vertebro- comb. form indicating an association with the vertebral column or a vertebra (e.g., vertebrocostal, pert. to a vertebra and a rib).

vertigo (vûr′tĭ-gō′) N. sensation that one's surroundings are spinning about; *compare* DIZZINESS.

vesical ADJ. pert. to the bladder, esp. the urinary bladder.

vesicant N. agent (e.g., a drug) that causes blistering of the skin.

vesicle (vĕs′ĭ-kəl) N.
1. blister; small thin-walled skin lesion containing fluid.
2. small, saclike part (e.g., seminal vesicle, which stores semen). ADJ. vesicular

vesico- comb. form indicating an association with the urinary bladder (e.g., vesicovaginal,

pert. to the urinary bladder and vagina).

vesicocele (vĕs′ĭ-kō-sēl′) N. bulging of the bladder into another part.

vesicourethral reflux N. abnormal backflow of urine from the bladder to the ureters, caused by congenital defect, obstruction of the bladder outlet, or urinary tract infection. Treatment depends on the cause.

vesiculitis (vĕ-sĭk′yə-lī′tĭs) N. inflammation of the seminal vesicle, usually occurring with prostatitis.

vessel (vĕs′əl) N. tubelike structure that carries fluids throughout the body. Major body vessels are arteries, veins, and lymph vessels.

vestibular gland (vĕ-stĭb′yə-lər) N. either of two pairs of glands at the vagina-vulva junction, the secretions of which lubricate the vagina during coitus. The posterior pair is also called Bartholin's glands.

vestibule (vĕs′tə-byōōl′) N. space at the entrance to a hollow organ or passageway (e.g., vestibule of the aorta, that part of the left ventricle where the aorta channels off). ADJ. vestibular

vestibulocochlear nerve (vĕ-stĭb′yə-lō-kŏk′lē-ər) *See* AUDITORY NERVE.

vestigial (vĕ-stĭj′ē-əl) ADJ. existing in a rudimentary form; pert. to a relatively useless organ that had a function in an earlier stage or a more primitive form of life, as the vermiform appendix in humans.

viable (vī′ə-bəl) ADJ. capable of surviving.

Viagra N. *See* TABLE OF COMMONLY PRESCRIBED DRUGS—TRADE NAMES.

Vibramycin N. trade name for the tetracycline antibiotic doxycycline.

vibrio (vĭb′rē-ō) N. genus of comma-shaped bacteria, some members of which produce disease in humans (e.g., *Vibrio cholerae*, the agent that causes cholera).

vibrissa N., *pl.* vibrissae, a stiff coarse hair, esp. that in the front part of the nostrils that helps filter inhaled air.

vicarious (vī-kâr′ē-əs) ADJ. in medicine, pert. to an action performed by an organ or part of the body not normally involved in that function (e.g., vicarious menstruation, a rare disorder in which monthly bleeding occurs from places other than the vagina, such as the nostrils or sweat glands).

Vicodin N. trade name for fixed combination of hydrocodone

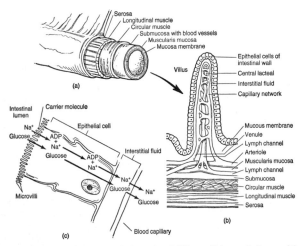

Structure of the small intestine and absorption. (a) The multiple muscle layers of the intestinal wall, (b) a single villus expanded to show its structure, and (c) absorption of sodium ions and glucose molecules.

and acetaminophen. *See* TABLE OF COMMONLY PRESCRIBED DRUGS—TRADE NAMES.

villus (vĭl′əs) N., *pl.* villi, one of many tiny projections, containing capillaries and a lacteal, occurring over the mucous membrane of the small intestine that function in the absorption of nutrients and fluids. ADJ. villous.

vinblastine (vĭn-blăs′tēn′) N. antineoplastic (trade name Velban) that disrupts cell division and is used to treat many cancers, esp. those of the lymphatic system. Adverse effects include a decrease in the number of white blood cells, nausea, vomiting, and hair loss.

Vincent's angina (vĭn′sənts ăn-jī′nə) *See* TRENCH MOUTH.

vincristine (vĭn-krĭs′tēn′) N. antineoplastic (trade name Oncovin) that disrupts cell division and is used to treat many cancers, esp. those of the lymphatic system. Adverse effects include a decrease in the number of white blood cells, nausea, vomiting, and hair loss.

viral (vī′rəl) ADJ. pert. to a virus.

viral hepatitis (hĕp′ə-tī′tĭs) N. form of hepatitis, inflammation of the liver, caused by one of the hepatitis viruses. Symptoms include anorexia (lack of appetite), headache, fever, pain in the region of the liver, malaise, jaundice, and diarrhea with clay-colored stools. Treatment includes rest, the avoidance of fatigue, and a low-fat, high-protein diet; the person is usually advised to abstain from alcohol for a year after the attack. Severe infection, esp. with hepatitis B, can cause permanent damage to liver tissue

and result in hepatic coma and death.

viral infection (ĭn-fĕk′shən) N. any disease caused by a virus pathogenic to humans. Some viral infections are serious diseases; others are mild, sometimes occurring with few or unnoticed symptoms. Among the common viral infections are measles, mumps, chicken pox, and some types of hepatitis and pneumonia.

viral load N. amount of virus present in a person's blood; usually measured by the polymerase chain reaction (PCR) method; measures severity of a viral infection. The result is given in number of virus particles per milliliter of blood. Currently, routine testing is available for HIV-1, cytomegalovirus, hepatitis B virus, and hepatitis C virus. Determination of viral load is part of the therapy monitoring during chronic viral infections and in immunocompromised patients (e.g., after bone marrow or solid organ transplantation). *See also* POLYMERASE CHAIN REACTION.

viral pneumonia (noo-mōn′yə) N. infection of the lung or lungs caused by a virus. *See also* PNEUMONIA.

viremia (vī-rē′mē-ə) N. presence of virus particles in the blood.

virilization (vĕr′ə-lĭ-zā′shən) N. production of secondary male sex characteristics (e.g., deeper voice, increased facial and body hair, greater muscle bulk) in a female, usually the result of adrenal malfunction or the intake of certain drugs, esp. hormones. *See also* MASCULINIZATION.

virion (vĭ′rē-ŏn′) N. virus particle, consisting of a protein coat called a capsid, and a nucleic acid core.

viroid N. tiny particle known to cause some plant diseases and suspected of causing some human diseases. It is much smaller than a virus and consists of a short ribonucleic acid (RNA) chain and no protective protein coat.

virologist N. specialist in virology.

virology (vī-rŏl′ə-jē) N. study of viruses, their growth, development, and relationship to diseases.

virulence (vĕr′yə-ləns) N. ability or power of a microorganism to produce disease. ADJ. virulent

virus (vī′rəs) N. small particle that is not living, does not exhibit signs of life, but can reproduce itself within a living cell. A virus particle is called a virion; it consists of a nucleic acid (DNA or RNA) core and a protein coat, called a capsid. A virus reproduces by infecting a host cell and taking over the nucleic acid of that host cell, making more virus nucleic acid and protein. As new virus particles develop, the host cell bursts, releasing the new virus particles. Viruses are responsible for many human diseases. *See also* VIRAL INFECTION.

viscera (vĭs′ər-ə) N. main internal organs within body cavities, esp. those in the abdominal cavity (e.g., the spleen and stomach). *sing.* viscus, ADJ. visceral

viscero- comb. form indicating an association with the internal organs (e.g., visceroperitoneal, pert. to the peritoneum and the internal organs of the abdominal cavity).

viscid (vĭs′ĭd) N., ADJ. sticky; gluelike.

viscous (vĭs′kəs) ADJ. adhesive-like; having a relatively high resistance to flow.

viscus N., *pl.* viscera, main internal organ.

vision (vĭzh′ən) N. ability to see; perception of things through the action of light on the eyes and optic centers in the brain. ADJ. visual

Visken N. trade name for the beta blocker pindolol.

Vistaril N. trade name for the tranquilizer hydroxyzine.

visual acuity (vĭzh′o͞o-əl ə-kyo͞o′ĭ-tē) N. sharpness of vision, most often determined by use of the Snellen chart.

visual field N. area in front of the eye, in which an object can be seen without moving the eye.

visual purple N. rhodopsin, the pigment in the cones of the retina.

vital (vīt′l) ADJ.
1. pert. to life or the living stage.
2. essential to maintaining life.

vital capacity (vīt′l kə-păs′ĭ-tē) N. maximum amount of air that

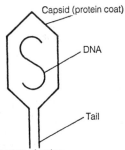

Capsid (protein coat)

DNA

Tail

Structure of a virus.

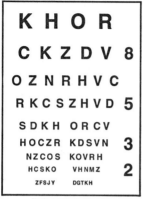

Typical eye chart used to measure visual acuity.

VISUAL PATHWAYS AND THE OPTIC CHIASMA

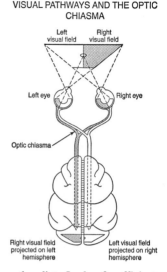

can be exhaled after a maximum inhalation, used in determining the status of lung tissue. One of several lung function tests collectively called pulmonary function tests or spirometry.

vital signs N. signs that show the overall health of a person, changes in which are often clues to disease or signs of alteration in a person's health. The vital signs are usually considered to be pulse rate, respiration rate, body temperature, and blood pressure.

vital statistics N. data relating to birth, death, disease, marriage, and health.

vitalism *See* TABLE OF ALTERNATIVE MEDICINE TERMS

vitamin (vī′tə-mĭn) N. any of a group of organic compounds that, in very small amounts, are essential for normal growth, development, and metabolism. They cannot be synthesized in the body (with a few exceptions) and must be supplied by the diet. Lack of sufficient quantities of any of the vitamins produces a specific deficiency disease. Vitamins are generally classified as water-soluble or fat-soluble. The water-soluble vitamins are the vitamin-B complex and vitamin C; the fat-soluble vitamins are vitamins A, D, E, and K. *See also* TABLE OF VITAMINS.

vitelline circulation (vĭ-tĕl′ĭn) N. circulation of blood and nutrients between the embryo and yolk sac through the vitelline artery and vitelline vein in the developing fetus.

vitellus N. yolk of an ovum.

vitiligo (vĭt′l-ī′gō) N. acquired, benign skin disease characterized by irregular patches of unpigmented skin, often surrounded by a hyperpigmented border, occurring most often on exposed areas of the skin. The cause is unknown, and there is no satisfactory treatment. (*Compare* LEUKODERMA.) ADJ. vitiliginous

vitreous humor (vĭt′rē-əs) N. transparent, semigelatinous substance that fills the cavity behind the lens and is closely applied to the retina. Also called vitreous body.

viviparous (vī-vĭp′ər-əs) ADJ. bearing live offspring, not eggs; it is characteristic of most mammals and also of some fishes and reptiles. N. viviparity

vocal cord (vō′kəl) N. either of two folds of tissue, each containing an elastic tissue known as the vocal ligament, that protrudes from the sides of the larynx forming a narrow slit in the larynx, called the glottis. As air is exhaled through the larynx, the vocal cords vibrate, producing sound. Movements of the tongue, lips, jaws, and accessory mouth structures mold the column of air passing through the glottis, producing sounds of different intensity and pitch.

voice box (vois) *See* LARYNX.

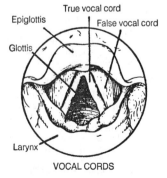

True vocal cord
Epiglottis
False vocal cord
Glottis
Larynx

VOCAL CORDS

void (void) V. to empty, as urine from the bladder.

volar ADJ. pert. to the palm or sole.

volition (və-lĭsh′ən) N. act or state of willing or choosing.

Voltaren N. trade name for the nonsteroidal anti-inflammatory agent, diclofenac sodium.

voluntary (vŏl′ən-tĕr′ē) ADJ. controlled or accomplished as the result of a person's free will, as a voluntary action.

voluntary muscle (vŏl′ən-tĕr′ē) *See* STRIATED MUSCLE.

volvulus (vŏl′vyə-ləs) N. twisting of the intestine, most often in the area of the ileum or sigmoid colon, resulting in intestinal obstruction. Severe pain, vomiting, nausea, a tense distended stomach, and the absence of bowel sounds usually occur. If not corrected surgically, the obstruction leads to peritonitis, rupture of the intestines, and death.

vomer (vō′mər) N. thin bone forming the lower and back part of the nasal septum.

vomit (vŏm′ĭt) V. to expel the contents of the stomach through the esophagus and mouth N. contents of the stomach ejected through the mouth; also called vomitus.

vomiting N. reflex action of ejecting the stomach contents through the mouth. Intestinal obstruction, irritation of the stomach, disease-producing organisms in the digestive tract, inner ear disturbances (e.g., in motion sickness), and certain drugs stimulate a special center in the brain that, in turn, produces contractions of the stomach and diaphragm musculature and relaxation of the sphincter muscle at the opening of the stomach, causing the stomach contents to be ejected through the mouth. Also called emesis.

von Recklinghausen's disease *See* NEUROFIBROMATOSIS.

vox N. voice.

voyeurism (voi-yŭr′ĭz′əm) N. disorder in which sexual excitement and gratification are obtained from viewing the naked bodies of others, esp. the genitalia, and from watching the sexual acts of others.

vulva (vŭl′və) N. external genitalia of the female. The labia majora and labia minora surround the openings of the vagina and urethra and extend to the clitoris. ADJ. vulvar.

vulvectomy (vŭl-věk′tə-mē) N. surgical removal of all or part of the vulva, usually done to treat malignant or premalignant neoplastic disease.

vulvitis (vŭl-vī′tĭs) N. inflammation of the vulva, usually producing a burning sensation and intense itching. It may be caused by infection (e.g., candidiasis) or by local irritation (e.g., from poorly fitting underwear).

vulvo- comb. form indicating an association with the vulva (e.g., vulvorectal, pert. to the vulva and rectum).

vulvovaginitis (vŭl′vō-văj′ə-nī′tĭs) N. inflammation of the vulva and the vagina.

FEMALE VULVA

Mons pubis — Glans clitoris
Labium majora — Urethra
Labium minora — Vagina
Vestibule —
Perineum — Anus

W

waist (wāst) N. narrowing of the body between the ribs and hips. In orthopedics, may refer to narrowing of a portion of a bone, such as the waist of the navicular bone in the wrist.

walker (wô′kər) N. light metal apparatus, about waist high with four sturdy legs, used as aid in walking, often by a person who has had a stroke.

wall (wôl) N. confining, limiting, or enclosing part, esp. a broad surface, as the wall of the abdominal cavity.

walleye (wôl′ī′) N. abnormal condition in which one or both eyes are off center and point outward; divergent strabismus.

warfarin N. anticoagulant (trade name Coumadin) used to prevent and treat thrombosis and embolism. Adverse effects include hemorrhage and the possibility of interaction with many other drugs. *See* TABLE OF COMMONLY PRESCRIBED DRUGS —GENERIC NAMES.

wart (wôrt) N. small, benign, often hard growth in the skin caused by a virus, and more common in children and young adults. Warts frequently disappear spontaneously but may be treated by cryosurgery (usually using liquid nitrogen), electrodesiccation, application of certain chemicals (e.g., salicylic acid), and removal by currette. Also called verruca.

    common wart N. benign growth, often with a rough surface.

juvenile wart N. benign, small growth, usually on the face and hands of children.

plantar wart N. small, benign growth on the sole, where subject to pressure, it often becomes covered with a callus.

venereal wart N. small benign growth on or around the genitalia and anus.

Wassermann test (wä′sər-mən) N. blood test to detect syphilis. A sample of blood is tested, using the complement fixation method, for antibodies to the syphilis organism *Treponema pallidum*; a positive reaction indicates the presence of antibodies and therefore syphilis infection. A false positive reaction also occurs in certain other diseases.

wasting (wā′stĭng) N. process of deterioration, in which there are weight loss and decreased strength, appetite, and activity.

water N. clear, colorless, odorless, and tasteless liquid; chemical formula H_2O.

water on the knee *See* HYDRARTHROSIS.

waterbed N. bed with a flexible waterproof mattress filled with water, used medically to prevent and treat bedsores.

Waterhouse-Friderichsen syndrome (wô′tər-hous′-frĭd′ə-rĭk′sən) N. severe systemic reaction associated with bacterial meningitis and characterized by sudden high fever, skin discoloration, petechiae, adrenal gland hemorrhage, and cardiovascular collapse. Treatment must be immediate and usually includes antibiotics, vasopressor drugs, corticosteroids, and fluids.

wax (wăks) *See* CERUMEN.

WBC *See* LEUKOCYTE.

wean (wēn) v. to induce a child to give up breast-feeding, or more generally, to detach a person from something he or she is dependent on. N. weaning

weed N. street name for marijuana.

Weil's disease (wīlz) N. serious form of leptospirosis, characterized by jaundice and liver and kidney damage.

Wellbutrin N. *See* TABLE OF COMMONLY PRESCRIBED DRUGS — TRADE NAMES.

wen N. small epidermal cyst of the scalp; also called pilar cyst.

Werdnig-Hoffman disease N. genetic disease (autosomal recessive disease) in which degeneration of spinal and brain nerve cells leads to progressive atrophy of skeletal muscles. Symptoms include flaccid paralysis, lack of sucking ability in the infant, lack of muscle tone, and absence of normal reflexes. Death from respiratory complications usually occurs in early childhood.

Wernicke's encephalopathy (vĕr′ nĭ-kēz ĕn-sĕf′ə-lŏp′ə-thē) N. inflammatory, degenerative disease of the brain, characterized by double vision, lack of muscular coordination, and decreased mental function. It is caused by thiamine deficiency, usually associated with alcoholism, occasionally with gastrointestinal disorder. (*Compare* KORSAKOFF'S PSYCHOSIS.)

wet dream *See* NOCTURNAL EMISSION.

wet lung N. condition characterized by cough and rales in the lung, occurring among persons exposed to irritants such as ammonia, chlorine, and corrosive chemical vapors. Treatment involves removal of the irritants and treatment of any possible lung damage.

wheal (wēl) N. individual lesion, usually with a red margin and pale center, of an itchy skin eruption, characteristic of many allergic reactions.

wheeze (wēz) N. abnormal high-pitched sound heard through a stethoscope in an airway blocked by mucus, neoplasm, muscle spasm, or pressure. It occurs in asthma, in chronic bronchitis, and unilaterally in the presence of a foreign body or neoplasm in the airway.

whiplash (wĭp′lăsh′) N. colloquial term for an injury to the cervical (neck) vertebrae and their associated ligaments and muscles, causing pain and stiffness; often the result of rapid acceleration or deceleration, as in a car accident. Also called cervical acceleration-deceleration syndrome.

white blood cell, white corpuscle (kôr′pə-səl) *See* LEUKOCYTE.

white matter N. nerve tissue of the spinal cord, surrounding the gray matter and made up mostly of myelinated and unmyelinated nerve fibers in a network of neuroglia cells. It is divided in each half of the spinal cord into columns containing tracts of closely related nerve fibers.

whitehead *See* MILIA.

whole blood N. blood that has not been modified or altered, except for the addition of an anticoagulant, used in blood transfusions. Various components of whole blood may be separated out and used to replace a missing or deficient clotting factor in the blood of persons with certain diseases (e.g., certain clotting factors separated out and given to those with hemophilia).

whooping cough (hoo′pĭng) *See* PERTUSSIS.

whorl (wôrl) N. something wound in a continuous series of loops so as to resemble a coil of rope; used in forensic medicine to describe types of fingerprints. May also refer to a spiral arrangement of heart muscle fibers.

Widal test (vē-däl′) N. test to detect typhoid fever and other salmonella infections.

Wilms tumor (vĭlms) N. malignant neoplasm of the kidney, occurring in young children; symptoms include hypertension, followed by pain, blood in the urine, and presence of a palpable mass. Treatment includes surgery, irradiation, and chemotherapy.

Wilson's disease N. rare, inherited disorder of copper metabolism in which copper accumulates in the liver and then in the erythrocytes (red blood cells) and brain, leading to anemia, tremors, dementia, and other symptoms. Treatment includes a diet low in copper and use of drugs to bind copper. Also called hepatolenticular degeneration.

windpipe (wĭnd′pīp′) *See* TRACHEA.

wisdom tooth (wĭz′dəm) N. any of the last 4 teeth on each side of the upper and lower jaws. They are the last teeth to erupt, usually between the ages of 16 and 21, and often cause pain and dental problems.

witch's milk N. milklike substance secreted from the breast of a newborn, caused by lactating hormones present in the maternal circulation.

withdrawal (wĭth-drô′əl) N. response to extreme stress or danger, characterized by apathy and depression, and, in extreme cases, sometimes associated with schizophrenia.

withdrawal method *See* COITUS INTERRUPTUS.

withdrawal symptoms N. unpleasant and sometimes life-threatening physiological changes that occur when a drug (e.g., narcotic, barbiturate, alcohol, stimulant) is withdrawn after the person became addicted to it during prolonged use. *See also* DELIRIUM TREMENS.

womb (woom) *See* UTERUS.

word blindness *See* ALEXIA.

word salad N. words combined in a way that has no meaning, as in the speech of some persons with schizophrenia.

Wormian bones N. any of several tiny, soft bones, found along the edges of the sutures between the cranial bones.

wound (woond) N. injury or break in the skin, usually caused by accident, not disease.

wrist (rĭst) N. joint between the forearm and the hand, formed of eight carpal bones; also called carpus. *See also* HAND.

writer's cramp (rītərz) N. *See* GRAPHOSPASM.

wryneck (rī′nĕk′) *See* TORTICOL-LIS.

Wytensin N. trade name for the antihypertensive guanabenz.

MAJOR BONES OF THE HAND

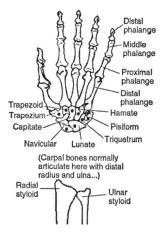

Distal phalange

Middle phalange

Proximal phalange

Distal phalange

Trapezoid
Trapezium
Capitate
Navicular   Lunate

Hamate
Pisiform
Triquetrum

(Carpal bones normally articulate here with distal radius and ulna...)

Radial styloid

Ulnar styloid

X–Y–Z

X chromosome (krō'mə-sōm') N. sex chromosome that in humans is present in both sexes—singly in males, in duplicate in females. The X chromosome is carried by all female gametes (ova) and by half of male gametes (sperm); it is larger than the Y chromosome and is associated with many sex-linked disorders (e.g., hemophilia, Hunter's syndrome).

Xalatan N. *See* TABLE OF COMMONLY PRESCRIBED DRUGS—TRADE NAMES.

Xanax N. trade name for the antianxiety agent alprazolam. *See* TABLE OF COMMONLY PRESCRIBED DRUGS—TRADE NAMES.

xanthelasma (zăn'thə-lăz'mə) N. condition marked by the formation of yellowish fatty deposits around the eyes, occurring chiefly in the elderly.

xanthemia (zăn-thē'mē-ə) *See* CAROTENE.

xanthine (zăn'thēn') N. byproduct of the metabolism of nucleoproteins, found in muscles, liver, and spleen. ADJ. xanthic

xantho- comb. form meaning yellow, yellowish (e.g., xanthochromia, a yellowish discoloration, as of the skin or cerebrospinal fluid).

xanthoma (zăn-thō'mə) N. benign, fatty, yellowish plaque, nodule, or tumor in the subcutaneous layers of the skin, usually due to accumulation of cholesterol and related compounds.

xanthoma disseminatum N. chronic condition in which orange or brownish papules develop on many surfaces of the body, esp. in the region of the mouth, in the upper respiratory tract, and on skin folds.

xanthomatosis (zăn'thō-mə-tō'sĭs) N. condition in which a disorder of lipid metabolism leads to the formation of yellowish fatty deposits in the skin and internal organs.

xanthopsia N. abnormality of vision in which objects appear to have a yellowish hue; sometimes occurring in jaundice or drug toxicity.

xanthosarcoma N. malignant neoplasm of tendon sheaths and aponeuroses, containing xanthoma cells.

xanthosis cutis N. yellow or orange-yellow coloring of the skin, usually resulting from consumption of excessive amounts of carotene-containing foods (yellow vegetables).

xanthosis diabetica N. yellowish tinge to the skin occurring in some persons with diabetes mellitus because of an excess of lipids in the blood.

xanthosis (zăn-thō'sĭs) N. abnormal yellowish discoloration.

xanthous ADJ. yellowish.

xeno- comb. form meaning strange and foreign (e.g., xenomenia, menstruation that occurs vicariously, as in bleeding from the nose).

xenograft (zĕn'ə-grăft') *See* HETEROGRAFT.

xenophobia (zĕn′ə-fō′bē-ə) N. irrational fear of strangers or unfamiliar situations. ADJ. xenophobic

xer-, xero- comb. forms indicating an association with dryness (e.g., xerocheilia, dryness of the lips).

xeroderma (zēr′ō-dûr′mə) N. abnormal dryness and roughness of the skin; also called xerodermia.

xeroma (zĭ-rō′mə) N. abnormally dry condition of the conjunctiva of the eye.

xerophthalmia (zēr′ŏf-thăl′mē-ə) N. dryness and inflammation of the conjutiva of the eye.

xeroradiography (zēr′ə-rā′dē-ŏg′rə-fē) N. photoelectric process for producing an X-ray image that uses lower radiation and shorter exposure time than conventional X-ray techniques; it is used chiefly to detect breast tumors.

xerostomia (zēr′ə-stō′mē-ə) N. dryness of the mouth caused by decreased saliva secretion; it may be a drug reaction or be caused by disease.

xiphoid process (zĭf′oid′) N. smallest of the three parts of the sternum (breastbone), articulating with the body of the sternum and with the seventh rib.

X-linked ADJ. pert. to genes, characteristics, or conditions carried on the X chromosome.

X-linked dominant inheritance (dŏm′ə-nənt ĭn-hĕr′ĭ-təns) N. hereditary pattern in which a dominant gene on the X chromosome causes a characteristic to be manifested. All of the daughters of an affected male will be affected, but none of the sons; half of all the offspring of an affected female will be affected.

X-linked recessive inheritance (rĭ-sĕs′ĭv ĭn-hĕr′ĭ-təns) N. hereditary pattern in which a recessive gene on the X chromosome results in the manifestation of characteristics of the given condition in males and a carrier state in females.

X ray N.
1. electromagnetic radiation of short wavelength used to penetrate tissues and record densities on film.
2. film produced by an X-ray procedure. ADJ. X-ray, V. x-ray

XX N. in genetics, normal sex chromosome complement in a female.

XXX N. in genetics, chromosomal aberration in which there are three X chromosomes (not the normal two) and an abnormal total chromosome number of 47 (not the normal 46). Affected persons are female with little or no symptoms, except usually some degree of mental retardation.

XXY N. in genetics, abnormal sex chromosome complement in males in which more than the normal single X chromosome is present and the total chromosome number of the body cell is abnormal also. See also KLEINFELTER'S SYNDROME.

XY N. in genetics, normal sex chromosome complement in a male.

Xylocaine N. trade name for the local anesthetic lidocaine.

XYY N. in genetics, abnormal sex chromosome complement in males in which there are more than the normal Y chromosome and an increased total chromosome complement. The condition is usually associated with tall stature and often with abnormal mental effects.

Y chromosome (krō′mə-sōm′) N. sex chromosome that in humans is present only in males, appearing singly (along with a single X chromosome). It is carried by one half of male gametes (sperm) and none of the female gametes (ova). It is smaller than the X chromosome and is not associated with many known sex-linked disorders.

yatobyo *See* TULAREMIA.

yawning N. reflex, usually triggered by boredom, fatigue, drowsiness, or seeing someone else yawn; the mouth is opened wide and air is drawn in and released slowly.

yaws (yôz) N. infection caused by the spirochete *Treponema pertenue,* transmitted by direct contact, chiefly among children, living in unsanitary conditions in tropical and subtropical areas. It is characterized by ulcerating sores on the body, leading to destruction of underlying tissue. Treatment is by penicillin. *See also* BEJEL; SYPHILIS.

yellow fever N. virus-caused disease, transmitted by mosquitoes, chiefly female Aëdes aegypti mosquitoes, found in tropical Africa and northern South America. Symptoms include fever, headache, pains in the back and limbs, reduced urine output, jaundice, and degeneration of liver and kidney tissue. There is no specific treatment, but the disease can be prevented by vaccination (which is advised for all who travel to areas where yellow fever is endemic); recovery from one attack usually confers subsequent immunity.

yellow marrow (măr′ō) *See under* BONE MARROW.

yolk (yōk) N. nutritive material, rich in protein and fats, found within the ovum to supply nourishment for the developing embryo. It is nearly absent in the ova of humans and other mammals, in whom the embryo receives nourishment from the mother, through the placenta.

yolk sac (săk) N. membranous sac that develops in the early embryo, providing part of the primitive gut, a site of blood cell formation, and a means for transporting nutrients to the early embryo. In humans it disappears in early embryonic development.

yolk stalk (stôk) N. narrow duct that connects the yolk sac and mid area of the embryonic gut during early development, usually disappearing in early embryonic growth.

zafirlukast N. *See* TABLE OF COMMONLY PRESCRIBED DRUGS—GENERIC NAMES.

Zantac N. trade name for the histamine blocker ranitidine. *See* TABLE OF COMMONLY PRESCRIBED DRUGS—TRADE NAMES.

Zarontin N. trade name for the anticonvulsant ethosuximide.

Zestoretic N. *See* TABLE OF COMMONLY PRESCRIBED DRUGS—TRADE NAMES.

Zestril N. trade name for the antihypertensive lisinopril. *See* TABLE OF COMMONLY PRESCRIBED DRUGS—TRADE NAMES.

Ziac N. *See* TABLE OF COMMONLY PRESCRIBED DRUGS—TRADE NAMES.

zinc (zĭngk) N. metallic element essential to normal body metabolism. Zinc compounds (e.g., zinc sulfate, zinc oxide) are also widely used as astringents in creams, ointments, and powders for skin irritations and minor wounds. *See also* TABLE OF IMPORTANT ELEMENTS.

zinc deficiency (dĭ-fĭsh′ən-sē) N. condition caused by inadequate zinc intake in the diet or by liver disease, cystic fibrosis, or certain other diseases that lead to inadequate zinc levels; symptoms include fatigue, mental dullness, poor appetite, and susceptibility to infection. Rich sources of zinc include meat, eggs, nuts, milk, peanut butter, and whole grains.

Zithromax N. trade name for the antibiotic zithromycin. *See* TABLE OF COMMONLY PRESCRIBED DRUGS—TRADE NAMES.

Zn symbol for the element zinc.

zoanthropy N. delusion that one has assumed the form of an animal.

Zocor N. trade name for simvastatin, an oral agent used in the treatment of hypercholesterolemia. *See* TABLE OF COMMONLY PRESCRIBED DRUGS—TRADE NAMES.

Zollinger-Ellison syndrome (zŏl′ĭn-jər-ĕl′ĭ-sən) N. condition in which excess gastric juice secretion leads to severe and recurrent peptic ulcers; it is usually caused by a tumor (often malignant) of the pancreas. Treatment may involve removal of the tumor, if possible; gastrectomy; and the use of antiulcer drugs (e.g., cimetidine).

Zoloft (zō′lôft′) N. trade name for the antidepressant sertraline HCl. *See* TABLE OF COMMONLY PRESCRIBED DRUGS—TRADE NAMES.

zolpidem N. *See* TABLE OF COMMONLY PRESCRIBED DRUGS—GENERIC NAMES.

zona (zō′nə) N., *pl.* zonae, bandlike area around a part or organ. Also called zone. ADJ. zonal

zona pellucida (pə-lōō′sĭ-də) N. thick membrane enclosing the mammalian ovum; it can be penetrated by one sperm in the fertilization process, and usually remains around the fertilized egg until its implantation in the wall of the uterus.

zonule (zōn′yōōl) N. small, bandlike area (e.g., zonule of Zinn, ligament holding the lens of the eye in place). Also called zonula.

zoo- comb. form indicating an association with nonhuman animals (e.g., zoograft, tissue from an animal transplanted to a person, as in the use of pig tissue to replace a damaged heart valve in a human).

zoonosis (zō-ŏn′ə-sĭs) N. disease of animals that can be transmitted to humans (e.g., brucellosis, leptospirosis, rabies).

zoophilism (zō-ŏf′ə-lĭz′əm) N. abnormal fondness for animals, esp. sexual attraction to animals. ADJ. zoophilic

zoophobia (zō′ə-fō′bē-ə) N. irrational and excessive fear of animals. ADJ. zoophobic

zoopsia N. visual hallucination of animals, sometimes occurring in delirium tremens.

zootoxin N. poisonous substance from an animal (e.g., snake venom).

Zovirax N. trade name for the antiviral acyclovir.

valproic acid (văl-prō′ĭk) N. anticonvulsant (trade name Depokene) used to prevent some types of seizures. Adverse effects include gastrointestinal disturbances, hair loss, headache, liver damage, and decreased blood-clotting ability. *See* TABLE OF COMMONLY PRESCRIBED DRUGS—GENERIC NAMES.

Valsartan N. *See* TABLE OF COMMONLY PRESCRIBED DRUGS—GENERIC NAMES.

valve (vălv) N. structure, usually a flap or fold of tissue, found in some tubes and tubular organs that restricts the flow of fluid in them in one direction only. Valves are important structures in the heart, veins, and lymph vessels. *See also* MITRAL VALVE; SEMILUNAR VALVE; TRICUSPID VALVE.

valvotomy (văl-vŏt′ə-mē) N. incision into a valve to correct a defect and permit its normal function of opening and closing to control the flow of a fluid.

valvular heart disease (văl′vyə-lər) N. disorder of heart valves caused by stenosis and obstructed blood flow or degeneration and blood regurgitation. Major types of valvular heart disease include aortic stenosis and mitral valve stenosis.

valvulitis (văl′vyə-lī′tĭs) N. inflammation of a valve, esp. a heart valve, usually resulting from rheumatic fever, sometimes from bacterial endocarditis or syphilis; stenosis and impaired blood flow commonly result.

Vancenase N. trade name for the inhaled corticosteroid drug, beclomethasone. *See* TABLE OF COMMONLY PRESCRIBED DRUGS—TRADE NAMES.

Vancocin N. trade name for the antibacterial vancomycin.

vancomycin (văng′kə-mī′sĭn) N. antibiotic (trade name Vancocin) used to treat some bacterial infections. Adverse effects include tinnitus, dizziness, and anaphylaxis.

Vantin N. trade name for the cephalosporin antibiotic, cefpodoxime.

varicella (văr′ĭ-sĕl′ə) *See* CHICKEN POX.

varicella zoster virus (VZV) (zŏs′tər) N. member of the herpes virus family that is responsible for varicella (chicken pox) and herpes zoster (shingles).

varicelliform ADJ. resembling the rash of chicken pox.

varicocele (văr′ĭ-kō-sēl′) N. dilatation or swelling of blood vessels associated with the spermatic cord in the testes.

varicose vein (văr′ĭ-kōs′) N. swollen, tortuous vein with abnormally functioning valves. It is a common condition, usually affecting the veins of the legs; it is more common in women than men and often associated with congenitally weak valves, pregnancy, obesity, or thrombophlebitis. Symptoms include pain, muscle cramps, and a feeling of heaviness in the legs. Elevation of the legs and the use of elastic stockings often help. Severe cases may require surgical intervention.

varicosis (văr′ĭ-kō′sĭs) N. condition characterized by one or more varicose veins.

varicosity (văr′ĭ-kŏs′ĭ-tē) N. abnormal condition in which a vein is swollen and tortuous.

variola (və-rī′ə-lə) *See* smallpox.

Zyban N. *See* TABLE OF COM-MONLY PRESCRIBED DRUGS—TRADE NAMES.

zygomatic (zī'gə-măt'ĭk) ADJ. pert. to the cheek region of the face.

zygomatic bone N. one of a pair of skull bones that form the lower part of the eye socket and prominence of the cheek.

zygote (zī'gōt') N. fertilized ovum.

Zyloprim N. trade name for allo-purinol.

zymoid ADJ. like an enzyme.

zymosis (zī-mō'sĭs) N. process of fermentation.

APPENDICES

OVERVIEW OF THE HUMAN BODY

Levels of Structure in the Human Body

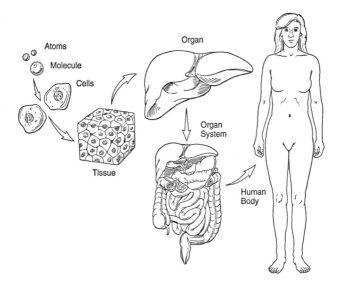

The human body from the submicroscopic level (atoms and molecules) to the microscopic level (cells and tissues) to the macroscopic level (organs, organ systems). The body is made up of several organ systems, each composed of several organs with related functions.

THE INTEGUMENTARY SYSTEM

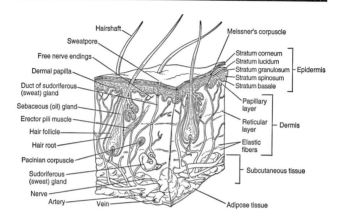

The integumentary system consists of the skin, hair, nails, and sweat glands.

THE SKELETAL SYSTEM

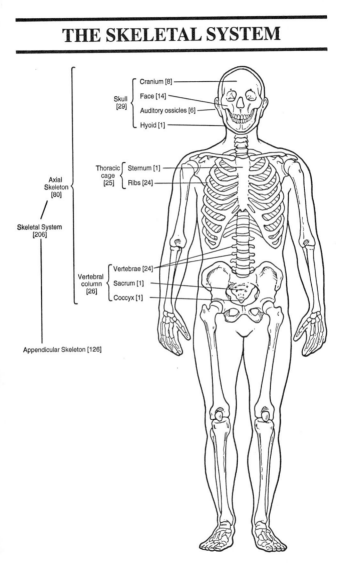

The bones of the axial skeleton.

THE SKELETAL SYSTEM

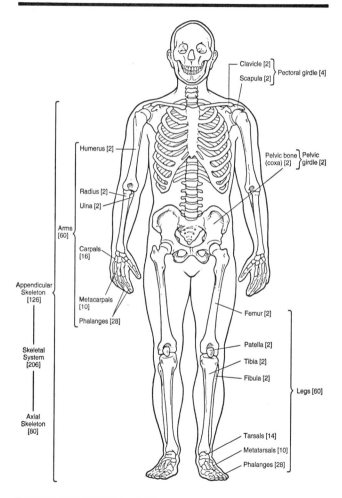

Clavicle [2]
Scapula [2]
Pectoral girdle [4]

Humerus [2]

Pelvic bone (coxa) [2]
Pelvic girdle [2]

Radius [2]
Ulna [2]

Arms [60]

Appendicular Skeleton [126]

Carpals [16]

Metacarpals [10]

Phalanges [28]

Femur [2]

Skeletal System [206]

Patella [2]
Tibia [2]
Fibula [2]

Axial Skeleton [80]

Legs [60]

Tarsals [14]
Metatarsals [10]
Phalanges [28]

The bones of the appendicular skeleton.

THE NERVOUS SYSTEM

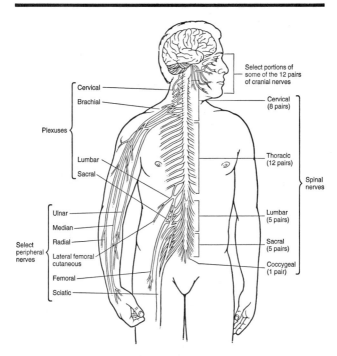

The central nervous system consists of the brain and spinal cord; the peripheral nervous system consists of 12 pairs of cranial nerves and 31 pairs of spinal nerves.

THE MAJOR ENDOCRINE GLANDS

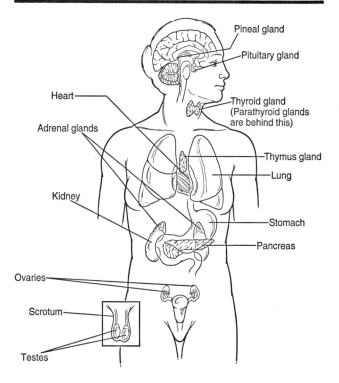

The endocrine system consists of pituitary, adrenal, thyroid, and other ductless glands.

THE MUSCULAR SYSTEM

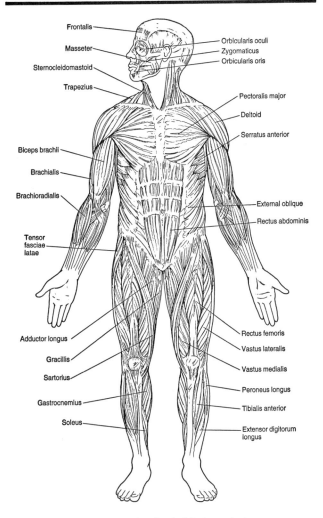

Frontalis

Masseter

Sternocleidomastoid

Trapezius

Orbicularis oculi

Zygomaticus

Orbicularis oris

Pectoralis major

Deltoid

Serratus anterior

Biceps brachii

Brachialis

Brachioradialis

External oblique

Rectus abdominis

Tensor fasciae latae

Adductor longus

Gracillis

Sartorius

Gastrocnemius

Soleus

Rectus femoris

Vastus lateralis

Vastus medialis

Peroneus longus

Tibialis anterior

Extensor digitorum longus

Major muscles of the anterior surface (front) of the human body.

THE MUSCULAR SYSTEM

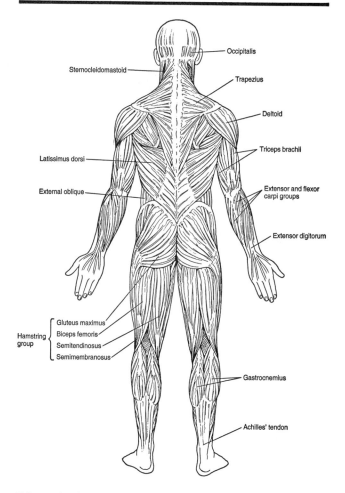

Major muscles of the posterior surface (back) of the human body.

THE DIGESTIVE SYSTEM

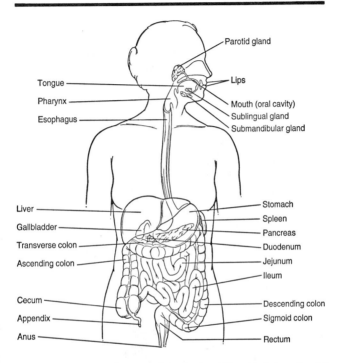

Parotid gland
Tongue
Pharynx
Esophagus
Lips
Mouth (oral cavity)
Sublingual gland
Submandibular gland
Liver
Gallbladder
Transverse colon
Ascending colon
Stomach
Spleen
Pancreas
Duodenum
Jejunum
Ileum
Cecum
Appendix
Anus
Descending colon
Sigmoid colon
Rectum

The function of the digestive system is to absorb soluble nutrients from digested foods.

THE RESPIRATORY SYSTEM

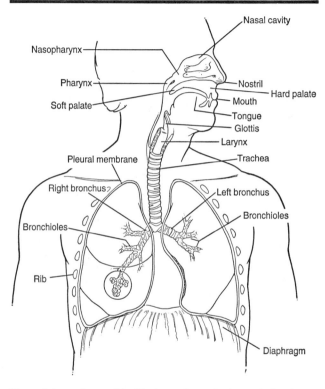

The respiratory system consists of the lungs, pharynx, trachea, and other air passageways.

THE CIRCULATORY SYSTEM

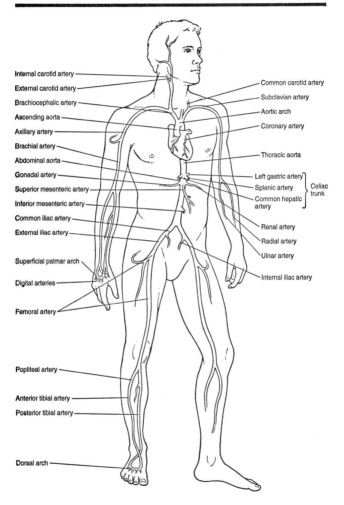

The major arteries of the human body, excluding the pulmonary arteries.

Internal carotid artery
External carotid artery
Brachiocephalic artery
Ascending aorta
Axillary artery
Brachial artery
Abdominal aorta
Gonadal artery
Superior mesenteric artery
Inferior mesenteric artery
Common iliac artery
External iliac artery
Superficial palmar arch
Digital arteries
Femoral artery
Popliteal artery
Anterior tibial artery
Posterior tibial artery
Dorsal arch

Common carotid artery
Subclavian artery
Aortic arch
Coronary artery
Thoracic aorta
Left gastric artery
Splenic artery
Common hepatic artery
Celiac trunk
Renal artery
Radial artery
Ulnar artery
Internal iliac artery

THE CIRCULATORY SYSTEM

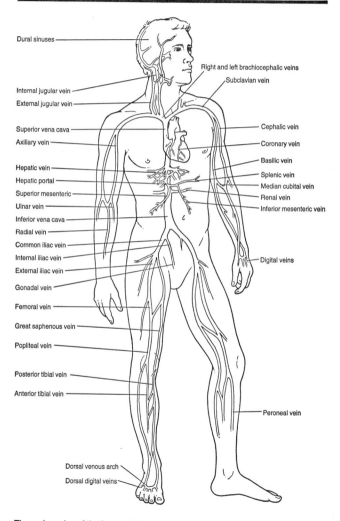

Dural sinuses

Right and left brachiocephalic veins

Subclavian vein

Internal jugular vein

External jugular vein

Superior vena cava

Axillary vein

Cephalic vein

Coronary vein

Basilic vein

Hepatic vein

Hepatic portal

Superior mesenteric

Ulnar vein

Inferior vena cava

Radial vein

Common iliac vein

Internal iliac vein

External iliac vein

Gonadal vein

Femoral vein

Great saphenous vein

Popliteal vein

Posterior tibial vein

Anterior tibial vein

Splenic vein

Median cubital vein

Renal vein

Inferior mesenteric vein

Digital veins

Peroneal vein

Dorsal venous arch

Dorsal digital veins

The major veins of the human body, excluding the pulmonary veins.

THE LYMPHATIC SYSTEM

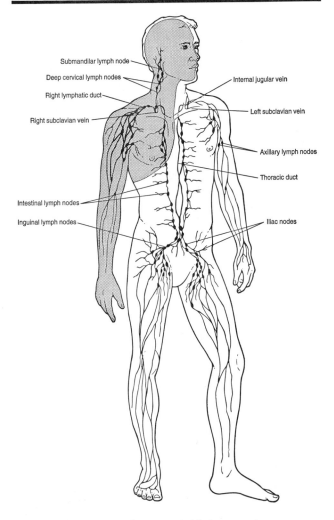

Submandilar lymph node

Deep cervical lymph nodes

Right lymphatic duct

Right subclavian vein

Intestinal lymph nodes

Inguinal lymph nodes

Internal jugular vein

Left subclavian vein

Axillary lymph nodes

Thoracic duct

Iliac nodes

The lymphatic system is a major component of the immune system.

THE URINARY SYSTEM

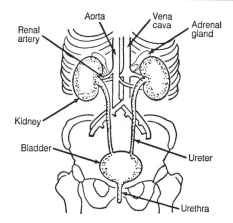

The kidney, bladder, and associated ducts make up the urinary system.

THE REPRODUCTIVE SYSTEM

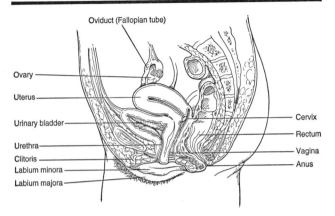

Oviduct (Fallopian tube)

Ovary

Uterus

Urinary bladder

Urethra

Clitoris

Labium minora

Labium majora

Cervix

Rectum

Vagina

Anus

Structures and organs of the female reproductive system.

Urinary bladder

Vas deferens

Prostate gland

Corpus cavernosa

Penis

Urethra

Corpus spongiosum

Prepuce

Glans penis

Seminal vesicle

Rectum

Ejaculatory duct

Anus

Epididymis

Testis

Scrotum

Structures and organs of the male reproductive system.

MAJOR ORGAN SYSTEMS

Organ System	Physiological Role	Components
Integumentary	Covers the body and protects it	Skin, hair, nails, and sweat glands
Skeletal	Protects the body and provides support for locomotion and movement	Bones, cartilage, and ligaments
Nervous	Receives stimuli, integrates information, and directs the body	Brain, spinal cord, nerves, and sense organs
Endocrine	Coordinates and integrates the activities of the body	Pituitary, adrenal, thyroid, and other ductless glands
Muscular	Produces body movement	Skeletal muscle, smooth muscle, and cardiac muscle
Digestive	Absorbs soluble nutrients from ingested food	Teeth, salivary glands, esophagus, stomach, intestines, liver, and pancreas
Respiratory	Collects oxygen and exchanges it for carbon dioxide	Lungs, pharynx, trachea, and other air passageways
Circulatory	Transports cells and materials throughout the body	Heart, blood vessels, blood, and lymph structures
Immune	Removes foreign chemicals and microorganisms from the bloodstream	T-lymphocytes, B-lymphocytes, and macrophages; lymph structures
Urinary	Removes metabolic wastes from the bloodstream	Kidney, bladder, and associated ducts
Reproductive	Produces sex cells for the next generation of organism	Testes, ovaries, and associated reproductive structures

POSITIONAL AND DIRECTIONAL TERMS

Term	Definition	Example
Anterior (ventral)	Nearer to or at the front of the body	Sternum is anterior to the heart
Posterior (dorsal)	Nearer to or at the back of the body	Esophagus is posterior to the trachea
Superior (cephalic or cranial)	Toward the head or the upper part of a structure; generally refers to structures in the trunk	Heart is superior to the liver
Inferior (caudal)	Away from the head or toward the lower part of the structure; generally refers to structures in the trunk	Stomach is inferior to the lungs
Medial	Nearer to the midline of the body or a structure	Ulna is on the medial side of the forearm
Lateral	Away from the midline of the body	Lungs are lateral to the heart
Ipsilateral	On the same side of the body	Gall bladder and ascending colon of the large intestine are ipsilateral
Contralateral	On the opposite side of the body	Ascending and descending colons of the large intestine are contralateral
Proximal	Nearer to the attachment of an extremity to the trunk or structure	Femur is proximal to the tibia
Distal	Farther from the attachment of an extremity to the trunk of a structure	Phalanges are distal to the carpals (wrist bones)
Superficial	Toward the surface of the body	Muscles of the thoracic wall are superior to the viscera in the thoracic cavity
Deep	Away from the surface of the body	Ribs are deep to the skin of the chest

TABLES OF WEIGHTS AND MEASURES

LENGTH

Name Equivalent)	Symbol	Equivalent in Meters (Common U.S.
ångström	Å	1/10,000,000,000 (one ten-billionth)
nanometer (millimicron)	nm (mμ)	1/1,000,000,000 (one billionth)
micrometer (micron)	μm (μ)	1/1,000,000 (one millionth)
millimeter	mm	1/1000 (one thousandth)
centimeter	cm	1/100 (one hundredth; 1 inch = 2.54 cm)
decimeter	dl	1/10 (one tenth)
meter	m	1 (1 yard = 0.91 m; 1 foot = 0.305 m)
decameter	dam	10
hectometer	hm	100
kilometer	km	1000 (1 mile = 1609 meters)

VOLUME

Name	Symbol	Equivalent in Liters (Common U.S. Equivalent)
microliter	μl	1/1,000,000 (one millionth)
milliliter	ml	1/1000 (one thousandth)
deciliter	dl	1/10 (one tenth)
liter	l	1 (1 US gallon = 3.79 liters)

MASS

Name	Symbol	Equivalent in Kilograms (Common U.S. Equivalent)
nanogram	ng	1/1,000,000,000 (one billionth)
microgram	μg	1/1,000,000 (one millionth)
gram	mg	1/1000 (one thousandth)
kilogram	kg	1 (1 pound = 0.45 kilograms)
metric ton	T	1000

COMMON ABBREVIATIONS USED IN MEDICINE

Abbreviation	Latin Derivation	Meaning
ā		before
āā	ana	of each
ac	ante cibum	before meals
AD	auris dextra	right ear
A and D		admission and discharge
ad	addi	let them be added
ad effect	ad effectum	until it is effective
ad lib	ad libitum	as desired, as much as patient desires
agit	agita	shake
AI		aortic insufficiency
ama		against medical advice
amb		ambulatory
amt		amount
AP	ante partum	before childbirth
ap	ante prandium	before dinner
APC		aspirin, phenacetin, caffeine
approx		approximately
aq	aqua	water
ARD		acute respiratory disease
AS	auris sinistra	left ear
AU	auris unitas	both ears
AV		arteriovenous, audiovisual
av		average
awa		as well as
B		black (race)
BCG		Bacillus Calmette-Guérin
bid	bis in die	twice each day
BMR		basal metabolism rate
BP		blood pressure
c̄		with
Ca		cancer, carcinoma
CBC		complete blood count
clin		clinical
CNS		central nervous system
CPR		cardiopulmonary resuscitation
CV		cardiovascular
CVA		cerebrovascular accident
dbl		double
DNA		deoxyribonucleic acid
DOA		dead on arrival
DT	delirium tremens	severe tremors
D/W		dextrose in water
Dx		diagnosis
ea		each

Abbreviation	Latin Derivation	Meaning
ECG		electrocardiogram
EEG		electroencephalogram
EENT		ear, eye, nose, and throat
EKG		electrocardiogram
EM		electron microscope
EMG		electromyogram
ENT		ear, nose, and throat
ER		emergency room
EST		electroshock therapy
et al.	et alii	and others
F		female
FACP		Fellow, American College of Physicians
FACS		Fellow, American College of Surgeons
FICS		Fellow, International College of Surgeons
FRCOG		Fellow, Royal College of Obstetricians and Gynecologists
FRCP		Fellow, Royal College of Physicians
FRCP(C)		Fellow, Royal College of Physicians of Canada
FRCP(E)		Fellow, Royal College of Physicians of Edinburgh
FRCP(I)		Fellow, Royal College of Physicians of Ireland
GI		gastrointestinal
GP		general practitioner
GSW		gunshot wound
GTT		glucose tolerance test
GU		genitourinary
Gyn		gynecology
h		height
hct		hematocrit
HG		hemoglobin
Hgb		hemoglobin
HID		headache, insomnia, and depression
HP		high power (microscope)
HPN		hypertension
HR		heart rate
hs	hora somni	at bedtime
HVL		half value layer
Hx		history
I and D		incision and drainage
I&O		intake and output
ID		identification
id	idem	the same
	in diem	during the day

Common Abbreviations (continued)

Abbreviation	Latin Derivation	Meaning
IM		intramuscular
		internal medicine
IOP		intraocular pressure
IQ		intelligence quotient
IST		insulin shock therapy
IUD		intrauterine (contraceptive) device
IV		intravenous
IVP		intravenous pyelogram
IVU		intravenous urogram
JND		just noticeable difference
k		constant
KUB		kidney, ureter, bladder
L		left
lab		laboratory
LD		lethal dose
LD_{50}		lethal dose in which 50% of the group survive
LE		lupus erythematosus
liq		liquid
LKS		liver, kidney, spleen
LM		light microscope
loc cit	loco citato	in the place cited
LP		low power, lumbar puncture, latent period
LPN		licensed practical nurse
M		male
MA		mental age
MAO		monoamine oxidase
mb	misce bene	mix well
MD	Medicinae Doctor	doctor of medicine
		muscular dystrophy
MDR		minimum daily requirement
MED		minimum effective dose
mEq		milliequivalent
M:F		male to female ratio
MFT		muscle function test
MI		mitral insufficiency
		myocardial infarction
mm Hg		millimeters of mercury (measure of blood pressure)
MS		multiple sclerosis
N		normal
		number
NA		not applicable
npo		nothing by mouth
NSA		no significant abnormality
ō		no
Ob-Gyn		obstetrics-gynecology
OBS		organic brain syndrome
OD	oculus dexter	right eye
		overdose

Abbreviation	Latin Derivation	Meaning
OR		operating room
OS	oculus sinister	left eye
OU	oculus uterque	each, both eyes
P		probability
$\bar{p}$		after
p		pulse
Pap		Papanicolaou
PBI		protein-bound iodine
pCO_2		carbon dioxide pressure, tension
PE		physical examination
PI		present illness
PM	post mortem	after death
po	per os	by mouth
pO_2		oxygen tension, pressure
prn	pro re nata	as circumstances may require
PT		physical therapy
		prothrombin time
pt		patient
Px		prognosis
qd	quaque die	every day
qh	quaque hora	every hour
qid	quater in die	four times each day
qq	quaque	each, every
qv	quantum vis	as much as you want
R		respiration
		response
r		roentgen
$\bar{s}$		without
RBC		red blood cell
RES		reticuloendothelial system
RNA		ribonucleic acid
RU		rat unit
Rx	recipe	prescription
		therapy
S		subject
S/S		signs and symptoms
sed		sedimentation (rate)
seq	sequela(e)	that which follows
SI		Système Internationale (metric units)
sig	signa	label
S-O-R		stimulus-organism-response
sp		species (singular)
sp g		specific gravity
spp		species (plural)
S-R		stimulus-response
Ss		subjects
STAT	statim	immediately
STP		standard temperature and pressure
sum	sumat	let it be taken

Common Abbreviations (continued)

Abbreviation	Latin Derivation	Meaning
T		temperature
t		time
T&A		tonsillectomy and adenoidectomy
TB		tuberculosis
tid	ter in die	three times each day
tinc		tincture
TLC		tender loving care
TPR		temperature, pulse, respiration
U		unit
UCS		unconditioned stimulus
UO		of undetermined origin
URI		upper respiratory infection
USP		United States Pharmacopoeia
USPHS		United States Public Health Service
ut dict	ut dictum	as directed
UV		ultraviolet
UVR		ultraviolet radiation
V		volume
VD		venereal disease
VDRL		Venereal Disease Research Laboratory
VHF		very high frequency
vid	vide	see
viz	videlicet	namely
VLF		very low frequency
V/O		verbal order
VPC		volume packed cells
v/v		percent volume in volume
W		white (race)
w		weight
w/		with
WBC		white blood cell(s)
WDWN		well developed, well nourished
wk		week
W/V		weight per volume
X		unknown, crossed

NAMING OPERATIONS

An operation may be named either for the person(s) who originated or perfected it (called an eponym, e.g., Blalock-Taussig operation) or for the anatomical part(s) involved and the specific action taken on it (them).

Other than eponymal terms, then, most operations have one of these appropriate roots:

Term	Meaning	Example
-centesis	needle puncture to draw fluid	amniocentesis (puncture of the fetal covering)
-desis	fusion, binding	arthrodesis (fusing joint surfaces)
-ectomy	to cut out	appendectomy (removal of appendix)
-nyxis	puncture	scleronyxis (puncture of the sclera of the eyeball)
-ostomy	making an opening	colostomy (making an artificial opening from the outside to the colon)
-pexy	fixing, fixation	gastropexy (stabilizing the stomach surgically)
-plasty	surgical repair	rhinoplasty (plastic surgery on the nose)
-rhaphy	surgical sewing	blepharorrhaphy (sewing the eyelids together)
-rhexis	fracturing a bone	anarrhexis (deliberate fracturing of a bone for restructuring)
-scopy	examination by use of instruments	laryngoscopy (examining the windpipe, larynx, with a special tube)
-tomy	cutting, making an incision	laparotomy (cutting through the abdominal wall)

TABLE OF IMPORTANT ELEMENTS

A chemical *element* is any one of over 100 fundamental substances whose atoms are of a single type. An element cannot be broken down into a simpler substance by ordinary chemical means. Most elements combine with other elements to form *compounds*. Elements of one *family* have similar properties (e.g., fluorine, chlorine, bromine, and iodine are members of the halogen family and have similar properties).

Common Name	Chemical Symbol	Atomic No.	Medical/Physiological Significance
aluminum	Al	13	Most abundant metal on earth's outer layer; used in compounds to treat excessive stomach acidity and as a disinfectant
arsenic	As	33	Highly poisonous element, present in many household and garden pesticides; formerly (but now used rarely) in compounds to treat certain skin diseases
barium	Ba	56	Compounds used for removing hair; as insoluble barium sulfate in contrast substances to show the form or action of stomach or intestinal parts on X-ray film
boron	B	5	Element believed necessary in trace amounts for cell-wall formation and in the production and breakdown of pectin; common compounds are borax and boric acid
bromine	Br	35	Compounds (bromides) used as sedatives; poisoning may result from prolonged use
calcium	Ca	20	An essential constituent of most animals and plants; a mineral nutrient, needed for formation and maintenance of bone and teeth; exchanges with sodium in some cell actions, as in retinal rod cells during vision
carbon	C	6	Chief element (in combination with hydrogen and oxygen) in organic compounds and, hence, all life forms (e.g., in forming glucose, an important sugar that fuels the cell)

Common Name	Chemical Symbol	Atomic No.	Medical/Physiological Significance
chlorine	Cl	17	Extremely pungent element, used as a disinfectant in water purification and in insecticides; toxic in high concentrations
cobalt	Co	27	Essential trace element in animal and plant metabolism; needed for formation of specific body chemicals; a radioactive isotope, Co-60, used in treatment of cancer
copper	Cu	29	An important trace element in animal and plant metabolism; needed in the synthesis of hemoglobin; involved in enzyme reactions
fluorine	F	9	Occurs in small amounts in bones and teeth; compounds are used in dentistry and derivatives added to drinking water in small amounts (three to four parts per million) to prevent decay of teeth (dental caries)
gold	Au	79	Formerly used in dental prostheses because of its inertness; used in compounds to treat arthritis; radioactive isotope (Au-198) used in cancer treatment and in liver scanning
hydrogen	H	1	Needed in formation of carbohydrates and thus essential to life forms; essential in metabolism and respiration cycles
iodine	I	53	Needed for thyroid gland to work normally; used in antiseptics and in treating goiter and cretinism
iron	Fe	26	Vital in helping to carry oxygen to cells; used in formation of hemoglobin and respiratory enzymes
lead	Pb	82	Used in shielding against radioactivity; a cumulative poison not excreted from the body; children often affected by eating dried paint containing one or more lead compounds

Table of Important Elements (continued)

Common Name	Chemical Symbol	Atomic No.	Medical/Physiological Significance
lithium	Li	3	Increases serotonin release in parts of the brain; compounds used in treating mental depression and mania
magnesium	Mg	12	Essential component of many enzymes; essential in photosynthesis; abundant in plants and animals (bones, chlorophyll); compounds used as antacids and mild laxatives (Epsom salts, milk of magnesia); needed for formation of bones, teeth
manganese	Mn	25	Trace element in plants and animals; involved in enzyme reactions
mercury	Hg	80	The only common metal that is liquid at normal temperatures; used in blood-pressure apparatuses and in mercury thermometers and as an amalgam in dentistry; implicated in environmental poisonings, esp. as a cumulative poison in fish
nitrogen	N	7	Makes up about 78% of atmosphere; important in forming proteins and nucleic acids; essential for all living cells and important in antibiotics; important to plant (food) growth through the nitrogen cycle
oxygen	O	8	Essential in respiration and in forming carbohydrates and proteins; most abundant of earth's elements in a free gas form in atmosphere and in combined forms in water and in inorganic and organic (e.g., proteins, carbohydrates) forms
phosphorus	P	15	Essential for formation of bones, teeth; needed by all living cells; used in fertilizers, detergents, toxic nerve gases, rodent and insect poisons; a component of proteins and nucleic acids; found in blood, muscles, and nerves

Common Name	Chemical Symbol	Atomic No.	Medical/Physiological Significance
plutonium	Pu	94	Artificially produced radioactive element manufactured in nuclear reactors; said to be the deadliest poison; collects in the bones; interferes with production of white blood cells
potassium	K	19	Essential to nervous system function; principal intracellular positively charged ion of most body tissues; probably plays a role in protein synthesis
radium	Ra	88	Radioactive; used in treatment of cancer and in radiography; releases radon, a radioactive gas
radon	Rn	86	Radioactive; produced during the decay of radium; used in radiotherapy for cancer treatment; suspected by some as causing lung cancer in persons exposed to the gas in homes or workplaces
silicon	Si	14	Second most abundant element in earth's outer layer (see oxygen); important in electronics (transistors) and silicone rubber implants
sodium	Na	11	Found in animals and most plants; sodium-ion pump is essential in transport of substances across cell membranes; compounds used in diuretics, function tests, detergents, antacids, gargles, anticoagulants; implicated as one cause of high blood pressure
sulfur	S	16	Important in forming proteins, used in fungicides, insecticides, and in compounds for treating skin diseases
zinc	Zn	30	Trace element in plants and animals; essential component of certain enzymes; low levels implicated in causing abnormalities in taste and smell functions

TABLE OF VITAMINS

Common Designation	Scientific Name (or Description)	Physiological Action	Source(s)
A	(either of 2 fat-soluble substances, vitamins A_1, A_2)	prevents drying and horny development (keratinization) of epithelial tissues	liver oils, egg yolk, dairy products
A_1	retinol	essential for normal vision	yellow fruits and vegetables
A_2	dehydroretinol	prevents "drying" of retina (xeropthalmia) and night blindness	leafy green vegetables
provitamin A	carotene	converts to vitamin A in the liver	
B complex	(originally thought to be one substance but now separated into several water-soluble "B" vitamins)		
B_1	thiamine	prevents beriberi (inflammation and degeneration of nerves with paralysis and muscle wasting); maintains appetite and growth	seed coats of cereal grains, meats (esp. pork), peas, beans, egg yolks
B_2	riboflavin	prevents skin lesions and weight loss	animal and plant tissue, milk
pellagra-preventing vitamin (PP)	niacin (nicotinic acid)	prevents pellagra (loss of vitality, diarrhea, mental disturbances); essential for proper enzyme function	yeast, veal, liver, pork, milk, eggs, whole wheat
B_6	pyridoxine, pyridoxal, pyridoxamine	essential for proper metabolism of amino acids and of starch (glycogen) to sugar (glucose)	most foods, but esp. liver, eggs, whole-grain cereals
B_{12}	cyanocobalamin	effective in treating pernicious anemia	eggs, fish, liver

Common Designation	Scientific Name (or Description)	Physiological Action	Source(s)
B_c	biotin (also: coenzyme R)	prevents paralysis and baldness in experimental animals	egg yolk, liver, tomatoes, yeast
	folic acid	may be essential for preventing anemia and an excess of iron deposits in the body (hemochromatosis)	yeast
C	ascorbic acid (water-soluble substance)	prevents scurvy (weakness, joint swelling, gum bleeding)	fresh fruit and vegetables, esp. citrus fruits (vitamin is rapidly destroyed by cooking)
D	calciferol (fat-soluble substance)	prevents rickets (bowed legs, crooked bones); essential for normal use of calcium and phosphorus in the body and for normal bone formation	fish-liver oil, egg yolk, butter and exposure to sunlight
E	tocopherols (fat-soluble substances)	essential for normal reproduction, muscle development, and other functions	wheat-germ oil, egg yolk, beef liver, cereals
K	group of fat-soluble substances	helps clot blood, increases prothrombin production in liver; prevents hemorrhages; used to treat jaundice; sometimes given to persons undergoing surgery	spinach, cabbage, egg yolk, liver

TABLE OF
MANAGED CARE TERMS

Term	Definition, Common Use
Capitation	Payment mechanism in which a provider is paid, in advance, a set fee for medical services regardless of the amount or intensity of medical services rendered to a patient. Typically, money left over at the end of a contract period is retained by the provider. On the other hand, any fees or costs that exceed the capitation amount must be absorbed by the provider without additional cost to the patient.
Diagnosis-Related Groups (DRG)	Federal system of classification of diseases into groups. This is used by Medicare Part A under the prospective payment system to determine the payment to hospitals for inpatient services. The prospective payment system involves payment of a fixed amount of money to the hospital, based on the patient's DRG. Like capitation, the DRG reimbursement is the total amount paid by Medicare for that particular hospitalization.
Fee-for-Service (FFS)	Payment mechanism in which a provider is paid for each service rendered to a patient. Payment may be made by either the insurer or by the patient.
Gatekeeper	Primary care or other health care provider who coordinates the utilization and delivery of medical services.
Health Maintenance Organization (HMO)	Managed care plan in which the patient must receive all medical services from within the plan's staff of employed providers or network of participating providers. Services outside of the HMO network are typically allowed only when similar services are not available by participating providers, in an emergency, or if the patient needs care outside of the plan's service area. Rules and regulations differ widely from plan to plan.
Managed Care Organization	Health insurance plan that relies on a gatekeeper to coordinate the utilization and delivery of medical services. The gatekeeper may be a nurse, clerk, or physician. Often, treatment approval algorithms are used by nonphysicians, with physician review as necessary.

Term	Definition, Common Use
Out-of-Network Provider	Provider who does not participate in the network of a managed care plan.
Participating Provider	Provider who contracts with a health insurance plan to provide medical services. The financial arrangement between patient, provider, and insurance plan varies with each individual plan.
Preferred Provider Organization (PPO)	Managed care plan in which the patient may receive medical services from the plan's network of participating providers, or may receive medical services from out-of-network providers. In the latter case, the patient may be responsible for a larger share of the bill.
Primary Care Provider (PCP)	Provider, often a general practitioner, family practitioner, or internist, responsible for the coordination and general medical care of a patient.
Provider	Hospital or health care facility, or a physician, nurse, physical therapist or other individual involved in providing medical care services to patients.

TABLE OF COMMONLY PRESCRIBED DRUGS—TRADE NAMES

Trade Name (®)	Generic Name	Type of Drug; Typical Uses
Abilify	Aripiprazole	Atypical antipsychotic drug indicated for the treatment of schizophrenia; sometimes used in the treatment of manic-depressive (bipolar) illness; hyperglycemia (elevated blood sugar), in some cases extreme, has been reported in patients treated with atypical antipsychotics
Accolate	Zafirlukast	Antiasthmatic; blocks action of leukotrienes, substances that cause airway inflammation in asthma
Accupril	Quinapril	Antihypertensive; works by inhibiting angiotensin converting enzyme (ACE; sometimes called ACE blockers), an enzyme that catalyzes the production of angiotensin II, a potent vasoconstrictor; common uses: congestive heart failure and hypertension
Actonel	Risedronate	Bisphosphonate drug that inhibits osteoclast-mediated bone resorption; used in the treatment of osteoporosis and to prevent development of osteoporosis-related fractures
Adalat	Nifedipine	Calcium channel blocker; blocks movement of calcium in various cells; common uses: angina, hypertension.
Adderall	Amphetamine Mixed Salts	Stimulant; common uses: attention deficit disorder
Advair	Fluticasone/ Salmeterol	Combination of inhaled steroid (fluticasone) and long-acting bronchodilator (salmeterol); the two act synergistically to improve lung function in asthma reducing the frequency of attacks, as well as the need for rescue inhaler use; intended for on-going treatment and prevention of symptoms, not as a rescue inhaler

Trade Name (®)	Generic Name	Type of Drug; Typical Uses
Agenerase	Amprenavir	Protease inhibitor—a class of anti-HIV drugs designed to inhibit the enzyme protease and interfere with virus replication; protease inhibitors prevent the cleavage of HIV precursor proteins into active proteins, a process that normally occurs when HIV replicates; used in therapy of AIDS and HIV infection
Alferon-N	Interferon	Antiviral protein that controls the immune response; naturally secreted by a virally infected cell; strengthens the defenses of nearby uninfected cells; the manufactured version is used for Kaposi sarcoma, hepatitis B, hepatitis C, and HIV infection
Allegra	Fexofenadine	Antihistamine; common uses: seasonal allergic rhinitis
Altace	Ramipril	Antihypertensive; works by inhibiting angiotensin converting enzyme (ACE; sometimes called ACE blockers), an enzyme that catalyzes the production of angiotensin II, a potent vasoconstrictor; common uses: congestive heart failure and hypertension
Amaryl	Glimepiride	Antidiabetic; oral blood-glucose-lowering drug of the sulfonylurea class; common uses: diabetes mellitus
Ambien	Zolpidem	Sedative hypnotic; common uses: insomnia
Amoxil	Amoxicillin	Antibiotic; common uses: various infections esp. *H. influenzae*
Anaprox	Naproxen sodium	Nonsteroidal anti-inflammatory (NSAID); common uses: arthritis, mild to moderate pain, various types of inflammation
Aricept	Donepezil	Reversible inhibitor of the enzyme acetylcholinesterase; indicated for the treatment of mild to moderate dementia of the Alzheimer's type (Alzheimer's disease)
Atacand	Candesartan	Antihypertensive; acts as angiotensin converting enzyme (ACE) inhibitor by blocking the specific angiotensin II AT_1 receptor subtype; common uses: hypertension, heart failure

Table of Commonly Prescribed Drugs — Trade Names (continued)

Trade Name (®)	Generic Name	Type of Drug; Typical Uses
Ativan	Lorazepam	Antianxiety; mild sedative; common uses: anxiety, insomnia
Atrovent	Ipratropium	Antiasthmatic; blocks parasympathetic receptors in lungs, leading to bronchodilation; common uses: asthma, chronic obstructive pulmonary disease (COPD)
Augmentin	Amoxicillin /Clavulanate	Antibiotic; common uses: various infections esp. upper respiratory
Axid	Nizatidine	Histamine blocker (H2); blocks H2 histamine receptors in the stomach, reducing the producing of gastric acid; common uses: acid/peptic disorder, esophageal reflux, peptic ulcer (gastric, duodenal)
Azmacort	Triamcinolone	Inhaled corticosteroid; common uses: asthma, COPD
Bactrim	Trimethoprim /Sulfa	Antibiotic; common uses: various infections esp. urinary tract
Bactroban	Mupirocin	Antibiotic ointment; used in impetigo
Biaxin	Clarithromycin	Antibiotic; common uses: various infections esp. upper respiratory, low grade pneumonia
BuSpar	Buspirone	Antianxiety; common uses: anxiety
Calan	Verapamil	Calcium channel blocker; blocks movement of calcium in various cells; common uses: angina, hypertension, cardiac dysrhythmias
Cardizem	Diltiazem	Calcium channel blocker; blocks movement of calcium in various cells; common uses: angina, hypertension, cardiac dysrhythmias
Cardura	Doxazosin	Mixed alpha receptor agonist/blocker; antihypertensive; used in benign prostatic hyperplasia (to increase urinary flow) and treat hypertension
Catapress	Clonidine	Antihypertensive; blocks alpha receptors of the autonomic nervous system; used in hypertension, also in narcotic withdrawal, Tourette's syndrome, attention deficit syndrome
Ceftin	Cefuroxime	Antibiotic; common uses: various moderate to severe infections

Trade Name (®)	Generic Name	Type of Drug; Typical Uses
Cefzil	Cefprozil	Antibiotic; common uses: various moderate to severe infections
Cialis	Tadalafil	Anti-impotence agent; indirectly enhances the action of nitric oxide (NO) in the corpus cavernosum of the penis, when combined with sexual stimulation, leading to inflow of blood and erection; this action, absent sexual stimulation, has no significant effect on erection; the mechanisms of tadalafil and organic nitrates (e.g., nitroglycerin) are similar; thus, the two drugs should never be given simultaneously; common uses: erectile dysfunction (male impotence; ED; a condition where the penis does not harden and expand when a man is sexually excited, or when he cannot keep an erection)
Cipro	Ciprofloxacin	Antibiotic; common uses: various infections esp. urinary tract, sexually transmitted diseases
Claritin	Loratadine	Antihistamine; common use: seasonal allergies
Claritin D 12HR	Loratidine/ Pseudoephedrine	Combination antihistamine (loratidine) and decongestant (pseudoephedrine); common use: seasonal allergies
Climara	Estradiol	Dermatologics (skin treatment); estrogens/progestins; common uses: vulvar/vaginal atrophy, breast cancer, prostate cancer, female hypogonadism, prevention of osteoporosis, ovarian failure, menopause
Clozaril	Clozapine	Atypical antipsychotic drug used in the treatment of schizophrenia; carries a significant risk of agranulocytosis (loss of infection-fighting granulocytes in the blood), a potentially life-threatening event; the drug should be reserved for severely ill patients with schizophrenia who fail to show an acceptable response to adequate courses of standard antipsychotic drug treatment or to reduce the risk of recurrent suicidal behavior; higher doses have also been associated with seizures; hyperglycemia (elevated blood sugar), in some cases extreme, has been reported in patients treated with atypical antipsychotics

Table of Commonly Prescribed Drugs — Trade Names (continued)

Trade Name (®)	Generic Name	Type of Drug; Typical Uses
Combivir	Zidovudine/ Lamivudine	Reverse transcriptase inhibitor—a drug that blocks viral replication by interfering with the reverse transcriptase enzyme, preventing synthesis of DNA from RNA; used in therapy of AIDS and HIV infection
Concerta	Methylphenidate	Amphetamine derivative; used in the treatment of attention deficit disorder (ADD)
Coumadin	Warfarin	Anticoagulant; common uses: prevention of recurrent blood clots
Cozaar	Losartan	Antihypertensive; acts as angiotensin converting enzyme (ACE) inhibitor by blocking the specific angiotensin II AT_1 receptor subtype; common use: hypertension
Crixivan	Indinavir	Protease inhibitor—a class of anti-HIV drugs designed to inhibit the enzyme protease and interfere with virus replication; protease inhibitors prevent the cleavage of HIV precursor proteins into active proteins, a process that normally occurs when HIV replicates; used in therapy of AIDS and HIV infection
Cymbalta	Duloxetine	Targets two chemicals, serotonin and norepinephrine, that are believed to play a role in how the brain and body affect mood and pain; indicated in the treatment of depression and the management of pain associated with diabetic peripheral neuropathy; sometimes used to treat bipolar disease
Cytovene	Gancyclovir	Interferes with viral synthesis of DNA; used in herpes virus infections
Darvocet N	Propoxyphene N/ Acetaminophen	Analgesic, narcotic; combination of the centrally acting narcotic analgesic agent, propoxyphene N and acetaminophen; common uses: mild to moderate pain
Daypro	Oxaprozin	Nonsteroidal anti-inflammatory (NSAID); common uses: arthritis, mild to moderate pain, various types of inflammation

Trade Name (®)	Generic Name	Type of Drug; Typical Uses
Deltasone	Prednisone	Adrenal corticosteroid; common uses: adrenal insufficiency, hemolytic anemia, inflammation (e.g., arthritis, bursitis), carditis, conjunctivitis, dermatitis, ulcerative colitis, enteritis, hypercalcemia, leukemia, allergic rhinitis, sarcoidosis, asthma, chronic obstructive pulmonary disease, thyroiditis, uveitis
Depakote	Valproic acid	Anticonvulsant; used in seizure disorders (epilepsy)
Desyrel	Trazodone	Antidepressant, serotonin-reuptake blocker; common use: depression
Detrol LA	Tolterodine	Blocks receptors in the parasympathetic nervous system, causing decreased contractions of the bladder; used in treatment of the treatment of overactive bladder with symptoms of urinary incontinence, urgency, and frequency
Diflucan	Fluconazole	Antifungal (synthetic) available for both oral and intravenous administration; common uses: candidiasis, cryptococcal meningitis; bone marrow transplantation adjunctive therapy
Dilantin	Phenytoin	Anticonvulsant; used in seizure disorders (epilepsy), occ. in cardiac dysrhythmias
Diovan	Valsartan	Antihypertensive; acts as angiotensin converting enzyme (ACE) inhibitor by blocking the specific angiotensin II AT_1 receptor subtype; common use: hypertension
Dyazide	Hydrochlorothiazide/ Triamterine	Antihypertensive; combination of the diuretic agents hydrochlorothiazide and triamterine; common uses: hypertension, edema
Effexor	Venlafaxine	Antidepressant; inhibits serotonin, norepinephrine, and dopamine reuptake; common uses: depression
Elavil	Amitriptyline	Tricyclic antidepressant; common uses: depression, enuresis, migraine headache prophylaxis

Table of Commonly Prescribed Drugs—Trade Names (continued)

Trade Name (®)	Generic Name	Type of Drug; Typical Uses
Endocet	Oxycodone/ Acetaminophen	Analgesic, narcotic; combination of the semisynthetic narcotic analgesic oxycodone (actions similar to those of morphine) and the nonnarcotic analgesic, acetaminophen; common uses: moderate to severe pain
Epivir	Lamivudine	Reverse transcriptase inhibitor—a drug that blocks viral replication by interfering with the reverse transcriptase enzyme, preventing synthesis of DNA from RNA; used in therapy of AIDS and HIV infection
Ery-Tab	Erythromycin	Antibiotic; common uses: various infections esp. upper respiratory
Esidrix	Hydrochloro-thiazide (HCTZ)	Antihypertensive, diuretic; exact antihypertensive mechanism unknown; hydrochlorothiazide increases excretion of sodium and chloride in approximately equivalent amounts; common uses: edema, hypertension
Estrace	Estradiol	Estrogen; common uses: vaginal/vulvar atrophy; breast/prostate cancer, female hypogonadism, menopause, osteoporosis prevention, ovarian failure, atrophic vaginitis
Estraderm	Estradiol	Estrogen; common uses: vaginal/vulvar atrophy; breast/prostate cancer, female hypogonadism, menopause, osteoporosis prevention, ovarian failure, atrophic vaginitis
Famvir	Famciclovir	Interferes with viral synthesis of DNA; use in herpes virus infections
Flexeril	Cyclobenzaprine	Antispasmodic; relieves skeletal muscle spasm of local origin without interfering with muscle function; ineffective in muscle spasm due to central nervous system disease; common uses: muscle spasm, esp. back or neck pain
Flonase	Fluticasone	Inhaled (nasal) corticosteroid; used in allergic rhinitis
Flovent	Fluticasone propionate	Inhaled corticosteroid; common uses: asthma, COPD
Flumadine	Rimantadine	Antiviral drug used to prevent or treat certain influenza (flu) infections (type A)

Trade Name (®)	Generic Name	Type of Drug; Typical Uses
Fortovase	Saquinavir	Protease inhibitor—a class of anti-HIV drugs designed to inhibit the enzyme protease and interfere with virus replication; protease inhibitors prevent the cleavage of HIV precursor proteins into active proteins, a process that normally occurs when HIV replicates; used in therapy of AIDS and HIV infection
Fosamax	Alendronate	Antiosteoporosis agent; acts as a specific inhibitor of osteoclast-mediated bone resorption; common uses: osteoporosis, Paget's disease
Geodon	Ziprasidone	Atypical antipsychotic indicated in the treatment of schizophrenia; sometimes used to treat bipolar disease; hyperglycemia (elevated blood sugar), in some cases extreme, has been reported in patients treated with atypical antipsychotics
Glucophage	Metformin	Antidiabetic; oral antihyperglycemic agent that improves glucose tolerance in non-insulin dependent patients; mechanisms of action are different from those of sulfonylureas; decreases hepatic glucose production, decreases intestinal absorption of glucose and improves insulin sensitivity (increases peripheral glucose uptake and utilization); rarely produces hypoglycemia in either diabetic or nondiabetic persons; common uses: non-insulin requiring diabetes mellitus
Glucotrol, Glucotrol XL	Glipizide	Antidiabetic; oral blood-glucose-lowering drug of the sulfonylurea class; common uses: non-insulin requiring diabetes mellitus
Hivid	Zalcitabine	Reverse transcriptase inhibitor—a drug that blocks viral replication by interfering with the reverse transcriptase enzyme, preventing synthesis of DNA from RNA; used in therapy of AIDS and HIV infection
Humulin N	Human Insulin-NPH	Blood glucose regulator; human recombinant NPH (intermediate-acting) insulin; used in diabetes mellitus

Table of Commonly Prescribed Drugs — Trade Names (continued)

Trade Name (®)	Generic Name	Type of Drug; Typical Uses
Humulin 70/30	Human Insulin 70/30	Blood glucose regulator; combinantion of human recombinant regular and NPH insulin; used in diabetes mellitus
Humulin R	Human Insulin Regular	Blood glucose regulator; human recombinant regular (short-acting) insulin; used in diabetes mellitus
Hytrin	Terazosin	Antihypertensive; mixed alpha receptor blocker and agonist; used in benign prostatic hyperplasia, hypertension
Hyzaar	Losartan/Hydrochlorothiazide	Antihypertensive, diuretic; combination of angiotensin II receptor (type AT_1) antagonist, losartan, and a diuretic, hydrochlorothiazide; common uses: edema, hypertension
Imdur	Isosorbide mononitrate	Antianginal, coronary vasodilator; an organic nitrate and the major biologically active metabolite of isosorbide dinitrate; vasodilator with effects on both arteries and veins; common uses: angina pectoris
Imitrex	Sumatriptan	Antimigraine; selective 5-hydroxytryptamine$_1$ receptor subtype agonist; common uses: migraine headache
Inderal	Propranolol	Antianginal, antiarrhythmics, antihypertensive, antimigraine, beta blocker; nonselective beta-adrenergic receptor blocking agent possessing no other autonomic nervous system activity; common uses: angina, arrhythmia, migraine headache, hypertension, pheochromocytoma, hypertrophic subaortic stenosis, tremor
K-Dur-20	Potassium chloride	Electrolyte supplement; oral replacement supplement for the essential mineral, potassium; uses: prevention/treatment of hypokalemia (low serum potassium), muscle cramps
Keflex	Cephalexin	Antibiotic; common uses: various infections esp. upper respiratory, skin

Trade Name (®)	Generic Name	Type of Drug; Typical Uses
Klonopin	Clonazepam	Antianxiety, anticonvulsant; enhances activity of gamma aminobutyric acid (GABA), the major inhibitory neurotransmitter in the central nervous system; common uses: anxiety, panic disorder, epilepsy
Klor-Con	Potassium chloride	Electrolyte supplement; oral replacement supplement for the essential mineral, potassium; uses: prevention/treatment of hypokalemia (low serum potassium), muscle cramps
Lamictal	Lamotrigine	Antiepileptic drug chemically unrelated to existing antiepileptic drugs; used in the treatment of seizure disorders and also, by some, to treat bipolar disorder; may result in life-threatening skin reactions
Lanoxin	Digoxin	Antiarrhythmic, cardiac glycoside; inhibits sodium-potassium ATPase, leading to an increase (by stimulation of sodium-calcium exchange) an increase in the intracellular concentration of calcium; the results are (1) an increase in the force and velocity of myocardial contraction (positive inotropic action); (2) a decrease in the degree of activation of the sympathetic nervous system and renin-angiotensin system (neurohormonal deactivating effect); and (3) slowing of the heart rate and decreased conduction velocity through the AV node (vagomimetic effect); common uses: atrial fibrillation (cardiac dysrhythmia), congestive heart failure (CHF)
Lasix	Furosemide	Antihypertensive, diuretic; common uses: edema, hypertension, pulmonary edema, congestive heart failure
Lescol	Fluvastatin	Antihyperlipidemic; inhibits HMG-CoA reductase, an enzyme that catalyzes an early and rate-limiting step in cholesterol biosynthesis; common uses: hypercholesterolemia, hyperlipidemia
Levaquin	Levofloxacin	Antibiotic; common uses: various infections esp. upper respiratory, urinary tract, skin

Table of Commonly Prescribed Drugs — Trade Names (continued)

Trade Name (®)	Generic Name	Type of Drug; Typical Uses
Levitra	Vardenafil	Anti-impotence agent; indirectly enhances the action of nitric oxide (NO) in the corpus cavernosum of the penis, when combined with sexual stimulation, leading to inflow of blood and erection; this action, absent sexual stimulation, has no significant effect on erection; the mechanisms of vardenafil and organic nitrates (e.g., nitroglycerin) are similar; thus, the two drugs should never be given simultaneously; common uses: erectile dysfunction (male impotence; ED; a condition where the penis does not harden and expand when a man is sexually excited, or when he cannot keep an erection)
Levoxyl	Levothyroxine	Thyroid medication; synthetic T4 (levothyroxine); common uses: goiter, hypothyroidism
Lipitor	Atorvastatin	Antihyperlipidemic; inhibits HMG-CoA reductase, an enzyme that catalyzes an early and rate-limiting step in cholesterol biosynthesis; common uses: hypercholesterolemia, hyperlipidemia
Lopid	Gemfibrozil	Antihyperlipidemic; lipid regulating agent that decreases serum triglycerides and very low density lipoprotein (VLDL) cholesterol, and increases high density lipoprotein (HDL) cholesterol; common uses: hypercholesterolemia, hyperlipidemia
LoPressor	Metoprolol succinate	Beta blocker, antihypertensive; beta$_1$-selective (cardioselective) adrenoceptor blocking agent for oral administration, available as extended release tablets; common uses: angina pectoris, hypertension
Lorabid	Loracarbef	Antibiotic; common uses: various infections esp. upper respiratory
Lotensin	Benazepril	Antihypertensive; works by inhibiting angiotensin converting enzyme (ACE; sometimes called ACE blockers), an enzyme that catalyzes the production of angiotensin II, a potent vasoconstrictor; common uses: congestive heart failure and hypertension

Trade Name (®)	Generic Name	Type of Drug; Typical Uses
Lotrel	Amlodipine/ Benazepril	Antihypertensive, ACE inhibitor; combination of calcium channel blocker amlodipine and ACE inhibitor benazepril; common uses: hypertension
Lotrisone	Clotrimoxazole/ Betamethasone	Antifungal; combination of clotrimazole, a synthetic antifungal agent, and betamethasone dipropionate, a synthetic corticosteroid, for dermatologic use; common uses: various forms of tinea-type rashes (e.g., *Tinea corporis*; *Tinea cruris*; *Tinea pedis*)
Macrobid	Nitrofurantoin	Antibiotic; common uses: urinary tract infections
Mevacor	Lovastatin	Antihyperlipidemic; inhibits HMG-CoA reductase, an enzyme that catalyzes an early and rate-limiting step in cholesterol biosynthesis; common uses: hypercholesterolemia, hyperlipidemia
Miacalcin	Calcitonin	Antiosteoporosis agent; synthetic calcitonin with same actions of mammalian calcitonin but more potent and with a greater duration of action; common uses: osteoporosis, Paget's disease
Micronase	Glyburide	Antidiabetic; oral blood-glucose-lowering drug of the sulfonylurea class; common uses: non-insulin requiring diabetes mellitus
Monopril	Fosinopril	Antihypertensive; works by inhibiting angiotensin converting enzyme (ACE; sometimes called ACE blockers), an enzyme that catalyzes the production of angiotensin II, a potent vasoconstrictor; common uses: congestive heart failure and hypertension
Motrin	Ibuprofen	Nonsteroidal anti-inflammatory (NSAID); common uses: arthritis, mild to moderate pain, various types of inflammation
Naproxyn	Naproxen	Nonsteroidal anti-inflammatory (NSAID); common uses: arthritis, mild to moderate pain, various types of inflammation

Table of Commonly Prescribed Drugs—Trade Names (continued)

Trade Name (®)	Generic Name	Type of Drug; Typical Uses
Neurontin	Gabapentin	Anticonvulsant; mechanism of action not known; common use: epilepsy, partial seizures
Nitrostat	Nitroglycerin	Antianginal, antihypertensive, coronary vasodilator; causes relaxation of vascular smooth muscle, primarily in veins and coronary arteries; common uses: angina, congestive heart failure, myocardial infarction, hypertension
Nolvadex	Tamoxifen	Antineoplastic (anticancer); nonsteroidal estrogen receptor binding agent; common uses: breast cancer
Norvasc	Amlodipine	Long-acting blocker; blocks movement of calcium in various cells; common uses: angina, hypertension
Norvir	Ritonavir	Protease inhibitor—a class of anti-HIV drugs designed to inhibit the enzyme protease and interfere with virus replication; protease inhibitors prevent the cleavage of HIV precursor proteins into active proteins, a process that normally occurs when HIV replicates; used in therapy of AIDS and HIV infection
OxyContin	Oxycodone	Pain medication containing oxycodone, a very strong narcotic pain reliever similar to morphine; designed so that the oxycodone is slowly released over time, allowing twice daily administration; the drug is intended to help relieve pain that is moderate to severe in intensity, when that pain is present all the time, and expected to continue for a long time; this level of pain severity may be caused by a variety of different medical conditions (e.g., metastatic cancer); has a very high abuse potential because breaking, chewing, or crushing the tablet causes a large amount of oxycodone to be released from the tablet all at once, causing a "high," and potentially resulting in a dangerous or fatal drug overdose
Paxil	Paroxetine	Antidepressant; blocks neuronal reuptake of serotonin; common uses: anxiety, panic disorder, depression, obsessive-compulsive disorder

Trade Name (®)	Generic Name	Type of Drug; Typical Uses
Pepcid	Famotidine	Histamine blocker (H2); blocks H2 histamine receptors in the stomach, reducing the producing of gastric acid; common uses: acid/peptic disorder, esophageal reflux, peptic ulcer (gastric, duodenal)
Percocet	Oxycodone/ Acetaminophen	Pain medication for moderate to severe pain of short duration (e.g., postsurgical). The potential for abuse and addiction exists, as with OxyContin, but is somewhat less since Percocet is not a sustained-release (long-acting) preparation; the combination of oxycodone and acetaminophen is synergistic—their combined effect is greater than the sum of either alone
Percodan	Oxycodone/ Aspirin	Pain medication for moderate to severe pain of short duration (e.g., postsurgical). The potential for abuse and addiction exists, as with OxyContin, but is somewhat less since Percodan is not a sustained-release (long-acting) preparation; the combination of oxycodone and aspirin is synergistic—their combined effect is greater than the sum of either alone
Phenergan	Promethazine	Antiemetic, antihistamine, antitussive; phenothiazine derivative, possesses antihistaminic, sedative, antimotion-sickness, antiemetic effects; common uses: anaphylaxis, allergies, motion sickness, nausea, vomiting, hives, mild sedation
Plendil	Felodipine	Antihypertensive, calcium channel blocker; blocks movement of calcium in various cells; common uses: hypertension
Pravachol	Pravastatin	Antihyperlipidemic; inhibits HMG-CoA reductase, an enzyme that catalyzes an early and rate-limiting step in cholesterol biosynthesis; common uses: hypercholesterolemia, hyperlipidemia

Table of Commonly Prescribed Drugs—Trade Names (continued)

Trade Name (®)	Generic Name	Type of Drug; Typical Uses
Precose	Acarbose	An oral agent that blocks the pancreatic enzyme alpha-glucosidase (breaks down sugars) resulting in delayed glucose absorption; this minimizes the rise in blood sugar after eating; used in the management of type 2 diabetes mellitus
Premarin	Conjugated estrogens	Adrenal corticosteroid; common uses: breast/prostate cancer, female hypogonadism, menopause, osteoporosis, ovarian failure, atrophic vaginitis
Prempro	Conjugated Estrogens/ Medroxy-progesterone	Adrenal corticosteroid; combination of conjugated estrogens and medroxy-progesterone acetate, a derivative of progesterone; common uses: menopause, osteoporosis, atrophic vaginitis
Prevacid	Lansoprazole	Antigastric secretory agent; suppresses gastric acid secretion by specific inhibition of an enzyme system at the surface of the gastric parietal cell (manufactures and secretes hydrochloric acid), blocking the final step of acid production; common uses: acid/peptic disorder, erosive esophagitis, duodenal ulcer, Zollinger-Ellison syndrome
Prilosec	Omeprazole	Antigastric secretory agent; suppresses gastric acid secretion by specific inhibition of an enzyme system at the surface of the gastric parietal cell (manufactures and secretes hydrochloric acid), blocking the final step of acid production; common uses: acid/peptic disorder, erosive esophagitis, duodenal ulcer, Zollinger-Ellison syndrome
Prinivil	Lisinopril	Antihypertensive; works by inhibiting angiotensin converting enzyme (ACE; sometimes called ACE blockers), an enzyme that catalyzes the production of angiotensin II, a potent vasoconstrictor; common uses: hypertension.
Procardia	Nifedipine	Calcium channel blocker; blocks movement of calcium in various cells; common uses: angina, hypertension

Table of Commonly Prescribed Drugs — Trade Names (continued)

Trade Name (®)	Generic Name	Type of Drug; Typical Uses
Propacet	Propoxyphene N/ Acetaminophen	Analgesic, narcotic; combination of the centrally acting narcotic analgesic agent, propoxyphene N and acetaminophen; common uses: mild to moderate pain
Propulsid	Cisapride	Antireflux agent; increases muscle tone of the sphincter between the esophagus and stomach, reducing acid reflux; common uses: gastrointestinal reflux
Proventil	Albuterol	Antiasthmatic/bronchodilator; relatively selective beta$_2$-adrenergic bronchodilator; common uses: acute exacerbations of asthma, chronic obstructive pulmonary disease (COPD)
Provera	Medroxy-progesterone	Progestin, contraceptive; derivative of progesterone active by both parenteral and oral routes of administration; common uses: amenorrhea, endometrial cancer, renal cancer, contraception, uterine hemorrhage
Prozac	Fluoxetine	Antidepressant, serotonin-reuptake blocker; common use: depression
Rebetron	Ribavirin/ Interferon	Combination of the antiviral drugs ribavirin and interferon; used in treatment of chronic hepatitis; the combination of ribavirin and interferon is synergistic — their combined effect is greater than the sum of either alone
Relafen	Nabumetone	Anti-inflammatory; nonsteroidal anti-inflammatory agent; common uses: arthritis (osteoarthritis, rheumatoid)
Relenza	Zanamivir	An antiviral drug, for persons aged 7 years and older for the treatment of uncomplicated influenza (flu) virus; this product is approved to treat type A and B influenza, the two types most responsible for flu epidemics; clinical studies showed that for the drug to be effective, patients needed to start treatment within two days of the onset of symptoms

Table of Commonly Prescribed Drugs—Trade Names (continued)

Trade Name (®)	Generic Name	Type of Drug; Typical Uses
Rescriptor	Delavirdine	Reverse transcriptase inhibitor—a drug that blocks viral replication by interfering with the reverse transcriptase enzyme, preventing synthesis of DNA from RNA; used in therapy of AIDS and HIV infection
Restoril	Temazepam	Sedative/hypnotic; benzodiazepine hypnotic agent; common uses: insomnia
Retin-A	Tretinoin	Acne products; retinoic acid (vitamin A acid) cream; common use: acne vulgaris
Retrovir	Zidovudine	Reverse transcriptase inhibitor—a drug that blocks viral replication by interfering with the reverse transcriptase enzyme, preventing synthesis of DNA from RNA; used in therapy of AIDS and HIV infection
Rezulin	Troglitazone	Antidiabetic; oral antihyperglycemic agent that acts primarily by decreasing insulin resistance; common uses: diabetes mellitus; rare cases of severe liver injury have been reported
Rhinocort	Budesonide	Adrenal corticosteroid (nasally inhaled); anti-inflammatory action; common uses: rhinitis (allergic and nonallergic)
Risperdal	Risperidone	Antipsychotics/antimanics; antipsychotic agent belonging to a new chemical class, the benzisoxazole derivatives, thought to work through a combination of dopamine type 2 (D_2) and serotonin type 2 ($5HT_2$) antagonism; common uses: psychosis, schizophrenia
Ritalin	Methylphenidate	Amphetamine derivative; used in the treatment of attention deficit disorder (ADD)
Septra	Trimethoprim/ Sulfamethoxazole	Antibiotic; common uses: various infections esp. urinary tract
Serevent	Salmeterol	Antiasthmatic; long-acting highly selective beta$_2$-adrenergic bronchodilator; common uses: prevention of asthma attacks; not indicated for emergency treatment of an acute exacerbation

Table of Commonly Prescribed Drugs—Trade Names (continued)

Trade Name (®)	Generic Name	Type of Drug; Typical Uses
Seroquel	Quetiapine	Psychotropic agent that blocks numerous neurotransmitter receptor sites in the brain; used to treat acute manic episodes associated with bipolar disorder
Serzone	Nefazodone	Antidepression; inhibits neuronal uptake of serotonin and norepinephrine; common uses: depression
Soma	Carisoprodol	Antispasmodic, particularly of skeletal muscle; used in muscle spasm of various types, esp. back pain
Spiriva	Tiotropium	Inhaled blocker of certain parasympathetic nervous system receptors in the lungs, leading to bronchodilation; used in the treatment of asthma—not intended for use as a rescue inhaler
Straterra	Atomoxetine	Selective norepinephrine (a neurotransmitter) reuptake inhibitor; indicated for the treatment of attention deficit disorder (ADD) in children, adolescents, and adults; recently, the FDA issued a Health Advisory requiring the manufacturer to add a black box warning that the drug could increase suicidal thoughts among youths
Sumycin	Tetracycline	Antibiotic; common uses: various infections esp. skin, sexually transmitted diseases
Sustiva	Efavirenz	Reverse transcriptase inhibitor—a drug that blocks viral replication by interfering with the reverse transcriptase enzyme, preventing synthesis of DNA from RNA; used in therapy of AIDS and HIV infection
Symmetrel	Amantadine	Antiviral drug used to prevent or treat certain influenza (flu) infections (type A); will not work for colds, other types of flu, or other virus infections
Synagis	Palivizumab	Antiviral drug indicated for the prevention of serious lower respiratory tract disease caused by respiratory syncytial virus (RSV) in pediatric patients at high risk of RSV disease
Synthroid	Levothyroxine	Thyroid medication; synthetic T4 (levothyroxine); common uses: goiter, hypothyroidism

Table of Commonly Prescribed Drugs — Trade Names (continued)

Trade Name (®)	Generic Name	Type of Drug; Typical Uses
Tagamet	Cimetidine	Histamine blocker (H2); blocks H2 histamine receptors in the stomach, reducing the production of gastric acid; common uses: acid/peptic disorder, esophageal reflux, peptic ulcer (gastric, duodenal)
Tamiflu	Oseltamivir	Oral antiviral drug for the treatment of uncomplicated influenza (flu) in patients one year and older whose flu symptoms have not lasted more than two days; this product is approved to treat type A and B influenza; also approved for the prevention of influenza in adults and adolescents older than 13 years
Tenormin	Atenolol	Antianginal, antihypertensive, beta blocker; synthetic, beta$_1$-selective (cardioselective) adrenoreceptor blocking agent; common uses: angina pectoris, hypertension, myocardial infarction
Timoptic	Timolol	Beta blocker; nonselective beta-adrenergic antagonist for ocular use; common uses: glaucoma
Tobradex	Tobramycin/ Dexamethasone	Antibiotic; combination creme of the aminoglycoside antibiotic tobramycin and the potent anti-inflammatory corticosteroid, dexamethasone; common uses: burns, conjunctivitis, dermatitis with secondary infection, foreign body, eye trauma, uveitis
Toprol	Metoprolol succinate	Beta blocker, antihypertensive; beta$_1$-selective (cardioselective) adrenoceptor blocking agent, for oral administration, available as extended release tablets; common uses: angina pectoris, hypertension
Trimox	Amoxicillin	Antibiotic; common uses: various infections esp. upper respiratory, urinary tract
Tylenol #3	Acetaminophen/ Codeine	Analgesic, narcotic; combination of the narcotic analgesic codeine with the nonnarcotic analgesic, acetaminophen; common uses: moderate to moderately severe pain

Table of Commonly Prescribed Drugs—Trade Names (continued)

Trade Name (®)	Generic Name	Type of Drug; Typical Uses
Ultram	Tramadol	Analgesic, nonnarcotic; centrally acting synthetic analgesic; mode of action not completely understood; common uses: pain, moderate to moderately severe
Valium	Diazepam	Antianxiety; mild sedative; common uses: anxiety, insomnia
Valtrex	Valacyclovir	Interferes with viral synthesis of DNA; use in herpes virus infections
Vancenase	Beclomethasone	Inhaled corticosteroid; common uses: asthma, chronic obstructive pulmonary disease (COPD)
Vasotec	Enalapril	Antihypertensive; works by inhibiting angiotensin converting enzyme (ACE; sometimes called ACE blockers), an enzyme that catalyzes the production of angiotensin II, a potent vasoconstrictor; common uses: congestive heart failure and hypertension
Veetids	Penicillin VK	Antibiotic; common uses: various infections esp. upper respiratory
Ventolin	Albuterol	Antiasthmatic/bronchodilator; relatively selective $beta_2$-adrenergic bronchodilator; common uses: acute exacerbations of asthma and chronic obstructive pulmonary disease (COPD)

TABLE OF COMMONLY PRESCRIBED DRUGS—GENERIC NAMES

Generic Name	Trade Name (®)	Type of Drug; Typical Uses
Abacavir	Ziagen	Reverse transcriptase inhibitor—a drug that blocks viral replication by interfering with the reverse transcriptase enzyme, preventing synthesis of DNA from RNA; used in therapy of AIDS and HIV infection
Acarbose	Precose	An oral agent that blocks the pancreatic enzyme alpha-glucosidase (breaks down sugars) resulting in delayed glucose absorption; this minimizes the rise in blood sugar after eating; used in the management of type 2 diabetes mellitus
Acetaminophen /Codeine	Tylenol #3	Analgesic, narcotic; combination of the narcotic analgesic codeine with the nonnarcotic analgesic, acetaminophen; common uses: moderate to moderately severe pain
Acyclovir	Zovirax	Interferes with viral synthesis of DNA; use in herpes virus infections
Albuterol	Proventil, Ventolin	Anti-asthmatic/bronchodilator; relatively selective beta$_2$-adrenergic bronchodilator; common uses: acute exacerbations of asthma, chronic obstructive pulmonary disease (COPD)
Alendronate	Fosamax	Antiosteoporosis agent; acts as a specific inhibitor of osteoclast-mediated bone resorption; common uses: osteoporosis, Paget's disease
Alprazolam	Xanax	Antianxiety agent; benzodiazepine class; common uses: anxiety, panic disorder
Amantadine	Symmetrel	Antiviral drug used to prevent or treat certain influenza (flu) infections (type A); will not work for colds, other types of flu, or other virus infections
Amitriptyline	Elavil	Tricyclic antidepressant; common uses: depression, enuresis, migraine headache prophylaxis

Table of Commonly Prescribed Drugs—Generic Names (continued)

Generic Name	Trade Name (®)	Type of Drug; Typical Uses
Amlodipine/ Benazepril	Lotrel	Antihypertensive, ACE inhibitor, combination of calcium channel blocker amlodipine and ACE inhibitor benazepril; common uses: hypertension
Amlodipine	Norvasc	Long-acting blocker; blocks movement of calcium in various cells; common uses: angina, hypertension
Amoxicillin	Amoxil, Trimox	Antibiotic; common uses: various infections esp. *H. influenzae*
Amoxicillin/ Clavulanate	Augmentin	Antibiotic; common uses: various infections esp. upper respiratory
Amphetamine Mixed Salts	Adderall	Stimulant; common uses: attention deficit disorder
Amprenavir	Agenerase	Protease inhibitor—a class of anti-HIV drugs designed to inhibit the enzyme protease and interfere with virus replication; protease inhibitors prevent the cleavage of HIV precursor proteins into active proteins, a process that normally occurs when HIV replicates; used in therapy of AIDS and HIV infection
Aripiprazole	Abilify	Atypical antipsychotic drug indicated for the treatment of schizophrenia; sometimes used in the treatment of manic-depressive (bipolar) illness; hyperglycemia (elevated blood sugar), in some cases extreme, has been reported in patients treated with atypical antipsychotics
Atenolol	Tenormin	Antianginal, antihypertensive, beta blocker; synthetic, $beta_1$-selective (cardioselective) adrenoreceptor blocking agent; common uses: angina pectoris, hypertension, myocardial infarction
Atomoxetine	Straterra	Selective norepinephrine (a neurotransmitter) reuptake inhibitor; indicated for the treatment of attention deficit disorder (ADD) in children, adolescents, and adults; recently, the FDA issued a Health Advisory requiring the manufacturer to add a black box warning that the drug could increase suicidal thoughts among youths

Table of Commonly Prescribed Drugs— Generic Names (continued)

Generic Name	Trade Name (®)	Type of Drug; Typical Uses
Atorvastatin	Lipitor	Antihyperlipidemic; inhibits HMG-CoA reductase, an enzyme that catalyzes an early and rate-limiting step in cholesterol biosynthesis; common uses: hypercholesterolemia, hyperlipidemia
Azithromycin	Zithromax	Antibiotic; common uses: various infections, esp. upper respiratory tract
Beclomethasone	Vancenase	Inhaled corticosteroid; common uses: asthma, chronic obstructive pulmonary disease (COPD)
Benazepril	Lotensin	Antihypertensive; works by inhibiting angiotensin converting enzyme (ACE; sometimes called ACE blockers), an enzyme that catalyzes the production of angiotensin II, a potent vasoconstrictor; common uses: congestive heart failure and hypertension
Bisoprolol/ Hydrochloro-thiazide	Ziac	Antihypertensive; combination of the synthetic beta$_1$-selective (cardioselective) adrenoceptor blocking agent (bisoprolol fumarate) and the diuretic hydrochlorothiazide; common uses: hypertension
Budesonide	Rhinocort	Adrenal corticosteroid (nasally inhaled); anti-inflammatory action; common uses: rhinitis (allergic and nonallergic)
Bupropion	Wellbutrin, Zyban	Antidepressant; mechanism of action unknown; common uses: depression, smoking cessation
Buspirone	BuSpar	Antianxiety; common uses: anxiety
Calcitonin	Miacalcin	Antiosteoporosis agent; synthetic calcitonin with same actions of mammalian calcitonin but more potent and with a greater duration of action; common uses: osteoporosis, Paget's disease
Candesartan	Atacand	Antihypertensive; acts as angiotensin converting enzyme (ACE) inhibitor by blocking the specific angiotensin II AT$_1$ receptor subtype; common uses: hypertension, heart failure
Carisoprodol	Soma	Antispasmodic, particularly of skeletal muscle; used in muscle spasm of various types, esp. back pain

Table of Commonly Prescribed Drugs— Generic Names (continued)

Generic Name	Trade Name (®)	Type of Drug; Typical Uses
Cefprozil	Cefzil	Antibiotic; common uses: various moderate to severe infections
Cefuroxime	Ceftin	Antibiotic; common uses: various moderate to severe infections
Celecoxib	Celebrex	Nonsteroidal anti-inflammatory drug that works somewhat differently from older agents (e.g., ibuprofen, naproxen) often resulting in a significantly decreased risk of stomach irritation and gastrointestinal bleeding; common uses: osteoarthritis, rheumatoid arthritis
Cephalexin	Keflex	Antibiotic; common uses: various infections esp. upper respiratory, skin
Cimetidine	Tagamet	Histamine blocker (H2); blocks H2 histamine receptors in the stomach, reducing the production of gastric acid; common uses: acid/peptic disorder, esophageal reflux, peptic ulcer (gastric, duodenal)
Ciprofloxacin	Cipro	Antibiotic; common uses: various infections esp. urinary tract, sexually transmitted diseases
Cisapride	Propulsid	Antireflux agent; increases muscle tone of the sphincter between the esophagus and stomach, reducing acid reflux; common uses: gastrointestinal reflux
Clarithromycin	Biaxin	Antibiotic; common uses: various infections esp. upper respiratory, low grade pneumonia
Clonazepam	Klonopin	Antianxiety, anticonvulsant; enhances activity of gamma aminobutyric acid (GABA), the major inhibitory neurotransmitter in the central nervous system; common uses: anxiety, panic disorder, epilepsy
Clonidine	Catapress	Antihypertensive; blocks alpha receptors of the autonomic nervous system; used in hypertension; also in narcotic withdrawal, Tourette's syndrome, attention deficit syndrome

Table of Commonly Prescribed Drugs—Generic Names (continued)

Generic Name	Trade Name (®)	Type of Drug; Typical Uses
Clotrimoxazole/ Betamethasone	Lotrisone	Antifungal; combination of clotrimazole, a synthetic antifungal agent, and besonezone tamethasone dipropionate, a synthetic corticosteroid, for dermatologic use; common uses: various forms of tinea-type rashes (e.g., *Tinea corporis, Tinea cruris, Tinea pedis*)
Clozapine	Clozaril	Atypical antipsychotic drug used in the treatment of schizophrenia; carries a significant risk of agranulocytosis (loss of infection-fighting granulocytes in the blood), a potentially life-threatening event; the drug should be reserved for severely ill patients with schizophrenia who fail to show an acceptable response to adequate courses of standard antipsychotic drug treatment or to reduce the risk of recurrent suicidal behavior; higher doses have also been associated with seizures; hyperglycemia (elevated blood sugar), in some cases extreme, has been reported in patients treated with atypical antipsychotics
Conjugated Estrogens	Premarin	Adrenal corticosteroid; common uses: breast/prostate cancer, female hypogonadism, menopause, osteoporosis, ovarian failure, atrophic vaginitis
Conjugated Estrogens/ Medroxy progesterone	Prempro	Adrenal corticosteroid; combination of conjugated estrogens and medroxyprogesterone acetate, a derivative of progesterone; common uses: menopause, osteoporosis, atrophic vaginitis
Cyclobenzaprine	Flexeril	Antispasmodic; relieves skeletal muscle spasm of local origin without interfering with muscle function; ineffective in muscle spasm due to central nervous system disease; common uses: muscle spasm, esp. back or neck pain
Delavirdine	Rescriptor	Reverse transcriptase inhibitor—a drug that blocks viral replication by interfering with the reverse transcriptase enzyme, preventing synthesis of DNA from RNA; used in therapy of AIDS and HIV infection

Table of Commonly Prescribed Drugs — Generic Names (continued)

Generic Name	Trade Name (®)	Type of Drug; Typical Uses
Diazepam	Valium	Antianxiety; mild sedative; common uses: anxiety, insomnia
Didanosine	Videx	Reverse transcriptase inhibitor — a drug that blocks viral replication by interfering with the reverse transcriptase enzyme, preventing synthesis of DNA from RNA; used in therapy of AIDS and HIV infection
Digoxin	Lanoxin	Antiarrhythmic, cardiac glycoside; inhibits sodium-potassium ATPase, leading to an increase (by stimulation of sodium-calcium exchange) an increase in the intracellular concentration of calcium; the results are (1) an increase in the force and velocity of myocardial contraction (positive inotropic action); (2) a decrease in the degree of activation of the sympathetic nervous system and renin-angiotensin system (neurohormonal deactivating effect); and (3) slowing of the heart rate and decreased conduction velocity through the AV node (vagomimetic effect); common uses: atrial fibrillation (cardiac dysrhythmia), congestive heart failure (CHF)
Diltiazem	Cardizem	Calcium channel blocker; blocks movement of calcium in various cells; common uses: angina, hypertension, cardiac dysrhythmias
Donepezil	Aricept	Reversible inhibitor of the enzyme acetylcholinesterase; indicated for the treatment of mild to moderate dementia of the Alzheimer's type (Alzheimer's disease)
Doxazosin	Cardura	Mixed alpha receptor agonist/blocker; antihypertensive; used in benign prostatic hyperplasia (to increase urinary flow) and to treat hypertension
Duloxetine	Cymbalta	Targets two chemicals, serotonin and norepinephrine, that are believed to play a role in how the brain and body affect mood and pain; indicated in the treatment of depression and the management of pain associated with diabetic peripheral neuropathy; sometimes used to treat bipolar disease

Table of Commonly Prescribed Drugs—Generic Names (continued)

Generic Name	Trade Name (®)	Type of Drug; Typical Uses
Efavirenz	Sustiva	Reverse transcriptase inhibitor—a drug that blocks viral replication by interfering with the reverse transcriptase enzyme, preventing synthesis of DNA from RNA; used in therapy of AIDS and HIV infection
Enalapril	Vasotec	Antihypertensive; works by inhibiting angiotensin converting enzyme (ACE; sometimes called ACE blockers), an enzyme that catalyzes the production of angiotensin II, a potent vasoconstrictor; common uses: congestive heart failure and hypertension
Erythromycin	Ery-Tab	Antibiotic; common uses: various infections esp. upper respiratory
Estradiol	Climara, Estraderm, Estrace	Dermatologics (skin treatment); estrogens/progestins; common uses: vulvar/vaginal atrophy; breast cancer, prostate cancer, female hypogonadism, prevention of osteoporosis, ovarian failure, menopause
Famciclovir	Famvir	Interferes with viral synthesis of DNA; use in herpes virus infections
Famotidine	Pepcid	Histamine blocker (H2); blocks H2 histamine receptors in the stomach, reducing the producing of gastric acid; common uses: acid/peptic disorder, esophageal reflux, peptic ulcer (gastric, duodenal)
Felodipine	Plendil	Antihypertensive, calcium channel blocker; blocks movement of calcium in various cells; common uses: hypertension
Fexofenadine	Allegra	Antihistamine; common uses: seasonal allergic rhinitis
Fluconazole	Diflucan	Antifungal (synthetic) available for both oral and intravenous administration; common uses: candidiasis, cryptococcal meningitis; bone marrow transplantation adjunctive therapy
Fluoxetine	Prozac	Antidepressant, serotonin-reuptake blocker; common use: depression
Fluticasone	Flonase	Inhaled (nasal) corticosteroid; used in allergic rhinitis

Table of Commonly Prescribed Drugs — Generic Names (continued)

Generic Name	Trade Name (®)	Type of Drug; Typical Uses
Fluticasone/ Salmeterol	Advair	Combination of inhaled steroid (fluticasone) and long-acting bronchodilator (salmeterol); the two act synergistically to improve lung function in asthma reducing the frequency of attacks, as well as the need for rescue inhaler use; intended for on-going treatment and prevention of symptoms, not as a rescue inhaler
Fluticasone propionate	Flovent	Inhaled corticosteroid; common uses: asthma, COPD
Fluvastatin	Lescol	Antihyperlipidemic; inhibits HMG-CoA reductase, an enzyme that catalyzes an early and rate-limiting step in cholesterol biosynthesis; common uses: hypercholesterolemia, hyperlipidemia
Fosinopril	Monopril	Antihypertensive; works by inhibiting angiotensin converting enzyme (ACE; sometimes called ACE blockers), an enzyme that catalyzes the production of angiotensin II, a potent vasoconstrictor; common uses: congestive heart failure and hypertension
Furosemide	Lasix	Antihypertensive, diuretic; common uses: edema, hypertension, pulmonary edema, congestive heart failure
Gabapentin	Neurontin	Anticonvulsant; mechanism of action not known; common use: epilepsy, partial seizures
Gancyclovir	Cytovene	Interferes with viral synthesis of DNA; use in herpes virus infections
Gemfibrozil	Lopid	Antihyperlipidemic; lipid regulating agent which decreases serum triglycerides and very low density lipoprotein (VLDL) cholesterol, and increases high density lipoprotein (HDL) cholesterol; common uses: hypercholesterolemia, hyperlipidemia
Glimepiride	Amaryl	Antidiabetic; oral blood-glucose-lowering drug of the sulfonylurea class; common uses: diabetes mellitus
Glipizide	Glucotrol XL, Glucotrol	Antidiabetic; oral blood-glucose-lowering drug of the sulfonylurea class; common uses: non-insulin requiring diabetes mellitus

Table of Commonly Prescribed Drugs — Generic Names (continued)

Generic Name	Trade Name (®)	Type of Drug; Typical Uses
Glyburide	Micronase	Antidiabetic; oral blood-glucose-lowering drug of the sulfonylurea class; common uses: non-insulin requiring diabetes mellitus
Human Insulin 70/30	Humulin 70/30	Blood glucose regulator; combinantion of human recombinant regular and NPH insulin; used in diabetes mellitus
Human Insulin-NPH	Humulin N	Blood glucose regulator; human recombinant NPH (intermediate-acting) insulin; used in diabetes mellitus
Human Insulin Regular	Humulin R	Blood glucose regulator; human recombinant regular (short-acting) insulin; used in diabetes mellitus
Hydrochloro-thiazide/ Triamterine	Dyazide	Antihypertensive; combination of the diuretic agents hydrochlorothiazide and triamterine; common uses: hypertension, edema
Hydrochloro-thiazide (HCTZ)	Esidrix	Antihypertensive, diuretic; exact antihypertensive mechanism unknown; hydrochlorothiazide increases excretion of sodium and chloride in approximately equivalent amounts; common uses: edema, hypertension
Hydrocodone w/Acetaminophen	Vicodin	Analgesic, narcotic; combination of the narcotic analgesic hydrocodone with the nonnarcotic analgesic, acetaminophen; common uses: moderate to moderately severe pain
Ibuprofen	Motrin	Nonsteroidal anti-inflammatory (NSAID); common uses: arthritis, mild to moderate pain, various types of inflammation
Indinavir	Crixivan	Protease inhibitor—a class of anti-HIV drugs designed to inhibit the enzyme protease and interfere with virus replication; protease inhibitors prevent the cleavage of HIV precursor proteins into active proteins, a process that normally occurs when HIV replicates; used in therapy of AIDS and HIV infection

Table of Commonly Prescribed Drugs — Generic Names (continued)

Generic Name	Trade Name (®)	Type of Drug; Typical Uses
Interferon	Alferon-N	Antiviral protein that controls the immune response. Naturally secreted by a virally infected cell; strengthens the defenses of nearby uninfected cells; the manufactured version is used for Kaposi sarcoma, hepatitis B, hepatitis C, and HIV infection
Ipratropium	Atrovent	Antiasthmatic; blocks parasympathetic receptors in lungs, leading to bronchodilation; common uses: asthma, chronic obstructive pulmonary disease (COPD)
Isosorbide mononitrate	Imdur	Antianginal, coronary vasodilator; an organic nitrate and the major biologically active metabolite of isosorbide dinitrate; vasodilator with effects on both arteries and veins; common uses: angina pectoris
Lamivudine	Epivir	Reverse transcriptase inhibitor — a drug that blocks viral replication by interfering with the reverse transcriptase enzyme, preventing synthesis of DNA from RNA; used in therapy of AIDS and HIV infection
Lamotrigine	Lamictal	Antiepileptic drug chemically unrelated to existing antiepileptic drugs; used in the treatment of seizure disorders and also, by some, to treat bipolar disorder; may result in life-threatening skin reactions
Lansoprazole	Prevacid	Antigastric secretory agent; suppresses gastric acid secretion by specific inhibition of an enzyme system at the surface of the gastric parietal cell (manufactures and secretes hydrochloric acid), blocking the final step of acid production; common uses: acid/peptic disorder, erosive esophagitis, duodenal ulcer, Zollinger-Ellison syndrome

Table of Commonly Prescribed Drugs— Generic Names (continued)

Generic Name	Trade Name (®)	Type of Drug; Typical Uses
Latanoprost	Xalatan	Antiglaucoma agent; selective analogue of prostaglandin F_{2alpha} which is believed to reduce the intraocular pressure by increasing the outflow of aqueous humor; may gradually change eye color, increasing the amount of brown pigment in the iris by increasing the number of melanosomes (pigment granules) in melanocytes; long-term effects of deposition of pigment granules to other areas of the eye is currently unknown; common uses: glaucoma
Levofloxacin	Levaquin	Antibiotic; common uses: various infections esp. upper respiratory, urinary tract, skin
Levothyroxine	Levoxyl, Synthroid	Thyroid medication; synthetic T4 (levothyroxine); common uses: goiter, hypothyroidism
Lisinopril	Prinivil, Zestril	Antihypertensive; works by inhibiting angiotensin converting enzyme (ACE; sometimes called ACE blockers), an enzyme that catalyzes the production of angiotensin II, a potent vasoconstrictor; common uses: hypertension.
Lisinopril/ Hydrochloro- thiazide	Zestoretic	Antihypertensive; combination of the diuretic hydrochlorothiazide and lisinopril; lisinopril works by inhibiting angiotensin converting enzyme (ACE; sometimes called ACE blockers), an enzyme that catalyzes the production of angiotensin II, a potent vasoconstrictor; common uses: congestive heart failure and hypertension
Loracarbef	Lorabid	Antibiotic; common uses: various infections esp. upper respiratory
Loratadine	Claritin	Antihistamine; common use: seasonal allergies
Loratidine/ Pseudoephedrine	Claritin D 12HR	Combination antihistamine (loratidine) and decongestant (pseudoephedrine); common use: seasonal allergies
Lorazepam	Ativan	Antianxiety; mild sedative; common uses: anxiety, insomnia

Table of Commonly Prescribed Drugs— Generic Names (continued)

Generic Name	Trade Name (®)	Type of Drug; Typical Uses
Losartan	Cozaar	Antihypertensive; acts as angiotensin converting enzyme (ACE) inhibitor by blocking the specific angiotensin II AT_1 receptor subtype; common use: hypertension
Losartan/ Hydrochloro- thiazide	Hyzaar	Antihypertensive, diuretic; combination of angiotensin II receptor (type AT_1) antagonist, losartan, and a diuretic, hydrochlorothiazide; common uses: edema, hypertension
Lovastatin	Mevacor	Antihyperlipidemic; inhibits HMG-CoA reductase, an enzyme that catalyzes an early and rate-limiting step in cholesterol biosynthesis; common uses: hypercholesterolemia, hyperlipidemia
Medroxy- progesterone	Provera	Progestin, contraceptive; derivative of progesterone active by both parenteral and oral routes of administration; common uses: amenorrhea, endometrial cancer, renal cancer, contraception, uterine hemorrhage
Metformin	Glucophage	Antidiabetic; oral antihyperglycemic agent which improves glucose tolerance in non-insulin dependent patients; mechanisms of action are different from those of sulfonylureas; decreases hepatic glucose production, decreases intestinal absorption of glucose and improves insulin sensitivity (increases peripheral glucose uptake and utilization); rarely produces hypoglycemia in either diabetic or nondiabetic persons; common uses: non-insulin requiring diabetes mellitus
Methylphenidate	Concerta, Ritalin	Amphetamine derivative; used in the treatment of attention deficit disorder (ADD)
Metoprolol succinate	LoPressor, Toprol	Beta blocker, antihypertensive; $beta_1$-selective (cardioselective) adrenoceptor blocking agent for oral administration, available as extended release tablets; common uses: angina pectoris, hypertension
Mupirocin	Bactroban	Antibiotic ointment; used in impetigo

Table of Commonly Prescribed Drugs — Generic Names (continued)

Generic Name	Trade Name (®)	Type of Drug; Typical Uses
Nabumetone	Relafen	Anti-inflammatory; nonsteroidal anti-inflammatory agent; common uses: arthritis (osteoarthritis, rheumatoid)
Naproxen	Naproxyn, Anaprox	Nonsteroidal anti-inflammatory (NSAID); common uses: arthritis, mild to moderate pain, various types of inflammation
Nefazodone	Serzone	Antidepression; inhibits neuronal uptake of serotonin and norepinephrine; common uses: depression
Nelfinavir	Viracept	Protease inhibitor—a class of anti-HIV drugs designed to inhibit the enzyme protease and interfere with virus replication; protease inhibitors prevent the cleavage of HIV precursor proteins into active proteins, a process that normally occurs when HIV replicates; used in therapy of AIDS and HIV infection
Nevirapine	Viramune	Reverse transcriptase inhibitor—a drug that blocks viral replication by interfering with the reverse transcriptase enzyme, preventing synthesis of DNA from RNA; used in therapy of AIDS and HIV infection
Nifedipine	Procardia, Adalat	Calcium channel blocker; blocks movement of calcium in various cells; common uses: angina, hypertension
Nitrofurantoin	Macrobid	Antibiotic; common uses: urinary tract infections
Nitroglycerin	Nitrostat	Antianginal, antihypertensive, coronary vasodilator; causes relaxation of vascular smooth muscle, primarily in veins and coronary arteries; common uses: angina, congestive heart failure, myocardial infarction, hypertension
Nizatidine	Axid	Histamine blocker (H2); blocks H2 histamine receptors in the stomach, reducing the producing of gastric acid; common uses: acid/peptic disorder, esophageal reflux, peptic ulcer (gastric, duodenal)

Table of Commonly Prescribed Drugs—Generic Names (continued)

Generic Name	Trade Name (®)	Type of Drug; Typical Uses
Olanzapine	Zyprexa	Atypical antipsychotic drug indicated in the treatment of schizophrenia; sometimes used to treat bipolar disorder; hyperglycemia (elevated blood sugar), in some cases extreme, has been reported in patients treated with atypical antipsychotics
Omeprazole	Prilosec	Antigastric secretory agent; suppresses gastric acid secretion by specific inhibition of an enzyme system at the surface of the gastric parietal cell (manufactures and secretes hydrochloric acid), blocking the final step of acid production; common uses: acid/peptic disorder, erosive esophagitis, duodenal ulcer, Zollinger-Ellison syndrome
Oseltamivir	Tamiflu	Oral antiviral drug for the treatment of uncomplicated influenza (flu) in patients one year and older whose flu symptoms have not lasted more than two days; this product is approved to treat type A and B influenza; also approved for the prevention of influenza in adults and adolescents older than 13 years
Oxaprozin	Daypro	Nonsteroidal anti-inflammatory (NSAID); common uses: arthritis, mild to moderate pain, various types of inflammation
Oxycodone	OxyContin	Pain medication containing oxycodone, a very strong narcotic pain reliever similar to morphine; designed so that the oxycodone is slowly released over time, allowing twice daily administration; the drug is intended to help relieve pain that is moderate to severe in intensity, when that pain is present all the time, and expected to continue for a long time; this level of pain severity may be caused by a variety of different medical conditions (e.g., metastatic cancer); has a very high abuse potential because breaking, chewing, or crushing the tablet causes a large amount of oxycodone to be released from the tablet all at once, causing a "high," and potentially resulting in a dangerous or fatal drug overdose

Table of Commonly Prescribed Drugs—Generic Names (continued)

Generic Name	Trade Name (®)	Type of Drug; Typical Uses
Oxycodone/ Acetaminophen	Percocet	Pain medication for moderate to severe pain of short duration (e.g., post-surgical); the potential for abuse and addiction exists, as with OxyContin, but is somewhat less since Percocet is not a sustained-release (long-acting) preparation; the combination of oxycodone and acetaminophen is synergistic— their combined effect is greater than the sum of either alone
Oxycodone/ Aspirin	Percodan	Pain medication for moderate to severe pain of short duration (e.g., post-surgical); the potential for abuse and addiction exists, as with OxyContin, but is somewhat less since Percodan is not a sustained-release (long-acting) preparation; the combination of oxycodone and aspirin is synergistic—their combined effect is greater than the sum of either alone
Palivizumab	Synagis	Antiviral drug indicated for the prevention of serious lower respiratory tract disease caused by respiratory syncytial virus (RSV) in pediatric patients at high risk of RSV disease
Phenytoin	Dilantin	Anticonvulsant; used in seizure disorders (epilepsy), occ. in cardiac dysrhythmias
Potassium chloride	K-Dur-20, Klor-Con	Electrolyte supplement; oral replacement supplement for the essential mineral, potassium; uses: prevention/treatment of hypokalemia (low serum potassium), muscle cramps
Pravastatin	Pravachol	Antihyperlipidemic; inhibits HMG-CoA reductase, an enzyme that catalyzes an early and rate-limiting step in cholesterol biosynthesis; common uses: hypercholesterolemia, hyperlipidemia
Prednisone	Deltasone	Adrenal corticosteroid; common uses: adrenal insufficiency, hemolytic anemia, inflammation (e.g., arthritis, bursitis), carditis, conjunctivitis, dermatitis, ulcerative colitis, enteritis, hypercalcemia, leukemia, allergic rhinitis, sarcoidosis, asthma, chronic obstructive pulmonary disease, thyroiditis, uveitis

Table of Commonly Prescribed Drugs — Generic Names (continued)

Generic Name	Trade Name (®)	Type of Drug; Typical Uses
Promethazine	Phenergan	Antiemetic, antihistamine, antitussive; phenothiazine derivative, possesses antihistaminic, sedative, antimotion-sickness, antiemetic effects; common uses: anaphylaxis, allergies, motion sickness, nausea, vomiting, hives, mild sedation
Propoxyphene N/ Acetaminophen	Propacet, Darvocet N	Analgesic, narcotic; combination of the centrally acting narcotic analgesic agent, propoxyphene N and acetaminophen; common uses: mild to moderate pain
Propranolol	Inderal	Antianginal, antiarrhythmics, antihypertensive, antimigraine, beta blocker; nonselective beta-adrenergic receptor blocking agent possessing no other autonomic nervous system activity; common uses: angina, arrhythmia, migraine headache, hypertension, pheochromocytoma, hypertrophic subaortic stenosis, tremor
Quetiapine	Seroquel	Psychotropic agent that blocks numerous neurotransmitter receptor sites in the brain; used to treat acute manic episodes associated with bipolar disorder
Quinapril	Accupril	Antihypertensive; works by inhibiting angiotensin converting enzyme (ACE; sometimes called ACE blockers), an enzyme that catalyzes the production of angiotensin II, a potent vasoconstrictor; common uses: congestive heart failure and hypertension
Ramipril	Altace	Antihypertensive; works by inhibiting angiotensin converting enzyme (ACE; sometimes called ACE blockers), an enzyme that catalyzes the production of angiotensin II, a potent vasoconstrictor; common uses: congestive heart failure and hypertension
Ranitidine	Zantac	Histamine blocker (H2); blocks H2 histamine receptors in the stomach, reducing the producing of gastric acid; common uses: acid/peptic disorder, esophageal reflux, peptic ulcer (gastric, duodenal)

Table of Commonly Prescribed Drugs — Generic Names (continued)

Generic Name	Trade Name (®)	Type of Drug; Typical Uses
Ribavirin	Virazole	Antiviral drug used to treat severe virus pneumonia in infants and young children; also used to treat hepatitis C, often in combination with either interferon or peginterferon
Ribavirin/ Interferon	Rebetron	Combination of the antiviral drugs ribavirin and interferon; used in treatment of chronic hepatitis; the combination of ribavirin and interferon is synergistic—their combined effect is greater than the sum of either alone
Rimantadine	Flumadine	Antiviral drug used to prevent or treat certain influenza (flu) infections (type A)
Risedronate	Actonel	Bisphosphonate drug that inhibits osteoclast-mediated bone resorption; used in the treatment of osteoporosis and to prevent development of osteoporosis-related fractures
Risperidone	Risperdal	Antipsychotics/antimanics; antipsychotic agent belonging to a new chemical class, the benzisoxazole derivatives, thought to work through a combination of dopamine type 2 (D_2) and serotonin type 2 ($5HT_2$) antagonism; common uses: psychosis, schizophrenia
Ritonavir	Norvir	Protease inhibitor—a class of anti-HIV drugs designed to inhibit the enzyme protease and interfere with virus replication; protease inhibitors prevent the cleavage of HIV precursor proteins into active proteins, a process that normally occurs when HIV replicates; used in therapy of AIDS and HIV infection
Saquinavir	Fortovase	Protease inhibitor—a class of anti-HIV drugs designed to inhibit the enzyme protease and interfere with virus replication; protease inhibitors prevent the cleavage of HIV precursor proteins into active proteins, a process that normally occurs when HIV replicates; used in therapy of AIDS and HIV infection

Table of Commonly Prescribed Drugs—Generic Names (continued)

Generic Name	Trade Name (®)	Type of Drug; Typical Uses
Sertraline	Zoloft	Antidepressant; blocks serotonin reuptake; common uses: anxiety, panic disorder, depression, obsessive-compulsive disorder
Sildenafil	Viagra	Anti-impotence agent; indirectly enhances the action of nitric oxide (NO) in the corpus cavernosum of the penis, when combined with sexual stimulation, leading to inflow of blood and erection; this action, absent sexual stimulation, has no significant effect on erection; the mechanisms of sildenafil and organic nitrates (enhancing the effect of NO) are similar; thus, the two drugs should never be given simultaneously; common uses: impotence
Simvastatin	Zocor	Antihyperlipidemic; inhibits HMG-CoA reductase, an enzyme that catalyzes an early and rate-limiting step in cholesterol biosynthesis; common uses: hypercholesterolemia, hyperlipidemia
Stavudine	Zerit	Reverse transcriptase inhibitor—a drug that blocks viral replication by interfering with the reverse transcriptase enzyme, preventing synthesis of DNA from RNA; used in therapy of AIDS and HIV infection
Sumatriptan	Imitrex	Antimigraine; selective 5-hydroxytryptamine$_1$ receptor subtype agonist; common uses: migraine headache
Tadalafil	Cialis	Anti-impotence agent; indirectly enhances the action of nitric oxide (NO) in the corpus cavernosum of the penis, when combined with sexual stimulation, leading to inflow of blood and erection; this action, absent sexual stimulation, has no significant effect on erection; the mechanisms of tadalafil and organic nitrates (e.g., nitroglycerin) are similar; thus, the two drugs should never be given simultaneously; common uses: erectile dysfunction (male impotence; ED; a condition where the penis does not harden and expand when a man is sexually excited, or when he cannot keep an erection)

Table of Commonly Prescribed Drugs—Generic Names (continued)

Generic Name	Trade Name (®)	Type of Drug; Typical Uses
Tamoxifen	Nolvadex	Antineoplastic (anticancer); non-steroidal estrogen receptor binding agent; common uses: breast cancer
Temazepam	Restoril	Sedative/hypnotic; benzodiazepine hypnotic agent; common uses: insomnia
Terazosin	Hytrin	Antihypertensive; mixed alpha receptor blocker and agonist; used in benign prostatic hyperplasia, hypertension
Tetracycline	Sumycin	Antibiotic; common uses: various infections esp. skin, sexually transmitted diseases
Timolol	Timoptic	Beta blocker; nonselective beta-adrenergic antagonist for ocular use; common uses: glaucoma
Tiotropium	Spiriva	Inhaled blocker of certain parasympathetic nervous system receptors in the lungs, leading to bronchodilation; used in the treatment of asthma—not intended for use as a rescue inhaler
Tobramycin/ Dexamethasone	Tobradex	Antibiotic; combination creme of the aminoglycoside antibiotic tobramycin and the potent anti-inflammatory corticosteroid, dexamethasone; common uses: burns, conjunctivitis, dermatitis with secondary infection, foreign body, eye trauma, uveitis
Tolterodine	Detrol LA	Blocks receptors in the parasympathetic nervous system, causing decreased contractions of the bladder; used in treatment of the treatment of overactive bladder with symptoms of urinary incontinence, urgency, and frequency
Tramadol	Ultram	Analgesic, nonnarcotic; centrally acting synthetic analgesic; mode of action not completely understood; common uses: pain, moderate to moderately severe
Trazodone	Desyrel	Antidepressant, serotonin-reuptake blocker; common use: depression
Tretinoin	Retin-A	Acne products; retinoic acid (vitamin A acid) cream; common use: acne vulgaris

Table of Commonly Prescribed Drugs — Generic Names (continued)

Generic Name	Trade Name (®)	Type of Drug; Typical Uses
Triamcinolone	Azmacort	Inhaled corticosteroid; common uses: asthma, COPD
Trimethoprim/ Sulfamethoxasole	Septra, Bactrim	Antibiotic; common uses: various infections esp. urinary tract
Troglitazone	Rezulin	Antidiabetic; oral antihyperglycemic agent that acts primarily by decreasing insulin resistance; common uses: diabetes mellitus; rare cases of severe liver injury have been reported
Valacyclovir	Valtrex	Interferes with viral synthesis of DNA; used in herpes virus infections
Valproic Acid	Depakote	Anticonvulsant; used in seizure disorders (epilepsy)
Valsartan	Diovan	Antihypertensive; acts as angiotensin converting enzyme (ACE) inhibitor by blocking the specific angiotensin II AT_1 receptor subtype; common use: hypertension
Vardenafil	Levitra	Anti-impotence agent; indirectly enhances the action of nitric oxide (NO) in the corpus cavernosum of the penis, when combined with sexual stimulation, leading to inflow of blood and erection; this action, absent sexual stimulation, has no significant effect on erection; the mechanisms of vardenafil and organic nitrates (e.g., nitroglycerin) are similar; thus, the two drugs should never be given simultaneously; common uses: erectile dysfunction (male impotence; ED; a condition where the penis does not harden and expand when a man is sexually excited, or when he cannot keep an erection)
Venlafaxine	Effexor	Antidepressant; inhibits serotonin, norepinephrine, and dopamine reuptake; common uses: depression
Verapamil	Calan	Calcium channel blocker; blocks movement of calcium in various cells; common uses: angina, hypertension, cardiac dysrhythmias
Warfarin	Coumadin	Anticoagulant; common uses: prevention of recurrent blood clots

Table of Commonly Prescribed Drugs — Generic Names (continued)

Generic Name	Trade Name (®)	Type of Drug; Typical Uses
Zafirlukast	Accolate	Antiasthmatic; blocks action of leukotrienes, substances that cause airway inflammation in asthma
Zalcitabine	Hivid	Reverse transcriptase inhibitor—a drug that blocks viral replication by interfering with the reverse transcriptase enzyme, preventing synthesis of DNA from RNA; used in therapy of AIDS and HIV infection
Zanamivir	Relenza	An antiviral drug, for persons aged 7 years and older for the treatment of uncomplicated influenza (flu) virus; this product is approved to treat type A and B influenza, the two types most responsible for flu epidemics; clinical studies showed that for the drug to be effective, patients needed to start treatment within two days of the onset of symptoms
Zidovudine	Retrovir	Reverse transcriptase inhibitor—a drug that blocks viral replication by interfering with the reverse transcriptase enzyme, preventing synthesis of DNA from RNA; used in therapy of AIDS and HIV infection
Zidovudine/ Lamivudine	Combivir	Reverse transcriptase inhibitor—a drug that blocks viral replication by interfering with the reverse transcriptase enzyme, preventing synthesis of DNA from RNA; used in therapy of AIDS and HIV infection
Ziprasidone	Geodon	Atypical antipsychotic indicated in the treatment of schizophrenia; sometimes used to treat bipolar disease; hyperglycemia (elevated blood sugar), in some cases extreme, has been reported in patients treated with atypical antipsychotics
Zolpidem	Ambien	Sedative hypnotic; common uses: insomnia

TABLE OF OVER-THE-COUNTER (OTC) MEDICATIONS

- All of the examples are either trademarks (™) or registered copyright (®) names. The relevant symbols are not shown in the table below.
- Not all available products are listed as examples below. Inclusion or exclusion of any particular product does not imply endorsement or lack thereof by either the author or the publishers.

Type of Medication	Examples	Comments
Acne	Clearasil, Stri-dex, Oxy-10, Neutrogena	Typically requires 4–8 weeks to see improvement. Once the acne clears, treatment must be continued to prevent new lesions from forming.
Allergy Prevention and Treatment	Benadryl, Sudafed, Actifed, Claritin	May cause drowsiness.
Analgesic/ antipyretic (pain and fever)	Advil, Aleve, Motrin, Nuprin, Excedrin, Tylenol, Bayer Aspirin	Acetaminophen (the active ingredient in Tylenol) overdose may result in fatal liver failure; ibuprofen (the active ingredient in Motrin and Nuprin) may increase the sensitivity of the skin to sunlight.
Antacids and Acid Reducing	Gas-X, Maalox, Mylanta, Tums, AXID AR, Pepcid AC, Prilosec OTC, Tagamet HB, Zantac 75	Persons with kidney disease should not take an antacid containing aluminum or magnesium.
Anti-arthritis	Glucosamine, Chondroitin	Relieve pain and may slow the rate of cartilage damage with mild to moderate osteoarthritis (OA).
Anti-baldness/ Hair Loss	Rogaine	Needs to be used for 2–4 months before results are noted.

Table of Over-the-Counter (OTC) Medications (continued)

Type of Medication	Examples	Comments
Antifungal Cremes	Lamisil AT, Lotramin AF, Micatin	Used for skin fungus, such as athlete's foot.
Anti-itch Lotions and Creams	Bactine, Caldecort, Cortaid, Hydro-cortisone, Lanacort, Calamine Lotion, Ben-adryl Cream, Caladryl	For athlete's foot, jock itch, bug bites, poison ivy.
Antibiotic (topical) Creams	Neosporin Ointment, Mycitracin, Tribiotic	Bacitracin, polymixin B, and neomycin are antibiotics commonly found in topical antibiotics. Products such as Neosporin Ointment, Mycitracin, and Tribiotic combine these ingredients into a single preparation.
Anticandial	Femstat 3, Gyne-Lotrimin, Mycelrx-7, Monistat 3, 7, Vagistat-1	Used for vaginal yeast infections.
Asthma	Primatene Mist, Asthmahaler Mist	Continued use can lead to tolerance.
Antidiarrheal and Laxatives	Ex-Lax, Pepto-Bismol, Immodium A.D., Kaopectate	Chronic laxative use can lead to bowel dysfunction.
Antihistamines	Actidil Syrup and Capsules, Actifed, Allerest, Benadryl, Claritin, Chlor-Trimeton, Contac, Dimetane, Drixoral, Nyquil, Sudafed, Tavist-1, Triaminic	May result in drowsiness; should not be combined with alcohol.
Cold Sore/ Fever Blister	Abreva Cream	Shortens healing time and duration of symptoms: tingling, pain, burning, and/or itching.

Table of Over-the-Counter (OTC) Medications (continued)

Type of Medication	Examples	Comments
Cough Suppressants	Robitussin, Vicks 44, Chloraseptic, Coricidin	Coricidin and Robitussin contain dextromethorphan, a narcotic derivative. When used as drugs of abuse, death has resulted.
Decongestant/ Nasal Decongestant and Cold Remedies	Advil Cold and Sinus, Afrin, Afrinol, Aleve Cold and Sinus, Children's Advil Cold, Duration, Dristan Long Lasting, Neo-Synephrine—12 Hour, Orrivin, Sudafed, Tavist-D, Tylenol Cold and Flu, Thera-flu, Alka Children's Advil Seltzer Cold and Flu, Nyquil, Actidil Syrup and Capsules, Actifed, Allerest, Benadryl, Claritin, Chlor-Trimeton, Contac	In November 2000, the Food and Drug Administration (FDA) issued a public health warning regarding phenyl-propanolamine (PPA) due to the risk of stroke. The FDA requested that manufacturers voluntarily discontinue marketing products that contain PPA. Avoid using PPA-containing medications that may have been purchased prior to November 2000.
Diaper Rash Ointments	Balmax, Desitin, A+D Ointment	Avoid steroid-containing cremes unless recommended by a health care professional.
Eye Drops for Allergy/Cold Relief	OcuHist, Naphcon A	Temporarily relieve itching and redness of the eyes caused by a variety of allergens (e.g., ragweed, animal hair).
Fiber Supplements	Benefiber, Metamucil	Cause an increase in the bulk of the stool. Used in the treatment of constipation, irritable bowel syndrome, and diverticulosis. People with difficulty swallowing should contact their health care provider prior to using these supplements.
Hemorrhoid Treatments	Preparation H, Hemorid, Tucks, Tronolane, Anusol HC-1	Avoid hemorrhoid creams that contain anesthetics such as benzocaine. These may temporarily relieve pain but can cause allergic side effects.

Table of Over-the-Counter (OTC) Medications (continued)

Type of Medication	Examples	Comments
Liniments	BenGay, Tiger Balm, Flexall	Used to treat minor muscle and joint aches.
Menstrual Cycle Medications	Midol, Pamprin, Premysyn PMS	May result in excessive sleepiness if combined with prescription tranquilizers (e.g., Valium) or sleeping aids (e.g., Halcion).
Migraine	Advil Migraine Liqui-gels, Excedrin Migraine, Motrin Migraine Pain	Taking for more than two days in a row may result in medication overuse headache (also called "rebound headache").
Motion Sickness	Dramamine, Marizine, Bonine, Antivert	May cause drowsiness.
Nicotine Gum or Patches and Smoking Cessation Aids	Commit, Nicorette, Nicotrol, Nicodin	Pieces of nicotine gum may have enough nicotine to make children and pets sick. Wrap used pieces of gum in paper and throw away in the trash.
Pediculicide (head lice)	Nix, Rid, Triple X	Treatment failures are common with any over-the-counter pediculicide.
Rehydration Solutions	Pedialyte, Infalyte, Rehydralyte	Oral rehydration solutions (ORSs) are used to prevent or correct dehydration in young children. They contain a mixture of salt, sugar, potassium, and other minerals to help replace body fluids and chemicals lost from diarrhea.
Sleep Prevention	No Doz, Vivarin	Used to help restore mental alertness or wakefulness when experiencing fatigue or drowsiness. May be abused as a substitute for amphetamines ("speed").
Sleep Aids	Sominex, Nytol, Unisom	Add to the sedative effects of alcohol and other medications that cause drowsiness.
Wart Removal	Tinamed	Should not be used on the face or genitals.

TABLE OF COMPLEMENTARY AND ALTERNATIVE MEDICINE TERMS

Name	Description
Alternative Medicine	Medical systems, professions, practices, interventions, modalities, therapies, applications, theories, or claims that are currently not part of the conventional medical system. These treatments and health care practices are not taught widely in medical schools, not generally used in hospitals, and are not usually reimbursed by medical insurance companies. Also known as complementary medicine, these health care options are classified into seven general areas: mind-body interventions (e.g., yoga, mental imaging), alternative systems of medical practice (e.g. Indian Ayurveda, Traditional Chinese Medicine, homeopathy, naturopathy), lifestyle and disease prevention, biologically-based therapies (e.g., herbalism, special diet therapies, orthomolecular medicine, pharmacological, biological and instrumental interventions), manipulative and body-based systems (e.g., chiropractic, massage and body work, unconventional physical therapies), biofield medicine (e.g. therapeutic touch, Reiki), and bioelectromagnetics. The Office of Alternative Medicine (OAM) was established by Congressional mandate in 1992 as a part of the National Institutes of Health (NIH). The Center's purpose is to facilitate the evaluation of alternative medical treatment modalities to determine their effectiveness as well as to serve as a public information clearinghouse and research training program.
Alternative Medical Systems	Complete systems of health care theory and practice that have been developed outside of the Western biomedical approach. Usually divided into four subcategories: Acupuncture and Oriental medicine, traditional Indigenous systems; unconventional Western systems, and Naturopathy.
Aromatherapy	Therapeutic use of essential oils extracted from plants. The technique uses a wide range of organic compounds of which the odor or fragrance play an important part. Essential oils are extracted from different parts of plants such as the roots, bark, stalks, flowers, or leaves, mostly by distillation. They may be applied to the body via massage, inhaled, used as a compress, mixed into an ointment, or inserted internally via the rectum, vagina, or mouth. Aromatherapy is one of the fastest growing complementary therapies in the United States. It has been used to treat a wide range of physical, mental,

Table of Complementary and Alternative Medicine Terms (continued)

Name	Description
	and emotional conditions including burns, bacterial infections, insomnia, depression, hypertension, and cardiac arrhythmias. Medical research in this area is currently in its infancy.
Ayurveda	Holistic system of natural health care that originated in the ancient Vedic civilization of India. According to Ayurveda, the universe is composed of earth, air, fire, water, and space. These interact, giving rise to all that exists. In humans, the five elements occur as three doshas (maintain health), seven dhatus (tissues responsible for sustaining the body), and three malas (waste products—urine, feces, and sweat). Ayurveda considers digestion to be the most important function in the human body and that abnormalities are the principal cause for all disease maladies. A recent revival of Ayurveda, Maharishi Ayurveda, is based on classical texts by Maharishi Mahesh Yogi and incorporates Transcendental Meditation into the healing process.
Biofield Medicine	Alternative medicine system that uses subtle energy fields in and around the body for medical purposes. Examples include Therapeutic Touch, Healing Touch, and Reiki.
Cupping	Traditional Chinese Medicine technique where a vacuum is induced in a small glass or bamboo cup, which is then promptly applied to the skin surface. The vacuum brings blood and lymph to the skin surface under the cup, increasing local circulation. It is used to drain or remove cold and damp "evils" from the body.
Curanderismo	Latin American healing tradition that has become popular in the United States. Considered a traditional healing system since biomedical beliefs, treatments, and practices are often used. It is not unusual for curanderos (healers) to recommend the use of prescription medications (which can often be purchased in Mexico across the counter) for infections and other illnesses. A parallel supernatural source of illness is also recognized, not amenable to treatment by traditional medicine. These may be repaired only by the supernatural manipulations of curanderos.
Folk Medicine	Generic term for "unofficial" health practices and beliefs found in all societies. These include both religious elements (e.g., prayers for healing) and material elements (e.g., "a hot breakfast" to prevent winter colds). Typically folk medicine is viewed as "unofficial" compared to "official" medicine that is authorized by a host of sources, such as the office of the Surgeon General and the bodies that accredit medical

Name	Description
	schools and hospitals. Folk health traditions are not given official standing by such agencies, and most lack formal authority structures of their own. Folk medicine carries authority, but it is the informal authority of life experience rather than the formal authority of licensure, certification, and accreditation. Therefore, folk medical belief and practice is much more variable and diverse than is official medical belief and practice.
Guided Imagery	Form of alternative and complementary medicine where the patient is taught to visualize, first, a familiar and comfortable place. The patient then forms an image representing the illness and receives suggestions that an inner healing force is acting on that symbolic representation of the illness to treat it. Guided imagery has been successfully used to treat depression, immune function, pain, anxiety, and sleep disorders.
Healing Touch	Type of alternative healing using hands-on and energy-based techniques to balance and align the human energy field. One of two commonly used hand-mediated energetic healing practices (see also Therapeutic Touch). The term refers specifically to approaches taught in the American Holistic Nurses' Associations's Certificate Program in Healing Touch for Health Care Professionals. Healing Touch is a complementary mode of facilitating the healing process, but functions from an energy perspective rather than only a physical one. The Healing Touch Practitioner re-aligns the patients' flow, re-activating the mind/body/spirit connection to eliminate blockages to self-healing.
Mind-Body Medicine	Combination of behavioral, psychological, social, and spiritual approaches to health. It is divided into four subcategories. Mind-body systems involve whole systems of mind-body practice that are used largely as primary interventions for disease. They are rarely delivered alone; instead, they are used in combination with lifestyle interventions, or are part of a traditional medical system. Mind-body methods contain individual modalities used in mind-body approaches to health. These approaches are often considered conventional practice and overlap with complementary and alternative medicine only when applied to medical conditions for which they are not usually used (e.g., hypnosis for genetic problems). Religion and spirituality deals with those nonbehavioral aspects of spirituality and religion that examine their relationship to biological function or clinical conditions. Social and contextual areas refers to so-

Table of Complementary and Alternative Medicine Terms (continued)

Name	Description
	cial, cultural, symbolic, and contextual interventions that are not covered in other areas.
Moxibustion	Form of Traditional Chinese Medicine were dried and powdered leaves of *Artemesia vulgaris* are burned either on or in proximity to the skin. The purpose is to affect movement of a person's energy or "qi" through a specific healing channel in the body. Often used in combination with acupuncture.
Naturopathy	Use of therapies that are primarily natural and nontoxic, including clinical nutrition, homeopathy, botanical medicine, hydrotherapy, physical medicine, and counseling. In the United States, the naturopathic medical profession's infrastructure is based on accredited educational institutions, professional licensing by a growing number of states, national standards of practice and care, peer review, and an ongoing commitment to state-of-the-art scientific research. Hippocrates is often considered the earliest predecessor of naturopathic physicians, particularly in terms of his teaching that "nature is healer of all diseases" and his formulation of the concept "vis medicatrix naturae"—"the healing power of nature." Naturopathic physicians also function within an integrated framework, for example referring patients to an appropriate medical specialist such as an oncologist or a surgeon. Naturopathic therapies can be employed within that context to complement the treatments used by conventionally trained medical doctors.
Orthomolecular Medicine	Type of complementary and alternative medicine where products are used as nutritional and food supplements for preventive or therapeutic purposes. They are usually used in combinations and at high doses. Examples include niacinamide for arthritis and melatonin to prevent breast cancer.
Qi	Traditional Asian Medicine term for the energy of life. This energy is felt to flow through the body concentrating along specific pathways called meridians. Traditional Asian Medicine views the body as an energetic expression of qi.
Qigong	Ancient Chinese healing discipline that is rapidly attracting attention throughout the world. It consists of breathing and mental exercises, often combined with physical exercise. The purpose is to balance the subtle energy system ("qi") within the body. Eighty million people in China get up early every morning to practice Qigong in groups in parks.
Reiki	Technique for stress reduction and relaxation that allows the patient to tap into an unlimited supply of

Name	Description
	"life force energy" to improve health and enhance the quality of life. The ability to use Reiki is not taught in the usual sense, but is transferred to the student by the Reiki Master. While Reiki is not a religion, for optimum well being in the light of Eastern medical theory that humans are a mind-body-spirit unity, the technique supports that it is necessary to live and act in a way that promotes harmony with others.
Therapeutic Touch	One of two hand-mediated energetic healing practices (see Healing Touch) also called the Krieger-Kunz Method of Therapeutic Touch. Practitioners use their hands to assess the patient's energy field. They provide treatment by moving the hands slowly in the space above the patient's body to direct energy to a specific location. Actual touching of the patient is not necessary. This technique has been taught to and used by many nurses in the United States.
Traditional Chinese Medicine	Multi-faceted group of techniques and beliefs regarding health care as practiced in China for many years. The philosophy of Chinese medicine begins with yin and yang—an expression of opposing, but complementary phenomena that exist in a state of dynamic equilibrium (e.g., light and dark). The most crucial concept is that of "qi," the energy of life. These forces pervade the body and cause most physiological functions and maintain the health and vitality of the individual. Techniques include acupuncture, moxibustion, cupping, bleeding, massage, manipulation, herbal medicines, and diet therapy.
Trancendental Meditation	Relaxation technique during which the mind goes beyond ("transcends") even the subtlest impulses of thought and settles down to the simplest state of awareness—the transcendental consciousness. Scientific data has demonstrated that during this time, the body's metabolism and EEG take on a unique pattern of profound rest and balance, with a reduction in metabolism significantly deeper than that during either sleep or eyes-closed rest.
Vitalism	Common principle in complementary and alternative medicine that more is needed to explain life than just physical or mechanical laws. Practitioners of most alternative healing believe that one source of their intervention is a kind of "vital energy" not appreciated by conventional biomedical science. Various alternative disciplines have different names for this energy (e.g., "spiritual vital force" in homeopathy, "universal intelligence" in chiropractic, "Mind" in New Thought, "qi" in acupuncture).

COMMON HERBAL MEDICINES

Herb	Use	Side Effects	Drug Interactions
Aloe vera	Burns, skin injuries, cosmetics (external use)	None known	None known
Cascara sagrada	Stimulant laxative	Intestinal cramping	Loss of potassium with chronic use may cause digitalis toxicity and cardiac arrhythmias
Capsium (Cayenne, hot pepper)	Pain relief in shingles, arthritis	Hypersensitivity	May interfere with MAO inhibitors; may increase liver metabolism of various drugs
Chamomile	Antispasmodic for indigestion, flatulence, GI tract inflammation	None known	None known
Cranberry	Prevention of urinary tract infection	None known	None known
Dandelion	Natural diuretic (leaves)	None known	None known
Dong quai	"Female tonic" to treat muscle cramps and pain during menstrual period	Contraindicated during pregnancy and lactation	Increases activity of blood thinning drugs (anticoagulants, antiplatelet drugs)

Herb	Use	Side Effects	Drug Interactions
Echinacea	Wound treatment, strengthening of immune system, treatment of colds and flu	Contraindicated in progressive systemic diseases (TB, MS)	May interfere with immunosuppressive therapy
Evening primose	Menstrual irregularities, arthritis pain	Mild headache, abdominal pain; not recommended for patients diagnosed with schizophrenia	Increased risk of temporal lobe epilepsy in schizophrenic patients being treated with phenothiazines (e.g., Thorazine)
Feverfew	Pain relief; menstrual cramps, migraine headache	Occasional mouth ulceration or gastric disturbance	None known
Garlic	Cardiovascular conditions, high cholesterol or triglycerides, prevention of colds and flu	Rare GI symptoms	May increase the activity of warfarin (Coumadin) anticoagulants
Ginger	Nausea, motion sickness, vomiting	Heartburn; may aggravate gallstone disease	Large doses may interfere with cardiac, antidiabetic, or anticoagulant therapy
Ginkgo	Conditions associated with aging (memory loss, poor-circulation), tinnitus (ringing in the ears), vertigo	Contraindicated in pregnancy and lactation	None known
Ginseng	Increase resistance to all types of stress; increase energy and endurance	None known; avoid in acute illness, hypertension	Stimulants, coffee, antipsychotic drugs, especially MAO inhibitors

COMMON HERBAL MEDICINES (CONTINUED)

Herb	Use	Side Effects	Drug Interactions
Goldenseal	Wound healing, colds and flu	Contraindicated during pregnancy and lactation; also in high blood pressure	May oppose the anticoagulant action of heparin
Hawthorn	Heart conditions (angina)	None known	None known
Kava kava root	Nervous anxiety, stress, restlessness; insomnia	Contraindicated in endogenous depression, pregnancy and lactation	May potentiate alcohol, barbiturates, and various psychopharmacological agents
Licorice	Inflammation, adrenal gland stimulation	Headache, lethargy, sodium and water retention, excessive loss of potassium, high blood pressure	Loss of potassium may increase sensitivity to digitalis glycosides
Milk thistle	Improvement of liver function	Mild laxative effect	None known
Passion flower	Mild sedative for insomnia	None known	None known
Peppermint	Antispasmodic action on stomach and intestinal tract	None known	None known
Psyllium	Major source of fiber; used as bulk laxative	Intestinal cramping	None known

Herb	Use	Side Effects	Drug Interactions
Saw palmetto	Benign prostatic hypertrophy (BPH); increases urine flow and reduces frequency of nightime urination	Headaches, diarrhea	None known
Senna	Laxative	Long-term dependence may develop	None known
St. John's wort	Mild to moderate depression	Photosensitization; contraindicated during pregnancy	May potentiate MAO inhibitors; should not be used at the same time as prescription antidepressants
Valerian	Sedative, sleep aid; said to be nonhabit forming	None known	None known

SOME HERBAL MEDICATIONS SUPPORTED BY RECENT MEDICAL DATA

Problem/Disease	Herbal Medication Reported as Useful
Arthritis	Capsaicin cream (osteoarthritis), evening primrose oil (rheumatoid arthritis) [reduced pain]
Benign prostatic hypertrophy (enlargement)	Saw palmetto (increase in urine flow; reduction in nightime bathroom trips)
Dementia (including Alzheimer's)	Ginkgo biloba (memory and concentration problems, headache, depression, dizziness)
Depression (mild to moderate)	St. John's wort
Diabetes	Ginseng (reduced fasting blood sugar level in some patients)
Fibromyalgia	Capsaicin cream (less tenderness at trigger points)
Hypercholesterolemia	Garlic (decreased total cholesterol, triglycerides and low density lipoprotein; increase in high density lipoprotein)
Liver disease	Milk thistle (silymarin) [helpful in Amanita mushroom poisoning, hepatitis, cirrhosis]
Malaria	Wormwood (quinghao, artemisinin)
Migraine headache	Feverfew leaves (reduced frequency and severity of headache)
Nausea, vomiting, motion sickness	Ginger
Neuropathy (diabetic, postherpetic)	Capsaicin cream (pain improvement)
Psoriasis	Aloe vera extract
Sexual dysfunction	Ginkgo biloba
Urinary tract infection	Cranberry juice (reduces incidence of infections by making the urine acidic; may inhibit bacteria from sticking to tissues)

Reference: Fugh-Berman, A., Clinical Trials of Herbs, Primary Care; Clinics in Office Practice. Volume 24, December 1997, p. 889, 1997 W.B. Saunders

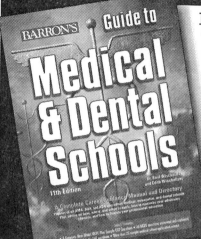